Memmler's

The Human Body
in Health
& Disease

Barbara Janson Cohen, BA, MSEd

Assistant Professor

Delaware County Community College
Media, Pennsylvania

Dena Lin Wood, RN, MS

Staff Nurse

VNA Care
Glendale, California

MEMMLER'S

The Human Body in Health & Disease

9th Edition

Barbara Janson Cohen

Dena Lin Wood

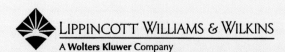

LIPPINCOTT WILLIAMS & WILKINS
A **Wolters Kluwer** Company
Philadelphia • Baltimore • New York • London
Buenos Aires • Hong Kong • Sydney • Tokyo

Acquisitions Editors: Margaret M. Biblis, John Butler
Editorial Assistant: Amy Amico
Managing Editor: Barbara Ryalls
Senior Production Manager: Helen Ewan
Production Coordinator: Mike Carcel
Art Director: Carolyn O'Brien
Indexer: Nancy Newman

9th Edition
Copyright © 2000 by Lippincott Williams & Wilkins

9   8   7   6   5   4   3   2   1

Library of Congress Cataloging-in-Publication Data

Cohen, Barbara J.
    Memmler's The human body in health & disease.—9th ed. / Barbara Janson
Cohen, Dena Lin Wood.
        p.   cm.
    Rev. ed. of: The human body in health & disease / Ruth L. Memmler,
Barbara Janson Cohen, Dena Lin Wood. 8th ed. c1996.
    Includes bibliographical references and index.
    ISBN 0-7817-2110-5 (alk. paper) (softbound)   ISBN 0-7817-2439-2 (casebound)
    1. Human physiology.   2. Physiology, Pathological.   3. Human
anatomy.   I. Wood, Dena Lin.   II. Memmler, Ruth Lundeen. Human
body in health & disease.   III. Title.   IV. Title: Human body in
health and disease.
    [DNLM: 1. Physiology.   2. Anatomy.   3. Pathology.   QT 104 C678h
2000]
QP34.5.M48   2000
612—dc21
DNLM/DLC
for Library of Congress   99–29504
                                                          CIP

Care has been taken to confirm the accuracy of the information presented and to describe generally accepted practices. However, the authors, editors, and publisher are not responsible for errors or omissions or for any consequences from application of the information in this book and make no warranty, express or implied, with respect to the contents of the publication.

The authors, editors and publisher have exerted every effort to ensure that drug selection and dosage set forth in this text are in accordance with current recommendations and practice at the time of publication. However, in view of ongoing research, changes in government regulations, and the constant flow of information relating to drug therapy and drug reactions, the reader is urged to check the package insert for each drug for any change in indications and dosage and for added warnings and precautions. This is particularly important when the recommended agent is a new or infrequently employed drug.

Some drugs and medical devices presented in this publication have Food and Drug Administration (FDA) clearance for limited use in restricted research settings. It is the responsibility of the health care provider to ascertain the FDA status of each drug or device planned for use in their clinical practice.

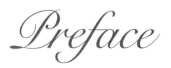
Preface

The ninth edition of *Memmler's The Human Body in Health and Disease* has built on the strong features of previous editions. It uses a systemic approach to study of the normal body and how it is affected by disease.

NEW FEATURES

1. Virtually all of the art has been redrawn to make the illustrations more appealing and modern. Figures have been revised for clarity and labeling has been enhanced. Some illustrations explaining physiologic concepts have been added.
2. The entire text has been updated, especially with regard to clinical advances, and additional material on physiology has been added.
3. The text has been reorganized and information is presented in smaller segments.
4. Checkpoints have been inserted at intervals in the text. These short questions require the student to pause and think about the previous section of text and answer a question on some highlight of the section. The answers to the checkpoints are at the end of each chapter.
5. The Special Interest Boxes have been updated, and each chapter on the body systems now contains an additional box on a related health topic.
6. Summary charts have been added to aid in learning. Some of these incorporate figures to illustrate materials in the chart.
7. Information on aging and its effects on each body system has been added where appropriate.

AIDS TO LEARNING

Many valuable student aids have been retained from previous editions. These include:

1. Each chapter begins with Behavioral Objectives that state the learning goals for the chapter.
2. Selected Key Terms are listed at the start of each chapter.
3. New terms are emphasized when introduced with **boldface italic** type and a phonetic pronunciation is given.
4. Abundant illustrations are included.
5. Summary charts help to organize material and to aid in review.
6. Each chapter is followed by a Summary outline for review. These summaries now more closely parallel the headings in the text for easy reference.
7. Questions for Study and Review are included at the end of each chapter.

8. There is a complete Glossary with definitions and pronunciations of all key terms and other important words used in the text.

9. Each chapter includes Special Interest Boxes that expand on the text or add related information. One box in each chapter centers on normal structure, another gives information on clinical matters, and a third in the systems chapters discusses a related health topic. Each type of box is identified with a logo as follows:

 represents a box focusing on normal function

 represents a box with a clinical focus

 represents a health box

10. Appendices provide information on the metric system, disease, and laboratory values.

11. A section on Medical Terminology shows how scientific words are built from prefixes, roots, and suffixes. Hearing these word parts will help the student remember terms and understand the meaning of new terms.

THE COMPLETE TEACHING–LEARNING PACKAGE INCLUDES

1. A Student Study Guide

   The Study Guide contains a variety of practice exercises that correlate directly with the text, including labeling exercises that correspond to illustrations. Practical Applications questions are based on clinical situations.

2. The Instructor's Manual and Testbank includes:

   Chapter Overviews, Topics for Emphasis, Suggestions for Additional Studies, Supplementary Reading Assignments, a list of Web resources, and more than 1,000 multiple-choice-type Testbank questions. The printed version of Testbank questions are perforated and drilled for ease of use. Answers to the Study Guide and Testbank questions and answers to the Chapter Questions for Review are also provided in the Instructor's Manual.

3. Computerized Testbank

   Available upon adoption are the exact same questions mentioned above in an automatic, test-authoring, test-generating program that allows instructors to select questions electronically and prepare and print a test. The test is completely customized and includes test (or question) instructions and an answer key. This test-generator (ParTEST for Windows) provides the ability to add, change, or sort questions by chapter, objective, subject area (anatomy, physiology, or clinical), and question type. Additional features of the program include the ability to manipulate questions to produce different versions of the same test. It can also generate feedback reports.

4. Overhead Transparencies

   A set of color transparencies of key illustrations in the text is available for classroom instruction.

GUIDE TO PRONUNCIATION

The stressed syllable in each word is shown with capital letters. The vowel pronunciations are as follows:

Any vowel at the end of a syllable is given a long sound, as follows:

a as in say
e as in be
i as in nice
o as in go
u as in true

A vowel followed by a consonant and the letter e (as in rate) also is given a long pronunciation.

Any vowel followed by a consonant receives a short pronunciation, as follows:

a as in absent
e as in end
i as in bin
o as in not
u as in up

Acknowledgments

Above all, the authors wish to pay tribute to Dr. Ruth L. Memmler, the original author of *The Human Body in Health and Disease*. She first envisioned a book that would serve the needs of so many students preparing for Allied Health careers and over the years contributed to their training, not only with this book but in many personal and direct ways as well. This edition of *The Human Body in Health and Disease* is dedicated to Dr. Memmler.

We thank the Lippincott Williams & Wilkins staff members who have contributed their skills to this effort: the editor, Margaret Biblis, editorial assistant Amy Amico, and Barbara Ryalls, Managing Editor. The art and design staff include Brett MacNaughton, Carolyn O'Brien, and Kathy Luedtke. We appreciate the comments of reviewers and especially Jim Rosack, who reviewed sections of the text and contributed to the health boxes. Special thanks to Peg Waltner, Developmental Editor, who guided this book from start to finish, and to Darlene Pedersen, who consulted in the early stages of development.

Brief Contents

Contents

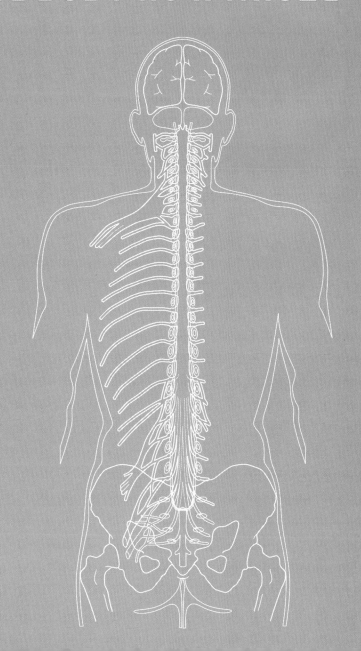

Unit I

THE BODY AS A WHOLE

This unit presents the basic levels of organization within the human body. Included is a description of the smallest units of life, called cells. Similar cells are grouped together as tissues, which are combined to form organs. Organs, in turn, work together in the various body systems, which together satisfy the needs of the entire organism. A short survey of chemistry, which deals with the composition of all matter and is important for the understanding of human physiology, is incorporated into this unit. These chapters should prepare the student for the more detailed study of individual body systems in the units that follow.

1

Organization of the Human Body

SELECTED KEY TERMS

The following terms are defined in the Glossary:

anabolism

anatomy

ATP

catabolism

cell

gram

homeostasis

liter

metabolism

meter

negative feedback

organ

pathology

physiology

system

tissue

BEHAVIORAL OBJECTIVES

After careful study of this chapter, you should be able to:

1. Define the terms *anatomy, physiology,* and *pathology*

2. Describe the organization of the body from chemicals to the whole organism

3. List 10 body systems and give the general function of each

4. Define *metabolism* and name the two phases of metabolism

5. Briefly explain the role of ATP in the body

6. Differentiate between extracellular and intracellular fluids

7. Define *homeostasis* and *negative feedback*

8. List and define the main directional terms for the body

9. List and define the three planes of division of the body

10. Name the subdivisions of the dorsal and ventral cavities

11. Name the basic metric units of length, weight, and volume

12. Name and locate the nine regions of the abdomen

13. Name the basic units of length, weight, and volume in the metric system

14. Define the metric prefixes *kilo-, centi-, milli-,* and *micro-*

STUDIES OF THE HUMAN BODY

Nearly everyone is interested in the human body and how it is affected by disease. Articles on health and medicine appear daily in newspapers and magazines. More and more, ordinary people not specifically trained in medicine are being asked to make decisions about medical treatments affecting their health and the health of their families.

The scientific term for the study of body structure is *anatomy* (ah-NAT-o-me). Part of this word means "to cut" because a fundamental way to learn about the human body is to cut it apart, or *dissect* it. *Physiology* (fiz-e-OL-o-je) is the term for the study of how the body functions, and the two sciences are closely related. They form the basis for all medical practice. Anything that upsets the normal structure or working of the body is considered a *disease* and is studied as the science of *pathology* (pah-THOL-o-je). It is hoped that from these studies you will gain an appreciation for the design and balance of the human body and for living organisms in general.

Levels of Organization

All living things are organized from very simple levels to more complex levels (Fig. 1-1). Living matter begins with simple chemicals. These chemicals are formed into the complex substances that make living *cells*—the basic units of all life. Specialized groups of cells form *tissues*, and tissues may function together as *organs*. Organs functioning together for the same general purpose make up organ *systems*. The organ systems work together to maintain the body.

✔ CHECKPOINT **1**:

In studying the human body, one may concentrate on either its structure or its function. What are these two studies called?

BODY SYSTEMS

Most of the studies of the body as a whole are organized according to the individual systems, as follows:

- The *integumentary* (in-teg-u-MEN-tar-e) *system.* The word *integument* (in-TEG-u-ment) means skin. The skin with its associated structures is considered a separate body system. The structures associated with the skin include the hair, the nails, and the sweat and oil glands.
- The *skeletal system.* The basic framework of the body is a system of more than 200 bones and the joints between them, collectively known as the *skeleton.*

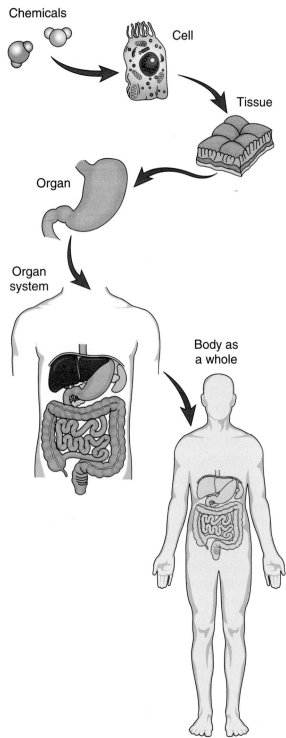

Chemicals

Cell

Tissue

Organ

Organ system

Body as a whole

FIGURE **1•1** Levels of organization.

- The ***muscular system.*** Body movements result from the action of the skeletal muscles, which are attached to the bones. Other types of muscles are present in the walls of body organs, such as the intestine and the heart.
- The ***nervous system.*** The brain, the spinal cord, and the nerves make up this complex system by which the body is controlled and coordinated. The organs of special sense (such as the eyes, ears, taste buds, and organs of smell), together with the receptors for touch and other senses, receive stimuli from the outside world. These stimuli are converted into impulses that are transmitted to the brain. The brain directs the body's responses to these outside messages and also to messages coming from within the body. Such higher functions as memory and reasoning also occur in the brain.
- The ***endocrine*** (EN-do-krin) ***system.*** The scattered organs known as ***endocrine glands*** are grouped together because they share a similar function. All produce special substances called ***hormones,*** which regulate such body activities as growth, food utilization within the cells, and reproduction. Examples of endocrine glands are the thyroid and the pituitary glands.
- The ***circulatory system.*** The heart and blood vessels make up the system that pumps blood to all the body tissues, bringing with it nutrients, oxygen, and other substances and carrying away waste materials. Lymphatic vessels play an important auxiliary role in circulation.
- The ***respiratory system.*** This system includes the lungs and the passages leading to the lungs. The purpose of this system is to take in air and conduct it to the areas designed for gas exchange. Oxygen passes from the air into the blood and is carried to all tissues by the circulatory system. In like manner, carbon dioxide, as a gaseous waste product, is taken by the circulation from the tissues back to the lungs to be expelled.
- The ***digestive system.*** This system comprises all the organs that are involved with taking in food and converting it into substances that body cells can use. Examples of these organs are the mouth, esophagus, stomach, intestine, liver, and pancreas.

- The ***urinary system.*** This system is also called the ***excretory system.*** Its main components are the kidneys, the ureters, the bladder, and the urethra. Its chief purpose is to rid the body of waste products and excess water. (Note that other waste products are removed by the digestive and respiratory systems and by the skin.)
- The ***reproductive system.*** This system includes the external sex organs and all related internal structures that are concerned with the production of offspring.

The number of systems may vary in different lists. Some, for example, show the sensory and lymphatic systems as separate entries. Others include the immune system, which protects the body from foreign matter. The immune system is identified by its function rather than its structure and includes elements of both the circulatory and lymphatic systems.

BODY PROCESSES

Metabolism

All the life-sustaining reactions that go on within the body systems together make up ***metabolism*** (meh-TAB-o-lizm). Metabolism can be divided into two types of activities:

- In ***catabolism*** (kah-TAB-o-lizm), complex substances are broken down into simpler compounds. The breakdown of the nutrients in food yields simple chemical building blocks and energy to power cell activities.
- In ***anabolism*** (ah-NAB-o-lizm), simple compounds are used to manufacture materials needed for growth, function, and repair of tissues. Anabolism is the building phase of metabolism.

The energy obtained from the breakdown of nutrients is used to form a compound often described as the "energy currency" of the cell. It has the long name of ***adenosine triphosphate*** (ah-DEN-o-sene tri-FOS-fate), but is commonly abbreviated ***ATP.*** Chapter 20 has more information on metabolism and ATP.

Fluid Balance

It is important to recognize that our bodies are composed of large amounts of fluids. The amount and composition of these fluids must be regulated at all times. Certain fluids bathe the cells, carry nutrient substances to and from the cells, and transport the nutrients into and out of the cells. This group of fluids is called ***extracellular fluid*** because it includes all body fluids outside the cells. A second type of fluid, ***intracellular fluid,*** is contained within the cells. Extracellular and intracellular fluids account for about 60% of an adult's weight.

Homeostasis

The purpose of metabolism is to maintain a state of balance within the organism, an important characteristic of all living things. Such conditions as body temperature, the composition of body fluids, heart rate, respiration rate, and blood pressure must be kept within set limits to maintain health. This steady state within the organism is called ***homeostasis*** (ho-me-o-STA-sis), which literally means "staying (stasis) the same (homeo)."

Feedback
Homeostasis is maintained by the feedback of information. Sensors throughout the body monitor internal conditions and bring them back to normal when they shift, much as a thermostat regulates the temperature of a house to a set level. Because each change, up or down, must be reversed to restore the norm, this mechanism is described as ***negative feedback.*** The main controllers in this self-regulation are the nervous and endocrine systems. You will find many examples of negative feedback throughout this book.

✔ CHECKPOINT **2**:

Metabolism is divided into a breakdown phase and a building phase. What are these two phases called?

DIRECTIONS IN THE BODY

Because it would be awkward and inaccurate to speak of bandaging the "southwest part" of the chest, a number of terms are used to designate position and directions in the body. They refer to the body in the ***anatomic position***—upright with face front, arms at the sides with palms forward, and feet parallel.

Directional Terms

The main terms for describing directions in the body are as follows (Fig. 1-2):

- ***Superior*** is a term meaning above, or in a higher position. Its opposite, ***inferior,*** means below, or lower. The heart, for example, is superior to the intestine.
- ***Ventral*** and ***anterior*** mean the same thing in humans: located toward the belly surface or front of the body. Their corre-

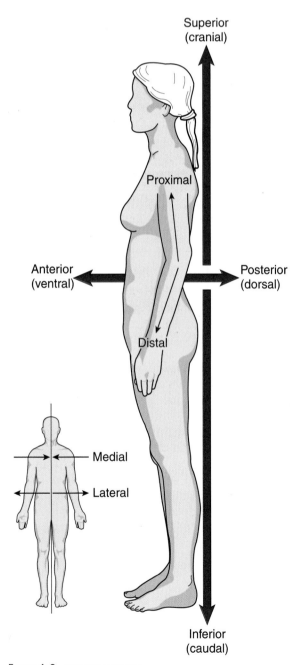

FIGURE **1•2**   Directional terms.

A Map of the Body

The body's surface landmarks provide a good introduction to body structure. These landmarks are also useful for orientation in surgery and other clinical procedures. For example, the lower tip of the sternum, the xiphoid process, is used as a reference point in the administration of CPR (cardiopulmonary resuscitation).

Feel for some of the other superficial markings to learn how your body is organized. The joint between the mandible and the temporal bone of the skull (the temporomandibular joint, or TMJ) can be felt in front of the ear canal as you move your lower jaw up and down. The pulse of the facial artery can be felt in a small depression about 1 inch in front of the angle of the lower jaw. The pulse of the carotid artery can be felt at the side of the neck.

Touch behind your neck for the spine of the 7th cervical vertebra, the prominent vertebra at the base of the neck. At the distal end of the forearm, you can feel the pulse of the radial artery at the lateral surface of the anterior wrist.

In the torso, you can feel the ribs and the lower margin of the rib cage. By placing your hands on your hips, you can feel the crest of the hip bone. When it hurts to sit on a hard chair, you become aware of the lower bone of the pelvic girdle on each side.

Many other features can be seen and felt at the surface to tell us about the structure and the condition of the body.

sponding opposites, **dorsal** and **posterior,** refer to locations nearer the back.

- **Cranial** means nearer to the head. **Caudal** means nearer to the sacral region of the spinal column (*i.e.,* where the tail is located in lower animals).
- **Medial** means nearer to an imaginary plane that passes through the midline of the body, dividing it into left and right portions. **Lateral,** its opposite, means farther away from the midline, toward the side.
- **Proximal** means nearer the origin of a structure; **distal,** farther from that point. For example, the part of your thumb where it joins your hand is its proximal region; the tip of the thumb is its distal region.

For additional information, see A Map of the Body.

Planes of Division

For convenience in visualizing the spatial relations of various body structures to each other, anatomists have divided the body into three imaginary planes, each of which is a cut through the body in a different direction (Fig. 1-3).

- The **sagittal** (SAJ-ih-tal) **plane.** If you were to cut the body in two from front to back, separating it into right and left portions, the sections you would see would be sagittal sections. A cut exactly down the midline of the body, separating it into equal right and left halves, is a **midsagittal** section.
- The **frontal plane.** If the cut were made in line with the ears and then down the middle of the body, creating a front and a rear portion, you would see a front (anterior or ventral) section and a rear (posterior or dorsal) section. Another name for this plane is *coronal plane.*
- The **transverse plane.** If the cut were made horizontally, across the other two planes, it would divide the body into an upper (superior) part and a lower (inferior) part. There could be many such cross-

Frontal
(coronal)
plane

Sagittal
plane

Transverse
(horizontal)
plane

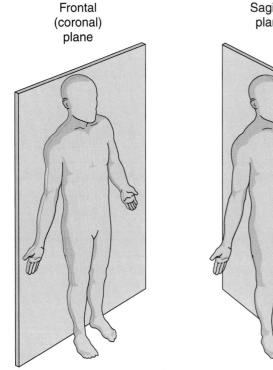
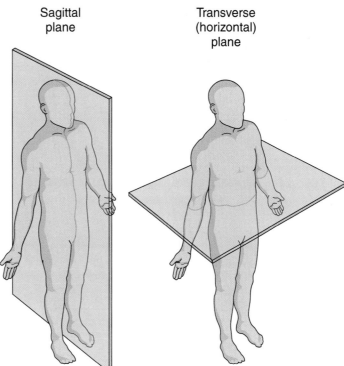

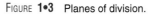

FIGURE **1•3** Planes of division.

sections, each of which would be on a transverse plane, also called a *horizontal plane.*

✔ CHECKPOINT **3**:

What are the three planes in which the body can be cut? What kind of a plane divides the body into two equal halves?

BODY CAVITIES

The body contains a few large internal spaces, or **cavities,** within which various organs are located. There are two main cavities: **dorsal** and **ventral** (Fig. 1-4).

Dorsal Cavity

The dorsal body cavity has two regions: the **cranial cavity,** containing the brain, and the **spinal canal,** enclosing the spinal cord. These two areas form one continuous space.

Ventral Cavity

The ventral cavity is much larger than the dorsal cavity. It has two main regions, which are separated by the **diaphragm** (DI-ah-fram), a muscle used in breathing. The **thoracic** (tho-RAS-ik) **cavity** is located above the diaphragm. Its contents include the heart, the lungs, and the large blood vessels that join the heart. The heart is contained in the pericardial sac; the lungs are in the pleural sacs (Fig. 1-5). The **abdominopelvic** (ab-dom-ih-no-PEL-vik) **cavity** is located below the diaphragm. This space is further subdivided into two regions. The uppermost **abdominal cavity** contains the stomach, most of the intestine, the kidneys, the liver, the gallbladder, the pancreas, and the spleen. The lower portion, set off by an imaginary line across the top of the hip bones, is the **pelvic cavity.** This cavity contains

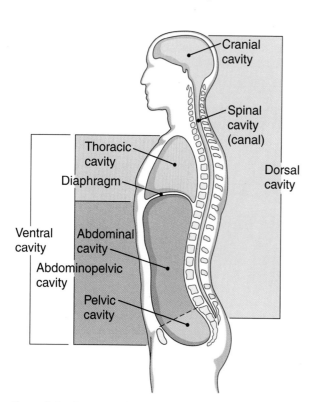

FIGURE **1•4**   Side view of the body cavities.

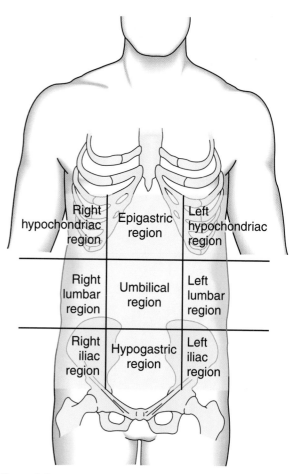

FIGURE **1•5**   The nine regions of the abdomen.

the urinary bladder, the rectum, and the internal parts of the reproductive system.

✔ CHECKPOINT **4**:

There are two main body cavities, one posterior and one anterior. Name these two cavities.

Regions of the Abdomen

Because the abdomen is so large, it is helpful to divide it for examination and reference into nine regions (see Fig. 1-5). The three central regions are the **epigastric** (ep-ih-GAS-trik) **region,** located just below the breastbone; the **umbilical** (um-BIL-ih-kal) **region** around the umbilicus (um-BIL-ih-kus), commonly called the *navel;* and the **hypogastric** (hi-po-GAS-trik) **region,** the lowest of all the midline regions.

At each side are the right and left **hypochondriac** (hi-po-KON-dre-ak) **regions,** just below the ribs; then the right and left **lumbar regions;** and finally the right and left **iliac,** or **inguinal** (IN-gwih-nal), **regions.**

A simpler but less precise division into four quadrants is sometimes used. These are the right upper quadrant (RUQ), left upper quadrant (LUQ), right lower quadrant (RLQ), and left lower quadrant (LLQ) (Fig. 1-6).

✔ CHECKPOINT **5**:

Name the three central regions and the three lateral regions of the abdomen.

See Imaging the Body.

THE METRIC SYSTEM

Now that we have set the stage for further study of the body and its structure and processes, a look at the metric system is in order because this is the system used for all scientific measurements. The drug industry and the health care industry already have converted to the metric system, so anyone who plans a career in health care should be acquainted with metrics.

The metric system is like the monetary sys-

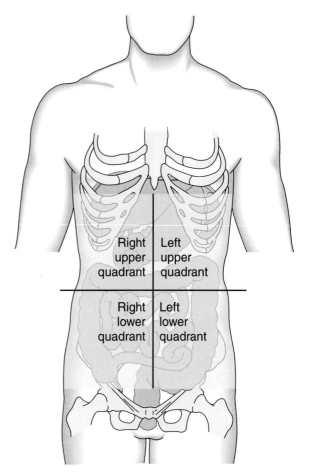

FIGURE **1•6** Quadrants of the abdomen showing the organs within each quadrant.

tem in the United States. Both are decimal systems based on multiples of the number 10. One hundred cents equal one dollar; one hundred centimeters equal one meter. Each multiple in the decimal system is indicated by a prefix:

kilo = 1000
centi = 1/100
milli = 1/1000
micro = 1/1,000,000

Units of Length

The basic unit of length in the metric system is the **meter.** Thus, 1 kilometer is equal to 1000 meters. A centimeter is 1/100 of a meter; stated another way, there are 100 centimeters in 1

Imaging the Body

Diagnostic imaging techniques are based on the physical properties of the human body and its response to forces such as ionizing radiation, magnetic fields, and sound waves. With diagnostic imaging, it is possible to view the interior of the body without resorting to exploratory surgery.

The oldest and most familiar method is radiography (ra-de-OG-rah-fe), which uses x-rays (a form of radiation) to produce a picture on a special type of film. The dark areas indicate where the beam passed through the body and exposed the film. The light areas show where the beam was blocked or deflected. Structures clearly visible on x-ray films are dense structures, such as bones. Structures not as dense as bone also deflect the rays but to a smaller extent. Sometimes, an opaque material is introduced to show outlines of soft tissue, as in a "barium swallow." X-rays are damaging to body tissues, but with modern equipment, extremely low doses can be used.

Newer methods for imaging include CT (computed tomography), which produces computerized images from a large number of x-rays passed at different angles through the body; MRI (magnetic resonance imaging), which uses a magnetic field and radiowaves to produce images; and ultrasound, which generates an image from the echoes of high-frequency sound waves traveling back from the tissues.

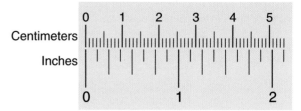

FIGURE **1•7** Comparison of centimeters and inches.

Units of Weight

The same prefixes used for linear measurements are used for weights and volumes. The *gram* is the basic unit of weight. Thirty grams are about equal to 1 ounce, and 1 kilogram to 2.2 pounds. Drug dosages are usually stated in grams or milligrams. One thousand milligrams equal 1 gram; a 500-milligram (mg) dose would be the equivalent of 0.5 gram (g), and 250 mg is equal to 0.25 g.

Units of Volume

The dosages of liquid medications are given in units of volume. The basic metric measurement for volume is the *liter* (LE-ter). There are 1000 milliliters (ml) in a liter. A liter is slightly greater than a quart, a liter being equal to 1.06 quarts. For smaller quantities, the milliliter is used most of the time. There are 5 ml in a teaspoon and 15 ml in a tablespoon. A fluid ounce contains 30 ml.

meter. A changeover to the metric system has been slow in coming to the United States. Often, measurements on packages, bottles, and yard goods are now given according to both scales. In this text, equivalents in the more familiar units of inches, feet, and so forth are included along with the metric units for comparison. There are 2.5 centimeters (cm) or 25 millimeters (mm) in 1 inch, as shown in Figure 1-7. Some equivalents that may help you to appreciate the size of various body parts are as follows:

1 mm = 0.04 inch, or 1 inch = 25 mm
1 cm = 0.4 inch, or 1 inch = 2.5 cm
1 m = 3.3 feet, or 1 foot = 30 cm

Temperature

The Celsius (centigrade) temperature scale, now in use by most countries and by scientists in this country, is discussed in Chapter 20.

A chart of all the common metric measurements and their equivalents is shown in Appendix 1. A Celsius-Fahrenheit temperature conversion scale appears in Appendix 2.

 CHECKPOINT **6**:

Name the basic units of length, weight, and volume in the metric system.

Summary

I. Studies of the human body
1. Anatomy—study of structure
2. Physiology—study of function
3. Pathology—study of disease

A. Levels of organization—chemicals, cell, tissue, organ, organ system, whole organism

II. Body systems
1. Integumentary system—skin and associated structures
2. Skeletal system—support
3. Muscular system—movement
4. Nervous system—reception of stimuli and control of responses
5. Endocrine system—production of hormones for regulation of growth, metabolism, reproduction
6. Circulatory system (includes lymphatic system)—transport
7. Respiratory system—intake of oxygen and release of carbon dioxide
8. Digestive system—intake and breakdown of food
9. Urinary system—elimination of waste and water
10. Reproductive system—production of offspring

III. Body processes
A. Metabolism—all the chemical reactions needed to sustain life
1. Catabolism—breakdown of complex substances into simpler substances; release of energy from nutrients
   a. ATP (adenosine triphosphate)—energy compound of cells
2. Anabolism—building of body materials

B. Fluid balance
1. Extracellular fluid—outside the cells
2. Intracellular fluid—inside the cells

C. Homeostasis
1. Steady state of body conditions
2. Maintained by negative feedback

IV. Directions in the body
1. Anatomic position—upright, palms forward, face front, feet parallel

A. Directional terms
1. Superior—above or higher; inferior—below or lower
2. Ventral (anterior)—toward belly or front surface; dorsal (posterior)—nearer to back surface
3. Cranial—nearer to head; caudal—nearer to sacrum
4. Medial—toward midline; lateral—toward side
5. Proximal—nearer to point of origin; distal—farther from point of origin

B. Planes of division
1. Sagittal—from front to back, dividing the body into left and right parts
   a. Midsagittal—exactly down the midline
2. Frontal (coronal)—from left to right, dividing the body into anterior and posterior parts
3. Transverse—horizontally, dividing the body into superior and inferior parts

V. Body cavities
A. Dorsal cavity—contains cranial and spinal cavities for brain and spinal cord

B. Ventral cavity
1. Thoracic—chest cavity
   a. Contains heart and lungs
   b. Divided from abdominal cavity by diaphragm
2. Abdominopelvic
   a. Abdominal—upper region containing stomach, most of intestine, kidneys, liver, spleen, and others
   b. Pelvic—lower region containing reproductive organs, urinary bladder, rectum
   c. Nine regions of the abdomen: epigastric, umbilical, hypogastric, right and left hypochondriac, right and left lumbar, right and left iliac (inguinal)

d. Quadrants—abdomen divided into four regions

VI. The metric system—based on multiples of 10
　　1. Basic units
　　　　a. Meter—length
　　　　b. Gram—weight
　　　　c. Liter—volume
　　2. Prefixes—indicate multiples of 10

a. Kilo—1000 times
b. Centi—1/100th (0.01)
c. Milli—1/1000th (0.001)
d. Micro—1/1,000,000 (0.000001)
A. Units of length
B. Units of weight
C. Units of volume
D. Temperature—measured in Celsius (centigrade) scale

Questions for Study and Review

1. List three types of study of the human body and define each.
2. List levels of organization in the body from the simplest to the most complex.
3. Define *cell, tissue, organ,* and *system.*
4. List 10 body systems and briefly describe the function of each.
5. Name and define the two phases of *metabolism.*
6. What is ATP?
7. Define the term *homeostasis* and give two examples. How is homeostasis maintained?
8. Stand in the anatomic position.
9. List the opposite term for each of the following body directions: *superior, ventral, anterior, cranial, medial,* and *proximal.* Define each term and its opposite.
10. Describe the location of the knee in relation to the ankle; in relation to the hip.
11. Describe the location of the stomach in relation to the heart; in relation to the urinary bladder.
12. Describe the location of the ears in relation to the nose.
13. What are the three main body planes? Explain the division each makes.
14. Name the cavities within the dorsal and ventral cavities. Name one organ found in each.
15. Make a rough sketch of the abdomen and label the nine divisions.
16. Name and locate the four quadrants of the abdomen.
17. Give some instances in which it would be helpful to identify subdivisions of the abdomen.
18. Why should you learn the metric system? What are its advantages?

✔ ANSWERS TO CHECKPOINTS

1. Study of body structure is anatomy; study of body function is physiology.
2. The breakdown phase of metabolism is catabolism; the building phase of metabolism is anabolism.
3. The three planes in which the body can be cut are sagittal, frontal (coronal), and transverse (horizontal). The midsagittal plane divides the body into two equal halves.
4. The posterior cavity is the dorsal cavity; the anterior cavity is the ventral cavity.
5. The three central regions of the abdomen are the epigastric, umbilical, and hypogastric regions; the three lateral regions of the abdomen are the hypochondriac, lumbar, and iliac (inguinal) regions.
6. The basic unit of length in the metric system is the meter; of weight, the gram; of volume, the liter.

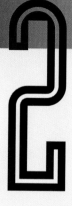

Chapter

2

Chemistry, Matter, and Life

SELECTED KEY TERMS

The following terms are defined in the Glossary:

acid

atom

base

buffer

carbohydrate

compound

covalent bond

electrolyte

electron

element

enzyme

ion

lipid

molecule

neutron

pH

protein

proton

solution

suspension

BEHAVIORAL OBJECTIVES

After careful study of this chapter, you should be able to:

1. Define an element
2. Describe the structure of an atom
3. Differentiate between molecules and compounds
4. Explain why water is so important to the body
5. Define *mixture*; list the three types of mixtures and give two examples of each
6. Differentiate between ionic and covalent bonds
7. Define the terms *acid, base,* and *salt*
8. Explain how the numbers on the pH scale relate to acidity and alkalinity
9. Define *buffer* and explain why buffers are important in the body
10. Define *radioactivity* and cite several examples of how radioactive substances are used in medicine
11. List three characteristics of organic compounds
12. Name the three main types of organic compounds and the building blocks of each
13. Define *enzyme*; describe how enzymes work

WHAT IS CHEMISTRY?

Great strides toward an understanding of living organisms, including humans, have come to us through *chemistry,* the science that deals with the composition of matter. Knowledge of chemistry and chemical changes helps us understand the normal and abnormal functioning of the body. The digestion of food in the intestinal tract, the production of urine by the kidneys, the regulation of breathing—all body processes—are based on chemical principles.

Chemistry also is important in *microbiology* (the study of microscopic plants and animals) and *pharmacology* (the study of drugs). The various solutions that are used to cleanse the skin before a surgical operation are chemicals, as are aspirin, penicillin, and all other drugs used in treating disease.

To provide some understanding of the importance of chemistry in the life sciences, this chapter briefly describes *elements, atoms* and *molecules, compounds,* and *mixtures,* which are fundamental forms of matter.

✔ CHECKPOINT **1**:

What is studied in the science of chemistry?

ELEMENTS

Elements are the substances from which all matter is made. Everything around us, everything we can see and touch, is made of elements—the food we eat, the atmosphere, all the water in the environment, the smoke coming out of a chimney. There are 92 naturally occurring elements. (Twenty additional elements have been created in the laboratory.) Examples of elements include various gases, such as hydrogen, oxygen, and nitrogen; liquids, such as the mercury used in thermometers and blood pressure instruments; and many solids, such as iron, aluminum, gold, silver, and carbon. Graphite (the so-called "lead" in a pencil), coal, charcoal, and diamonds are examples of the element carbon.

Elements can be identified by their names or their chemical symbols, which are abbreviations of the modern or Latin names of the element. Each element is also identified by its own number, which is based on the structure of the atoms that compose it. Table 2-1 lists some elements found in the human body along with their functions.

ATOMS

The subunits of elements are *atoms.* These are the smallest complete units of matter. They cannot be broken down or changed into another

Table 2•1	Some Common Chemical Elements*	
NAME	SYMBOL	FUNCTION
Oxygen	O	Part of water; needed to metabolize nutrients for energy
Carbon	C	Basis of all organic compounds; in carbon dioxide, the waste gas of metabolism
Hydrogen	H	Part of water; participates in energy metabolism, acid–base balance
Nitrogen	N	Present in all proteins, ATP (the energy compound), and nucleic acids (DNA and RNA)
Calcium	Ca	Builds bones and teeth; needed for muscle contraction, nerve impulse conduction, and blood clotting
Phosphorus	P	Active ingredient in the energy-storing compound ATP; builds bones and teeth; in cell membrane and nucleic acids
Potassium	K	Nerve impulse conduction; muscle contraction; water balance and acid–base balance
Sulfur	S	Part of many proteins
Sodium	Na	Active in water balance, nerve impulse conduction, and muscle contraction
Chlorine	Cl	Active in water balance and acid–base balance; found in stomach acid
Iron	Fe	Part of hemoglobin, the compound that carries oxygen in red blood cells

*The elements are listed in decreasing order by weight in the body.

form by ordinary chemical and physical means. These subunits are so small that millions of them could fit on the sharpened end of a pencil.

Atomic Structure

Despite the fact that the atom is such a tiny particle, it has been carefully studied and has been found to have a definite structure. At the center of the atom is a nucleus, which contains positively charged electrical particles called **protons** and noncharged particles called **neutrons.** Together, the protons and neutrons contribute nearly all of the atom's weight.

Outside the nucleus, in regions called orbitals, are **electrons** (Fig. 2-1). These nearly weightless particles are negatively charged. The protons and electrons always are equal in number, so that the atom as a whole is electrically neutral. The atomic number of an element is equal to the number of protons that are present in the nucleus of each of its atoms. Because the number of protons is equal to the number of electrons, the atomic number also represents the number of electrons whirling around the nucleus.

The positively charged protons keep the negatively charged electrons in the orbital area around the nucleus by means of the opposite charges on the particles. Positively (+) charged protons attract negatively (–) charged electrons. It is the electrons that determine how the atom will react chemically.

Energy Levels

Most atoms have several orbitals of electrons. Each orbital, however, can hold only two electrons. The orbitals are arranged into energy levels. Their distance from the nucleus of the atom identifies energy levels. The first energy level, the one closest to the nucleus, is composed of one orbital. The second energy level, the next in distance away from the nucleus, can have four orbitals. Because each orbital contains two electrons, the second energy level has the capacity to hold eight electrons.

The electrons farthest away from the nucleus are the particles that give the atom its chemical

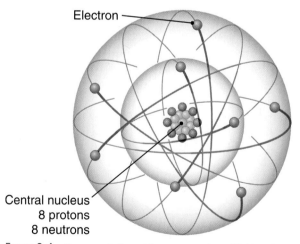

Electron

Central nucleus
8 protons
8 neutrons

FIGURE **2•1** Representation of the oxygen atom. Eight protons and eight neutrons are tightly bound in the central nucleus, around which the eight electrons revolve.

characteristics. If the outermost energy level has more than four electrons but less than its capacity of eight, the atom normally completes this level by gaining electrons. In the process, it becomes negatively charged because it has more electrons than protons. Such an atom is called a **nonmetal.** The oxygen atom illustrated in Figure 2-1 has six electrons in its second, or outermost, level. When oxygen enters into chemical reactions, it gains two electrons. The oxygen atom then has two more electrons than protons.

If the outermost shell has fewer than four electrons, the atom normally loses those electrons to attain a complete outer energy level. In so doing, it becomes positively charged. Such an atom is called a **metal.**

MOLECULES AND COMPOUNDS

When, on the basis of electron structure, two or more atoms unite, a **molecule** is formed. A molecule can be made of like atoms—the oxygen molecule is made of two identical atoms—but more often it is made of two or more different atoms. For example, a molecule of water (H_2O) contains 1 atom of oxygen (O) and 2 atoms of hydrogen (H) (Fig. 2-2).

Substances that contain molecules formed by the union of two or more different atoms are called **compounds.** Some compounds are made of a few elements in a simple combination. For example, the gas carbon monoxide (CO) contains 1 atom of carbon (C) and 1 atom of oxygen (O). Other compounds are very large and complex. Such complexity characterizes many of the compounds found in living organisms. Some proteins, for example, have thousands of atoms.

It is interesting to observe how different a compound is from any of its constituents. For example, a molecule of liquid water is formed from oxygen and hydrogen, both of which are gases. Another example is a crystal sugar, glucose ($C_6H_{12}O_6$). Its constituents include 12 atoms of the gas hydrogen, 6 atoms of the gas oxygen, and 6 atoms of the solid element carbon. In this case, the component gases and the solid carbon do not in any way resemble the glucose.

✔ CHECKPOINT **2**:

What is the difference between atoms and molecules?

More About Water

Water is the most abundant compound in the body. No plant or animal, including the human, can live very long without it. Water is of critical importance in all physiologic processes in body tissues. Water carries substances to and from the cells and makes possible the essential processes of absorption, exchange, secretion, and excretion. What are some of the properties of water that make it such an ideal medium for living cells?

- Water can dissolve many different substances in large amounts. For this reason, it is called the **universal solvent.** All the materials needed by the body, such as gases, minerals, and nutrients, dissolve in water to be carried from place to place.
- Water is stable as a liquid at ordinary temperatures. Water does not freeze until the temperature drops to 0°C (32°F) and does

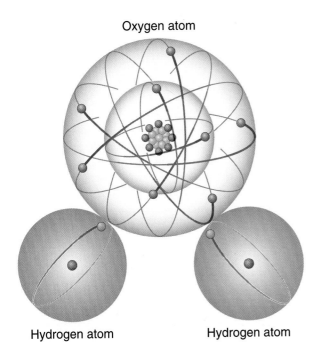

Oxygen atom

Hydrogen atom   Hydrogen atom

FIGURE **2•2**   Molecule of water.

not boil until the temperature reaches 100°C (212°F). This stability provides a constant environment for body cells. Water can also be used to distribute heat throughout the body and to cool the body by evaporation of sweat from the body surface.

- Water participates in chemical reactions in the body. It is needed directly in the process of digestion and in many of the metabolic reactions that occur in the cells.

✔ CHECKPOINT **3**:

What is the most abundant compound in the body?

Mixtures: Solutions and Suspensions

Not all elements or compounds combine chemically when brought together. The air we breathe every day is a mixture of gases, largely nitrogen, oxygen, and carbon dioxide, along with smaller percentages of other substances. The constituents in the air maintain their identity, although the proportions of each may vary. Blood plasma is also a mixture in which the various components maintain their identity. The many valuable compounds in the plasma remain separate entities with their own properties. Such combinations are called *mixtures*— blends of two or more substances.

A mixture, such as salt water, in which the component substances remain evenly distributed, is called a *solution.* The dissolving substance, in this case water, is the *solvent;* the substance dissolved, in this case salt, is the *solute.* Solutions of glucose, salts, or both in water are used for intravenous fluid treatments.

In some mixtures, the material distributed in the solvent settles out unless the mixture is constantly shaken; this type of mixture is called a *suspension.* Settling occurs in a suspension because the particles in the mixture are large and heavy. Examples of suspensions are milk of magnesia, finger paints, and, in the body, red blood cells suspended in blood plasma.

One other type of mixture is of importance in the body. Some organic compounds form *col-*

loidal suspensions, in which the molecules do not dissolve yet remain distributed in the solvent. The particles have electrical charges that repel each other, and the molecules are small enough to stay in suspension. The fluid that fills the cells (cytoplasm) is a colloidal suspension, as is blood plasma.

Many mixtures are complex, with properties of solutions, suspensions, and colloidal suspensions. Blood plasma has dissolved compounds, making it a solution. The red blood cells and other formed elements give blood the property of a suspension. The proteins in the plasma give it the property of a colloidal suspension. Chocolate milk also has all three properties.

✔ CHECKPOINT **4**:

Both solutions and suspensions are types of mixtures. What is the difference between them?

CHEMICAL BONDS

Ionic Bonds

When discussing the structure of the atom, we mentioned the positively charged (+) protons that are located in the nucleus, with the corresponding number of negatively charged (−) electrons found in the surrounding space that neutralize the protons. This neutrality is altered in chemical reactions. Atoms interact to reach a stable number of electrons in the outermost energy level. The sodium atom, for example, tends to lose the single electron in its outermost shell (Fig. 2-3). Removal of a single electron from the sodium atom leaves one more proton than electrons, and the atom then has a single net positive charge. The sodium atom in this form is symbolized as Na^+.

Similarly, atoms can gain electrons so that there are more electrons than protons. Chlorine, which has seven electrons in its outermost energy level, tends to gain one electron to fill the level to its capacity. Such an atom of chlorine is negatively charged (Cl^-) (see Fig. 2-3A).

An atom or group of atoms with a positive or negative charge is called an *ion* (I-on). An ion that is positively charged is a *cation*

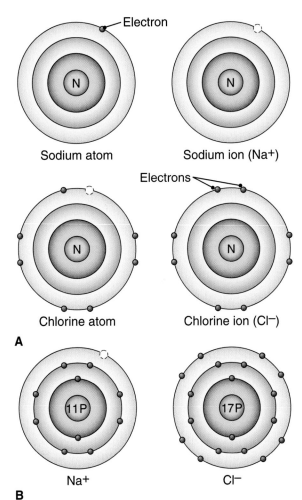

A

B

FIGURE **2•3** **(A)** Formation of sodium cation (Na⁺) and chlorine anion (Cl⁻). Only the electrons in the outermost energy level are shown. **(B)** A sodium ion with 11 protons in the nucleus and 10 electrons in orbitals is attracted to a chlorine ion with 17 protons in the nucleus and 18 electrons in oribitals to form the compound sodium chloride.

(CAT-i-on), whereas a negatively charged ion is an **anion** (AN-i-on).

Let us imagine a sodium atom coming in contact with a chlorine atom. The chlorine atom gains an electron from the sodium atom, and the two newly formed ions (Na^+ and Cl^-), because of their opposite charges, which attract each other, cling together and produce the compound sodium chloride, ordinary table salt. A bond formed by this method of electron transfer is called an **ionic bond** (see Fig. 2-3*B*).

Electrolytes

Ionically bonded molecules, when they go into solution, separate into charged particles. Compounds formed by ionic bonds that release ions when they are in solution are called **electrolytes** (e-LEK-tro-lites). (In practice, the term *electrolytes* is also used to refer to the ions themselves in body fluids.) Electrolytes are responsible for the acidity and the alkalinity of solutions. They also include a variety of salts, such as sodium chloride and potassium chloride. Electrolytes must be present in exactly the right quantities in the fluid within the cell (intracellular fluid) and the fluid outside the cell (extracellular fluid), or very damaging effects will result, preventing the cells in the body from functioning properly.

Ions in the Body

Many different ions are found in body fluids. Calcium ions (Ca^{++}) are necessary for the clotting of blood, the contraction of muscle, and the health of bone tissue. Bicarbonate ions (HCO_3^-) are required for the regulation of acidity and alkalinity of body fluids. The stable condition of the normal organism, homeostasis, is influenced by ions.

Because ions are charged particles, electrolyte solutions can conduct an electric current. Records of electric currents in tissues are valuable indications of the functioning or malfunctioning of tissues and organs. The **electrocardiogram** (e-lek-tro-KAR-de-o-gram) and the **electroencephalogram** (e-lek-tro-en-SEF-ah-lo-gram) are graphic tracings of the electric currents generated by the heart muscle and the brain, respectively (see Chaps. 10 and 14).

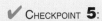 CHECKPOINT **5**:

Ionically bonded substances are called electrolytes. What happens when an electrolyte goes into solution?

Covalent Bonds

Although ionic bonds form many chemical compounds, a much larger number of compounds are formed by another type of chemical bond.

This bond involves not the exchange of electrons but a sharing of electrons between the atoms in the molecule and is called a *covalent bond.* The electrons orbit around both of the atoms, making both of them stable. Sometimes, the electrons are equally shared, as in the case of a hydrogen molecule (H_2), as well as other molecules composed of atoms of the same element. More commonly, the electrons are held closer to one atom than the other, as in the case of water (H_2O), shown in Figure 2-2. These bonds are called *covalent bonds.* Covalently bonded compounds do not conduct an electric current in solution. Carbon, the element that is the basis of organic chemistry, forms covalent bonds. Thus, the compounds that are characteristic of living things are covalently bonded compounds. These bonds may involve the sharing of one, two, or three pairs of electrons between atoms.

✔ CHECKPOINT **6**:

What type of chemical bond is formed by the sharing of electrons?

TYPES OF COMPOUNDS

Acids

An *acid* is a chemical substance capable of donating a hydrogen ion (H^+) to another substance. A common example is hydrochloric acid, the acid found in stomach juices:

$$HCl \rightarrow H^+ + Cl^-$$
(hydrochloric acid) (hydrogen ion) (chlorine ion)

Bases

A *base* is a chemical substance, usually containing a hydroxide ion (OH^-), that can accept a hydrogen ion. Sodium hydroxide, which releases hydroxide ion in solution, is an example of a base:

$$NaOH \rightarrow Na^+ + OH^-$$
(sodium hydroxide) (sodium ion) (hydroxide ion)

Salts

A reaction between an acid and a base produces a *salt,* such as sodium chloride:

$$HCl + NaOH \rightarrow NaCl + H_2O$$

THE pH SCALE

The greater the concentration of hydrogen ions in a solution, the greater is the acidity of that solution. As the concentration of hydrogen ions becomes less than it is in pure water, the more alkaline (basic) the solution becomes. Acidity is indicated by *pH* units, which represent the concentration of hydrogen ions in a solution. These units are listed on a scale from 0 to 14, with 0 being the most acidic and 14 being the most basic (Fig. 2-4).

A pH of 7.0 is neutral, having an equal number of hydrogen and hydroxide ions. Solutions that measure less than 7.0 are acidic; those that measure above 7.0 are alkaline (basic).

Each pH unit on the scale represents a 10-fold change in the number of hydrogen and hydroxide ions present. A solution registering 5.0 on the scale has 10 times the number of hydrogen ions as a solution that registers 6.0. A solution registering 9.0 has one tenth the number of hydrogen ions and 10 times the number of hydroxide ions as one registering 8.0. Thus, the lower the pH rating, the greater is the acidity, and the higher the pH, the greater is the alkalinity. Blood and other body fluids are close to neutral but are slightly on the alkaline side,

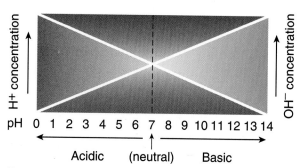

FIGURE **2•4** The pH scale measures degree of acidity or alkalinity.

with a pH range of 7.35 to 7.45, or nearly neutral. Figure 2-5 shows the pH of some other common substances.

Buffers

A delicate balance exists in the acidity or alkalinity of body fluids. If a person is to remain healthy, these chemical characteristics must remain within narrow limits. This balanced chemical state is maintained in large part by **buffers.** Chemicals that serve as buffers form a system that prevents sharp changes in hydrogen ion concentration and thus maintains a relatively constant pH. Buffers are important in maintaining the stability of body fluids.

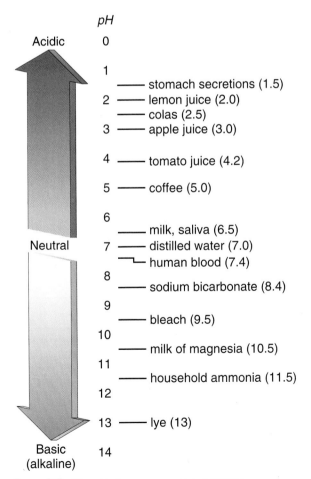

FIGURE **2•5**   The pH of some common substances.

> ✓ CHECKPOINT **7**:
>
> The pH scale is used to measure acidity of fluids. What number is neutral on the pH scale? What kind of compound measures lower than this number? Higher?

ISOTOPES AND RADIOACTIVITY

No discussion of atoms is complete without reference to the part some play in the diagnosis and treatment of disease. Atoms of an element may exist in several forms, called *isotopes.* These forms are alike in their chemical reactions but different in weight (*e.g.,* heavy oxygen and regular oxygen). The greater weight of the heavier isotopes is due to the presence of one or more additional neutrons in the nucleus. Some isotopes are stable and maintain constant characteristics. Others disintegrate (fall apart) and give off rays of atomic particles. These isotopes are said to be *radioactive.* Radioactive elements may occur naturally, as is the case with isotopes of the very heavy elements radium and uranium. Others may be produced artificially by bombarding the atoms of lighter, nonradioactive elements in accelerators that smash their nuclei together.

Use of Radioactive Isotopes

The rays given off by some radioactive elements, also called radioisotopes, are used in the treatment of cancer because they have the ability to penetrate and destroy tissues. Radiation therapy is often given by means of machines that are able to release tumor-destroying particles. The sensitivity of the younger, dividing cells in a growing cancer allows selective destruction of these abnormal cells with minimal damage to normal tissues. Modern radiation instruments produce tremendous amounts of energy (in the multimillion electron-volt range) and yet can destroy deep-seated cancers without causing serious skin reactions.

Radioactive isotopes, such as cobalt 60, in the form of pellets, may be sealed in stainless steel cylinders. These cylinders are mounted on arms or cranes that permit the proper alignment for directing the beams through a porthole to the area to be treated. In the form of needles, seeds, or tubes, implants containing radioactive isotopes are widely used in the treatment of many types of cancer.

In addition to its therapeutic values, irradiation is extensively used in diagnosis. X-rays penetrate tissues and produce an impression of their interior on a photographic plate. Radioactive iodine and other "tracers" taken orally or injected into the bloodstream are used to diagnose abnormalities of several body organs. Rigid precautions must be followed by health care personnel to protect themselves and the patient when using radiation in diagnosis or therapy because the rays can destroy both healthy and diseased tissues.

✔ CHECKPOINT **8**:

Some isotopes are stable; others break down to give off atomic particles. What word is used to describe isotopes that give off radiation?

Trace Elements

Trace elements are required in very small amounts by the body but are absolutely essential for health. Many are used in enzymes and vitamins.

Iodine is needed for the manufacture of thyroid hormones. Selenium is an antioxidant; that is, it helps to prevent damage to cells caused by the chemical process of oxidation. A deficiency of selenium leads to muscular disorders. Growth is impaired if the body lacks chromium. This element works with insulin, the hormone that helps the cells to take up glucose from the blood. Copper is needed for the proper use of iron, and cobalt is a part of vitamin B_{12} needed for blood cell formation. Zinc is used in energy metabolism, protein manufacture, immunity, and wound healing.

Other elements that are needed in trace amounts include silicon, nickel, fluorine, tin, and manganese. The diet must contain adequate sources of trace elements, which may be missing in refined and processed foods. More information on trace elements may be discovered as nutrition studies continue.

CHEMISTRY OF LIVING MATTER

Of the 92 elements that exist in nature, only 26 have been found in living organisms. Most of these are the elements that are light in weight. Not all are present in large quantity. Hydrogen, oxygen, carbon, and nitrogen are the elements that make up about 96% of the cells. Calcium, sodium, potassium, phosphorus, sulfur, chlorine, and magnesium are the seven elements that make up most of the remaining 4% of the elements in living cells. A number of others are present in trace amounts, such as iron, copper, iodine, and fluorine (see Trace Elements).

Organic Compounds

The chemical compounds that characterize living things are called *organic compounds.* All of these contain the element *carbon.* Because carbon can combine with a variety of different elements and can even bond to other carbon atoms to form long chains, most organic compounds consist of large, complex molecules. The starch found in potatoes, the fat in the tissue under the skin, and many drugs are examples of organic compounds. These large molecules are often formed from simpler molecules called *building blocks,* which bond together in long chains. The main types of organic compounds are carbohydrates, lipids, and proteins. All three contain carbon, hydrogen, and oxygen as their main ingredients.

✔ CHECKPOINT **9**:

Where are organic compounds found?

Carbohydrates

Carbohydrates are the simple sugars, called *monosaccharides* (mon-o-SAK-ah-rides), or are molecules made from simple sugars linked together. Carbohydrates in the form of sugars and starches are important sources of energy in the diet. Examples of carbohydrates in the body are the glucose that circulates in the blood as a nutrient for the cells and a storage form of glucose called ***glycogen*** (GLI-ko-jen).

Lipids

Lipids are a class of organic compounds mainly found in the body as ***fat.*** Fats are made from a substance called ***glycerol*** (glycerin) in combination with fatty acids. Fats provide insulation for the body and protection for organs. In addition, they are the main form in which energy is stored.

A group of complex lipids, called ***phospholipids*** (fos-fo-LIP-ids) because they contain the element phosphorus, is of importance. Among other functions, phospholipids make up a major part of the membrane around living cells. ***Cholesterol,*** found in cell membranes and also needed for the metabolism of fats, is derived from lipid, as are certain hormones.

Proteins

All ***proteins*** contain, in addition to carbon, hydrogen, and oxygen, the element ***nitrogen.*** They may also contain sulfur or phosphorus. Proteins are composed of building blocks called ***amino*** (ah-ME-no) ***acids.*** Although there are only about 20 different amino acids found in the body, a vast number of proteins can be made by linking them together in different combinations.

Proteins are the structural materials of the body, found in muscle, bone, and connective tissue. They also make up the pigments that give hair, eyes, and skin their color. It is protein that makes each individual physically distinct from others. All three categories of organic compounds, in addition to minerals and vitamins, must be taken in as part of a normal diet. These compounds are discussed further in Chapters 19 and 20.

✔ CHECKPOINT **10**:

What are the three main categories of organic compounds?

Enzymes

Enzymes are proteins that are essential for metabolism. They serve as catalysts in the hundreds of reactions that take place within cells. Without these catalysts, which speed the rate of chemical reactions, metabolism would not occur at a fast enough rate to sustain life. Because each enzyme works only on a specific substance and does only one specific chemical job, many different enzymes are needed. Their production is determined by genes (see Enzymes and Disease).

Like all catalysts, enzymes take part in reactions only temporarily; they are not used up or changed by the reaction. Therefore, they are needed in very small amounts. Many of the vitamins and minerals required in the diet are parts of enzymes.

The shape of the enzyme is important in its action. The form of the enzyme must match the shape of the substance or substances the enzyme combines with in much the same way as a key fits a lock. This so-called "lock-and-key" mechanism is illustrated in Figure 2-6. Harsh conditions, such as extremes of temperature or pH, can alter the shape of an enzyme and stop its action. Such an event is always harmful to the cells.

You can usually recognize the names of enzymes because, with few exceptions, they end

Enzymes and Disease

A hereditary unit called a gene controls the production of each enzyme. By controlling the manufacture of enzymes, genes govern all cell activities. Many hereditary disorders result from defects in the genes that control specific enzymes. These include PKU (phenylketonuria), a disorder in the ability to metabolize the amino acid phenylalanine. Some others are Gaucher (go-SHA) disease and Tay-Sachs disease, in which abnormal byproducts of metabolism accumulate in the tissues.

A more common example of enzyme deficiency occurs in people who are described as "lactose intolerant." These people lack the enzyme lactase used to digest the sugar in milk (lactose). Eating dairy products causes cramps, diarrhea, and gas. Someone with lactose intolerance must avoid milk products, buy lactose-free milk, or add lactase to their milk.

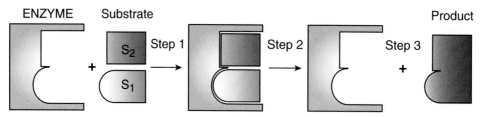

FIGURE **2•6** Diagram of enzyme action. The enzyme combines with substance 1 (S_1) and substance 2 (S_2). When a new product is formed, the enzyme is released unchanged.

with the suffix -*ase*. Examples are amylase, lipase, and oxidase. The first part of the name usually refers to the substance acted on or the type of reaction in which the enzyme is involved.

> ✔ CHECKPOINT **11**: _____
>
> Enzymes are proteins that act as catalysts. What is a catalyst?

Summary

I. What is chemistry?
  1. Science that deals with composition of matter
  2. Important in study of life sciences

II. Elements—substances from which all matter is made

III. Atoms—subunits of elements
  A. Atomic structure
    1. Protons—positively charged particles in the nucleus
    2. Neutrons—neutral particles in the nucleus
    3. Electrons—negatively charged particles in energy levels around the nucleus

IV. Molecules and compounds
  1. Molecules—combinations of two or more atoms
  2. Compounds—combinations of different atoms
  A. More about water—solvent; essential for metabolism

  B. Mixtures: solutions and suspensions
    1. Mixtures: blend of two or more substances
    2. Solution: substance (solute) remains evenly distributed in solvent (*e.g.,* salt in water)
    3. Suspension—material settles out of mixture on standing (*e.g.,* red cells in blood plasma)
    4. Colloidal suspension—particles do not dissolve but remain suspended (*e.g.,* cytoplasm)

V. Chemical bonds
  A. Ionic bonds—formed by transfer of electrons from one atom to another
    1. Electrolytes
      a. ionically bonded substances
      b. separate in solution into charged particles (ions)
      c. conduct electric current
  B. Covalent bonds—formed by sharing of electrons between atoms

VI. Types of compounds
  A. Acids—donate hydrogen ions
  B. Bases—accept hydrogen ions
  C. Salts—formed by reaction between acid and base

VII. The pH scale
  1. Measure of acidity or alkalinity of a solution
  2. Scale goes from 0 to 14
    a. 7 is neutral; below 7 is acidic; above 7 is alkaline (basic)
  A. Buffer—maintains constant pH of a solution

VIII. Isotopes and radioactivity
  A. Use of radioactive isotopes
    1. Diagnosis
    2. Cancer therapy
    3. X-ray films

IX. Chemistry of living matter
  A. Organic compounds—all contain carbon
    1. Carbohydrates (*e.g.,* sugars, starches)
    2. Lipids (*e.g.,* fats)
    3. Proteins (*e.g.,* structural materials, enzymes)
  B. Enzymes—organic catalysts

Questions for Study and Review

  1. Define *chemistry* and tell something about what is included in this study.
  2. Define an atom and describe the basic structure of an atom.
  3. Define *molecule, element, compound,* and *mixture.*
  4. What is an element and what are some examples of elements?
  5. Why is water so important to life?
  6. How does a mixture differ from a compound? Give two examples of each.
  7. Dissolve a teaspoon of sugar in a cup of tea. Which is the solute? The solvent?
  8. What are ions and how are they related to electrolytes? What are some examples of ions and of what importance are they in the body?
  9. Explain how covalent bonds are formed. Give two examples of covalently bonded compounds.
  10. What would a pH reading of 6.5 indicate about a solution? 8.5? 7.0?
  11. What is meant by *radioactivity* and what are some of its practical uses?
  12. What are organic compounds and what element is found in all of them?
  13. What elements are found in the largest amounts in living cells?
  14. What are the building blocks of carbohydrates? fats? proteins?
  15. What are enzymes? What type of organic compound are they?
  16. Why is the shape of an enzyme important to its action?

✔ ANSWERS TO CHECKPOINTS

  1. The composition of matter is studied in the science of chemistry.
  2. Atoms are the building blocks of elements; molecules are formed by the union of two or more atoms.
  3. Water is the most abundant compound in the body.
  4. In a solution, the components remain evenly distributed; in a suspension, the particles settle out unless the mixture is shaken.
  5. When an electrolyte goes into solution, it separates into charged particles called ions.
  6. A covalent bond is formed by the sharing of electrons.
  7. A value of 7.0 is neutral on the pH scale. An acid measures lower than 7.0; a base measures higher than 7.0.
  8. Isotopes that break down to give off radiation are termed radioactive.
  9. Organic compounds are found in living things.
  10. The three main categories of organic compounds are carbohydrates, lipids, and proteins.
  11. A catalyst is a compound that speeds up the rate of a chemical reaction.

3

Cells and Their Functions

SELECTED KEY TERMS

The following terms are defined in the Glossary:

active transport

cancer

cell membrane

centriole

chromosome

cytoplasm

diffusion

DNA

interphase

isotonic

micrometer

mitochondria

mitosis

mutation

nucleotide

nucleus

organelle

osmosis

phagocytosis

ribosome

RNA

BEHAVIORAL OBJECTIVES

After careful study of this chapter, you should be able to:

1. List three types of microscopes used to study cells

2. Describe the function and composition of the plasma membrane and the cytoplasm

3. Name and describe the main organelles in the cell

4. Give the composition, location, and function of DNA in the cell

5. Give the composition, location, and function of RNA in the cell

6. Explain briefly how cells make proteins

7. Name and briefly describe the stages in cell division

8. Define six methods by which substances enter and leave cells

9. Explain what will happen if cells are placed in solutions with the same or different concentrations than the cell fluids

10. Define *cancer*

11. List several risk factors for cancer

STUDIES OF CELLS

The cell is the basic unit of all life. It is the simplest structure that shows all the characteristics of life, including organization, metabolism, responsiveness, homeostasis, growth, and reproduction. In fact, it is possible for a single cell to live independently of other cells. Examples of some free-living cells are microscopic organisms such as protozoa and bacteria, some of which produce disease. All the activities of the human body, which is composed of millions of cells, result from the activities of individual cells. Cells produce all the materials manufactured within the body.

Microscopes

The scientific study of cells began more than 300 years ago with the invention of the microscope by Anton van Leeuwenhoek. In time, his single-lens microscope was replaced by the modern compound light microscope, which has two sets of lenses. This is the type of microscope most commonly used in laboratories. A great boon to cell biologists has been the development of the *transmission electron microscope,* which uses an electron beam instead of visible light to magnify an image up to 1 million times

(Fig. 3-1). Another type, the *scanning electron microscope,* does not magnify as much (×100,000) but gives a three-dimensional view of an object.

The metric unit used for microscopic measurements is the *micrometer* (MI-kro-me-ter). This unit is 1/1000 of a millimeter and is symbolized with the Greek letter for m, as μm.

Before they are examined under the microscope, cells and tissues usually are colored with special dyes called *stains* to aid in viewing. These stains produce the variety of colors you see when looking at pictures of cells and tissues taken under a microscope.

✔ CHECKPOINT **1**:

The cell is the basic unit of life. What characteristics of life does it show?

STRUCTURE OF THE CELL

Just as people may look different but still have certain features in common—two eyes, a nose, and a mouth, for example—all cells share certain characteristics. A typical animal cell is shown in Figure 3-2.

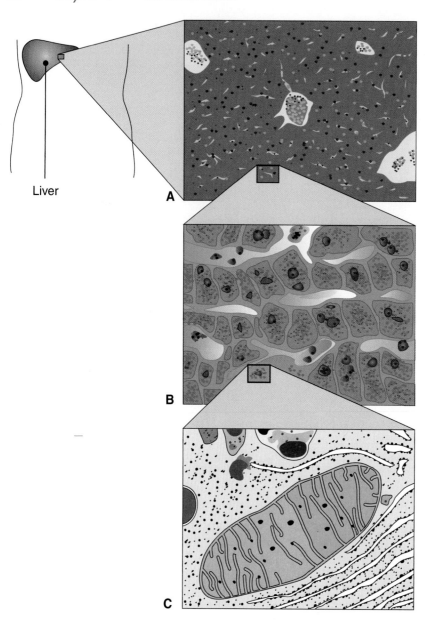

Liver

A

B

C

FIGURE **3•1** Liver tissue shown at three different magnifications. **(A)** Low power of the compound light microscope—100X. **(B)** Highest power of the compound light microscope—1000X. **(C)** Portion of a cell seen with a transmission electron microscope—48,000X.

Plasma Membrane

The outer limit of the cell is the ***plasma membrane,*** also called the *cell membrane* (Fig. 3-3). A double layer of lipid molecules makes up the main substance of this membrane. Because these lipids contain the element phosphorus, they are called ***phospholipids.*** Some molecules of cholesterol, another type of lipid, are located between the phospholipids. Cholesterol strengthens the membrane.

A variety of different proteins float within the phospholipids. Some proteins act as receptors, that is, as points of attachment for materials coming to the cell in the blood or tissue fluid. Others are enzymes, participating in reactions occurring at the plasma membrane. Some are transporters, shuttling materials into or out of the cell, and some form channels through which selected substances can pass. The plasma membrane is important in regulating what can enter and leave the cell.

3

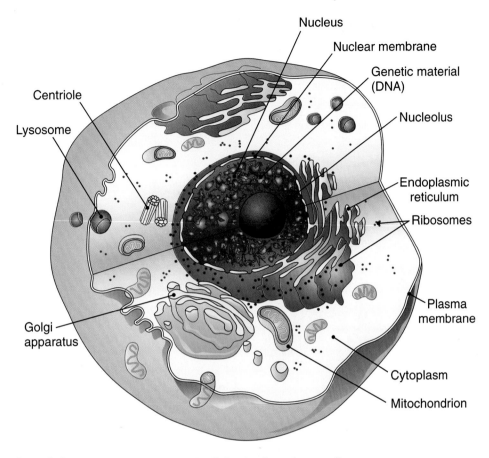

FIGURE **3•2**   Diagram of a typical animal cell showing the main organelles.

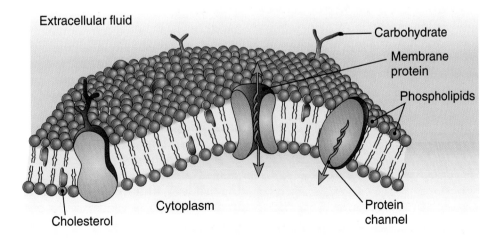

FIGURE **3•3**   Current concept of the structure of the plasma membrane.

Carbohydrates are present in small amounts, combined either with proteins or with lipids. These carbohydrates help cells to recognize each other and to stick together (see Cell Junctions).

Cytoplasm

The main substance that fills the cell and holds the cell contents is the *cytoplasm* (SI-to-plazm). This is a suspension of nutrients, minerals, enzymes, and other specialized materials in water. Although the composition of the cytoplasm has been analyzed, no one has been able to produce it in a laboratory; there must be

something about the organization of these substances that has not yet been discovered.

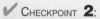

> ✔ CHECKPOINT **2**:
> _____
>
> The outer limit of the cell is a complex membrane. What are the three main ingredients in this plasma membrane?

Organelles

Just as the body has different organs to carry out special functions, the cell contains specialized subdivisions that perform different tasks. These structures are called *organelles,* which means "little organs." Each of these is examined next (see Fig. 3-2).

Nucleus

The largest organelle is the *nucleus* (NU-kle-us). This is often called the *control center* of the cell because it contains the genetic material, which governs all the activities of the cell, including protein manufacture and cell reproduction. Within the nucleus is a smaller globule called the *nucleolus* (nu-KLE-o-lus), which means "little nucleus." Its functions are not entirely understood, but it is believed to act in the manufacture of proteins within the cell.

Organelles in the Cytoplasm

The actual formation of proteins occurs on small bodies called *ribosomes* (RI-bo-somz). These are attached to a network of membranes throughout the cell called the *endoplasmic reticulum* (en-do-PLAS-mik re-TIK-u-lum). The name literally means "network" (reticulum) "within the cytoplasm" (endoplasmic), but for ease, it is almost always called simply the *ER.*

The *mitochondria* (mi-to-KON-dre-ah) are large organelles. They are round or bean-shaped structures with folded membranes on the inside. Within the mitochondria, the energy from nutrients is converted to energy for the cell in the form of ATP. These are the "power plants" of the cell. Active cells need lots of energy and thus have large numbers of mitochondria.

Cell Junctions

Some cells, for example, blood cells floating in plasma, are not in fixed contact with other cells. Most cells, however, are held in position with surrounding cells. What keeps cells together? First, the cell membranes contain complex substances that are sticky and tend to bind cells to each other. Second, there are special intercellular junctions, which vary according to the functions of the cells.

A *tight junction* is formed when the membranes cf adjacent cells actually become fused. This type of junction is found in the lining of the digestive tract and acts to keep digestive juices and other harmful substances from damaging the organs. One substance that can seep through the tight junctions of the stomach and damage the deeper tissues is alcohol.

Connections can form between adjacent cells where tissues are under great stress, for example, in the skin. Protein filaments extend from the cells; bridging the space between the membranes and anchoring cells to each other. These junctions are called *desmosomes* (DES-mo-somz).

Gap junctions allow materials to pass between cells. Small tubes made of protein connect the cells and act as channels for exchange of chemicals. These are found where cells need to communicate easily, as in the nervous system.

Other organelles in a typical cell include the *Golgi* (GOL-je) *apparatus,* which formulates special substances, such as mucus, released from cells; *lysosomes* (LI-so-somes), which contain digestive enzymes (see Lysosomes); and the *centrioles,* rod-shaped bodies near the nucleus that function in cell division. The features of all these cell structures are summarized in Table 3-1 for easy study.

Although the basic structure of all body cells is the same, individual cells may vary widely in size, shape, and composition according to the function of each. In size, they may range from the 7 μm of a red blood cell to the 200 μm or more of a muscle cell. A neuron with its long fibers is different in appearance from a muscle cell or from a transparent cell in the clear lens of the eye. Most human cells have all the organelles described, but these may vary in number.

Cilia and Flagellum

Some cells have small, hairlike projections from the surface called *cilia* (SIL-e-ah), which wave to create movement around the cell. Examples are the cells that line the passageways of the respiratory and reproductive tracts. A long, whiplike extension from the cell is a *flagellum*

Lysosomes

Lysosomes are small sacs in the cytoplasm of the cell that break down waste and foreign matter. They are most apparent in phagocytes, cells that engulf impurities in tissues and body fluids. They are also needed to dispose of cell debris in normal repair and remodeling of tissues.

Lysosomes contain digestive enzymes that would be harmful if they escaped into the cell. Normally, these enzymes are held safely within the membrane of the lysosome. If the membrane breaks or weakens, however, the cell begins to digest itself in a process called *autolysis* (aw-TOL-ih-sis), literally "self-destruction." Some investigators believe that autolysis is involved in cell aging and in a group of disorders described as *autoimmune diseases,* in which the body develops an immune response to its own tissues. Rheumatoid arthritis, a disorder of the joints, is one example of such a disease.

(flah-JEL-lum). Each human sperm cell has a flagellum that is used for locomotion. Thus, each cell is specialized for its particular function.

Table 3•1   Cell Structures

NAME	DESCRIPTION	FUNCTION
Cell membrane	Outer layer of the cell; composed mainly of lipids and proteins	Limits the cell; regulates what enters and leaves the cell
Cytoplasm	Colloidal suspension that fills cell	Holds cell contents
Nucleus	Large, dark-staining body near the center of the cell, composed of DNA and proteins	Contains the chromosomes with the genes (the hereditary material that directs all cell activities)
Nucleolus	Small body in the nucleus; composed of RNA, DNA, and protein	Needed for protein manufacture
Endoplasmic reticulum (ER)	Network of membranes in the cytoplasm	Used for storage and transport; holds ribosomes
Ribosomes	Small bodies attached to the ER; composed of RNA and protein	Manufacture proteins
Mitochondria	Large organelles with folded membranes inside	Convert energy from nutrients into ATP
Golgi apparatus	Layers of membranes	Put together special substances such as mucus
Lysosomes	Small sacs of digestive enzymes	Digest substances within the cell
Centrioles	Rod-shaped bodies (usually two) near the nucleus	Help separate the chromosomes in cell division
Cilia	Short, hairlike projections from the cell	Create movement around the cell
Flagellum	Long, whiplike extension from the cell	Moves the cell

✔ CHECKPOINT **3**:

What are cell organelles?

✔ CHECKPOINT **4**:

What are the two types of organelles used for movement, and what do they look like?

CELL FUNCTIONS

Protein Synthesis

Because protein molecules play an indispensable part in the body's activities, we need to identify the cellular substances that direct the production of protein. In the cytoplasm and in the nucleus are chemicals called ***nucleic*** (nu-KLE-ik) ***acids.*** The two nucleic acids important in protein production are ***deoxyribonucleic*** (de-ok-se-RI-bo-nu-kle-ik) ***acid,*** or ***DNA,*** and ***ribonucleic*** (RI-bo-nu-kle-ik) ***acid,*** abbreviated ***RNA.*** Both of these are large, complex molecules composed of subunits called ***nucleotides*** (NU-kle-o-tides) (Fig. 3-4). There are four nucleotides in DNA and four in RNA, but only three of these are common to both.

DNA

DNA molecules are found mostly in the nucleus of the cell, where they make up the ***chromosomes*** (KRO-mo-somes), which are dark-staining, threadlike bodies. Looking at Figure 3-4, you can see that DNA exists as a double strand. The two strands are matched according to the pattern of the nucleotides. The adenine (A) nucleotide always pairs with the thymine (T) nucleotide; the guanine (G) nucleotide always pairs with the cytosine (C) nucleotide. The two strands of DNA are held together by weak bonds. The doubled strands then coil into a spiral, giving DNA the descriptive name of the *double helix.*

Specific regions of the DNA in the chromosomes make up the ***genes,*** the hereditary factors of each cell. It is the genes that carry the messages for the development of particular in-

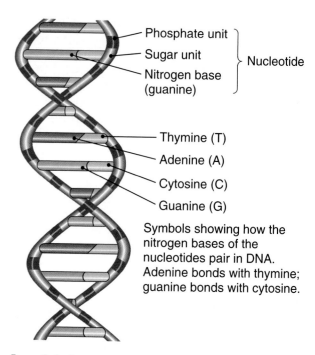

FIGURE **3•4** Schematic representation of the basic structure of a DNA molecule. Each structural unit, or nucleotide, consists of a phosphorus-containing unit and a sugar unit to which is attached a nitrogen base. There are four different nucleotides. Their arrangement "spells out" the genetic instructions that control all activities of the cell. The symbols in the upper right show how the nucleotides pair in DNA.

herited characteristics, such as brown eyes, curly hair, or blood type. Their message is actually contained in the pattern of the four nucleotides in the DNA (see DNA Fingerprinting in Chapter 6, page 81). These subunits code for the building of amino acids into the various cellular proteins. Remember that all enzymes are proteins, and enzymes are essential for cellular reactions. DNA is thus considered the master blueprint for the cell.

✔ CHECKPOINT **5**:

What category of compounds does DNA code for in the cell?

The Role of RNA

A blueprint is only a map. The information it illustrates must be translated by appropriate actions. RNA is the substance needed for this step. RNA is much like DNA except that it is a single strand and has a nucleotide called *thymine* (T) instead of cytosine (C). By pairing of nucleotides, RNA picks up the message of the DNA, which has by now broken its weak bonds and uncoiled into single strands. This *messenger RNA* travels into the cytoplasm to the ribosomes attached to the ER. Ribosomes are the organelles responsible for protein manufacture. They are so named because they are composed mainly of RNA. At the ribosomes, the genetic message is decoded to build amino acids into the long chains that form proteins.

Cell Division

For growth, repair, and reproduction, cells must multiply to increase their numbers. To ensure that every cell in the body has the same genetic information, cell division must be precise. In this process of cell division, or mitosis (mi-TO-sis), each original parent cell divides to form two identical daughter cells. Before mitosis can occur, however, the genetic information (DNA) in the parent cell must be doubled. DNA duplicates during interphase, the period between one mitosis and the next. While DNA is uncoiled from its double-stranded form, each strand duplicates itself according to the pattern of the nucleotides.

Stages of Mitosis

Mitosis itself is described as occurring in four stages, during which distinct changes can be seen in the dividing cell (Fig. 3-5).

- In **prophase** (PRO-faze), the doubled strands return to their spiral organization and become visible under the microscope as dark, threadlike chromosomes. Meanwhile, in the cytoplasm, the two centrioles move to opposite ends of the cell, trailing thin, threadlike substances that form a structure resembling a spindle stretched across the cell.
- In **metaphase** (MET-ah-faze), the chromosomes line up across the threadlike spindle.
- Then, in **anaphase** (AN-ah-faze), the duplicated chromosomes separate and begin to move toward opposite ends of the cell.
- As mitosis continues into **telophase** (TEL-o-faze), the nuclear area becomes pinched in the middle until two new nuclei have formed.

A similar pinching off occurs in the plasma membrane during telophase, making the cell resemble a dumbbell. The midsection between the two halves of the dumbbell becomes progressively smaller until, finally, the cell splits in two. There are now two identical daughter cells, which are themselves identical to, but smaller

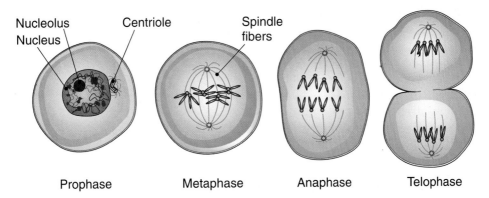

Nucleolus   Centriole   Spindle fibers
Nucleus

Prophase   Metaphase   Anaphase   Telophase

FIGURE **3•5**   The stages of mitosis. The cell shown is for illustration only. It is not a human cell, which has 46 chromosomes.

than, the parent cell. The two new cells grow and mature and continue to carry out life functions.

During mitosis, all the organelles, except those needed for the division process, temporarily disappear. After the cell splits, these organelles reappear in each daughter cell. Also at this time, the centrioles usually duplicate in preparation for the next cell division.

Body cells differ in the rate at which they reproduce. Some, such as nerve cells and muscle cells, stop dividing at some point in development and are not replaced if they die. They remain in interphase. Others, such as skin cells, multiply rapidly to replace cells destroyed by injury, disease, or natural wear-and-tear. As a person ages, characteristic changes in the overall activity of his or her body cells take place. One example of these changes is the slowing down of repair processes. A bone fracture, for example, takes considerably longer to heal in an aged person than in a young person.

> ✔ CHECKPOINT **6**:
>
> Cells must divide to allow for growth, repair, and reproduction. What is the scientific name for cell division?

Movement of Substances Across the Plasma Membrane

Cells constantly need nutrients and other materials from their environment to function. How to receive these nutrients would seem to be a problem because a protective membrane surrounds cells. However, if a cell is bathed in water containing dissolved nutrients, an interesting thing happens: the water with the dissolved nutrient particles passes through the plasma membrane. Not only do these molecules pass in, but also waste products pass out of the cell in the opposite direction, enabling the cell to perform the function of elimination. Thus, exchanges of some substances can occur between the cell and its environment through the plasma membrane. For this reason, the plasma membrane is described as **semipermeable** (sem-e-PER-me-ah-bl). It is permeable or passable to some molecules but impassable to oth-

ers. Some particles, for example, proteins, are simply too large to travel through the membrane unaided.

Water, a tiny molecule, is always able to penetrate the membrane with ease. Foods, however, must be split into small molecules by the process of digestion so that they can travel through the plasma membrane. For example, sucrose (table sugar) is converted to glucose, a smaller molecule that enters the cell to serve as a major source of energy.

Various physical processes are responsible for exchanges through plasma membranes. These are grouped according to whether they require cellular energy.

Movement That Does Not Require Cellular Energy

- **Diffusion** is the constant movement of molecules from a region of relatively higher concentration to one of lower concentration. Molecules, especially those in solution, tend to spread throughout an area until they are equally concentrated in all parts of a container (Figs. 3-6 and 3-7). When substances diffuse through a membrane, such as the intact plasma membrane, passage is limited to those particles small enough to pass through spaces in the membrane. A large-scale example is shown in Figure 3-8.

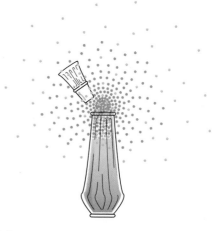

FIGURE **3•6** Diffusion of gaseous molecules throughout a given space. When a solution vaporizes, the molecules tend to spread throughout the area. Common examples are the diffusion of perfumes, oils, and cleaning solutions.

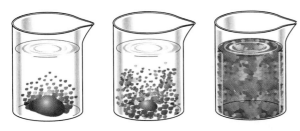

FIGURE **3•7** Diffusion of a solid in a liquid. Here, a solid diffuses into water. The molecules of the solid tend to spread evenly throughout the water.

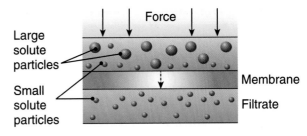

FIGURE **3•9** Filtration. A mechanical force pushes a substance through a membrane.

• ***Osmosis.*** Of all substances, water moves most rapidly through the cell membrane. The term *osmosis* means specifically the diffusion of water through a semipermeable membrane. The water molecules move, as expected, from an area where they are in higher number to an area where they are in lower number. That is, they move from a more dilute solution into a more concentrated solution. The tendency of a solution to draw water into it is called the **osmotic pressure** of the solution. This force is directly related to concentration: the higher the concentration of a solution, the greater is its tendency to draw water in.

• ***Filtration*** is the passage of water containing dissolved materials through a membrane as a result of a mechanical ("pushing") force on one side (Fig. 3-9). One example of filtration in the body is the formation of urine in the kidney (see Chap. 22). Another is the movement of materials out of the capillaries under the force of blood pressure (see Chap. 15).

These three processes are described as *passive* because they do not require cellular energy. They depend on the natural energy of the molecules for movement.

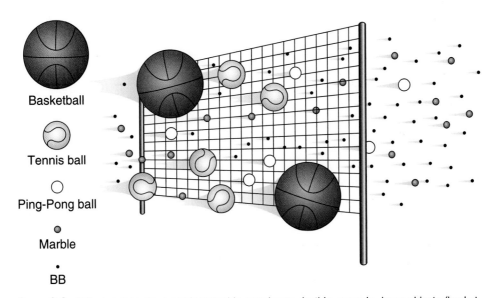

FIGURE **3•8** Diffusion through a semipermeable membrane. In this example, large objects (basketballs and tennis balls) cannot pass through the net. In the human body, large particles (proteins and blood cells) do not pass through intact membranes, such as the walls of the blood capillaries.

Movement That Requires Cellular Energy

- **Active transport.** Molecules often move into or out of a living cell in a direction opposite to the way they would normally flow by diffusion. That is, they move from an area where they are in relatively lower concentration to an area where they are in higher concentration. This movement, because it is against the natural flow, requires energy in the form of ATP. It also requires proteins in the cell membrane that act as **transporters** for the molecules.

  This process, called **active transport,** is a function of the living cell membrane. It allows the cell to take in what it needs from the surrounding fluids and to release materials from the cell. Because the cell membrane can carry on active transport, it is most accurately described as **selectively permeable.** It regulates what can enter and leave the cell based on its needs.

- **Phagocytosis** (fag-o-si-TO-sis) is the engulfing of relatively large particles by the cell membrane and the movement of these particles into the cell. Certain white blood cells carry out phagocytosis to rid the body of foreign material and dead cells.

- In **pinocytosis** (pi-no-si-TO-sis), droplets of fluid are engulfed by the cell membrane. This is a way for large protein molecules in suspension to travel into the cell. The word *pinocytosis* means "cell drinking."

> ✔ CHECKPOINT **7**:
>
> Substances are constantly moving into and out of cells through the plasma membrane. What types of movement do not require cellular energy and what types of movement do require cellular energy?

How Osmosis Affects Cells

As stated earlier, water moves easily through the cell membrane. Therefore, for a normal fluid balance to be maintained, all cells must be kept in solutions that have the same concentration of dissolved substances (solutes) as the fluids within the cell (Fig. 3-10). If not, water will

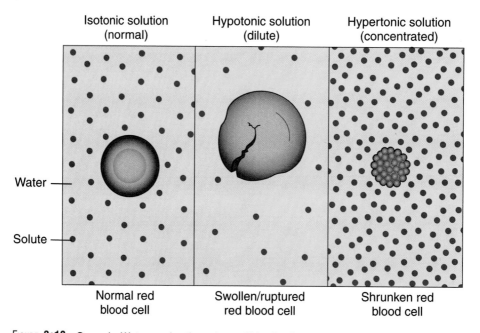

Isotonic solution   Hypotonic solution   Hypertonic solution
(normal)   (dilute)   (concentrated)

Water —

Solute —

Normal red   Swollen/ruptured   Shrunken red
blood cell   red blood cell   blood cell

FIGURE **3•10** Osmosis. Water moving through a red blood cell membrane in solutions with three different concentrations of solute. *(Left)* The isotonic (normal) solution has the same concentration as the cell, and the water moves into and out of the cell at the same rate. *(Center)* The hypotonic (dilute) solution causes the cell to swell and eventually hemolyze (burst) because of the large amount of water moving into the cell. *(Right)* The hypertonic (concentrated) solution draws water out of the cell, causing it to shrink.

move rapidly into or out of the cell by osmotic pressure. Solutions with concentrations equal to the concentration of the cytoplasm are described as *isotonic.*

Tissue fluids and blood plasma are isotonic for body cells. Manufactured solutions that are isotonic for the cells and can thus be used to replace body fluids include 0.9% salt or *normal saline* and 5% dextrose (glucose).

A solution that is less concentrated than the intracellular fluid is described as *hypotonic.* A cell placed in a hypotonic solution draws water in, swells, and may burst. When a red blood cell draws in water and bursts in this way, the cell is said to *hemolyze* (HE-mo-lize). If a cell is placed in a *hypertonic* solution, which is more concentrated than the cell fluid, it loses water to the surrounding fluids and shrinks (see Fig. 3-10).

Fluid balance is an important facet of homeostasis and must be properly regulated for health. You can figure out in which direction water will move through the plasma membrane if you remember the saying "water follows salt," salt meaning any dissolved material (solute). The total amount and distribution of body fluids is discussed in Chapter 21.

✔ CHECKPOINT **8**:

The concentration of fluids in and around the cell is important in homeostasis. What term describes a fluid that is the same concentration as the fluid within the cell (intracellular fluid)? What type of fluid is less concentrated? More concentrated?

CELLS AND CANCER

Through the study of cells, we gain some insight into the laws of growth. Based on the working of their DNA, cells develop various forms. Those that are of the same kind then congregate to form one of the basic tissues. These tissues, in turn, become the specialized organs. In the early stages of development, cells multiply rapidly, and the body grows to a maximum point. Thereafter, cell division is usually less frequent. It continues, however, at a rate sufficient to replace cells that wear out or have

been damaged. In this manner, the tissues are maintained, and every cell and formation of cells has its purpose.

Occasionally, some change occurs in the genetic material (DNA) of a cell. Such a change, termed a *mutation,* may cause a cell to reproduce without control. If these cells do not die naturally or get destroyed by the immune system, they will continue to multiply and may spread to other tissues, producing *cancer.* Cancer cells form tumors, which interfere with normal functions, crowding out normal cells and robbing them of nutrients. There is more information on the various types of tumors in Chapter 4.

Cancer Risk Factors

The causes of cancer are complex, involving the interaction of factors in the cell and the environment. Because cancer may take a long time to develop, it is often difficult to identify its cause or causes. Certain forces increase the chances of developing the disease and are considered risk factors. These include the following:

* *Heredity.* Certain types of cancer occur more frequently in some families than in others, indicating that there is some inherited predisposition to the development of cancer.
* *Chemicals.* Certain industrial and environmental chemicals are known to increase the risk of cancer. Any chemical that causes cancer is called a *carcinogen* (kar-SIN-o-jen). The most common carcinogens in our society are those present in cigarette smoke. Carcinogens are also present, both naturally and as additives, in foods. Certain drugs may be carcinogenic.
* *Ionizing radiation.* Certain types of radiation can produce damage to cellular DNA that may lead to cancer. These include x-rays, rays from radioactive substances, and ultraviolet rays. For example, the ultraviolet rays received from exposure to the sun are very harmful to the skin.
* *Physical irritation.* Continued irritation, such as the intake of hot foods or the con-

3

tact of a hot pipestem on the lip, increases cell division and thus increases the chance of mutation.

- **Diet.** It has been shown that diets high in fats and total calories are associated with an increased occurrence of certain forms of cancer. A general lack of fiber and insuffi-

cient amounts of certain fruits and vegetables in the diet can leave one susceptible to cancers of the digestive tract.

- **Viruses** have been implicated in cancers of the liver, the blood (leukemias), and lymphatic tissues (lymphomas).

Summary

I. Studies of cells
1. Cell is basic unit of life
   a. Has all characteristics of life
   b. Is responsible for all body activities
   A. Microscopes
   1. Types
      a. Compound light microscope
      b. Transmission electron microscope—magnifies up to 1 million times
      c. Scanning electron microscope—gives three-dimensional image
   2. Micrometer—metric unit commonly used for microscopic measurements
   3. Stains—dyes used to aid in viewing cells under the microscope

II. Structure of the cell
   A. Plasma membrane—regulates what enters and leaves cell
   B. Cytoplasm—colloidal suspension that holds organelles
   C. Organelles—subdivisions that carry out special functions
   1. Nucleus
      a. Controls cell activities
      b. Contains nucleolus
   2. Ribosomes, ER, mitochondria, Golgi apparatus, lysosomes, centrioles
   3. Cilia, flagellum—used for movement

III. Cell functions
   A. Protein synthesis—carried out by nucleic acids
   1. DNA
      a. Double strand of nucleotides
      b. Located in the nucleus
      c. Carries the genetic message
   2. RNA
      a. Single strand of nucleotides
      b. Located in the cytoplasm
      c. Translates DNA message into proteins
      d. Ribosomes—site of protein synthesis
   B. Cell division
   1. Duplication of chromosomes during interphase
   2. Mitosis
      a. Separation of chromosomes
      b. Division of cell into two identical daughter cells
      c. Four stages—prophase, metaphase, anaphase, telophase
   C. Movement of substances across plasma membrane
   1. Movement that does not require cellular energy
      a. Diffusion—molecules move from area of higher concentration to area of lower concentration
      b. Osmosis—diffusion of water through semipermeable membrane
      c. Filtration—movement of materials through cell membrane under mechanical force
   2. Movement that requires cellular energy

a. Active transport—movement of molecules from area of lower concentration to area of higher concentration
b. Phagocytosis—engulfing of large particles by plasma membrane
c. Pinocytosis—intake of droplets of fluid
3. How osmosis affects cells
   a. Isotonic solution—same concentration as cell fluids; cell remains the same
   b. Hypotonic solution—lower concentration than cell fluids; cell swells and may hemolyze (burst)
c. Hypertonic solution—higher concentration than cell fluids; cell shrinks

IV. Cells and cancer
1. Mutation
   a. Change in DNA
   b. May produce cancer
A. Cancer risk factors
1. Heredity
2. Chemicals—carcinogens
3. Ionizing radiation
4. Physical irritation
5. Diet
6. Viruses

Questions for Study and Review

1. Why is the study of cells so important in the study of the body?
2. Why is the plasma membrane so important to the cell?
3. Define the term *organelle.* List 10 organelles found in cells and give the function of each.
4. Compare DNA and RNA with respect to location in the cell and composition.
5. What are chromosomes? Where are they located in the cell and what is their function?
6. Explain the role of each of the following in protein synthesis: DNA, nucleotide, RNA, ribosomes.
7. Name the stage between one mitosis and the next.
8. Name the process of cell division. Name the stages of cell division and describe what happens during each.
9. Explain why it is necessary to reduce large molecules to smaller molecules by the process of digestion.
10. List and define six methods by which materials cross the cell membrane. Which of these requires cellular energy?
11. What substance moves most rapidly through the cell membrane?
12. Why is the cell membrane described as selectively permeable?
13. What is meant by the term *isotonic?* Name four isotonic solutions.
14. What will happen to a red blood cell placed in a 5.0% salt solution? in distilled water?
15. Define *mutation.*
16. List six risk factors associated with cancer.

✔ ANSWERS TO CHECKPOINTS

1. The cell shows organization, metabolism, responsiveness, homeostasis, growth, and reproduction.
2. The three main ingredients in the plasma membrane are phospholipids (lipids), proteins, and carbohydrates.
3. The cell organelles are specialized subdivisions that perform different tasks.
4. The two types of organelles used for movement are the cilia, which are small and hairlike, and the flagellum, which is long and whiplike.
5. DNA codes for proteins in the cell.
6. Mitosis is the scientific name for cell division.
7. Diffusion, osmosis, and filtration do not require cellular energy; active transport, phagocytosis, and pinocytosis require cellular energy.
8. An isotonic solution is the same concentration as the fluid within the cell; a hypotonic solution is less concentrated; a hypertonic solution is more concentrated

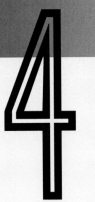

4

Tissues, Glands, and Membranes

SELECTED KEY TERMS

The following terms are defined in the Glossary:

adipose

areolar

benign

cartilage

collagen

endocrine

epithelium

exocrine

fascia

histology

malignant

matrix

membrane

metastasis

mucosa

myelin

neoplasm

neuroglia

neuron

serosa

BEHAVIORAL OBJECTIVES

After careful study of this chapter, you should be able to:

1. Name the four main groups of tissues and give the location and general characteristics of each

2. Describe the difference between exocrine and endocrine glands and give examples of each

3. Give examples of soft, fibrous, hard, and liquid connective tissues

4. Describe three types of epithelial membranes

5. List several types of connective tissue membranes

6. Explain the difference between benign and malignant tumors and give several examples of each type

7. List five methods of diagnosing cancer

8. List three methods of treating cancer

Tissues are groups of cells similar in structure, arranged in a characteristic pattern, and specialized for the performance of specific tasks. The study of tissues is known as *histology* (his-TOL-o-je). The tissues in our bodies might be compared with the different materials used to construct a building. Think for a moment of the great variety of building materials used according to need—wood, stone, steel, plaster, insulation, and so forth. Each of these has different properties, but together they contribute to the building as a whole. The same may be said of tissues in the body.

TISSUE CLASSIFICATION

The four main groups of tissue are the following:

- *Epithelial* (ep-ih-THE-le-al) *tissue* covers surfaces, lines cavities, and forms glands.
- *Connective tissue* supports and forms the framework of all parts of the body.
- *Muscle tissue* contracts and produces movement.
- *Nervous tissue* conducts nerve impulses.

This chapter concentrates mainly on epithelial and connective tissues; muscle and nervous tissues receive more attention in later chapters.

Epithelial Tissue

Epithelial tissue, or *epithelium* (ep-ih-THE-le-um), forms a protective covering for the body and all the organs. It is the main tissue of the outer layer of the skin. It forms the lining of the intestinal tract, the respiratory and urinary passages, the blood vessels, the uterus, and other body cavities.

Structure of Epithelial Tissue

Epithelium has many forms and many purposes, and the cells of which it is composed vary accordingly. Epithelial tissue is classified according to the shape and the arrangement of its cells (Fig. 4-1). In shape, the cells may be referred to as follows:

- *Squamous* (SKWA-mus)—flat and irregular
- *Cuboidal*—square
- *Columnar*—long and narrow.

The cells may be arranged in a single layer, described as *simple,* or in many layers, termed *stratified.* Thus, a single layer of flat, irregular cells would be described as *simple squamous epithelium,* whereas tissue with many layers of these same cells would be described as *stratified squamous epithelium.*

Some organs, such as the urinary bladder, must vary a great deal in size during the course

4

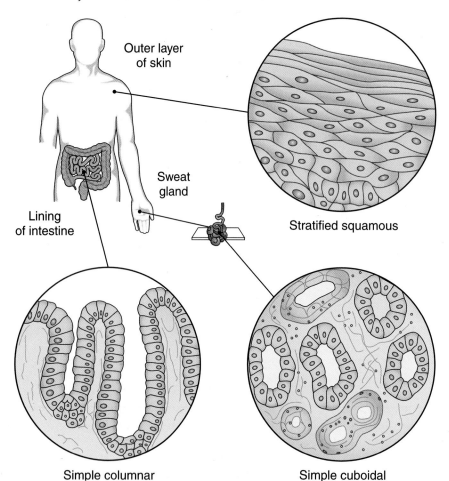

Outer layer
of skin

Sweat
gland

Lining
of intestine

Stratified squamous

Simple columnar

Simple cuboidal

FIGURE **4•1** Three types of epithelium.

of their work. For this purpose, there is a special wrinkled, crepe-like tissue, called ***transitional epithelium,*** which is capable of great expansion yet returns to its original form once tension is relaxed—as when, in this case, the bladder is emptied.

Functions of Epithelial Tissue

The cells of some kinds of epithelium produce secretions, such as ***mucus*** (MU-kus) (a clear, sticky fluid), digestive juices, sweat, and other substances. The digestive tract is lined with a special kind of epithelium, the cells of which not only produce secretions but also are designed to absorb digested foods. The air that we breathe passes over yet another form of epithelium that lines the passageways of the respiratory (breathing) system. This lining secretes mucus

and is provided with tiny hairlike projections called ***cilia.*** Together, the mucus and the cilia help trap bits of dust and other foreign particles that could otherwise reach the lungs and damage them.

Certain areas of the epithelium that form the outer layer of the skin are capable of modifying themselves for greater strength whenever they are subjected to unusual wear and tear; the growth of calluses is a good example of this response.

Epithelium repairs itself quickly after it is injured. If, for example, there is a cut, the cells near and around the wound immediately form daughter cells, which grow until the cut is closed. Epithelial tissue reproduces frequently in areas of the body subject to normal wear and tear, such as the skin, the inside of the mouth, and the lining of the intestinal tract.

Glands

The active cells of many glands are epithelial cells. A gland is an organ specialized to produce a substance that is sent out to other parts of the body. These secretions are manufactured from blood constituents.

Glands are divided into two categories:

- ***Exocrine*** (EK-so-krin) ***glands*** have ducts or tubes to carry secretions away from the gland. The secretions may be carried to another organ, to a body cavity, or to the body surface. They are effective in a limited area near their source. Examples include the digestive juices, the secretions from the sebaceous (oil) glands of the skin, and tears from the lacrimal glands. These glands are discussed in the chapters on specific systems.
- ***Endocrine*** (EN-do-krin) ***glands*** depend on blood flowing through the gland to carry the secretion to another organ. These substances, called ***hormones,*** have specific effects on other tissues. Endocrine glands are the so-called ductless glands.

Exocrine glands vary in design from simple depressions resembling tiny dimples to more complex structures. Simple, tubelike glands are found in the stomach wall and in the intestinal lining. Complex glands composed of treelike groups of ducts are found in the liver, the pancreas, and the salivary glands. Most glands are made largely of epithelial tissue with a framework of connective tissue. There may be a tough connective tissue capsule (a fibrous envelope) enclosing the gland, with extensions into the organ that form partitions. Between the partitions are groups of cells that unite to form lobes.

Endocrine glands produce secretions that are carried to all parts of the body by the blood. These substances often affect tissues at a considerable distance from the point of origin. Endocrine glands, because they secrete directly into the blood stream, have an extensive blood vessel network. The organs believed to have the richest blood supply in the body are the tiny adrenal glands located near the upper part of the kidneys. Some glands, such as the pancreas, have both endocrine and exocrine functions and therefore have both ducts and a rich blood supply. Hormones and the glands that produce them are discussed in Chapter 12.

CONNECTIVE TISSUE

The supporting fabric of all parts of the body is connective tissue (Fig. 4-2). This is so extensive and widely distributed that if we were able to dissolve all the tissues except connective tissue, we would still be able to recognize the contours of the entire body.

Connective tissue has large amounts of nonliving material between the cells. This intercellular background material or ***matrix*** (MA-trix) contains varying amounts of water, fibers, and hard minerals. Connective tissue may be classified simply according to its degree of hardness:

- Soft connective tissue—loosely held together with semi-liquid material between the cells; includes adipose (fat) tissue and areolar (loose) connective tissue
- Fibrous connective tissue—most connective tissue contains some fibers, but this type is densely packed with them. Cells called fibroblasts produce the fibers in connective tissue. (The word ending -*blast* refers to a young and active cell). Examples of structures composed of fibrous connective tissue are ligaments, tendons, and the capsules (coverings) around certain organs.
- Hard connective tissue—has a very firm consistency, as in cartilage, or is hardened by minerals in the matrix, as in bone.

SOFT AND LIQUID CONNECTIVE TISSUE

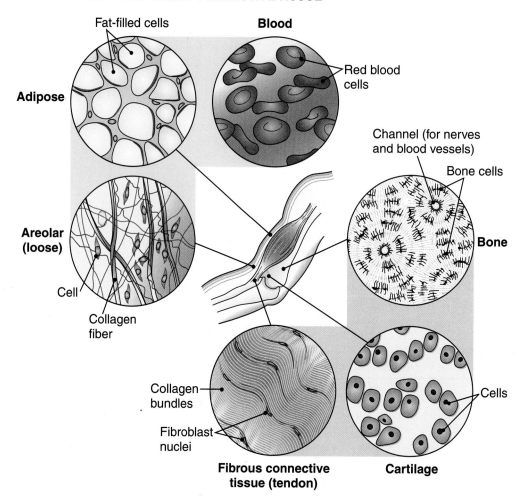

FIGURE **4•2** Connective tissue.

• Liquid connective tissue—Blood and lymph (the fluid that circulates in the lymphatic system) are examples of liquid connective tissues. The cells in liquid connective tissue are suspended in a fluid environment.

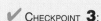

✔ CHECKPOINT **3**:

Connective tissue varies according to the composition of the material that is between the cells. What is the general name for this intercellular material?

Soft Connective Tissue

The *areolar* (ah-RE-o-lar) or loose form of connective tissue (see Fig. 4-2) is found in membranes around vessels and organs, between muscles, and under the skin. It is the most common type of connective tissue in the body. It contains cells and fibers in a very loose, jellylike background material.

Adipose (AD-ih-pose) *tissue* (see Fig. 4-2) contains cells that are able to store large amounts of fat. The fat in this tissue is used as a reserve energy supply for the body. Adipose tissue also serves as a heat insulator and as protective padding for organs and joints.

Fibrous Connective Tissue

Fibrous connective tissue (see Fig. 4-2) is very dense and has large numbers of fibers that give it strength and flexibility. The main type of fiber in this and other connective tissues is *collagen* (KOL-ah-jen), a flexible white protein (see Collagen: The Body's Scaffolding).

Some fibrous connective tissue contains large amounts of elastic fibers that allow the tissue to stretch and then return to its original length. This type of elastic connective tissue appears in the vocal cords, the passageways of the respiratory tract, and the walls of the large arteries (blood vessels).

This tissue makes up the fibrous membranes that cover various organs, as described later in this chapter. Particularly strong forms make up the tough *capsules* around certain organs, such as the kidneys, liver, and glands. If the fibers in the connective tissue are all arranged in the same direction, like the strands of a cable, the tissue can pull in one direction. Examples are the cordlike *tendons,* which connect muscles to bones, and the *ligaments,* which connect bones to other bones.

Tissue Repair

Like epithelial tissue, fibrous connective tissue can repair itself easily. Repair begins after blood has clotted and a scab has formed at the surface to protect underlying tissue. From damaged capillaries, new vessels branch and grow into the injured tissue. Fibroblasts (cells that produce fibers) manufacture collagen to close the gap made by the wound. A large wound requires extensive growth of new connective tissue, which forms a *scar*. After the upper layer of epithelium has regenerated, the scab is released. The underlying scar tissue may then continue to show at the surface as a white line.

Suturing (sewing) the edges of a clean wound together, as is done in the case of operative wounds, decreases the amount of connective tissue needed for repair and thus reduces the size of the resulting scar. Scar tissue is strong but is not as flexible as normal tissue and does not function like the tissue it replaces.

Excess production of collagen in the formation of a scar may result in the development of *keloids* (KE-loyds), sharply raised areas on the surface of the skin. These are not dangerous but may be removed for the sake of appearance.

Hard Connective Tissue

The hard connective tissues, which as the name suggests are more solid than the other groups, include cartilage and bone (see Fig. 4-2).

Cartilage

Because of its strength and flexibility, cartilage is used as a shock absorber and as a bearing surface that reduces friction between moving parts. A common form of cartilage is the tough, elastic, translucent material, popularly called *gristle*, that covers the ends of the long bones. Another form of cartilage is found between seg-

Collagen: The Body's Scaffolding

The most abundant protein in the body, making up about 25% of total protein, is the tough, flexible, white material known as *collagen*. Its name comes from a Greek word meaning "glue," indicating that it is the main structural substance in the body. Collagen is the major ingredient in all connective tissue.

The arrangement of the fibers in collagen gives this substance its different properties. It may form a fibrous connective tissue, as in the heart valves; a cord of great strength, as in tendons and ligaments; or a tough, transparent tissue, as in the cornea of the eye. It is collagen that gives strength and resilience to the skin.

The varied properties of collagen are evident in the preparation of a gelatin dessert. Gelatin is a collagen extract made by boiling animal bones and other connective tissue. It is a viscous (thick) liquid in hot water but forms a semisolid gel on cooling.

ments of the spine. Cartilage is also used as structural material and reinforcement, such as at the tip of the nose, the outer ear, and parts of the larynx ("voicebox") and trachea ("windpipe").

Bone

The tissue of which bones are made, called ***osseous*** (OS-e-us) ***tissue***, is much like cartilage in its cellular structure (see Fig. 4-2). In fact, the skeleton of the fetus in the early stages of development is made almost entirely of cartilage. This tissue gradually becomes impregnated with salts of calcium and phosphorus that make bone characteristically solid and hard. Within the bones are nerves, blood vessels, bone-forming cells, and a special form of tissue, bone marrow, in which blood cells are manufactured.

The liquid connective tissues, blood and lymph, are discussed in Chapters 13 and 16, respectively.

✔ CHECKPOINT **4**:

Connective tissue is the supportive and protective material found throughout the body. What are some examples of soft, fibrous, hard, and liquid connective tissue?

MUSCLE TISSUE

Muscle tissue is designed to produce movement by contraction of its cells, which are called ***muscle fibers*** because most of them are long and threadlike. If a piece of well-cooked meat is pulled apart, small groups of these muscle fibers may be seen. Muscle tissue is usually classified as follows (Fig. 4-3):

*   ***Skeletal muscle,*** which works with tendons and bones to move the body. This type of tissue is also known as ***voluntary***

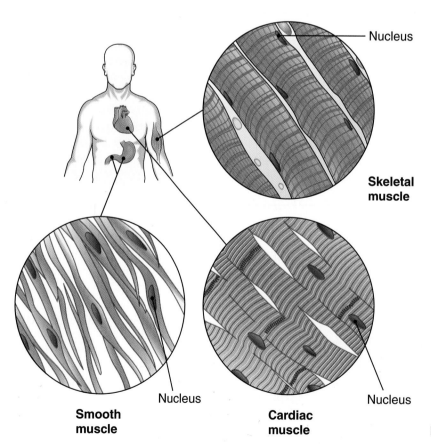

Nucleus

Skeletal muscle

Nucleus

Smooth muscle

Nucleus

Cardiac muscle

FIGURE **4•3** Muscle tissue.

muscle because it can be made to contract by conscious thought.

The next two types of muscle tissue are described as ***involuntary muscle*** because they typically contract independently of thought. Most of the time we are not aware of their actions at all.

- ***Cardiac muscle,*** which forms the bulk of the heart wall and is known also as ***myocardium*** (mi-o-KAR-de-um). This is the muscle that produces the regular contractions known as *heartbeats.*
- ***Smooth muscle,*** known also as ***visceral muscle,*** which forms the walls of the ***viscera*** (VIS-er-ah), or organs of the ventral body cavities (with the exception of the heart). Some examples of visceral muscles are those that move food and waste materials along the digestive tract. Visceral muscle is also found in the walls of many tubular structures, such as the blood vessels and the tubes that carry urine from the kidneys. A smooth muscle is attached to the base of each body hair. Contraction of these muscles causes the skin condition we call *gooseflesh.* Other structures containing visceral muscle are discussed under the various body systems.

Muscle tissue, like nervous tissue, repairs itself only with difficulty or not at all once an injury has been sustained. When injured, muscle tissue is frequently replaced with connective tissue.

Chapter 8 has more detail on muscles.

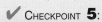 CHECKPOINT **5**:

What are the three types of muscle tissue?

NERVOUS TISSUE

The human body is made up of countless structures, both large and small, each of which contributes something to the action of the whole organism. This aggregation of structures might be compared to an army. For all the members of the army to work together, there must be a central coordinating and order-giving agency somewhere; otherwise, chaos would ensue. In the body, this central agency is the ***brain.*** Each structure of the body is in direct communication with the brain by means of its own set of "wires," called ***nerves.*** The nerves from even the most remote parts of the body all come together and form a great trunk cable called the ***spinal cord,*** which in turn leads directly into the central switchboard of the brain. Here, messages come in and orders go out 24 hours a day. This entire communication system, brain and all, is made of nervous tissue.

The Neuron

The basic unit of nervous tissue is the ***neuron*** (NU-ron), or nerve cell (Fig. 4-4). A neuron consists of a nerve cell body plus small branches, like those of a tree, called *fibers.* One type of fiber, the ***dendrite*** (DEN-drite), carries nerve impulses, or messages, to the nerve cell body. A single fiber, the ***axon*** (AK-son), carries impulses away from the nerve cell body. Neurons may be quite long; their fibers can extend for several feet. A nerve is a bundle of nerve cell fibers held together with connective tissue.

Just as wires are insulated to keep them from being short-circuited, some axons are insulated and protected by a coating of material called ***myelin*** (MI-eh-lin). Groups of myelinated fibers form "white matter," so called because of the color of the myelin, which is much like fat in appearance and consistency. Not all neurons have myelin, however; some axons are unmyelinated, as are all dendrites and all cell bodies. These areas appear gray in color. Because the outer layer of the brain has large collections of cell bodies and unmyelinated fibers, the brain is popularly termed *gray matter.*

Neuroglia

Nervous tissue is supported by special connective tissue cells known as ***neuroglia*** (nu-ROG-le-ah) or *glial* (GLI-al) *cells,* which are named from the Greek word *glia* meaning "glue." Some of these cells protect the brain from harmful substances; others get rid of foreign organisms

4

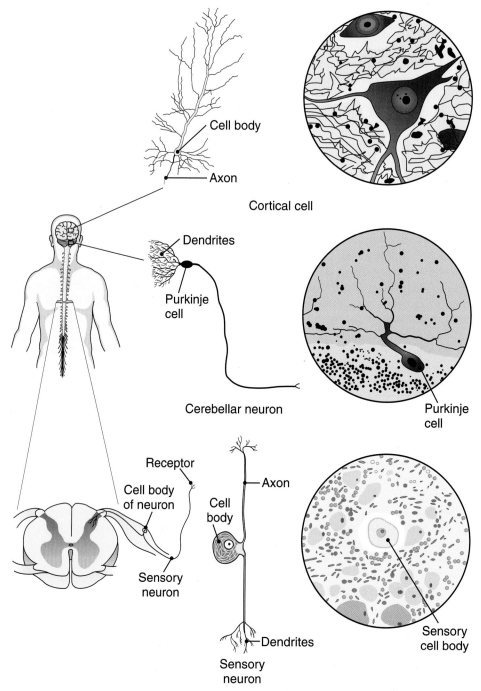

Cell body

Axon

Cortical cell

Dendrites

Purkinje
cell

Cerebellar neuron

Purkinje
cell

Receptor

Cell body
of neuron

Axon

Cell
body

Sensory
neuron

Dendrites

Sensory
neuron

Sensory
cell body

FIGURE **4•4** Nervous tissue.

and cellular debris; still others form the myelin sheath around axons. They do not, however, transmit nerve impulses.

A more detailed discussion of nervous tissue and the nervous system can be found in Chapters 9 and 10.

✔ CHECKPOINT **6**:
_____

What is the basic cellular unit of the nervous system and what is its function?

✔ CHECKPOINT **7**:
_____

What are the nonconducting support cells of the nervous system called?

MEMBRANES

Membranes are thin sheets of tissue. Their properties vary: some are fragile, others tough; some are transparent, others opaque (*i.e.,* they cannot be seen through). Membranes may cover a surface, may serve as a dividing partition, may line a hollow organ or body cavity, or may anchor an organ. They may contain cells that secrete lubricants to ease the movement of organs, such as the heart and lung, and the movement of joints.

Epithelial Membranes

An *epithelial membrane* is so named because its outer surface is made of epithelium. Underneath, however, there is a layer of connective tissue that strengthens the membrane, and in some cases, there is a thin layer of smooth muscle under that. Epithelial membranes are made of closely packed active cells that manufacture lubricants and protect the deeper tissues from invasion by microorganisms. Epithelial membranes are of several types:

- *Serous* (SE-rus) *membranes* line the walls of body cavities and are folded back onto the surface of internal organs, forming their outermost layer.
- *Mucous* (MU-kus) *membranes* line tubes

and other spaces that open to the outside of the body.
- The *cutaneous* (ku-TA-ne-us) *membrane,* commonly known as the *skin,* has an outer layer of epithelium. This membrane is complex and is discussed in detail in Chapter 6 on the integumentary system.

Because they consist mainly of epithelial and connective tissue, serous and mucous membranes are described here.

Serous Membranes

Serous membranes line the closed ventral body cavities and do not communicate with the outside of the body. They secrete a thin, watery lubricant that allows organs to move with a minimum of friction. The thin epithelium of serous membranes is a smooth, glistening kind of tissue called *mesothelium* (mes-o-THE-le-um). The membrane itself may be referred to as the *serosa* (se-RO-sah).

There are three serous membranes:

- The *pleurae* (PLU-re) or *pleuras* (PLU-rahs) line the thoracic cavity and cover each lung.
- The *pericardium* (per-ih-KAR-de-um) is a sac that encloses the heart, which is located in the chest between the lungs.
- The *peritoneum* (per-ih-to-NE-um) is the largest serous membrane. It lines the walls of the abdominal cavity, covers the organs of the abdomen, and forms supporting and protective structures within the abdomen (see Fig. 19-3 in Chap. 19).

Serous membranes are so arranged that one portion forms the lining of the closed cavity while another part folds back to cover the surface of an organ. The serous membrane attached to the wall of a cavity or sac is known as the *parietal* (pah-RI-eh-tal) *layer;* the word *parietal* refers to a wall. Parietal pleura lines the chest wall, and parietal pericardium lines the sac that encloses the heart. Because internal organs are called *viscera,* the membrane attached to the organs is the *visceral layer.* On the surface of the heart is visceral pericardium, and each lung surface is covered by visceral pleura. To visualize this, think of pushing your hand into a soft balloon. The balloon is continuous, but has been folded into two layers. The outer layer is the parietal layer; the inner layer, against your hand, is the visceral layer.

The area between the layers of a serous membrane is a **potential space.** It is *possible* for a space to exist there, but normally the membrane surfaces are in direct contact, with a minimal amount of lubricant between them. Only if substances accumulate between the layers, as when inflammation causes the production of excessive amounts of fluid, is there an actual space.

Mucous Membranes

Mucous membranes are so named because they produce a thick and sticky substance called **mucus** (MU-kus). (Note that the adjective *mucous* contains an "o," whereas the noun *mucus* does not). These membranes form extensive continuous linings in the digestive, respiratory, urinary, and reproductive systems, all of which are connected with the outside of the body. They vary somewhat in both structure and function. The cells that line the nasal cavities and the passageways of the respiratory tract are supplied with tiny, hairlike extensions called *cilia,* as described in Chapter 3. The microscopic cilia move in waves that force secretions outward. In this way, foreign particles, such as bacteria, dust, and other impurities trapped in the sticky mucus, are prevented from entering the lungs and causing harm. Ciliated epithelium is also found in certain tubes of both the male and the female reproductive systems.

The mucous membranes that line the digestive tract have special functions. For example, the mucous membrane of the stomach serves to protect the deeper tissues from the action of powerful digestive juices. If for some reason a portion of this membrane is injured, these juices begin to digest a part of the stomach itself—as in the case of peptic ulcers. Mucous membranes located farther along in the digestive system are designed to absorb food materials, which are then transported to all the cells of the body.

The noun **mucosa** (mu-KO-sah) is used in referring to the mucous membrane of an organ.

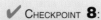

✔ CHECKPOINT **8**:

Epithelial membranes have an outer layer of epithelium. Which are the three type of epithelial membranes?

Connective Tissue Membranes

The following list is an overview of membranes that consist of connective tissue with no epithelium. These membranes are described in greater detail in later chapters.

* **Synovial** (sin-O-ve-al) **membranes** are thin connective tissue membranes that line the joint cavities. They secrete a lubricating fluid that reduces friction between the ends of bones, thus permitting free movement of the joints. Synovial membranes also line small cushioning sacs near the joints called **bursae** (BUR-se).
* The **meninges** (men-IN-jeze) are several layers of membranes covering the brain and the spinal cord.

Fascia (FASH-e-ah) refers to fibrous bands or sheets that support organs and hold them in place. Fascia is found in two regions:

* **Superficial fascia** is the continuous sheet of tissue that underlies the skin and contains adipose (fat) tissue to insulate and protect the skin.
* **Deep fascia** covers, separates, and protects skeletal muscles

Finally, there are membranes whose names all start with the prefix *peri-* because they are around organs:

* The **pericardium** (per-e-KAR-de-um) is the fibrous sac that encloses the heart.
* **Periosteum** (per-e-OS-te-um) is around bones.
* **Perichondrium** (per-e-KON-dre-um) is around cartilage (*chondro* is the word root for cartilage).

Membranes and Disease

We are all familiar with a number of diseases that directly affect membranes. These range from the common cold, which is an inflammation of the mucosa of the nasal passages, to the sometimes fatal condition known as *peritonitis,* an infection of the peritoneum, which can follow rupture of the appendix and other mishaps.

Although membranes usually help to prevent the spread of infection from one area of the body to another, they may sometimes act as pathways along which disease may spread. In general, epithelial membranes appear to have more resistance to infections than do layers made of connective tissue. Lowered resistance, however, may allow the transmission of infection along any membrane. For example, infections may travel along the lining of the tubes of the reproductive system into the urinary system in males. In females, an infection may travel up the tubes and spaces of the reproductive system into the peritoneal cavity (see Fig. 23-12 in Chap. 23).

The connective tissue or collagen diseases, such as *systemic lupus erythematosus* (LU-pus er-ih-them-ah-TO-sus) (SLE) and *rheumatoid arthritis,* may affect many parts of the body because collagen is the major intercellular protein in solid connective tissue. In systemic lupus erythematosus, serous membranes, such as the pleura, pericardium, and peritoneum, are often involved. In rheumatoid arthritis, the synovial membrane becomes inflamed and swollen, and the cartilage in the joints is gradually replaced with fibrous connective tissue.

BENIGN AND MALIGNANT TUMORS

For a variety of reasons, the normal pattern of cell and tissue growth may be broken by an upstart formation of cells having no purpose whatsoever in the body. Any abnormal growth of cells is called a *tumor,* or *neoplasm.* If the tumor is confined to a local area and does not spread, it is called a *benign* (be-NINE) tumor. If the tumor spreads to neighboring tissues or to distant parts of the body, it is called a *malignant* (mah-LIG-nant) tumor. The general term

for any type of malignant tumor is *cancer.* The process of tumor cell spread is called *metastasis* (meh-TAS-tah-sis).

Tumors are found in all kinds of tissue, but they occur most frequently in those tissues that repair themselves most quickly, specifically epithelium and connective tissue, in that order.

Benign Tumors

Benign tumors, theoretically at least, are not dangerous in themselves; they do not spread. Their cells stick together, and often they are encapsulated, that is, surrounded by a containing membrane. Benign tumors grow as a single mass within a tissue, lending them neatly to complete surgical removal. Of course, some benign tumors can be quite harmful; they may grow within an organ, increase in size, and cause considerable mechanical damage. A benign tumor of the brain, for example, can kill a person just as a malignant one can because it grows in an enclosed area and compresses vital brain tissue. Some examples of benign tumors are given below (note that most of the names end in *-oma,* which means "tumor").

- *Papilloma* (pap-ih-LO-mah)—a tumor that grows in epithelium as a projecting mass. One example is a wart.
- *Adenoma* (ad-eh-NO-mah)—an epithelial tumor that grows in and about the glands (*adeno-* means "gland")
- *Lipoma* (lip-O-mah)—a connective tissue tumor originating in fatty (adipose) tissue
- *Osteoma* (os-te-O-mah)—a connective tissue tumor that originates in the bones
- *Myoma* (mi-O-mah)—a tumor of muscle tissue. Rare in voluntary muscle, it is common in some types of involuntary muscle, particularly in the uterus (womb). When found in the uterus, however, it is ordinarily called a *fibroid.*
- *Angioma* (an-je-O-mah)—a tumor that usually is composed of small blood or lymphatic vessels; an example is a birthmark
- *Nevus* (NE-vus)—a small skin tumor of one of a variety of tissues. Some nevi are better known as moles; some are angiomas. Ordinarily, these tumors are harmless, but they can become malignant.

• **Chondroma** (kon-DRO-mah)—a tumor of cartilage cells that may remain within the cartilage or develop on the surface, as in the joints.

Malignant Tumors

Malignant tumors, unlike benign tumors, can cause death no matter where they occur. The word *cancer* means "crab," and this is descriptive: a cancer sends out clawlike extensions into neighboring tissue. A cancer also spreads "seeds," which plant themselves in other parts of the body. These seeds are, of course, cancer cells, and they are transported everywhere by either the blood or the lymph (another circulating fluid). When the cancer cells reach their destination, they immediately form new (secondary) growths, or **metastases** (meh-TAS-tah-seze). Malignant tumors, moreover, grow much more rapidly than benign tumors.

Malignant tumors are classified into two main categories according to whether they originate in epithelial or connective tissue:

• **Carcinoma** (kar-sih-NO-mah). This type of cancer originates in epithelium and is by far the most common form of cancer. Usual sites of carcinoma are the skin, mouth, lung, breast, stomach, colon, prostate, and uterus. Carcinomas are usually spread by the lymphatic system (see Chap. 16).
• **Sarcoma** (sar-KO-mah). These are cancers of connective tissue of all kinds and hence may be found anywhere in the body. Their cells are usually spread by the blood stream, and they often form secondary growths in the lungs.

Cancers of the nervous system, lymphatic system, and blood are classified differently according to the cells in which they originate as well as other clinical features. A **neuroma** (nu-RO-mah) is a tumor that arises from a nerve. Because nervous tissue does not multiply throughout life, however, it is rarely involved in cancer. Usually, a tumor of the nervous system originates in the connective tissue of the brain or spinal cord and is called a **glioma** (gli-O-mah). A malignant neoplasm of lymphatic tissue is called a **lymphoma** (lim-FO-mah), and cancer of white blood cells is **leukemia** (lu-KE-me-ah).

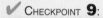

> ✔ CHECKPOINT **9**:
>
> What is the difference between a benign and a malignant tumor?

Symptoms of Cancer

Everyone should be familiar with certain signs that may be indicative of early cancer and should report these signs for further investigation by their health care provider. Early symptoms may include unusual bleeding or discharge, persistent indigestion, chronic hoarseness or cough, changes in the color or size of moles, a sore that does not heal in a reasonable time, the presence of an unusual lump, and the presence of white patches inside the mouth or white spots on the tongue. Late symptoms of cancer include weight loss and pain. Many cases of cancer are now diagnosed by routine screening tests that are part of the standard physical examination.

Diagnosis of Cancer

Improved methods of cancer detection lead to earlier and more successful treatment. These methods include the following:

• **Biopsy** (BI-op-se) is the removal of living tissue for the purpose of microscopic examination of the cells (see Biopsy).
• **Ultrasound** is the use of reflected high-frequency sound waves to differentiate various kinds of tissue.
• **Computed tomography** (CT) is the use of x-rays to produce a cross-sectional picture of body parts, such as the brain (see Fig. 10-8 in Chap. 10).
• **Magnetic resonance imaging** (MRI) is the use of magnetic fields and radio waves to show changes in soft tissues.
• **Blood tests** are the newest approach to cancer diagnosis. A few types of cancer

Biopsy

A valuable tool of the pathologist, one who studies disease, is the examination of tissue under the microscope. The process of sampling tissue for examination is known as *biopsy* (BI-op-se). Tissue samples may be removed either surgically or through a needle in an *aspiration biopsy.*

Often, a biopsy is performed to examine tissue for signs of cancer, as in the lung, breast, or lining of the uterus. A change in the size, shape, and arrangement of cells in the specimen, a condition known as *dysplasia* (dis-PLA-ze-ah), may signal early stages of cancer. Later stages of tumor formation show more extreme and irreversible changes in the tissue.

Biopsy may also reveal infection or degenerative disease, for example, in muscle, kidney, or liver tissue. Bone marrow is sampled to identify changes in blood cells, as in leukemia, which involves an overgrowth of white blood cells. Biopsy is also used to follow any adverse effects of radiation therapy or chemotherapy on the blood-forming tissue in bone marrow. Certain birth defects can be found by examining amniotic fluid from around the fetus or tissue taken from the placenta during pregnancy.

have been found to secrete substances into the blood that can be tested for in the laboratory. The first and most widely used of these screenings is for prostate-specific antigen (PSA), a protein produced in large quantity by prostate tumors. Similar tests for other types of cancer have been developed, and more are probably forthcoming.

Diagnostic studies are used for a process called *staging,* which means the classification of a tumor based on size and extent of invasion. Staging helps the physician select appropriate treatment and predict the outcome of the disease.

Treatment of Cancer

Some standard forms of treatment are described here.

Surgery

Benign tumors usually can be removed completely by surgery. Malignant tumors cannot be treated so easily, for a number of reasons. If cancerous tissue is removed surgically, there is always the probability that a few hidden cells will be left behind to grow anew. If the cells have spread to distant parts of the body, predicted outcome is usually grim.

The *laser* (LA-zer), a device that produces a highly concentrated and intense beam of light, may sometimes successfully destroy the tumor or may be employed as a cutting device for removing the growth. Important advantages of the laser are its ability to coagulate blood, so that bleeding is largely prevented, and the capacity to direct a narrow beam of light accurately to attack harmful cells and avoid normal cells.

Radiation

Sometimes, surgery is preceded or followed by radiation. Radiation therapy is administered by x-ray machines or by the placement of small amounts of radioactive material within the involved organ. Radiation destroys the more rapidly dividing cancer cells while causing less damage to the more slowly dividing normal cells. Methods are being developed that will permit more accurate focusing of the beam of radiation and thus reduce the damage to normal body structures.

Chemotherapy

Drugs used for the treatment of cancer include those that act selectively on tumor cells. Known as *antineoplastic* (an-ti-ne-o-PLAS-tik) *agents,* these drugs are most effective when used in combination. The treatment of cancer with antineoplastic agents is one form of *chemotherapy* (ke-mo-THER-ah-pe) (see Chap. 5). Certain types of leukemia and various cancers of the lymphatic system often are treated effectively by this means. Research continues to develop new drugs and more effective drug combinations.

✔ CHECKPOINT **10**:

What are three standard approaches to the treatment of cancer?

4

Summary

I. **Tissue classification**—epithelial tissue, connective tissue, muscle tissue, nervous tissue
   A. Epithelial tissue—covers surfaces, lines cavities
      1. Cells—squamous, cuboidal, columnar
      2. Arrangement—simple or stratified
   B. Glands—active cells are epithelial cells
      1. Exocrine
         a. Secrete through ducts
         b. Produce external secretions
      2. Endocrine
         a. Secrete into bloodstream
         b. Produce hormones

II. **Connective tissue**—supports, binds, forms framework of body
   A. Soft—jellylike intercellular material
      1. Areolar (loose)
      2. Adipose—stores fat
   B. Fibrous—dense tissue with collagenous or elastic fibers between cells
      1. Examples
         a. Tendons—attach muscle to bone
         b. Ligaments—connect bones
         c. Capsules—around organs
         d. Fascia—bands or sheets that support organs
      2. Tissue repair—epithelium and fibrous connective tissue repair easily
   C. Hard—firm and solid
      1. Cartilage—found at ends of bones, nose, outer ear, trachea, etc.
      2. Bone—contains mineral salts
   D. Liquid
      1. Blood
      2. Lymph

III. **Muscle tissue**—contracts to produce movement
      1. Skeletal muscle—voluntary; moves skeleton
      2. Cardiac muscle—forms the heart
      3. Smooth muscle—involuntary; forms visceral organs

IV. **Nervous tissue**
   A. Neuron—nerve cell
      1. Cell body—contains nucleus
      2. Dendrite—fiber carrying impulses toward cell body
      3. Axon—fiber carrying impulses away from cell body
         a. Myelin—fatty material that insulates some axons
            (1) Myelinated fibers—make up white matter
            (2) Unmyelinated cells and fibers—make up gray matter
   B. Neuroglia—support and protect nervous tissue

V. **Membranes**—thin sheets of tissue
   A. Epithelial membranes—outer layer epithelium
      1. Serous membrane—secretes watery fluid
         a. Parietal layer—lines body cavity
         b. Visceral layer—covers internal organs
         c. Examples—pleurae, pericardium, peritoneum
      2. Mucous membrane
         a. Secretes mucus
         b. Lines tube or space that opens to the outside (*e.g.,* respiratory, digestive, reproductive tracts)
      3. Cutaneous membrane—skin
   B. Connective tissue membranes
      1. Synovial membrane—lines joint cavity
      2. Meninges—around brain and spinal cord
      3. Fascia—under skin and around muscles
      4. Pericardium—around heart; periosteum—around bone; perichondrium—around cartilage
   C. Membranes and disease

VI. **Benign and malignant tumors**—tumor (neoplasm) results from uncontrolled growth of cells
   A. Benign tumor—localized
   B. Malignant tumor—invades tissue and spreads to other parts of the body (metastasizes)

1. Carcinoma—originates in epithelim
2. Sarcoma—cancer of connective tissue
3. Others—cancers of nervous system, lymphatic system, blood

C. Symptoms of cancer—bleeding, persistent indigestion, hoarseness or cough, change in mole, lump, nonhealing sore, pain, weight loss

D. Diagnosis of cancer
   1. Biopsy (study of tissue), ultrasound, CT, MRI, blood tests
   2. Staging—classification based on size of tumor and extent of invasion

E. Treatment of cancer
   1. Surgical removal
   2. Radiation
   3. Chemotherapy—drugs

Questions for Study and Review

1. Define *tissue.* Give a few general characteristics of tissues.
2. Define *epithelium* and give three examples of epithelium.
3. Describe the difference between endocrine and exocrine glands and give examples of each.
4. Define *connective tissue.* Name the main kinds of connective tissue and give an example of each.
5. What kinds of fibers are found in connective tissue?
6. Name three kinds of muscle tissue and give an example of each.
7. What is the difference between voluntary and involuntary muscle?
8. What is the main purpose of nervous tissue? What is its basic structural unit called?
9. Define *myelin.* Where is it found?
10. What are some general characteristics of epithelial membranes?
11. Compare serous and mucous membranes.
12. Name and describe the two layers of serous membranes.
13. List five examples of connective tissue membranes.
14. What is an infection of the peritoneum called? What is a possible cause of this condition?
15. What is the relation between membranes and disease?
16. What is a tumor? In what kinds of tissue are tumors most commonly found?
17. What is the difference between a benign and a malignant tumor?
18. Name four examples of benign tumors and tell where each is found.
19. Name the two main categories of malignant tumor. In what kinds of tissue are these tumors found? Which kind is the most common?
20. Name some early symptoms of cancer.
21. In what ways is cancer diagnosed?
22. In what ways is cancer treated?
23. What is staging and how is it used?

✔ ANSWERS TO CHECKPOINTS

1. The three basic shapes of epithelium are squamous (flat and irregular), cuboidal (square), and columnar (long and narrow).
2. Exocrine glands secrete through ducts; endocrine glands do not have ducts and secrete directly into the bloodstream.
3. The intercellular material in connective tissue is the matrix.
4. Examples of soft connective tissue are areolar (loose) and adipose tissue; fibrous connective tissue makes up capsules, tendons, and ligaments; hard connective tissue is cartilage and bone; liquid connective tissue is blood and lymph.
5. The three types of muscle tissue are skeletal (voluntary), cardiac, and smooth (visceral) muscle.
6. The basic cellular unit of the nervous system is the neuron and it carries nerve impulses.
7. The nonconducting support cells of the nervous system are neuroglia (glial cells).
8. The three types of epithelial membranes are the cutaneous membrane (skin), serous membranes, and mucous membranes.
9. A benign tumor does not spread; a malignant tumor spreads (metastasizes) to other tissues.
10. The three standard approaches to treatment of cancer are surgery, radiation, and chemotherapy.

The two chapters in this unit incorporate a discussion of deviations from the normal, which is the basis for disease. One chapter is devoted largely to the most common causes of disease. These are the microorganisms, including bacteria, viruses, and protozoa, and larger organisms, such as worms. The most important defense against the multitude of causes of disease is the skin, the first line of defense. The skin, as well as being classified as a system, is the largest organ of the body. Its properties and functions are discussed in this unit.

Unit II

DISEASE AND THE FIRST LINE OF DEFENSE

Disease and Disease-Producing Organisms

SELECTED KEY TERMS

The following terms are defined in the Glossary:

acute

asepsis

chemotherapy

chronic

diagnosis

disease

epidemic

etiology

microorganism

pathogen

pathophysiology

prognosis

sign

spore

sterilization

symptom

systemic

toxin

BEHAVIORAL OBJECTIVES

After careful study of this chapter, you should be able to:

1. Define disease and list seven causes of disease

2. List six predisposing causes of disease

3. Define terminology used in describing and treating disease

4. List four types of organisms studied in microbiology and give the characteristics of each

5. List some diseases caused by each type of microorganism

6. Describe the three types of bacteria according to shape

7. List several diseases in humans caused by worms

8. Describe how microorganisms may be spread

9. Describe several public health measures taken to prevent the spread of disease

10. Differentiate *sterilization, disinfection,* and *antisepsis*

11. Describe standard precautions

12. Define *chemotherapy*

13. Describe several methods used to identify microorganisms in the laboratory

WHAT IS DISEASE?

Disease may be defined as abnormality of the structure or function of a part, organ, or system. The effects of a disease may be felt by a person or observed by others. A disease may be of known or unknown cause with marked variation in severity and its effect on the individual.

Categories of Diseases

Diseases fall into a number of different, but often overlapping, categories. These include the following:

- *Infection.* Infectious organisms are believed to play a part in at least half of all human illnesses. Disease-producing organisms are discussed in this chapter. Other forms of illness mentioned below are discussed in later chapters.
- *Degenerative diseases.* These are disorders that involve degeneration (breaking down) of tissues in any system of the body. Examples are muscular dystrophy, cirrhosis of the liver, Alzheimer's disease, osteoporosis, and arthritis. Some of these disorders are hereditary; that is, they are passed on by parents through their reproductive cells. Others are due to infection, injury, substance abuse, or normal "wear and tear." Still others, such as multiple sclerosis, have no known cause.
- *Nutritional disorders.* Most of us are familiar with diseases caused by a dietary lack of essential vitamins, minerals, proteins, or other substances required for health: scurvy due to a lack of vitamin C, beriberi due to a lack of thiamine, rickets due to a lack of calcium for bone development, kwashiorkor, a disease of children in underdeveloped countries due to protein deficiency. This category also includes problems caused by excess intake, such as alcoholism, overdosing on vitamins or minerals, consuming excess protein, or intake of too many calories leading to obesity (see Chap. 19 and 20).
- *Metabolic disorders.* These include any disruption of the reactions involved in cellular metabolism, such as diabetes, gout (a disorder of the joints), digestive disorders, and hereditary dysfunctions. Hormones regulate many metabolic reactions. The glands that produce hormones and the diseases caused by excess or deficiency of hormones are the subject of Chapter 12. Hereditary errors of metabolism result from genetic changes that affect enzymes. The basics of heredity are described in Chapter 25.
- *Immune disorders.* These relate to the system that protects us against infectious

diseases (see Chap. 17). Some deficiencies in the immune system are inherited; some, such as AIDS, are the result of infection. This category also includes allergies, in which the immune system is overactive, and autoimmune diseases, which occur when the immune system becomes active against one's own tissues.

- *Neoplasms.* The word *neoplasm* means "new growth" and refers to cancer and other types of tumors (see Chap. 4).
- *Psychiatric disorders.* Psychiatry is the medical field that specializes in the treatment of mental disorders. The brain and the nervous system as a whole are discussed in Chapters 9 and 10. Note, however, that it is often impossible to separate mental from physical factors in any discussion of disease.

Predisposing Causes

Other factors that enter into the production of a disease are known as *predisposing causes.* Although a predisposing cause may not in itself give rise to a disease, it increases the probability of a person's becoming ill. Examples of predisposing causes include the following:

- *Age.* Tissues degenerate with age, becoming less active and less capable of performing normal functions. Decline may be speeded by the normal "wear and tear" of life, by continuous infection, or by repeated minor injuries. Age may also be a factor in the incidence of specific diseases. For example, measles is more common in children than in adults. Other diseases may appear most commonly in young adults or people in middle years.
- *Sex.* Certain diseases are more characteristic of one gender than the other. Men are more susceptible to early heart disease, whereas women are more likely to develop diabetes.
- *Heredity.* Some individuals inherit a "tendency" to acquire certain diseases—particularly diabetes, many allergies, and certain forms of cancer.
- *Living conditions and habits.* Individuals who habitually fail to get enough sleep

or who pay little attention to diet and exercise are highly vulnerable to disease. The abuse of drugs, alcohol, and tobacco also can lower vitality and predispose to disease. Overcrowding and poor sanitation invite epidemics.

- *Emotional disturbance.* Some physical disturbances have their basis in emotional upsets, stress, and anxiety in daily living. Headaches and so-called "nervous indigestion" are examples.
- *Physical and chemical damage.* Injuries that cause burns, cuts, fractures, or crushing damage to tissues predispose to infection and degeneration. Some chemicals that may be poisonous, carcinogenic, or otherwise injurious if present in excess are lead compounds (in paint), pesticides, solvents, carbon monoxide and other pollutants in air, and a wide variety of other environmental toxins.

  Exposure to radiation is associated with an increased incidence of cancer. Many of the so-called "occupational diseases" that have appeared throughout history have been caused by exposure to environmental agents. For example, inhalation of coal dust or other types of dusts or asbestos fibers has caused lung damage.

- *Preexisting illness.* Any preexisting illness, especially a chronic disease such as high blood pressure or diabetes, increases one's chances of contracting another disease.

✔ CHECKPOINT **1**:

What is the definition of a predisposing cause of disease?

THE STUDY OF AND TREATMENT OF DISEASE

The modern approach to the study of disease emphasizes the close relationship of the pathologic and physiologic aspects of any disorder and the need to understand the fundamentals of each in treatment. The term used for this combined study in medical science is *pathophysiology.*

Underlying the basic medical sciences are the still more fundamental disciplines of physics and chemistry. Knowledge of both of these is essential to any real understanding of the life processes (see The CDC).

Disease Terminology

The study of the cause of any disease, or the theory of its origin, is *etiology* (e-te-OL-o-je). Any study of a disease usually includes some indication of *incidence,* which means its range of occurrence and its tendency to affect certain groups of individuals more than other groups. Information about the geographic distribution of a disease and its tendency to appear in one sex, age group, or race more or less frequently than another is usually included in any study on disease incidence.

Diseases are often classified on the basis of severity and duration as follows:

- *Acute.* These diseases are relatively severe but usually last a short time.
- *Chronic.* These diseases are often less severe but are likely to be continuous or recurring for long periods.
- *Subacute.* These diseases are intermediate between acute and chronic, not being as severe as acute infections nor as long-lasting as chronic disorders.

A term used in describing a disease without known cause is *idiopathic* (id-e-o-PATH-ik), which means "self-originating." Such diseases have no explanation at this time.

A *communicable* disease is one that can be transmitted from one person to another. If many people in a given region acquire a certain disease at the same time, that disease is said to be *epidemic.* If a given disease is found to a lesser extent but continuously in a particular region, the disease is *endemic* to that area. A disease that is prevalent throughout an entire country or continent, or the whole world, is said to be *pandemic.*

The CDC

In any article on infectious diseases in the United States, the initials CDC are likely to appear. This federal agency, the full name of which is the Centers for Disease Control and Prevention, is located in Atlanta, Georgia. Since its establishment in 1946, it has traced the origins and spread of infectious diseases and has gradually expanded its role to include the prevention of injury and disease.

The CDC participated in the fight against polio, which has virtually been eliminated in the United States, and joined the World Health Organization in efforts to eradicate smallpox worldwide. More recently, it has led in efforts to study and treat toxic shock syndrome, Legionnaire's disease, AIDS, and tuberculosis. In 1993, researchers at the CDC, working with local health agencies, rapidly identified the strain of hantavirus that caused a serious and often fatal pulmonary disease in people in the Southwest. The CDC currently coordinates efforts at laboratories throughout the country to identify organisms that may be involved in causing unexplained illnesses. Modern techniques of DNA and RNA analysis are used in these studies to search for evidence of new pathogens.

The CDC employs about 6900 people working in more than 170 occupations. Many are assigned to various state, federal, and foreign locations, where they investigate health problems, conduct research, and promote public health policies. Their stated goal is "healthy people in a healthy world—through prevention."

✔ CHECKPOINT **2**:

What two sciences are involved in any study of disease?

Steps in Treatment

To treat a patient, a physician must first reach a conclusion as to the nature of the illness—that is, make a *diagnosis.* To do this, the physician must know the *symptoms,* which are the conditions of disease noted by the patient, and the *signs,* which are the evidence (objective manifestations) the physician or other health care professional can observe. A characteristic group of symptoms and signs accompanies each disease. Such a group is called a **syndrome** (SIN-drome). Frequently, the physician uses laboratory tests to help establish the diagnosis. A **prognosis** (prog-NO-sis) is a prediction of the probable outcome of a disease based on the condition of the patient and the physician's knowledge about the disease.

Nurses and other health care professionals play an extremely valuable role in this process by observing closely for signs, collecting and organizing information from the patient about his or her symptoms, and then reporting this information to the physician. Once a patient's disorder is known, the physician prescribes a course of treatment, known as **therapy.** Specific measures in a course of treatment include those carried out by the nurse and other health care providers under the physician's orders.

Prevention of Disease

In recent years, physicians, nurses, and other health care workers have taken on increasing responsibilities in **prevention.** Throughout most of medical history, the physician's aim has been to cure patients of existing diseases. The modern concept of prevention, however, seeks to stop disease before it actually happens—to keep people well through the promotion of health. A vast number of organizations exist for this purpose, ranging from the World Health Organization (WHO) on an international level to local private and community health programs. A rapidly growing responsibility of all people in health occupations is educating individual patients on the maintenance of total health, both physical and mental.

✔ Checkpoint **3**:

A physician uses signs and symptoms to identify an illness. What is this identification called?

Infectious Disease

The predominant cause of disease in humans is the invasion of the body by disease-producing **microorganisms** (mi-kro-OR-gan-izms). The word *organism* means "anything having life"; *micro* means "small." Hence, a microorganism is a tiny living thing, too small to be seen by the naked eye. Other terms for microorganism are *microbe* and, more popularly, *germ*. A microbe, or any other organism, that lives on or within a living **host** and at the host's expense is called a **parasite.**

Although most microorganisms are harmless to humans, and many are beneficial, a few types cause illness; that is, they are **pathogenic** (path-o-JEN-ic). Any disease-causing organism is a **pathogen** (PATH-o-jen). If the body is invaded by pathogens, with adverse effects, the condition is called an **infection.** If the infection is restricted to a relatively small area of the body, it is **local.** A generalized, or **systemic** (sis-TEM-ik), infection is one in which the whole body is affected. The blood frequently spreads systemic infections.

An infection that takes hold because the host has been weakened by disease is described as an **opportunistic infection.** For example, people with depressed immune systems, such as those with AIDS (acquired immunodeficiency syndrome), become infected with organisms that are ordinarily harmless.

Modes of Transmission

Microorganisms may be transmitted from an infected human, insect, or animal host to a susceptible human; this transfer may be by direct or indirect contact. For example, infected human hosts may transfer their microorganisms to other individuals through direct personal contact, such as shaking hands, kissing, or having sexual intercourse. An insect bite may introduce infectious organisms into the body. An insect or other animal that transmits a disease-causing organism from one host to another is termed a **vector** (VEK-tor) (see Fig. 5-4).

Indirect contact includes touching objects that have been contaminated by an infected person or breathing in droplets containing organisms. For example, microorganisms may be transferred indirectly through bedding, toys, food, and dishes. Also, insects may deposit infectious material on food, skin, or clothing. Pets may be an indirect source of some infections. (See How to Avoid the Common Cold).

Avoiding the Common Cold

The term "common cold" does not precisely define any specific disease. However, it generally refers to a viral infection of the mucous membranes of the upper respiratory tract that may include a variety of symptoms. The cause of this syndrome is infection by one of many different families of viruses. Indeed, several hundred strains of virus have been linked to the common cold. One of the characteristics of these viruses is a high rate of genetic mutation. Because of the extreme variability in the agents that cause the common cold, immunologists have not been able to develop a broadly effective vaccine. However, research conclusively shows that several simple precautions help reduce the chances of catching a cold.

Colds are primarily spread through direct contact with a contaminated surface. When an infected individual coughs or sneezes, small droplets of water filled with viral particles are propelled through the air. One unshielded sneeze may spread hundreds of thousands of viral particles several feet. Ventilation systems may then spread them further. Depending upon temperature and humidity, these particles may live on surfaces for as long as 3 to 6 hours. They are then picked up on the hands of someone who touches the contaminated surface.

The following measures help prevent the transmission of cold viruses:

- *Wash hands frequently.* This directly reduces cross-contamination.
- *Avoid putting your hands to your face.* Touching or rubbing your eyes, nose, or mouth with contaminated hands may transmit enough viral particles to infect your mucous membranes.
- *Avoid close contact with someone who is sneezing or coughing.* If you can't keep your distance, shield yourself from the person.
- *Force fluids.* This helps to keep mucous membranes moist and lubricated so they can trap and eliminate the viral particles from your system.
- *Use saline nasal sprays.* Again, this helps to flush the mucous membranes and keep mucus thin enough to encourage drainage.
- *Turbo-charge your immune system.* Both vitamin C and zinc have been shown to increase immune system function in mucous membranes that may help to prevent infection, and both have been conclusively shown to decrease the duration of a cold once infection does occur.

Portal of Entry and Exit

There are several avenues through which microorganisms may enter the body: the skin, respiratory tract, and digestive system as well as the urinary and reproductive systems. These portals of entry may also serve as exit routes, leading to the spread of infection. For example, discharges from the respiratory and intestinal tracts may spread infection through air, by contamination of hands, and by contamination of food and water supplies.

Control of infectious disease involves breaking the "chain of infection" by which microorganisms spread through a population. Microbial control is discussed later in this chapter.

✔ CHECKPOINT **4**:

What is the relationship between a parasite and a host?

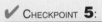

✔ CHECKPOINT **5**:

What are some factors involved in the spread of infectious disease organisms?

MICROORGANISMS

Microorganisms are simple, usually single-cell forms of life (Fig. 5-1). The study of these microscopic organisms is ***microbiology*** (mi-kro-bi-OL-o-je). Other sciences have grown up within the science of microbiology, and each has become a specialty in itself. Some examples of these more specialized sciences include the following:

- ***Bacteriology*** (bak-te-re-OL-o-je) is the study of bacteria, both beneficial and disease producing. It includes the study of rickettsias and chlamydias, which are extremely small bacteria that multiply within living cells.
- ***Mycology*** (my-KOL-o-je) is the study of fungi, which include yeasts and molds.
- ***Virology*** (vi-ROL-o-je) is the study of viruses, extremely small infectious agents that can multiply only within living cells.
- ***Protozoology*** (pro-to-zo-OL-o-je) is the

5

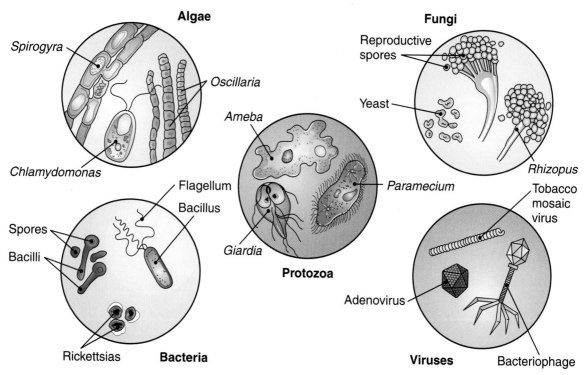

Algae
Spirogyra
Oscillaria
Chlamydomonas

Fungi
Reproductive spores
Yeast
Rhizopus

Ameba
Flagellum
Bacillus
Spores
Bacilli
Giardia
Paramecium
Protozoa

Tobacco mosaic virus
Adenovirus
Viruses
Bacteriophage

Rickettsias **Bacteria**

FIGURE **5•1**   Some examples of microorganisms.

study of single-cell animals called *protozoa.* Although the term **parasitology** (par-ah-si-TOL-o-je) is the study of parasites in general, in practice, it usually refers to the study of protozoa and worms (helminths).

Despite the fact that this discussion centers on pathogens, most microorganisms are harmless to humans and are even essential to the continuation of all life on earth. It is through the actions of microorganisms that dead animals and plants are decomposed and transformed into substances that enrich the soil. Sewage is rendered harmless by microorganisms. Several groups of bacteria transform the nitrogen of the air into a form usable by plants, a process called *nitrogen fixation.* Farmers take advantage of this capacity by allowing a field to lie fallow (untilled) so that the nitrogen of its soil can be replenished. Certain bacteria and fungi produce the antibiotics that make our lives safer. Others produce the fermented products that make our lives more enjoyable, such as beer, wine, cheeses, and yogurt.

Normal Flora

We have a population of microorganisms that normally grows on and within our bodies. We live in balance with these organisms, known as the **normal flora.** These populations are beneficial because they crowd out and prevent the growth of other harmful varieties of organisms. Some microorganisms that are normally harmless may become pathogenic if the normal flora is destroyed, as by the administration of antibiotics that act on a wide range of microoganisms.

✔ CHECKPOINT **6**:

What term refers to the microorganisms that normally live in or on the body?

Bacteria

Bacteria are single-cell organisms that are among the most primitive forms of life on earth. They can be seen only with a microscope; from 10 to 1000 bacteria (depending on the species) would, if lined up, span a pinhead. Staining of the cells with dyes helps make their structures more visible and reveals information about their properties.

Bacteria are found everywhere: in soil, in hot springs, in polar ice, and on and within plants and animals. Their requirements for water, nutrients, oxygen, temperature, and other factors vary widely according to species. Some are capable of carrying out photosynthesis, like green plants; others must take in organic nutrients, as do animals. Some, described as *anaerobic* (an-air-O-bik), can grow in the absence of oxygen; others, called *aerobic* (air-O-bik), require oxygen.

Some bacteria can produce *spores,* resistant forms that can tolerate long periods of dryness or other adverse conditions. Because these spores become airborne easily and are resistant to ordinary methods of disinfection, pathogenic organisms that form spores are particularly dangerous. Other bacteria are capable of swimming rapidly by themselves by means of threadlike appendages called *flagella* (flah-JEL-ah).

Bacteria comprise the largest group of pathogens. Not surprisingly, these pathogenic bacteria are most at home within the "climate" of the human body. When living conditions are ideal, the organisms reproduce by binary fission (simple cell division) with unbelievable rapidity. If they succeed in overcoming the body's natural defenses, they can cause damage in two ways: by producing poisons, or *toxins,* and by entering the body tissues and growing within them. Table 1 in Appendix 4 lists some typical pathogenic bacteria and the diseases they cause.

Main Types of Bacteria

There are so many different types of bacteria that their classification is complicated. For our purposes, a convenient and simple grouping is based on the shape and arrangement of these organisms as seen with a microscope (Figs. 5-2 and 5-3):

- *Rod-shaped cells—bacilli* (bah-SIL-i). These cells are straight and slender. Some are cigar shaped, with tapering ends. Typical diseases caused by bacilli include tetanus, diphtheria, tuberculosis, typhoid fever, and Legionnaire's disease.

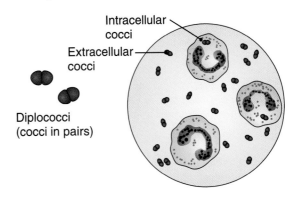

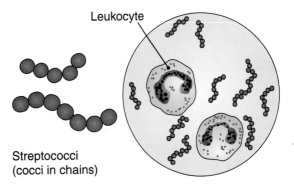

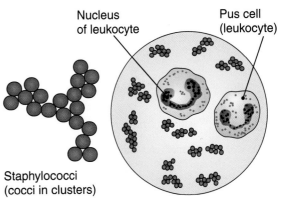

FIGURE **5•2**   Spherical bacteria (Gram stained).

- *Spherical cells—cocci* (KOK-si). These cells are round and are seen in characteristic arrangements. Those that are in pairs are called *diplococci* (*diplo-* means "double"). Those that are arranged in chains, like a string of beads, are called *streptococci* (*strepto-* means "chain"). A third group, seen in large clusters, is known as *staphylococci* (staf-ih-lo-KOK-si) (*staphylo-* means "bunch of grapes"). Among the diseases caused by diplococci are gonorrhea and meningitis; streptococci

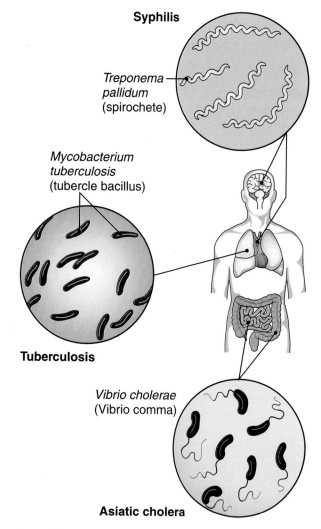

Syphilis

Treponema pallidum (spirochete)

Mycobacterium tuberculosis (tubercle bacillus)

Tuberculosis

Vibrio cholerae (Vibrio comma)

Asiatic cholera

FIGURE **5•3** Rod-shaped and curved bacteria. The illustrations show areas of the body invaded by these pathogens.

and staphylococci are responsible for a wide variety of infections, including pneumonia, rheumatic fever, and scarlet fever.

- *Curved rods.* One type of bacteria, which has only a slight curvature, like a comma, is called *vibrio* (VIB-re-o). Cholera is caused by a vibrio. Another form, which resembles a corkscrew, is known as *spirillum* (spi-RIL-um). (The plural is *spirilla.*)
- Bacteria similar to the spirilla, but capable of waving and twisting motions, are called *spirochetes* (SPI-ro-ketes). One infection caused by a spirochete is syphilis. In syphilis, the spirochetes enter the body at the point of contact, usually through the

genital skin or mucous membranes. They then travel into the bloodstream and set up a systemic infection. (See Table 1 in Appendix 4 for a summary of the three stages of syphilis.)

A spirochete is also responsible for Lyme disease, which has increased in the United States since it first appeared in the early 1960s. People who walk in or near woods are advised to wear white protective clothing that covers their ankles. They should examine their bodies for the freckle-sized ticks that carry the disease.

Other Bacteria

Members of the genus *Rickettsia* (rih-KET-se-ah) and the genus *Chlamydia* (klah-MID-e-ah) are classified as bacteria, although they are considerably smaller. These microorganisms can exist only inside living cells. Because they exist at the expense of their hosts, they are parasites; they are referred to as *obligate intracellular parasites* because they must grow within living cells.

The rickettsias are the cause of a number of serious diseases in humans, such as typhus and Rocky Mountain spotted fever. In almost every instance, these organisms are transmitted through the bites of insects, such as lice, ticks, and fleas. A few common diseases caused by rickettsias are listed in Table 1 in Appendix 4.

The chlamydias are smaller than the rickettsias. They are the causative organisms in trachoma (a serious eye infection that ultimately causes blindness), parrot fever or psittacosis, the sexually transmitted disease lymphogranuloma venereum, and some respiratory diseases (see Table 1 in Appendix 4).

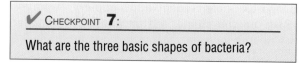

✔ CHECKPOINT **7**:

What are the three basic shapes of bacteria?

Fungi

The true *fungi* (FUN-ji) are a large group of simple plantlike organisms. Only a few types are pathogenic. Although fungi are much larger and more complicated than bacteria, they are a simple form of life. They differ from the higher plants in that they lack the green pigment chlorophyll, which enables most plants to use the energy of sunlight to manufacture food. Like bacteria, fungi grow best in dark, damp places. Fungi reproduce in several ways, including by simple cell division and by production of large numbers of reproductive spores. Single-cell forms of fungi are generally referred to as *yeasts;* the fuzzy, filamentous forms are called *molds.* Familiar examples of fungi are mushrooms, puffballs, bread molds, and the yeasts used in baking and brewing.

Fungal Diseases

Diseases caused by fungi are called *mycotic* (mi-KOT-ik) infections (*myco-* means "fungus"). Examples of these are athlete's foot and ringworm. *Tinea capitis* (TIN-e-ah KAP-ih-tis), which involves the scalp, and *tinea corporis* (kor-PO-ris), which may be found almost anywhere on the nonhairy parts of the body, are common types of ringworm.

One yeast-like fungus that may infect a weakened host is *Candida.* This is a normal inhabitant of the mouth and digestive tract that may produce skin lesions, an oral infection called *thrush,* digestive upset, or inflammation of the vaginal tract (vaginitis) as an opportunistic infection in a weakened host.

Although fungi cause few systemic diseases, some diseases they cause are very dangerous, and all are difficult to cure. Pneumonia can be caused by the inhalation of fungal spores contained in dust particles. Table 2 in Appendix 4 is a list of typical fungal diseases.

Viruses

Although bacteria seem small, they are enormous in comparison with *viruses.* Viruses are comparable in size to large molecules, but unlike other molecules, they contain genetic material and are able to reproduce. Viruses are so tiny that they are invisible with a light microscope; they can be seen only with an electron microscope. Because of their small size and the difficulties associated with growing them in the laboratory, viruses were not studied with much success until the middle of the 20th century.

Viruses are the smallest known infectious agents. They have some of the fundamental properties of living matter, but they are not cellular, and they have no enzyme system. Like the rickettsias and the chlamydias, they can grow only within living cells—they are obligate intracellular parasites; unlike these other organisms, however, the viruses are not usually susceptible to antibiotics.

There is no universally accepted classification of viruses. For our purposes, it is appropriate to think of them in relation to the diseases they cause. There are a considerable number of them—measles, poliomyelitis, hepatitis, chickenpox, and the common cold, to name a few. *AIDS* is a very serious viral disease discussed in Chapter 17. The virus that causes AIDS and other representative viruses are listed in Table 3 in Appendix 4.

Protozoa

With the *protozoa* (pro-to-ZO-ah), we come to the only group of microbes that can be described as animal-like. Although protozoa are also single-cell organisms, they are much larger than bacteria.

Protozoa are found all over the world in the soil and in almost any body of water from moist grass to mud puddles to the sea. There are four main divisions of protozoa:

- *Amebas* (ah-ME-bas). An ameba is an irregular mass of cytoplasm that propels itself by extending part of its cell (a pseudopod, or "false foot") and then flowing into the extension. Amebic dysentery is caused by a pathogen of this group.
- *Ciliates* (SIL-e-ates). This type of protozoon is covered with tiny hairs called *cilia* that produce a wave action to propel the organism.
- *Flagellates* (FLAJ-eh-lates). Long, whiplike filaments called flagella propel these organisms. One of this group, a *trypanosome* (tri-PAN-o-some), causes African sleeping sickness (Fig. 5-4).
- *Sporozoa* (spor-o-ZO-ah). Unlike other protozoa, sporozoa cannot propel themselves. They are obligate parasites, unable

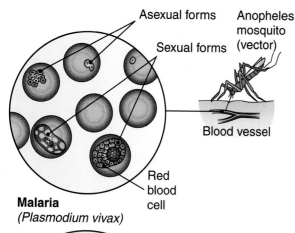

Malaria
(Plasmodium vivax)

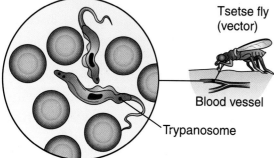

African sleeping sickness
(Trypanosoma gambiense)

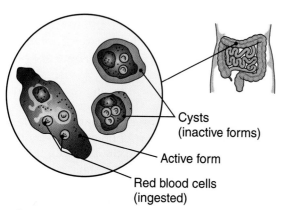

Amebic dysentery
(Entamoeba histolytica)

FIGURE **5•4** Pathogenic protozoa.

to grow outside a host. Members of the genus *Plasmodium* (plaz-MO-de-um) cause malaria. These protozoa, carried by a type of mosquito, cause much serious illness in the tropics, resulting in up to 3 million deaths each year.

Two other members of this group have emerged as opportunistic infections in people suffering from AIDS and in those whose immune system is working poorly. *Pneumocystis carinii* causes a previously rare pneumonia. A *Cryptosporidium* causes severe and prolonged diarrhea.

Figure 5-4 illustrates some of the pathogenic protozoa and their portals of entry. Table 4 in Appendix 4 presents a list of typical pathogenic protozoa with the diseases they cause.

✔ CHECKPOINT **8**:

What group of microorganisms is most animal-like?

PARASITIC WORMS

Many species of worms, also referred to as *helminths*, are parasitic by nature and select the human organism as their host. The study of worms, particularly parasitic worms, is called *helminthology* (hel-min-THOL-o-je). Whereas invasion by any form of organism is usually called an *infection,* the presence of parasitic worms in the body also can be termed an *infestation* (Fig. 5-5). A microscope is required to see the eggs or larval forms of most worm infestations.

Roundworms

Intestinal Roundworms

Many human parasitic worms are classified as roundworms, one of the most common of which is the large worm ***ascaris*** (AS-kah-ris). This worm is prevalent in many parts of Asia, where it is found mostly in larval form. In the United States, it is found especially frequently in children (ages 4 to 12 years) of the rural South.

Ascaris is a long, white-yellow worm pointed at both ends. It may infest the lungs or the intestines, producing intestinal obstruction if present in large numbers. The eggs produced by the adult worms are deposited with excreta (feces) in the soil. These eggs are very resistant;

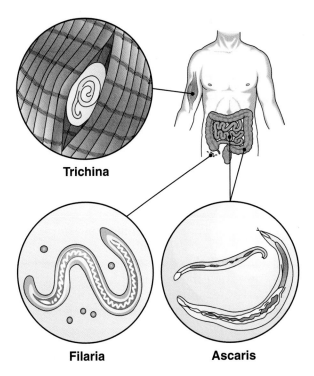

Trichina

Filaria   **Ascaris**

FIGURE **5•5**   Common parasitic worms.

they can live in soil during either freezing or hot, dry weather and cannot be destroyed even by strong antiseptics. New worms develop within the eggs and later reach the digestive system of a host by means of contaminated food. This condition may be diagnosed by a routine stool examination.

Pinworms

Another fairly common infestation, particularly in children, is the seat worm, or pinworm (*Enterobius vermicularis*), which is also hard to control and eliminate. The worms average 12 mm (somewhat less than ½ inch) in length and live in the large intestine. The adult female moves outside the vicinity of the anus to lay its thousands of eggs. A child's fingers often transfer these eggs from the itching anal area to the mouth. In the digestive system of the host, the eggs develop to form new adult worms, and thus a new infestation is begun.

The child also may infect others by this means. In addition, pinworm eggs that are expelled from the body constitute a hazard because they may live in the external environ-

ment for several months. Patience and every precaution, with careful attention to medical instructions, are necessary to rid the patient of the worms. Washing the hands, keeping the fingernails clean, and avoiding finger sucking are all essential.

Hookworms

Hookworms are parasites that live in the small intestine. They are dangerous because they suck blood from the host, causing such a severe anemia (blood deficiency) that the victim becomes sluggish, both physically and mentally. Most victims become susceptible to various chronic infections because of extremely reduced resistance following great and continuous blood loss.

Hookworms lay thousands of eggs, which are distributed in the soil by contaminated excreta. The eggs develop into small larvae, which are able to penetrate the intact skin of bare feet. They enter the blood and, by way of the circulating fluids, the lungs and the upper respiratory tract, finally reaching the digestive system. Proper disposal of body wastes, attention to sanitation, and wearing shoes in areas where the soil is contaminated best prevent this infestation.

Other Roundworms

Excreta transmit most roundworms; however, the small **trichina** (trik-I-nah), found mainly in pork, is an exception. These tiny roundworms become enclosed in cysts, or sacs, inside the muscles of rats, pigs, and humans. If undercooked pork is eaten, the host's digestive juices dissolve the cysts in it, and the tiny worms mature and travel to the host's muscles, where they again become encased. This disease is known as **trichinosis** (trik-ih-NO-sis).

Biting insects, such as flies and mosquitoes, transmit the tiny, threadlike worm that causes **filariasis** (fil-ah-RI-ah-sis). The worms grow in large numbers, causing various body disturbances. If they clog the lymphatic vessels, a condition called **elephantiasis** (el-eh-fan-TI-ah-sis) results, in which the lower extremities and the scrotum may become tremendously enlarged. Filariasis is most common in tropical and subtropical lands, such as southern Asia and many of the South Pacific islands.

Flatworms

Some flatworms resemble long ribbons, whereas others have the shape of a leaf. Tapeworms may grow in the intestinal tract to a length of 1.5 to 15 meters (5 to 50 feet). They are spread by infected, improperly cooked meats, including beef, pork, and fish. Like that of most intestinal worm parasites, the flatworm's reproductive system is highly developed, so that each worm produces an enormous number of eggs, which may then contaminate food, water, and soil. Leaf-shaped flatworms, known as *flukes,* may invade various parts of the body, including the blood, lungs, liver, and intestine.

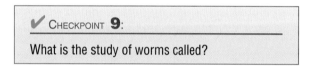

✔ CHECKPOINT **9**:

What is the study of worms called?

MICROBIAL CONTROL

Spread of Microorganisms

There is scarcely a place on earth that is naturally free of microorganisms. One exception is the interior of normal body tissue. However, body surfaces and passageways leading to the outside of the body, such as the mouth, throat, nasal cavities, and large intestine, harbor an abundance of both harmless and potentially pathogenic microbes. As explained in Chapter 17, the body has natural defenses against these organisms. If these natural defenses are sound, a person may harbor many microbes without ill effect. If that person's resistance becomes lowered, however, an infection can result.

Microbes are spread in innumerable ways. The simplest means is by person-to-person contact. The more crowded the living conditions, the greater are the chances of epidemics. The atmosphere is a carrier of microorganisms. Although microbes cannot fly, the dust of the air is alive with them. In close quarters, bacteria-laden droplets discharged by sneezing, coughing, and even normal conversation further contaminate the atmosphere. Pathogens also are spread by such pests as rats, mice, fleas, lice, flies, and mosquitoes. Dirty conditions and a lack of sunlight abet microbial growth. In poor areas throughout the world, there is often a combination of crowded conditions and poor sanitation. Many inhabitants do not receive immunizations and have lowered resistance because of poor nutrition. As a result, epidemics are apt to begin in these districts.

Microbes and Public Health

All societies establish and enforce measures designed to protect the health of their populations. Most of these practices are concerned with preventing the spread of infectious organisms. A few examples of fundamental public health considerations are listed below:

- *Sewage and garbage disposal.* In times past, when people disposed of the household "slops" by the simple expedient of throwing them out the window, great epidemics were inevitable. Modern practice is to divert sewage into a processing plant in which harmless microbes are put to work destroying the pathogens. The resulting noninfectious "sludge" makes excellent fertilizer.
- *Purification of the water supplies.* Drinking water that has become polluted with untreated sewage may be contaminated with such dangerous pathogens as typhoid bacilli, the viruses of polio and hepatitis, and dysentery amebas. A filtering process usually purifies the municipal water supply, and a close and constant watch is kept on its microbial population. Industrial and chemical wastes, such as asbestos fibers, acids and detergents from homes and from industry, and pesticides used in agriculture, complicate the problem of obtaining pure drinking water.
- *Prevention of food contamination.* Various national, state, and local laws seek to prevent outbreaks of disease through contaminated food. Certain animal diseases (*e.g.,* tuberculosis and tularemia) can be passed on, and food is also a natural breeding place for many dangerous pathogens.

Some of the organisms that cause food poisoning are the botulism bacillus (*Clostridium botulinum*) that grows in improperly canned foods, so-called staph (*Staphylococcus aureus*), and species of *Salmonella* transmitted in eggs, poultry, dairy products, and poultry. In recent years, a variety of the normally harmless intestinal bacillus *Escherichia coli* has caused outbreaks of food poisoning from undercooked meat and from produce. For further information, see Table 1 in Appendix 4.

Most cities have sanitary regulations requiring, among other things, compulsory periodic inspection of food-handling establishments.

- *Milk pasteurization.* Milk is rendered free of pathogens by pasteurization, a process in which the milk is heated to 63°C (145°F) for 30 minutes and then cooled rapidly before being packaged. Sometimes, slightly higher temperatures are used for a much shorter time with satisfactory results. The entire pasteurization process, including the cooling and packing, is accomplished in a closed system, without any exposure to air. Pasteurized milk still contains microbes, but no harmful ones. Pasteurization is also used to preserve other beverages and dairy products.

Aseptic Methods

In the practice of medicine, surgery, nursing, and other health fields, specialized procedures are performed for the purpose of reducing to a minimum the influence of pathogenic organisms. The word *sepsis* means "poisoning due to pathogens"; *asepsis* (a-SEP-sis) is its opposite—a condition in which no pathogens are present. Procedures that are designed to kill, remove, or prevent the growth of microbes are called *aseptic methods*.

There are a number of terms designating aseptic practices. These are often confused with one another. Some of the more commonly used terms and their definitions are as follows (Fig. 5-6):

- *Sterilization.* To sterilize an object means to kill *every* living microorganism on it. In operating rooms and delivery rooms espe-

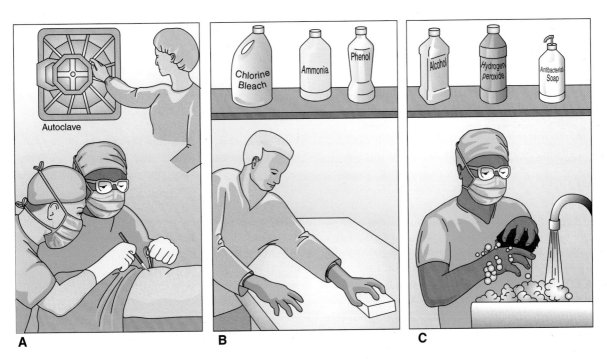

A   B   C

FIGURE 5•6   Aseptic methods. **(A)** Sterilization. **(B)** Disinfection. **(C)** Antisepsis.

cially, as much of the environment as possible is kept sterile, including the gowns worn by operating room personnel and the instruments used.

The usual sterilization agent is live steam under pressure in an **autoclave.** Dry heat is also used. Ethylene oxide, a gas, is used to sterilize supplies and equipment not able to withstand high temperatures. Most pathogens can be killed by exposure to boiling water for 4 minutes. However, the time and temperature required to ensure the destruction of all spore-forming organisms in sterilization are much greater than those required to kill most pathogens.

- *Disinfection.* Disinfection refers to any measure that kills all pathogens (except spores) but does not necessarily kill all harmless microbes. Most **disinfectants** (disinfecting agents) are chemicals that can be applied directly to nonliving surfaces. Examples are chlorine compounds, such as household bleach, phenol compounds, and mercury compounds. Commercial products for disinfection contain more than one chemical agent in order to kill a variety of organisms. Two other terms for bacteria-killing agents, synonymous with disinfectant, are **bactericide** and **germicide,** agents that kill bacteria and germs.
- *Antisepsis.* This term refers to any process in which pathogens are not necessarily killed but are prevented from multiplying, a state called **bacteriostasis** (bak-te-re-o-STA-sis). (*Stasis* means "steady state.") **Antiseptics** are less powerful than disinfectants and are safe to use on living tissues. Examples are alcohol, organic iodine solutions, and hydrogen peroxide.

Standard Precautions

Special measures must be taken to prevent the spread of infection when handling body fluids, such as blood, semen, urine, saliva, or any other moist body substance. Standard precautions are applied to all situations involving body fluids even if no blood is visible.

These precautions were originally directed at controlling the spread of the blood-borne diseases hepatitis and AIDS. Now, standard precautions treat all clients the same to prevent disease transmission.

Barriers such as gloves, masks, goggles, and gowns are used for protection. Needles and other sharp instruments must be handled safely and disposed of in puncture-proof containers. **Needles are never recapped.** All waste and laundry from health care facilities is treated as if contaminated.

Additional isolation precautions are instituted for patients infected with pathogens according to the way in which that pathogen is spread.

Handwashing

Handwashing is the single most important measure for preventing the spread of infection in all settings. Thorough washing promptly after patient contact and after contact with any body secretions is of utmost importance in infection control. Standard precautions include handwashing after removal of gloves due to the rapid multiplication of normal flora inside the gloves. Gloves are not considered a substitute for handwashing because they may have small defects, they may be torn, or hands may become contaminated when the gloves are removed.

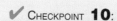 CHECKPOINT **10**:

Aseptic practices are intended to eliminate pathogens. What are the three levels of asepsis?

CHEMOTHERAPY

Chemotherapy (ke-mo-THER-ah-pe) means the treatment of a disease by the administration of a chemical agent. The chemical may be either a natural or artificial (synthetic) substance and is usually referred to as a *drug.* Two categories of drugs used in chemotherapy are described here. Other examples of chemotherapy are given in later chapters.

Antibiotics

An *antibiotic* is a chemical substance produced by living cells. It has the power to kill or arrest the growth of pathogenic microorganisms by upsetting vital chemical processes within them. Antibiotics that are relatively nontoxic to the host are used for the treatment of infectious diseases. Most antibiotics are derived from fungi (molds) and soil bacteria. Penicillin, the first widely used antibiotic, is made from a common blue mold, *Penicillium.* Often, the drugs derived from penicillin can be recognized by the ending *-cillin* in the name. Other fungi that produce a large number of antibiotics are members of the group *Cephalosporium.* The soil bacteria *Streptomyces* produce a number of frequently used antibiotics. These drug names often end in *-mycetin.*

The development of antibiotics has been of incalculable benefit to humanity. Since the time that penicillin saved many lives on the battlefields of World War II in the 1940s, antibiotics have been considered miracle drugs. Enthusiasm for their use, however, has given rise to some undesirable effects.

One danger is the development of opportunistic infections. As noted, there is a normal flora of microorganisms in the body that competes with pathogens. Antibiotics, especially those that kill a wide variety of bacteria (broad-spectrum antibiotics), eliminate these competitors and allow pathogens to thrive. For example, antibiotics often destroy the normal flora of the vaginal tract and allow a troublesome yeast infection to develop.

The widespread use of antibiotics has resulted in the natural evolution of strains of pathogens that are resistant to these medications. Some strains of common organisms, such as streptococci, staphylococci, pneumococci, *E. coli* (an intestinal organism), and tuberculosis are now resistant to most antibiotics (see Appendix 4 for diseases caused by these microorganisms). When taking antibiotics, it is important to complete the entire course of treatment to guarantee the destruction of all pathogens, or the more resistant cells will be able to survive and grow.

One of the greatest problems in hospitals today is the prevalence of antibiotic-resistant pathogens. These pathogens may cause serious infections that are unresponsive to chemotherapy. About 5% of acute care hospital patients contract one or more of these infections. Patients who are elderly or severely debilitated are most susceptible to these **nosocomial** (nos-o-KO-me-al) diseases (hospital-acquired diseases).

Pharmaceutical companies continue to search for new antibiotics. We may even be able to reverse the trend toward resistance by prescribing these drugs less often. (Antibiotics are also used in agriculture to protect farm animals from infections that cut down on productivity.) There is some evidence that susceptibility to a given drug will reappear when a bacterial population is no longer exposed to it (see Plasmids and Antibiotic Resistance).

Antineoplastic Agents

Antineoplastic agents are a group of chemotherapeutic drugs extensively employed to treat cancers. These agents are toxic to tumor cells but are also damaging to normal cells and should be administered by health care personnel who understand the complications

Plasmids and Antibiotic Resistance

Antibiotic resistance usually develops over time as exposure to a given drug gradually selects out cells that can survive in its presence. This public health problem is made worse by the fact that bacteria can sometimes transfer their resistance directly to other cells. Although bacteria are considered to be asexual (they do not need to mate in order to reproduce), they do sometimes transfer genetic information (DNA) to other cells.

Plasmids are small pieces of DNA in the cytoplasm of the cell that can carry genes for antibiotic resistance as well as other traits. Copies of plasmid can be transferred to sensitive cells, causing them to become resistant, sometimes to multiple antibiotics. When plasmids are involved, multiple-drug resistance develops at a faster rate in bacterial populations than it does when the slower selection process is at work. Plasmids that carry genes for antibiotic resistance have been found among many pathogenic bacteria, including organisms that cause dysentery (an intestinal infection), pneumonia, and a number of opportunistic infections.

caused by these drugs. Because of their weakened state, patients who receive these drugs are subject to the development of opportunistic infections.

✔ CHECKPOINT **11**:

What is chemotherapy?

LABORATORY IDENTIFICATION OF PATHOGENS

The nurse, physician, or laboratory worker may obtain specimens from patients to identify bacteria and other organisms. Specimens most frequently studied are blood, spinal fluid, feces, urine, and sputum along with swabbings from other areas. Swabs are used to collect specimens from the nose, throat, eyes, and cervix as well as from ulcers or other infected areas.

Staining Techniques

There are so many different kinds of bacteria requiring identification that the laboratory must use a number of procedures for determining which organisms are present in the material obtained from a patient. One of the most frequently used methods for beginning the process of identification involves the application of colored dyes, known as *stains,* to a thin smear of the specimen on a glass slide.

The most commonly used staining procedure is known as the *Gram stain* (see Fig. 5-2). A bluish purple dye (such as crystal violet) is applied, and then a weak solution of iodine is added. This causes a colorfast combination within certain organisms, so that washing with alcohol does not remove the dye. These bacteria are said to be *gram positive* and appear bluish purple under the microscope. Examples are the pathogenic staphylococci and streptococci; the cocci that cause certain types of pneumonia; and the bacilli that produce diphtheria, tetanus, and anthrax. Other organisms are said to be

gram negative because the coloring can be removed from them by the use of a solvent. These are then stained for visibility, usually with a red dye. Examples of gram-negative organisms are the diplococci that cause gonorrhea and epidemic meningitis and the bacilli that produce typhoid fever, influenza, and one type of dysentery. The colon bacillus (*E. coli*) normally found in the bowel is also gram negative, as is the cholera vibrio.

Another stain used to identify organisms is the *acid-fast stain.* After being stained with a reddish dye (carbolfuchsin), the smear is treated with acid. Most bacteria quickly lose their stain upon application of the acid, but the organisms that cause tuberculosis and leprosy remain colored. Such organisms are said to be *acid fast.*

A few organisms, such as the spirochetes of syphilis and the rickettsias, do not stain with any of the commonly used dyes. Special techniques must be used to identify these organisms.

Other Methods

In addition to the various staining procedures, laboratory techniques for identifying bacteria include: (1) growing cells in cultures, a process using substances called *media* (such as nutrient broth or agar) that bacteria can use as food; (2) studying the ability of bacteria to act on (ferment) various carbohydrates (sugars); (3) observing reactions to various test chemicals; (4) inoculating animals and analyzing their reactions to the injections; and (5) studying bacteria by serologic (immunologic) tests based on the antigen–antibody reaction (see Chap. 17).

These are only a few of the many laboratory procedures that play a vital part in the process of diagnosing disease.

✔ CHECKPOINT **12**:

One way of identifying microorganisms is to examine them under a microscope. Before examination, the cells are colored so they can be seen. What are the dyes used to color the cells called?

Summary

I. What is disease?

A. Categories of disease—infection, degenerative disease, nutritional disorders, metabolic disorders, immune disorders, neoplasms, psychiatric disorders

B. Predisposing causes—age, sex, heredity, living conditions and habits, emotional disturbance, physical and chemical damage, preexisting illness

II. The study of and treatment of disease

A. Disease terminology
1. Pathophysiology—study of pathologic and physiologic aspects of a disorder
2. Etiology—study of causation
3. Incidence—range of occurrence
4. Terms related to severity and duration
   a. Acute—severe, of short duration
   b. Chronic—less severe, of long duration
   c. Subacute—intermediate between acute and chronic
5. Idiopathic—of unknown cause
6. Communicable—transmissible
   a. Epidemic—widespread in a given region
   b. Endemic—characteristic of a given region
   c. Pandemic—prevalent throughout an entire country or the world

B. Steps in treatment
1. Diagnosis—determination of the nature of the illness
   a. Symptom—change in body function felt by the patient
   b. Sign—change in body function observable by others
   c. Syndrome—characteristic group of signs and symptoms

2. Prognosis—prediction of probable outcome of disease
3. Therapy—course of treatment

C. Prevention of disease—removal of potential causes of disease

D. Infectious disease
1. Terms
   a. Parasite—organism that lives on or within a host at host's expense
   b. Pathogenic—causing disease
   c. Opportunistic—taking hold in a weakened host
2. Modes of transmission
   a. Direct or indirect
   b. Portals of entry and exit- skin, respiratory, digestive, urinary, and reproductive systems

III. Microorganisms—single-cell organisms visible only with a microscope

1. Microbiology—study of microorganisms
   a. Bacteriology—study of bacteria
   b. Mycology—study of fungi
   c. Virology—study of viruses
   d. Protozoology—study of protozoa
2. Normal flora—population of microorganisms normally growing on and within the body

A. Bacteria
1. Bacilli—straight rods; may produce spores (resistant forms)
2. Cocci—spheres
   a. Diplococci—pairs
   b. Streptococci—chains
   c. Staphylococci—clusters
3. Curved rods
   a. Vibrios—comma shaped
   b. Spirilla—corkscrew or wavy
   c. Spirochetes—flexible spirals
4. Other types of bacteria—obligate intracellular parasites
   a. Rickettsias
   b. Chlamydias

B. Fungi—simple, plantlike organisms, including yeasts and molds

C. Viruses—smallest infectious agents; obligate intracellular parasites

D. Protozoa—single-cell, animal-like organisms, including amebas, ciliates, flagellates, sporozoa

have potential for transmission of disease

IV. Parasitic Worms—helminths
  A. Roundworms—ascaris, pinworms, trichina, filaria, hookworms
  B. Flatworms—tapeworms, flukes

V. Microbial control
  A. Spread of microorganisms
  B. Microbes and public health: sewage disposal, water purification, food inspection, milk pasteurization
  C. Aseptic methods
    1. Sterilization—killing of all organisms
    2. Disinfection—destruction of all pathogens except spores
    3. Antisepsis—pathogens killed or prevented from multiplying (bacteriostasis); safe for living tissues
    4. Standard precautions—used on assumption that all body fluids

VI. Chemotherapy—treatment with a chemical agent (drug)
  A. Antibiotics
    1. Produced by living cells
    2. Kill or arrest growth of pathogens
  B. Antineoplastic agents—used for treatment of cancer

VII. Laboratory identification of pathogens
    1. Collection of specimens
  A. Staining techniques
    1. Gram stain—most commonly used stain
    2. Acid-fast stain—used to identify tuberculosis
  B. Other methods—cultivation, sugar fermentation, chemical reactions, animal tests, immunologic tests, and others

Questions for Study and Review

1. What is disease? List five direct and five indirect causes of disease.
2. List seven categories of disease.
3. Define a *predisposing cause*. List six predisposing causes of disease.
4. Explain the difference between the terms in each of the following pairs:
    a. *etiology* and *incidence*
    b. *acute* and *chronic*
    c. *idiopathic* and *communicable*
    d. *epidemic* and *endemic*
    e. *diagnosis* and *prognosis*
    f. *symptom* and *sign*
    g. *prevention* and *therapy*
    h. *pathogen* and *parasite*
    i. *aerobic* and *anaerobic*
5. Name the portals of entry for disease.
6. In what ways are microorganisms beneficial to humans?
7. What are spores? Why are they important in the study of disease?
8. What are the three characteristic shapes of bacterial cells? Name a typical disease caused by each group.
9. How do the rickettsias and the chlamydias differ from other bacteria in size and living habits?
10. Name two diseases caused by rickettsias and two due to chlamydias.

11. What is the typical mode of transmission of rickettsias?
12. Name two types of pathogenic fungi and one common fungal infection.
13. List four viral diseases. What does the acronym (abbreviation) *AIDS* mean?
14. What microbial group is described as animal-like? Name three diseases these microbes cause.
15. List several types of parasitic worms.
16. What are the most common ways by which disease organisms are spread?
17. What measures do communities take to prevent outbreaks of disease?
18. Define the term *asepsis.*
19. Compare the terms *sterilization, disinfection,* and *antisepsis.* How is each accomplished?
20. Why are standard precautions followed? What measures are included in the use of standard precautions?
21. Define *chemotherapy.* Name two types of chemotherapeutic agents.
22. What are some of the disadvantages of the use of antibiotics?
23. Who would be subject to a nosocomial infection?
24. What are laboratory stains and how are they used?
25. Give examples of gram-positive, gram-negative, and acid-fast organisms.
26. List some techniques used to study bacteria.

✔ ANSWERS TO CHECKPOINTS

1. A predisposing cause of disease is a factor that may not in itself give rise to a disease but that increases the probability of a person's becoming ill.
2. The two sciences that are involved in study of disease are pathology (study of disease) and physiology (study of function).
3. Signs and symptoms are used to make a diagnosis of disease.
4. A parasite is an organism that lives on or within a host and at the host's expense.
5. Some factors involved in the spread of infectious disease organisms are the mode of transmission, the portal of entry, and the portal of exit.
6. The term normal flora refers to the microorganisms that normally live in or on the body.
7. The three basic shapes of bacteria are rod-shaped (bacilli), spherical (cocci), and curved rods.
8. The protozoa are most animal-like.
9. Helminthology is the study of worms.
10. Three levels of asepsis are sterilization, disinfection, and antisepsis.
11. Chemotherapy is the treatment of disease by administration of a chemical agent.
12. Stains are used to color cells so that they can be examined under the microscope.

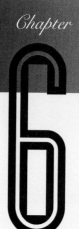

Chapter

6

The Skin in Health and Disease

SELECTED KEY TERMS

The following terms are defined in the Glossary:

dermatitis

dermis

epidermis

erythema

integument

keratin

lesion

melanin

sebaceous

sebum

subcutaneous

sudoriferous

BEHAVIORAL OBJECTIVES

After careful study of this chapter, you should be able to:

1. Name and describe the layers of the skin
2. Describe the subcutaneous tissue
3. Give the location and function of the appendages of the skin
4. List the main functions of the skin
5. Summarize the information to be gained by observation of the skin
6. List the main disorders of the skin

The skin is easily observed. It is the one organ that can be inspected in its entirety without requiring surgery or special equipment. The skin not only gives clues to its own health but also reflects the health of other body systems. Although the skin may be viewed simply as a membrane enveloping the body, it is far more complex than the other epithelial membranes described in Chapter 4.

The skin is associated with structures known as *appendages,* which include glands, hair, and nails. Together with blood vessels, nerves, and sensory organs, the skin and its appendages form the ***integumentary*** (in-teg-u-MEN-tar-e) ***system.*** This name is from the word *integument* (in-TEG-u-ment), which means "covering." The term *cutaneous* (ku-TA-ne-us) also refers to the skin. The functions of this system are discussed later in the chapter after a description of its structure.

STRUCTURE OF THE SKIN

The skin consists of two layers (Fig. 6-1):

- The ***epidermis*** (ep-ih-DER-mis), the outermost portion, which itself is subdivided into thin layers called ***strata*** (STRA-tah). The epidermis is composed entirely of epithelial cells and contains no blood vessels.
- The ***dermis,*** or true skin, which has a framework of connective tissue and contains many blood vessels, nerve endings, and glands.

Epidermis

The epidermis is the surface layer of the skin, the outermost cells of which are constantly lost through wear and tear. Because there are no blood vessels in the epidermis, the only living cells are in its deepest layer, the ***stratum germinativum*** (jer-min-a-TI-vum), where nourishment is provided by capillaries in the underlying dermis. The cells in this layer are constantly dividing and producing daughter cells, which are pushed upward toward the surface. As the surface cells die from the gradual loss of nourishment, they undergo changes. Mainly, they develop large amounts of a protein called ***keratin*** (KER-ah-tin), which serves to thicken and protect the skin.

By the time epidermal cells reach the surface, they have become flat and horny, forming the uppermost layer of the epidermis, the ***stratum corneum*** (KOR-ne-um). Between the stratum germinativum and the stratum corneum there are additional layers that vary in number and quantity depending on the thickness of the skin. Cells in the deepest layer of the epidermis produce ***melanin*** (MEL-ah-nin), a dark pigment that colors the skin; irregular patches of melanin are called *freckles.*

6

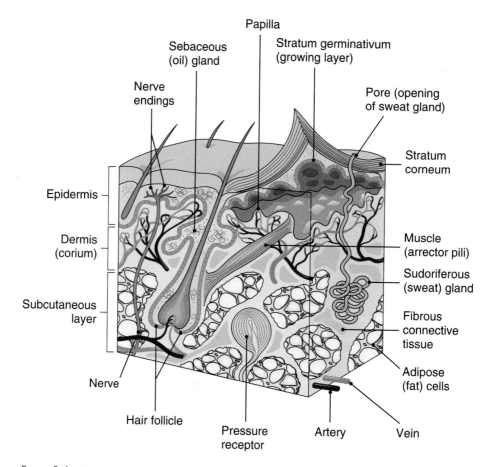

FIGURE **6•1** Cross section of the skin.

Dermis

The ***dermis,*** or ***corium*** (KO-re-um), the so-called "true skin," has a framework of elastic connective tissue and is well supplied with blood vessels and nerves. Because of its elasticity, the skin can stretch, even dramatically as in pregnancy, with little damage. Most of the appendages of the skin, including the sweat glands, the oil glands, and the hair, are located in the dermis and may extend into the subcutaneous layer under the skin.

The thickness of the dermis also varies in different areas. Some places, such as the soles of the feet and the palms of the hands, are covered with very thick layers of skin, whereas others, such as the eyelids, are covered with very thin and delicate layers.

Portions of the dermis extend upward into the epidermis, allowing blood vessels to get closer to the surface cells (see Fig. 6-1). These extensions, or ***papillae,*** form a distinct pattern of ridges on the surface of thick skin, which help to prevent slipping, such as when grasping an object. The unchanging patterns of the ridges are determined by heredity. Because they are unique to each person, fingerprints and footprints can be used for identification (see DNA Fingerprinting).

Subcutaneous Layer

The dermis rests on the subcutaneous (sub-ku-TA-ne-us) layer, sometimes referred to as the *hypodermis* or the *superficial fascia* (see Fig. 6-1). This layer connects the skin to the surface muscles. It consists of loose connective tissue and large amounts of adipose (fat) tissue. The fat serves as insulation and as a reserve supply for energy. Continuous bundles of elastic fibers connect the subcutaneous tissue with the der-

DNA Fingerprinting

Alike only in name, DNA fingerprinting is totally different from the traditional method of identification using raised patterns of the skin on the fingertips. This newer method starts with any tissue specimen, such as a sample of skin, hair, blood, or semen, and analyzes the pattern of the DNA (the genetic material) in the cells. Even very small quantities suffice because the DNA can be multiplied in the laboratory for the test. The DNA is first extracted from the cells. Enzymes are then used to cut the DNA into fragments based on specific patterns of bases (subunits) of the molecules. After the fragments are marked with radioactive labels, their picture can be taken with x-ray film. When these fragments are sorted and organized by length, they give a unique pattern that looks much like a labeling bar code.

DNA fingerprinting has been used to link suspects to the scene of a crime. When the DNA pattern of an unknown sample matches that of the suspect, the chances are extremely low that they came from different individuals. The method can also be used to identify missing persons or to analyze the closeness of relationship, as in establishing paternity of a child. The DNA patterns of related individuals show many matching bars.

mis, so there is no clear boundary between the two.

The blood vessels that supply the skin and help to regulate body temperature run through the subcutaneous layer. This tissue is also rich in nerves and nerve endings, including those that supply the dermis and epidermis. The thickness of the subcutaneous layer varies in different parts of the body; it is thinnest on the eyelids and thickest on the abdomen.

Figure 6-2 is a photograph of the skin and its appendages as seen through a microscope.

> ✔ CHECKPOINT **1**:
>
> The skin and all its associated structures comprise a body system. What is the name of this system?

> ✔ CHECKPOINT **2**:
>
> The skin itself is composed of two layers. Moving from the superficial to the deeper layer, what are the names of these layers?

APPENDAGES OF THE SKIN

Sweat Glands

The *sudoriferous* (su-do-RIF-er-us) *glands,* or sweat glands, are coiled, tubelike structures located in the dermis and the subcutaneous tissue (see Fig. 6-1). Each gland has an excretory tube that extends to the surface and opens at a pore. The slant at which the excretory tube joins the skin serves as a valve. Sudoriferous glands function to regulate body temperature through the evaporation of sweat from the body surface. Sweat consists of water with small amounts of mineral salts and other wastes.

Another type of sweat gland is located mainly in the armpits and the groin area. These glands release their secretions through the hair follicles in response to emotional stress and sexual stimulation. The secretions contain cellular material that is broken down by bacteria, producing body odor.

Several types of glands associated with the skin are modified sweat glands. These are the *ceruminous* (seh-RU-min-us) *glands* in the ear canal that produce ear wax, or *cerumen;* the *ciliary* (SIL-e-er-e) *glands* at the edges of the eyelids; and the *mammary glands.*

Sebaceous Glands

The *sebaceous* (se-BA-shus) *glands* are saclike in structure, and their oily secretion, *sebum* (SE-bum), lubricates the skin and hair and prevents drying. The ducts of the sebaceous glands open into the hair follicles.

Babies are born with a covering produced by these glands that resembles cream cheese; this secretion is called the *vernix caseosa* (VERniks ka-se-O-sah).

Blackheads consist of a mixture of dried sebum and keratin that may collect at the open-

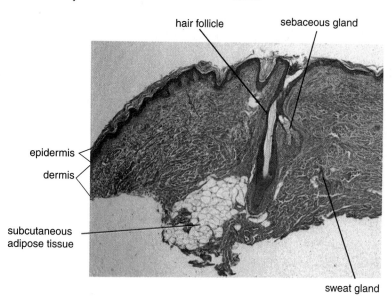

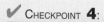

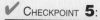

FIGURE **6•2** Microscopic view of thin skin showing tissue layers and some appendages. (Adapted from Cormack DH: Essential Histology, Plate 12-1B. Philadelphia, JB Lippincott, 1993)

ings of the sebaceous glands. If these glands become infected, pimples result. If sebaceous glands become blocked by accumulated sebum, a sac of this secretion may form and gradually increase in size. These sacs are referred to as ***sebaceous cysts.*** Usually, it is not difficult to remove such tumorlike cysts by surgery.

✔ CHECKPOINT **3**:

What is the scientific name for the sweat glands?

✔ CHECKPOINT **4**:

Some skin glands produce an oily secretion called sebum. What is the name of these glands?

Hair

Almost all of the body is covered with hair, which in most areas is soft and fine. Hair is composed mainly of keratin and is not living. Each hair develops within a sheath called a ***follicle,*** and new hair is formed from cells at the bottom of the follicles (see Fig. 6-1). Attached to most hair follicles is a thin band of involuntary muscle. When this muscle contracts, the hair is

raised, forming "goose bumps" on the skin. (The name of this muscle is *arrector pili*, which literally means "hair raiser.") This response is of no importance to humans but helps animals with furry coats to conserve heat. As this muscle contracts, it presses on the sebaceous gland associated with the hair follicle, causing the release of sebum to lubricate the skin.

Nails

Nails are protective structures made of hard keratin produced by cells that originate in the outer layer of the epidermis (stratum corneum). New cells form continuously at the proximal end of the nail in an area called the ***nail root.***

Nails of both the toes and the fingers are affected by general health. Changes in nails, including abnormal color, thickness, shape, or texture (*e.g.,* grooves or splitting), occur in chronic diseases such as heart disease, peripheral vascular disease, malnutrition, and anemia.

✔ CHECKPOINT **5**:

Each hair develops within a sheath. What is this sheath called?

FUNCTIONS OF THE SKIN

Although the skin has many functions, the following are its four major functions:

- Protection against infection
- Protection against dehydration (drying)
- Regulation of body temperature
- Collection of sensory information

Protection Against Infection

Intact skin forms a primary barrier against invasion of pathogens. The cells of the stratum corneum, the outermost layer of the epidermis, form a tight interlocking pattern that is resistant to penetration. The surface cells are constantly being shed, causing the mechanical removal of pathogens. Rupture of this barrier, as in cases of wounds or burns, invites infection of deep tissues (see Burns). The skin also protects against bacterial toxins (poisons) and other harmful chemicals in the environment.

Protection Against Dehydration

The function of the epidermis in preventing water loss is vital to maintenance of the wet environment required by all cells. In addition to keratin, the sebum that serves as a lubricant for the skin is also waterproof and helps to prevent loss by evaporation.

Regulation of Body Temperature

Both the loss of excess heat and protection from cold are important functions of the skin. Indeed, most of the blood supply to the skin is concerned with temperature regulation. The skin forms a large surface for radiating body heat to the surrounding air. When the blood vessels dilate (widen), more blood is brought to the surface so that heat can be dissipated.

The other mechanism for cooling the body involves the sweat glands. The evaporation of perspiration from the surface of the skin draws heat from the body. A person feels uncomfortable on a hot and humid day because water does not evaporate as readily from the skin into the surrounding air. A dehumidifier makes one more comfortable even though the temperature remains high.

In cold conditions, vessels in the skin become

Burns

Burns of the skin may have serious consequences because they destroy the body's outer protective layer and may lead to infection, dehydration, and other complications.
Burns are classified according to the depth of the damage.

- First-degree burns involve the outermost layer of the skin—the epidermis—which becomes red and painful. Most sunburns are first-degree burns. Pain and damage from a first-degree burn can be reduced by bathing the wound in cold water.
- Second-degree burns penetrate into deeper layers and often cause the formation of blisters. Severe sunburns or scalding with hot water are examples of this type.
- Third-degree burns are the most serious and involve the full thickness of the skin, and often the underlying tissues, such as muscle and connective tissues.

The percentage of the body's total skin area damaged by a burn is used as a measure of the seriousness of the injuries and the chances for the patient's survival. Skin grafts are used in the treatment of serious burns. Such grafts may be taken from uninjured areas of the body or may be grown in the laboratory from a small sample of skin obtained from the patient.

narrower (constrict) to reduce the flow of blood to the surface and diminish heat loss. The skin may become visibly pale under these conditions. Special vessels that directly connect arteries and veins in the skin of the ears, nose, and other exposed locations provide the volume of blood flow needed to prevent freezing. As is the case with so many body functions, temperature regulation is complex and involves several parts of the body, including certain centers in the brain.

Collection of Sensory Information

Because of the many nerve endings and other special receptors for pain, touch, pressure, and temperature, which are located mostly in the dermis, the skin may be regarded as one of the chief sensory organs of the body. Many of the reflexes that make it possible for humans to adjust themselves to the environment begin as sensory impulses from the skin. Here, too, the skin works with the brain and the spinal cord to make these important functions possible.

Other Activities of the Skin

Substances can be absorbed through the skin in limited amounts. Some drugs, for example, estrogens and medications to control motion sickness, can be absorbed from patches placed on the skin (see Using Medication Patches). Most medicated ointments used on the skin, however, are for the treatment of local conditions only. Injection of medication into the subcutaneous tissues is limited by the slow absorption that occurs here.

There is also a minimal amount of excretion through the skin. A mixture of water and electrolytes (salts) is excreted in perspiration. Some nitrogen-containing wastes are also eliminated through the skin, but even in disease, the amount of waste products excreted by the skin is small.

Vitamin D needed for the development and maintenance of bone tissue is manufactured in the skin under the effects of ultraviolet radiation in sunlight (see Vitamin D in Chap. 7).

Note that the human skin does not "breathe." The pores of the epidermis serve only as outlets for perspiration from the sweat glands and sebum (oil) from the sebaceous glands. They are not used for exchange of gases.

✔ CHECKPOINT **6**:

What two mechanisms are used to regulate temperature through the skin?

OBSERVATION OF THE SKIN

What can the skin tell you? What do its color, texture, and other attributes indicate? Is there any damage? Much can be learned by an astute observer. In fact, the first indication of a serious systemic disease (such as syphilis) may be a skin disorder.

Color

The color of the skin depends on a number of factors, including the following:

- Amount of pigment in the epidermis
- Quantity of blood circulating in the surface blood vessels
- Composition of the circulating blood
  - Quantity of oxygen
  - Concentration of hemoglobin
  - Presence of bile, silver compounds, or other chemicals

Pigment

The main pigment of the skin, as we have noted, is called ***melanin.*** This pigment is also found in the hair, the middle coat of the eyeball, the iris of the eye, and certain tumors. Melanin is common to all races, but darker people have a much larger quantity in their tissues. The melanin in the skin helps to protect against damaging ultraviolet radiation from the sun. Thus, skin that is exposed to the sun shows a normal increase in this pigment, a response we call *tanning.*

Using Medication Patches

Some medications are given by means of patches placed on the skin. Here is some information on how these patches work and how long they last.

Most medications in patches are not, in themselves, in a sustained release form. Instead, delivery is regulated by the slow absorption of the medication through the skin. First, the drug must pass through the epidermis. Then, it must diffuse deeply enough to be absorbed into capillaries and enter the bloodstream.

The diffusion process leaves a deposit of medication under the skin, so that removing the patch does not entirely remove the medicine. The body continues slowly to absorb what has been left behind. In using medication patches, it is important to know how long the patch must be in place before it is effective. In regulating dosage, it is also important to know how long it takes for the effects of the medication to disappear after removal of the patch.

Sometimes, there are abnormal increases in the quantity of melanin, which may occur either in localized areas or over the entire body surface. For example, diffuse spots of pigmentation may be characteristic of some endocrine disorders.

Discoloration

Pallor (PAL-or) is paleness of the skin, often caused by reduced blood flow. Pallor is most easily noted in the lips, nail beds, and mucous membranes. ***Flushing*** is redness of the skin, often related to fever. Signs of flushing are most noticeable in the face and neck.

When there is not enough oxygen in circulating blood, the skin may take on a bluish discoloration termed ***cyanosis*** (si-ah-NO-sis). This is a symptom of heart failure and of breathing problems, such as asthma or respiratory obstruction.

A yellowish discoloration of the skin may be due to the presence of excessive quantities of bile pigment (bilirubin) in the blood. This condition, called ***jaundice*** (JAWN-dis), may be a symptom of a number of disorders, such as the following:

- A tumor pressing on the common bile duct or a stone within the duct, either of which would obstruct the flow of bile into the small intestine
- Inflammation of the liver (hepatitis)
- Certain diseases of the blood in which red blood cells are rapidly destroyed

Another possible cause of a yellowish discoloration of the skin is the excessive intake of carrots and other deeply colored vegetables. This condition is known as ***carotenemia*** (kar-o-te-NE-me-ah).

Chronic poisoning may cause gray or brown discoloration of the skin. A peculiar bronze cast is present in Addison's disease (malfunction of the adrenal gland). Many other disorders cause discoloration of the skin, but their discussion is beyond the scope of this chapter.

Lesions

A ***lesion*** (LE-zhun) is any wound or local damage to tissue. In examining the skin for lesions, it is important to make note of their type, arrangement, and location. Lesions may be flat or raised or may extend below the surface of the skin (Fig. 6-3).

Surface Lesions

A surface lesion is often called a ***rash*** or, if raised, an ***eruption*** (e-RUP-shun). Skin rashes may be localized, as in diaper rash, or generalized, as in measles and other systemic infections. Often, these lesions are accompanied by

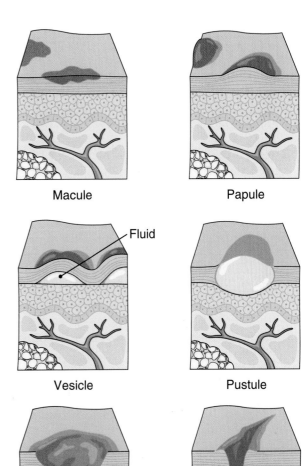

Macule

Papule

Fluid

Vesicle

Pustule

Ulcer

Fissure (laceration)

Figure **6•3** Some common skin lesions.

erythema (er-eh-THE-mah), or redness of the skin. The following are some terms used to describe surface skin lesions:

- *Macules* (MAK-ules). These spots are neither raised nor depressed. They are typical of measles and descriptive of freckles.
- *Papules* (PAP-ules). These are firm, raised areas, as in some stages of chickenpox and in the second stage of syphilis. Pimples are papules. A large firm papule is called a *nodule* (NOD-ule).
- *Vesicles* (VES-ih-klz). These are blisters or small sacs that are full of fluid, such as may be found in some of the eruptions of chickenpox or shingles.
- *Pustules* (PUS-tules). These are vesicles filled with pus. They may develop in chickenpox if the vesicles become infected.

Deeper Lesions

A deeper lesion of the skin may develop from a surface lesion or may be caused by *trauma* (TRAW-mah), that is, a wound or injury (see Fig. 6-3). Because such breaks may be followed by infection, wounds should be cared for to prevent the entrance of pathogens and toxins into deeper tissues and body fluids. Deeper injuries to the skin include the following:

- *Excoriation* (eks-ko-re-A-shun), which is a scratch of the skin surface
- *Laceration* (las-er-A-shun), which is a rough, jagged wound made by tearing of the skin
- *Ulcer* (UL-ser), which is a sore associated with disintegration and death of tissue
- *Fissure* (FISH-ure), which is a crack in the skin as seen in athlete's foot

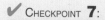

✔ CHECKPOINT **7**:

Disorders are sometimes associated with discoloration of the skin. What is the name for any substance that gives color to the skin?

✔ CHECKPOINT **8**:

What is a lesion?

Effects of Aging on the Integumentary System

As people age, wrinkles, or crow's feet, develop around the eyes and mouth owing to the loss of fat and collagen in the underlying tissues. The dermis becomes thinner, and the skin may become transparent and lose its elasticity, the effect of which is sometimes called "parchment skin." The formation of pigment decreases with age. However, there may be localized areas of extra pigmentation in the skin with the formation of brown spots ("liver spots"), especially on areas exposed to the sun (*e.g.* the back of the hands).

The hair does not replace itself as rapidly as before and thus becomes thinner. Lack of pigment causes the hair to become gray or white. The sweat glands decrease in number, so there is less output of perspiration and lowered ability to withstand heat. The elderly are also more sensitive to cold because of less fat in the skin and poor circulation. Lack of sebum causes dryness of the hair and skin. The fingernails may flake, become brittle, or develop ridges, and toenails may become discolored or abnormally thickened.

CARE OF THE SKIN

The most important factors in caring for the skin are those that ensure good general health. Proper nutrition and adequate circulation are vital to the maintenance of the skin. Regular cleansing removes dirt and dead skin debris and sustains the slightly acid environment that inhibits bacterial growth on the skin. Careful handwashing with soap and water, with attention to the undernail areas, is a simple measure that reduces the spread of disease.

The skin needs protection from continued exposure to sunlight to prevent premature aging and cancerous changes. Appropriate applications of sunscreens before and during time spent in the sun can prevent skin damage (see Protection From the Sun).

SKIN DISORDERS

Dermatosis and Dermatitis

Dermatosis (der-mah-TO-sis) is a general term referring to any skin disease. Inflammation of the skin is called **dermatitis** (der-mah-TI-tis). It may be due to many kinds of irritants, such as the oil of poison oak or poison ivy plants, detergents, and strong acids, alkalis, or other chemicals. Prompt removal of the irritant is the most effective method of prevention and treatment. A thorough soap-and-water bath taken as soon as possible after contact with plant oils may prevent the development of itching eruptions.

Atopic Dermatitis

Atopic dermatitis (ah-TOP-ik der-mah-TI-tis) or **eczema** (EK-ze-mah) is characterized by intense itching and skin inflammation. The affected areas show redness (erythema), blisters (vesicles), pimplelike lesions (papules), and scaling and crusting of the skin surface. Scratching of the skin can lead to a secondary bacterial infection. This disorder commonly first occurs in early childhood, with the recurrence of acute episodes throughout life. The skin may be excessively sensitive to many soaps, detergents, rough fabrics, or perspiration. The person with atopic dermatitis may also be subject to allergic disorders, such as hay fever, asthma, and food allergies.

Sunburn

Sunlight may cause chemical and biologic changes in the skin. The skin first becomes reddened (erythematous) and then may become swollen and blistered. Some people suffer from severe burns and become seriously ill. Continued excessive exposure to the sun is a risk factor in skin cancer. Tanning requires the skin to

Protection from the Sun

Each of the three most common forms of skin cancer, basal cell carcinoma, squamous cell carcinoma, and malignant melanoma, share a common risk factor—exposure to the ultraviolet radiation found in sunlight. Excessive exposure to the sun may not only cause cancer, it may also cause premature aging of the skin, including the production of wrinkles, discoloration, and changes in texture.

The damaging radiation found in sunlight occurs in two different forms, ultraviolet-A (UVA) and ultraviolet-B (UVB). UVA damages the deeper layers of the skin, resulting in a loss of elasticity and a general decrease in blood flow to the skin. UVA also causes damage to the skin cells' ability to repair themselves, thereby increasing the risk of the cells becoming cancerous. UVB damages the outermost layers of the skin. Exposure leads to the redness, swelling, and peeling common to the average "sunburn." Repeated, excessive exposure leads to changes in the texture of the skin such as wrinkling and thickening, as well as a change in texture most often referred to as "leathery skin."

The best way to reduce the risks of damage caused by UVA and UVB is to limit exposure to them. This is especially important between the hours of 10 AM and 4 PM when the level of radiation from the sun is at its highest. You can significantly reduce your exposure to UVA and UVB even during exposure to the midday sun, by doing the following:

- Always apply a sunscreen with an SPF (sun protection factor) of at least 15. The SPF generally indicates the amount of time you are protected relative to using no sunscreen at all (therefore, an SPF of 15 allows you to stay in the sun 15 times longer than without SPF-rated protection.) Always follow the specific products' directions. However, generally, all sunscreens should be applied at least 15–20 minutes before exposure and should be reapplied periodically during continued exposure.
- Take advantage of the protection offered by clothing. Hats, long pants, and long-sleeve shirts can protect much of the skin. Special fabrics continue to be developed that effectively block both UVA and UVB.
- Take advantage of the shade. Although shaded areas are still exposed to both UVA and UVB, shade can significantly decrease overall exposure.
- Drink plenty of fluids during and after prolonged exposure to the sun. This can help keep the skin fully hydrated, which promotes the skin's own natural defenses.

6

protect itself by producing considerably more than usual amounts of melanin. This increase in pigmentation may reduce the body's ability to profit from smaller amounts of sun available during some parts of the year.

Cancer

Skin cancer is the most common form of cancer in the United States. Basal cell and squamous cell carcinomas arise in the epidermis and generally appear on the face and neck. Early detection and treatment in these cases usually results in cure, although squamous cell carcinoma is the more likely to metastasize.

A malignant tumor of melanin-forming cells is *melanoma* (mel-ah-NO-mah), the fastest growing form of cancer in the United States. This cancer originates in a mole or birthmark anywhere in the body. Exposure to sunlight predisposes to development of skin cancer, which, in the United States, is most common among people who have fair skin and who live in the Southwest, where exposure to the sun is consistent and may be intense.

Common Acne

Acne (AK-ne) is a disease of the sebaceous (oil) glands connected with the hair follicles. The common type, called *acne vulgaris* (vul-GA-ris), is found most often in people between the ages of 14 and 25 years. The infection of the oil glands takes the form of pimples, which generally surround blackheads. Acne is usually most severe at adolescence, when certain endocrine glands in the body that control the secretions of the sebaceous glands are particularly active.

Impetigo

Impetigo (im-peh-TI-go) is an acute contagious disease of staphylococcal or streptococcal origin that may be serious enough to cause death in newborn infants. It takes the form of blisterlike lesions that become filled with pus and contain millions of virulent bacteria. It is found most frequently among poor and undernourished

children. Affected people may reinfect themselves or infect others.

Alopecia (Baldness)

Alopecia (al-o-PE-she-ah), or baldness, may be due to a number of factors. The most common type, known as male pattern baldness, is an expression of heredity and aging; it is influenced by male sex hormones. Topical applications of the drug minoxidil (used as an oral medication to control blood pressure) have produced growth of hair in this type of baldness. Alopecia may be the result of a systemic disease, such as uncontrolled diabetes, thyroid disease, or malnutrition; in such cases, control of the disease results in regrowth of hair. A growing list of drugs has been linked with baldness, including the chemotherapeutic drugs used in treating neoplasms.

Athlete's Foot

Fungi are the usual cause of athlete's foot, also known as *epidermophytosis* (ep-ih-der-mo-fi-TO-sis). The disease most commonly involves the toes and the soles but occasionally affects the fingers, the palms, and the groin region. In acute cases, the lesions may include vesicles, fissures, and ulcers. Predisposition to fungal infection varies. Some people may be exposed to pathogenic fungi with no ill effects, whereas others develop severe skin infections with only mild exposure. Those who perspire a great deal are particularly susceptible to athlete's foot.

Other Disorders of the Skin

In addition to those discussed previously, other skin lesions include the following:

- *Furuncle* (FU-rung-kl), or boil, which is a localized collection of pus in a cavity formed by the disintegration of tissue. They are caused by bacteria that enter hair follicles or sebaceous glands.
- *Carbuncle* (KAR-bung-kl), which is a pus-producing lesion that results from the ex-

tension of an infectious process, such as a boil. They involve both the skin and subcutaneous tissues and have numerous drainage channels that extend to the skin surface.

- *Psoriasis* (so-RI-ah-sis), which is characterized by sharply outlined, red, flat areas (plaques) covered with silvery scales. The cause of this chronic, recurrent skin disease is unknown.
- *Herpes* (HER-peze) *simplex virus,* which is characterized by the formation of watery vesicles (cold sores, fever blisters) on the skin and mucous membranes, including the genital area (see Table 3 in Appendix 4).
- *Shingles* (herpes zoster virus), which is seen in adults and is caused by the same virus that causes chickenpox. Infection follows nerve pathways, producing small lesions on the skin. Vesicular lesions may be noted along the course of a nerve. Pain, increased sensitivity, and itching are common symptoms that usually last longer than a year. Prompt treatment with antiviral drugs decreases the severity of this disease.

- *Urticaria* (ur-tih-KA-re-ah), or hives, which is an allergic reaction characterized by the temporary appearance of elevated red patches (wheals) often accompanied by severe *pruritus* (pru-RI-tus), or itching.
- *Scleroderma* (skle-ro-DER-mah), which together with some of the metabolic diseases, such as certain forms of lupus erythematosus, causes thickening of the dermis.
- *Decubitus* (de-KU-bih-tus) *ulcer* (bedsore, pressure ulcer), which is an ulcerous area seen in bedridden, poorly nourished patients with decreased circulation. The immediate cause is impaired blood supply of an area of skin that is pressed between bone and the bed by the patient's weight. Prevention of decubitus ulcer by frequent position change and adequate nutrition is far easier than treatment of an established ulcer.

 CHECKPOINT **9**:

What is the difference between dermatosis and dermatitis?

Summary

I. Structure of the skin
- **A.** Epidermis—surface layer of the skin
- **B.** Dermis—deeper layer of the skin
  1. Subcutaneous layer—under the skin

II. Appendages of the skin
- **A.** Sweat glands—sudoriferous glands
- **B.** Sebaceous glands—oil glands
- **C.** Hair
- **D.** Nails

III. Functions of the skin
1. Protection against infection
2. Protection against dehydration
3. Regulation of body temperature
4. Collection of sensory information
5. Other activities of the skin—absorption, excretion, manufacture of vitamin D

IV. Observation of the skin
- **A.** Color
  1. Pigment—main one is melanin
  2. Discoloration—pallor, flushing, cyanosis, jaundice, poisoning
- **B.** Lesions—wound or local damage
  1. Surface lesions—rash, eruption
  2. Deeper lesions—trauma, ulcer, fissure
- **C.** Effects of aging on the integumentary system

V. Care of the skin

VI. Skin disorders
- **A.** Dermatosis and dermatitis
  1. Dermatosis—skin disease

2. Dermatitis—inflammation
B. Atopic dermatitis (eczema)
C. Sunburn—may lead to skin cancer
D. Cancer—basal cell and squamous cell carcinomas, melanoma
E. Acne—disease of sebaceous glands related to increased endocrine secretions
F. Impetigo—infectious disease of infants and children
G. Alopecia—baldness
H. Athlete's foot—fungal infection
I. Other disorders of the skin—psoriasis, herpes simplex virus, shingles, scleroderma, etc.

Questions for Study and Review

1. Of what type of cells is the epidermis composed? Name the deepest and the uppermost layers.
2. Explain how the outermost cells of the epidermis are replaced.
3. Describe the structure of the dermis.
4. Describe the contents and functions of the subcutaneous layer.
5. Describe the location and function of the two types of skin glands.
6. Explain the four most important functions of the skin.
7. What are the most important contributors to the color of the skin, normally?
8. Define melanin and explain its function.
9. Name and describe four types of surface skin lesions.
10. Name and describe four types of deeper skin lesions.
11. What changes may occur in the skin with age?
12. List some factors involved in proper care of the skin.
13. What is the difference between the terms *dermatosis* and *dermatitis*?
14. What are some examples of irritants that frequently cause dermatitis?
15. What are the dangers of overexposure to the sun, and what precautions against it need to be considered?
16. Name the common forms of skin cancer.
17. Define *acne.* When is it usually most severe? Why?
18. What are the most common causes of baldness?
19. What are the best measures to take to prevent and control athlete's foot?
20. Define *pruritus, urticaria, psoriasis, atopic dermatitis, shingles.*
21. What is a decubitus ulcer? List the two best measures for preventing decubitus ulcers.

✔ ANSWERS TO CHECKPOINTS

1. The skin and all its associated structures make up the integumentary system.
2. The superficial layer of the skin is the epidermis; the deeper layer is the dermis.
3. The sweat glands are the sudoriferous glands.
4. The sebaceous glands produce an oily secretion called sebum.
5. Each hair develops within a sheath called the follicle.
6. Temperature is regulated through the skin by changes in the size of blood vessels and by evaporation of perspiration from the surface of the body.
7. Any substance that gives color to the skin is a pigment.
8. A lesion is any wound or local damage to tissue.
9. Dermatosis is any skin disease; dermatitis is inflammation of the skin.

This unit deals with the skeletal and muscular systems. It covers the functions of the skeletal system, going beyond support purposes and including those purposes related to blood formation and to the storage and metabolism of certain mineral salts. The important muscles and their functions in various movements, as well as their ability to produce heat and to aid in the circulation of body fluids, are noted in Chapter 8, The Muscular System.

Unit III

MOVEMENT AND SUPPORT

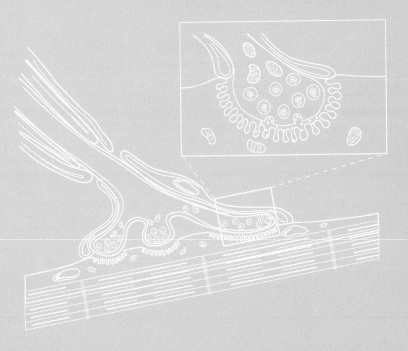

The Skeleton: Bones and Joints

SELECTED KEY TERMS

The following terms are defined in the Glossary:

amphiarthrosis

arthritis

bursa

circumduction

diaphysis

diarthrosis

endosteum

epiphysis

fontanel

joint

osteoblast

osteoclast

osteocyte

osteoporosis

periosteum

resorption

synarthrosis

synovial

BEHAVIORAL OBJECTIVES

After careful study of this chapter, you should be able to:

1. List the functions of bones
2. Describe the structure of a long bone
3. Differentiate between compact bone and spongy bone with respect to structure and location
4. Differentiate between red and yellow marrow with respect to function and location
5. Name the three different types of bone cells and describe the functions of each
6. Explain how a long bone grows
7. Name and describe various markings found on bones
8. List the bones in the axial skeleton
9. List the bones in the appendicular skeleton
10. Describe the normal curves of the spine
11. Describe five bone disorders
12. Describe how the skeleton changes with age
13. List and define six types of fractures
14. Describe the three types of joints
15. Describe the structure of a synovial joint and give six examples of synovial joints
16. Define six types of movement that occur at synovial joints
17. Describe four types of arthritis
18. List some causes of backache

The skeleton is the strong framework on which the body is constructed. Much like the frame of a building, the skeleton must be strong enough to support and protect all the body structures. Bones work with muscles to produce movement at the joints. The bones and joints, together with supporting connective tissue, form the skeletal system.

BONES

Main Functions of Bones

Bones have a number of functions, several of which are not evident in looking at the skeleton. Some of these are listed below:

- To serve as a firm framework for the entire body
- To protect such delicate structures as the brain and the spinal cord
- To serve as levers, working with attached muscles to produce movement
- To serve as a storehouse for calcium salts, which may be resorbed into the blood if there is not enough calcium in the diet
- To produce blood cells (in the red marrow)

Bone Structure

The complete bony framework of the body, known as the *skeleton* (Fig. 7-1), consists of 206 bones. These bones have several differ-

ent shapes. They may be flat (rib, skull), cube shaped (wrist, ankle), or irregular (vertebrae, face). The most familiar shape, however, is the *long bone,* the type of bone that makes up almost all of the arms and legs. This bone has a long narrow shaft, called the *diaphysis* (di-AF-ih-sis), which has a central marrow cavity, and two irregular ends, each called an *epiphysis* (eh-PIF-ih-sis) (Fig. 7-2).

Bone Tissue

Bones are not lifeless. Even though the spaces between the cells of bone tissue are permeated with stony deposits of calcium salts, the bone cells themselves are very much alive. Bones are organs, with their own system of blood vessels, lymphatic vessels, and nerves.

There are two types of bone tissue, known as *osseous* (OS-e-us) *tissue* (see Fig. 7-2).

One type is *compact bone,* which is hard and dense. This makes up the main shaft of a long bone and the outer layer of other bones. The osteocytes in this type of bone are located in rings of bone tissue around a central *haversian* (ha-VER-shan) *canal* containing nerves and blood vessels. The second type, called *spongy bone,* has more spaces than compact bone. It is made of a meshwork of small, bony plates filled with red marrow and is found at the ends of the long bones and at the center of other bones.

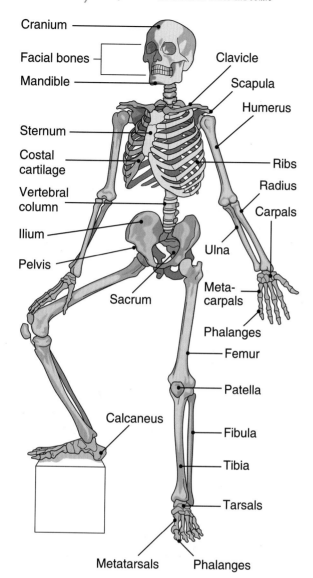

FIGURE **7•1** The skeleton.

Labels (top to bottom, left side): Cranium, Facial bones, Mandible, Sternum, Costal cartilage, Vertebral column, Ilium, Pelvis, Sacrum, Calcaneus, Metatarsals

Labels (right side): Clavicle, Scapula, Humerus, Ribs, Radius, Carpals, Ulna, Meta-carpals, Phalanges, Femur, Patella, Fibula, Tibia, Tarsals, Phalanges

Bone Marrow

Bones contain two kinds of marrow. **Red marrow** is found at the ends of the long bones and at the center of other bones. Red bone marrow manufactures blood cells. **Yellow marrow** is found chiefly in the central cavities of the long bones. Yellow marrow is composed largely of fat.

Bone Membranes

Bones are covered on the outside (except at the joint region) by a membrane called the **periosteum** (per-e-OS-te-um). The inner layer of this membrane contains cells (osteoblasts, which are essential in bone formation, not only during growth but also in the repair of fractures. Blood vessels and lymphatic vessels in the periosteum play an important role in the nourishment of bone tissue. Nerve fibers in the periosteum make their presence known when one suffers a fracture, or when one receives a blow, such as on the shinbone. A thinner membrane, the **endosteum** (en-DOS-te-um), lines the marrow cavity of a bone; it too contains cells that aid in the growth and repair of bone tissue.

> ✔ CHECKPOINT **1**:
>
> A long bone has a long narrow shaft and two irregular ends. What are the scientific names for the shaft and the ends of a long bone?

> ✔ CHECKPOINT **2**:
>
> What are the two types of osseous (bone) tissue and where is each type found?

Bone Growth and Repair

Bone Cells and Their Actions

In the embryo (the early developmental stage of a baby), most of the "bones to be" are composed of cartilage. (Portions of the skull develop from fibrous connective tissue.) Bone formation, known as **ossification,** begins during the second and third months of embryonic life. At this time, bone-building cells, called **osteoblasts** (OS-te-o-blasts), become active. First, they begin to manufacture the **matrix,** which is the material located between the cells. This intercellular substance contains large quantities of **collagen,** a fibrous protein that gives strength and resilience to the tissue. Then, with the help of enzymes, calcium compounds are deposited within the matrix. Once this intercellular material has hardened around the cells, they are known as **osteocytes** (OS-te-o-sites). These cells are still living and continue to maintain the bone, but they do not produce new bone tissue. Other cells, called **osteoclasts** (OS-te-o-klasts), are responsible for the process of **resorption,**

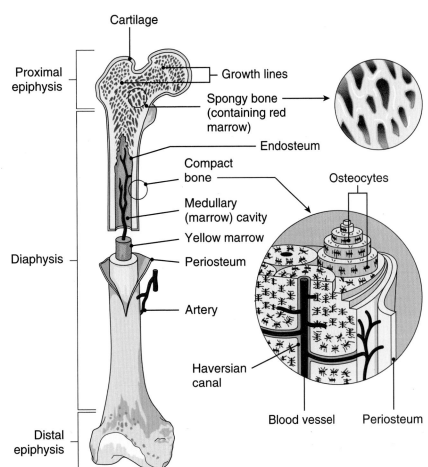

Cartilage

Proximal
epiphysis

Growth lines

Spongy bone
(containing red
marrow)

Endosteum

Compact
bone

Osteocytes

Medullary
(marrow) cavity

Yellow marrow

Diaphysis

Periosteum

Artery

Haversian
canal

Blood vessel   Periosteum

Distal
epiphysis

FIGURE **7•2** The structure of a long bone; the composition of compact bone.

7

or the breakdown of bone, which is necessary for remodeling and repair. The formation and resorption of bone tissue are regulated by several hormones, including vitamin D (see Vitamin D).

Formation of a Long Bone

In a long bone, the transformation of cartilage into bone begins at the center of the shaft. Later, secondary bone-forming centers develop across the ends of the bones. The long bones continue to grow in length at these centers through childhood and into the late teens. Finally, by the late teens or early 20s, the bones stop growing in length. Each bone-forming region hardens and can be seen in x-ray films as a thin line across the end of the bone. Physicians can judge the future growth of a bone by the appearance of these lines on x-ray films.

As a bone grows in length, the shaft is remodeled so that it grows wider as the central marrow cavity increases in size. Thus, alterations in the shape of the bone are a result of the addition of bone tissue to some surfaces and its resorption from others.

The processes of bone resorption and bone formation continue throughout life, more actively in some places than in others, as bones are subjected to "wear and tear" or injuries. The bones of small children are relatively pliable because they contain a larger proportion of cartilage and are undergoing active bone formation. In elderly people, there is a slowing of the processes that continually renew bone tissue. As a result, the bones are weaker and more fragile. Elderly people also have a decreased ability to form the protein framework on which calcium salts are deposited. Fractures in elderly

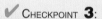

Vitamin D

Vitamin D is necessary for the formation and maintenance of bone. This "vitamin" is actually a group of related fat-soluble compounds that aids in the intestinal absorption of calcium from foods. It is manufactured from a substance in the skin that is activated by the ultraviolet (UV) radiation in sunlight. Enzymes in the liver and kidneys then modify it into its most active form. Because it is manufactured in the body and carried in the blood to the tissues on which it acts, vitamin D is now considered to be a hormone.

A lack of vitamin D results in bone malformation. This condition is called rickets in children and osteomalacia (literally, "bone softening") in adults. The requirement for vitamin D is easily met by even moderate exposure to sunlight. Exposure of the arms and face fo only 1 hour per week is enough to avoid a deficiency. As a safeguard, all milk sold in the United States is fortified with vitamin D. Only people who stay mostly indoors and drink little or no milk are at risk for developing a deficiency in this vitamin.

people heal more slowly because of these decreases in bone metabolism.

✔ CHECKPOINT **3**:

As the embryonic skeleton is converted from cartilage to bone, the intercellular matrix becomes hardened. What compounds are deposited in the matrix to harden it?

Bone Markings

In addition to their general shape, bones have other distinguishing features, or **bone markings.** These markings include raised areas and depressions that help to form joints or serve as points for muscle attachments and various holes that allow the passage of nerves and blood vessels. Some of these identifying features are described next.

Projections

- **Head**—a rounded, knoblike end separated from the rest of the bone by a slender region, the neck
- **Process**—a large projection of a bone, such as the upper part of the ulna in the forearm that creates the elbow
- **Crest**—a distinct border or ridge, often rough, such as over the top of the hip bone
- **Spine**—a sharp projection from the surface of a bone, such as the spine of the scapula (shoulder blade)

Depressions or Holes

- **Foramen** (fo-RA-men)—a hole that allows a vessel or a nerve to pass through or between bones. The plural is **foramina** (fo-RAM-ih-nah).
- **Sinus** (SI-nus)—an air space found in some skull bones
- **Fossa** (FOS-sah)—a depression on a bone surface. The plural is fossae (FOS-se).
- **Meatus** (me-A-tus)—a short channel or passageway, such as the channel in the temporal bone of the skull that leads to the inner ear

---

✔ CHECKPOINT **4**:

Bones have a number of projections, depressions, and holes. What are the purposes of these markings?

Examples of these and other markings can be seen on the bones illustrated in this chapter.

DIVISIONS OF THE SKELETON

The skeleton may be divided into two main groups of bones (see Fig. 7-1):

- The **axial** (AK-se-al) **skeleton** consists of 80 bones and includes the bony framework of the head and the trunk.
- The **appendicular** (ap-en-DIK-u-lar) **skeleton** consists of 126 bones and forms

the framework for the *extremities* (limbs) and for the shoulders and hips.

We describe the axial skeleton first and then proceed to the appendicular skeleton. Table 7-1 provides an outline of all the bones included in this discussion.

Bones of the Axial Skeleton

Framework of the Skull

The bony framework of the head, called the *skull,* is subdivided into two parts: the cranium and the facial portion. Refer to Figures 7-3 through 7-6, which show different views of the skull, as you study the following descriptions.

Cranium

This rounded chamber that encloses the brain is composed of eight distinct cranial bones.

- The *frontal bone* forms the forehead, the front of the skull's roof, and the roof of the

eye socket. The *frontal sinuses* (air spaces) communicate with the nasal cavities. These sinuses and others near the nose are described as *paranasal sinuses.*

- The two *parietal* (pah-RI-eh-tal) bones form most of the top and the side walls of the cranium.
- The two *temporal bones* form part of the sides and some of the base of the skull. Each one contains *mastoid sinuses* as well as the ear canal, the eardrum, and the entire middle and internal ears. The *mastoid process* of the temporal bone projects downward immediately behind the external part of the ear. It contains the mastoid air cells and serves as a place for muscle attachment.
- The *ethmoid* (ETH-moyd) *bone* is a light, fragile bone located between the eyes. It forms a part of the medial wall of the eye sockets, a small portion of the cranial floor, and most of the nasal cavity roof. It contains several air spaces, comprising some of

Table 7•1	**Bones of the Skeleton**	
REGION	BONES	DESCRIPTION
Axial Skeleton		
Skull		
Cranium	Cranial bones (8)	Chamber enclosing the brain; houses the ear and forms part of the eye socket
Facial portion	Facial bones (14)	Form the face and chambers for sensory organs
Hyoid		U-shaped bone under lower jaw; used for muscle attachments
Ossicles	Ear bones (3)	Transmit sound waves in inner ear
Trunk		
Vertebral column	Vertebrae (26)	Encloses the spinal cord
Thorax	Sternum	Anterior bone of the thorax
	Ribs (12 pair)	Enclose the organs of the thorax
Appendicular Skeleton		
Upper Division		
Shoulder girdle	Clavicle	Anterior; between sternum and scapula
	Scapula	Posterior, anchors muscles that move arm
Upper extremity	Humerus	Proximal arm bone
	Ulna	Medial bone of forearm
	Radius	Lateral bone of forearm
	Carpals (8)	Wrist bones
	Metacarpals (5)	Bones of palm
	Phalanges (14)	Bones of fingers
Lower Division		
Pelvis	Os coxae (2)	Join sacrum and coccyx to form the bony pelvis
Lower extremity	Femur	Thigh bone
	Patella	Kneecap
	Tibia	Medial bone of leg
	Fibula	Lateral bone of leg
	Tarsal bones (7)	Ankle bones
	Metatarsals (5)	Bones of instep
	Phalanges (14)	Bones of toes

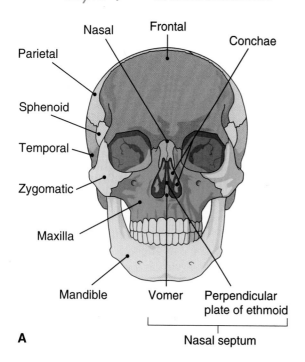

A

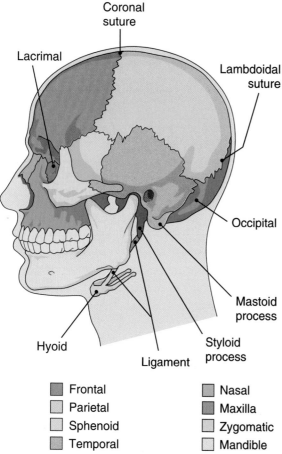

B

FIGURE **7•3**   The skull **(A)** from the front and **(B)** from the left.

FIGURE **7•4**   The skull from below, lower jaw removed.

the paranasal sinuses. A thin, platelike, downward extension of this bone (the perpendicular plate) forms much of the nasal septum, a midline partition in the nose.

- The ***sphenoid*** (SFE-noyd) ***bone,*** when seen from above, resembles a bat with its wings extended. It lies at the base of the skull in front of the temporal bones and forms part of the eye socket. The sphenoid contains a saddlelike depression, the ***sella turcica*** (SEL-a-TUR-sih-ka), that holds and protects the pituitary gland (Fig. 7-5).

- The ***occipital*** (ok-SIP-ih-tal) ***bone*** forms the back and a part of the base of the skull. The ***foramen magnum***, located at the base of the occipital bone, is a large opening through which the spinal cord commu-

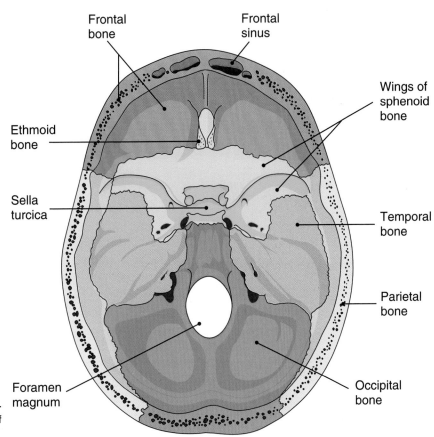

FIGURE **7•5**   Floor of cranium showing the internal surfaces of some of the cranial bones.

nicates with the brain (see Figs. 7-4 and 7-5).

Facial Bones

The facial portion of the skull is composed of 14 bones (see Fig. 7-3).

* The *mandible* (MAN-dih-bl), or lower jaw bone, is the only movable bone of the skull.
* The two *maxillae* (mak-SIL-e) fuse in the midline to form the upper jaw bone, including the front part of the hard palate (roof of the mouth). Each maxilla contains a large air space, called the *maxillary sinus,* that communicates with the nasal cavity.
* The two *zygomatic* (zi-go-MAT-ik) *bones,* one on each side, form the prominences of the cheeks.
* Two slender *nasal bones* lie side by side, forming the bridge of the nose.
* The two *lacrimal* (LAK-rih-mal) *bones,* each about the size of a fingernail, lie near the inside corner of the eye in the front part of the medial wall of the orbital cavity.
* The *vomer* (VO-mer), shaped like the blade of a plow, forms the lower part of the nasal septum (see Fig. 7-4).
* The paired *palatine bones* form the back part of the hard palate (see Figs. 7-4 and 7-6).
* The two *inferior nasal conchae* (KON-ke) extend horizontally along the lateral wall (sides) of the nasal cavities. The paired superior and middle conchae are part of the ethmoid bone (see Figs. 7-3A and 7-6).

In addition to the bones of the cranium and the facial bones, there are three tiny bones, or *ossicles* (OS-sik-ls), in each middle ear (see Chap. 11) and a single horseshoe, or U-shaped, bone just below the skull proper, called the *hyoid* (HI-oyd) *bone,* to which the tongue and other muscles are attached.

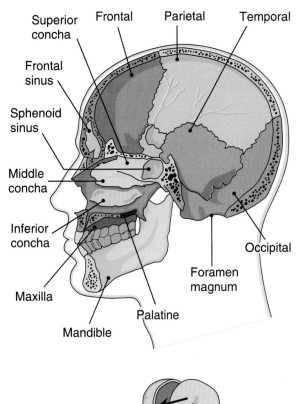

NELS). Although there are a number of these, the largest and best known is near the front of the skull at the junction of the two parietal bones and the frontal bone. This ***anterior fontanel*** usually does not close until the child is about 18 months old (Fig. 7-7).

Framework of the Trunk

The bones of the trunk include the spine, or ***vertebral*** (VER-teh-bral) ***column,*** and the bones of the chest, or ***thorax*** (THO-raks).

Vertebral Column

This bony sheath for the spinal cord is made of a series of irregularly shaped bones. These number 33 or 34 in the child, but because of fusions that occur later in the lower part of the spine, there usually are just 26 separate bones in the adult spinal column (Figs. 7-8 and 7-9).

The ***vertebrae*** (VER-teh-bre) have a drum-shaped body (centrum) located toward the front

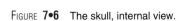

Figure **7•6**   The skull, internal view.

Openings in the base of the skull provide spaces for the entrance and exit of many blood vessels, nerves, and other structures. Projections and slightly elevated portions of the bones provide for the attachment of muscles. Some portions contain delicate structures, such as the part of the temporal bone that encloses the middle and internal sections of the ear. The sinuses provide lightness and serve as resonating chambers for the voice (which is why your voice sounds better to you as you are speaking than it sounds when you hear it played back as a recording).

Infant Skull

The skull of the infant has areas in which the bone formation is incomplete, leaving so-called ***soft spots,*** properly called ***fontanels*** (fon-tah-

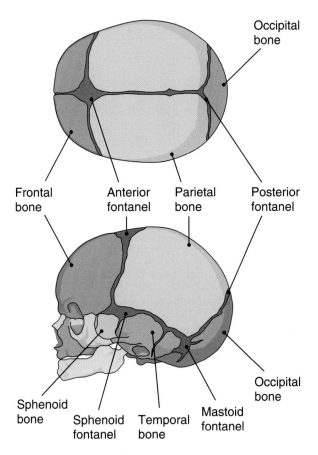

Figure **7•7**   Infant skull showing fontanels.

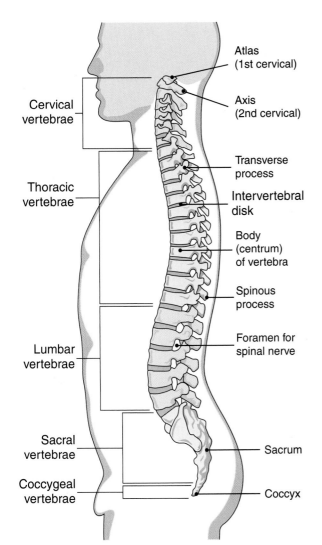

Figure **7•8** Vertebral column from the side.

through which spinal nerves emerge as they leave the spinal cord.

The bones of the vertebral column are named and numbered from above downward, on the basis of location:

- The ***cervical*** (SER-vih-kal) ***vertebrae,*** seven in number, are located in the neck. The first vertebra, called the ***atlas,*** supports the head; when one nods the head, the skull rocks on the atlas at the occipital bone. The second cervical vertebra, called the ***axis,*** serves as a pivot when the head is turned from side to side. The absence of a body in these vertebrae allows for the extra movement.
- The ***thoracic vertebrae,*** 12 in number, are located in the chest. The posterior ends of the 12 pairs of ribs are attached to these vertebrae.
- The ***lumbar vertebrae,*** five in number, are located in the small of the back. They are larger and heavier than the other vertebrae to support more weight.
- The ***sacral*** (SA-kral) ***vertebrae*** are five separate bones in the child. They eventually fuse to form a single bone, called the ***sacrum*** (SA-krum), in the adult. Wedged between the two hip bones, the sacrum completes the posterior part of the bony pelvis.
- The ***coccyx*** (KOK-siks), or tail bone, consists of four or five tiny bones in the child. These fuse to form a single bone in the adult.

Curves of the Spine

When viewed from the side, the vertebral column can be seen to have four curves, corresponding to the four groups of vertebrae (see Fig. 7-8). In the newborn infant, the entire column is concave forward (curves away from a viewer facing the infant), as seen in Figure 7-10. This is the primary curve.

When the infant begins to assume an erect posture, secondary curves develop. These curves are convex (curve toward the viewer). The cervical curve appears when the head is held up at about 3 months of age; the lumbar curve appears when the child begins to walk. The thoracic and sacral curves remain the two

(anteriorly) that serves as the weight-bearing part; disks of cartilage between the vertebral bodies act as shock absorbers and provide flexibility.

In the center of each vertebra is a large hole, or foramen (see Fig. 7-9). When all the vertebrae are linked in series by strong connective tissue bands (ligaments), these spaces form the spinal canal, a bony cylinder that protects the spinal cord. Projecting backward from the bony arch that encircles the spinal cord is the ***spinous process,*** which usually can be felt just under the skin of the back. When viewed from the side, the vertebral column can be seen to have a series of ***intervertebral foramina***

7

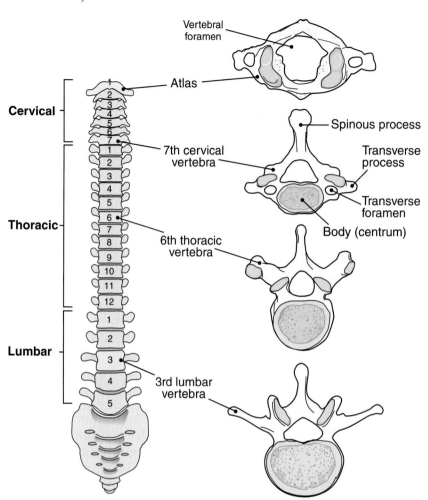

Vertebral foramen

Atlas

Cervical

7th cervical vertebra

Spinous process

Transverse process

Transverse foramen

Body (centrum)

Thoracic

6th thoracic vertebra

Lumbar

3rd lumbar vertebra

Front view of vertebral column

Vertebrae from above

FIGURE **7•9**   Front view of the vertebral column; vertebrae from above.

primary curves. These curves of the vertebral column provide some of the resilience and spring so essential in balance and movement.

Thorax

The bones of the ***thorax*** (Fig. 7-11) form a cone-shaped cage. Twelve pairs of ***ribs*** form the bars of this cage, completed by the ***sternum*** (STER-num), or breastbone, anteriorly. These bones enclose and protect the heart and lungs and other organs of the thorax.

The top portion of the sternum is the broadly T-shaped ***manubrium*** (mah-NU-bre-um) that joins at the top on each side with the clavicle (collarbone) and joins laterally with the first pair of ribs. The ***body*** of the sternum is long

and bladelike. It joins along each side with ribs two through seven. Where the manubrium joins the body of the sternum, there is a slight elevation, the ***sternal angle,*** which easily can be felt as a surface landmark.

The lower end of the sternum consists of a small tip that is made of cartilage in youth but becomes bone in the adult. This is the ***xiphoid*** (ZIF-oyd) ***process.*** It is used as a landmark for CPR (cardiopulmonary resuscitation) to locate the region for chest compression. The thorax protects the heart, lungs, and other organs.

All 12 of the ribs on each side are attached to the vertebral column posteriorly. However, variations in the *anterior* attachment of these slender, curved bones have led to the following classification:

- ***True ribs,*** the first seven pairs, are those that attach directly to the sternum by means of individual extensions called ***costal*** (KOS-tal) ***cartilages.***
- ***False ribs*** are the remaining five pairs. Of these, the 8th, 9th, and 10th pairs attach to the cartilage of the rib above. The last two pairs have no anterior attachment at all and are known as ***floating ribs.***

The spaces between the ribs, called ***intercostal spaces,*** contain muscles, blood vessels, and nerves.

✔ CHECKPOINT **5**:
What division of the skeleton consists of the bones of the skull and trunk?

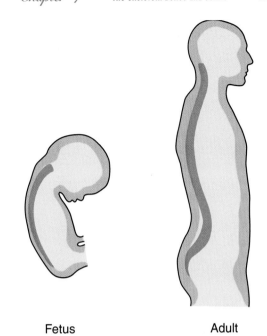

Fetus   Adult

FIGURE **7•10**   Curves of the infant spine and adult spine.

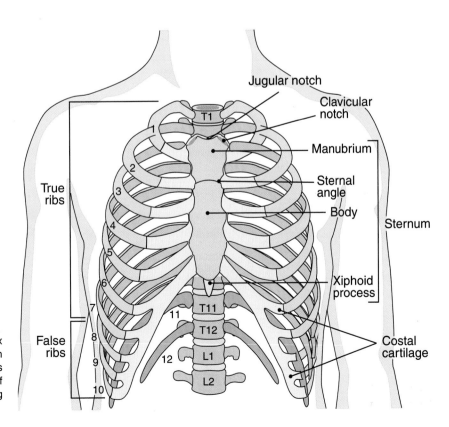

FIGURE **7•11** Bones of the thorax (anterior view). The first seven pairs of ribs are the true ribs; pairs 8 through 12 are the false ribs, of which the last two pairs are floating ribs.

Bones of the Appendicular Skeleton

The appendicular skeleton may be considered in two divisions: upper and lower. The upper division on each side includes the shoulder, the arm (between the shoulder and the elbow), the forearm (between the elbow and the wrist), the wrist, the hand, and the fingers. The lower division includes the hip (part of the pelvic girdle), the thigh (between the hip and the knee), the leg (between the knee and the ankle), the ankle, the foot, and the toes.

The Upper Division of the Appendicular Skeleton

The bones of the upper division may be divided into two groups:

The Shoulder Girdle

The shoulder girdle consists of two bones (Fig. 7-12):

- The *clavicle* (KLAV-ih-kl), or collarbone, is a slender bone with two shallow curves. It joins the sternum anteriorly and the scapula laterally and helps to support the shoulder. Because it often receives the full force of falls on outstretched arms or of blows to the shoulder, it is the most frequently broken bone.
- The *scapula* (SKAP-u-lah), or shoulder blade, is shown from a posterior view in

Figure 7-12*B*. The *spine* of the scapula is the raised ridge that can be felt behind the shoulder in the upper portion of the back. Muscles that move the arm attach to the fossae (depressions) above and below the scapular spine. The *acromion* (ah-KRO-me-on) is the process that joins the clavicle. This can be felt as the highest point of the shoulder. Below the acromion there is a shallow socket, the *glenoid cavity,* that forms a ball-and-socket joint with the arm bone (humerus). Medial to the glenoid cavity is the *coracoid process,* to which muscles attach.

The Upper Extremity

Also referred to as the upper limb, or simply the arm, the upper extremity consists of the following bones:

- The proximal bone, the *humerus* (HU-mer-us), or arm bone, forms a joint with the scapula above and with the two forearm bones at the elbow (Fig. 7-13).
- The forearm bones are the *ulna* (UL-nah), which lies on the medial side, in line with the little finger, and the *radius* (RA-de-us), on the lateral side, above the thumb. When the palm is up, or forward, the two bones are parallel; when the palm is turned down, or back, the lower end of the radius rotates around the ulna so that the shafts of the

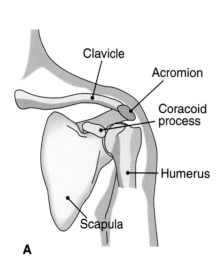

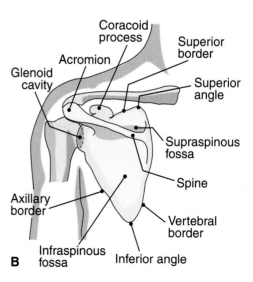

FIGURE **7•12** **(A)** Bones of the shoulder girdle. **(B)** Left scapula (posterior view)

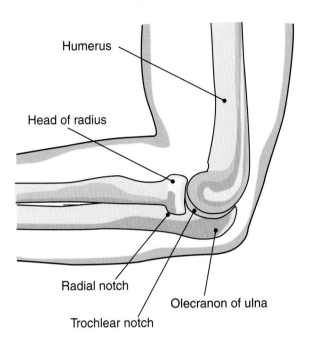

Figure **7•13**   Lateral view of the right elbow.

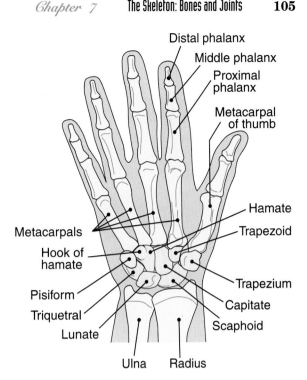

Figure **7•14**   Bones of the right hand, anterior view.

two bones are crossed. In this position, a distal projection of the ulna (the styloid process) pops up at the outside of the wrist.

- The top of the ulna has the large *olecranon* (o-LEK-rah-non) that forms the point of the elbow (see Fig. 7-13). The pulley-shaped *trochlea* (TROK-le-ah) of the distal humerus fits into the deep *trochlear notch* of the ulna, allowing a hinge action at the elbow joint. This depression, because of its deep half-moon shape, is also known as the *semilunar notch*.
- The wrist contains eight small *carpal* (KAR-pal) *bones* arranged in two rows of four each. The names of these eight different bones are given in Figure 7-14.
- Five *metacarpal bones* are the framework for the palm of each hand. Their rounded distal ends form the knuckles.
- There are 14 *phalanges* (fah-LAN-jeze), or finger bones, in each hand, two for the thumb and three for each finger. Each of these bones is called a *phalanx* (FA-lanx). They are identified as the first, or proximal, which is attached to a metacarpal; the second, or middle; and the third, or distal. Note that the thumb has only two phalanges, a proximal and a distal (see Fig. 7-14).

The Lower Division of the Appendicular Skeleton

The bones of the lower division are grouped together in a similar fashion.

The Pelvic Bones

The hip bone, or *os coxae,* begins its development as three separate bones that later fuse (Fig. 7-15):

- The *ilium* (IL-e-um), which forms the upper, flared portion. The *iliac* (IL-e-ak) *crest* is the curved rim along the upper border of the ilium. It can be felt just below the waist. At either end of the crest are two bony projections. The most prominent of these is the *anterior superior iliac spine*, which is often used as a surface landmark in diagnosis and treatment.
- The *ischium* (IS-ke-um), which is the lowest and strongest part. The *ischial* (IS-ke-al) *spine* at the back of the pelvic outlet is used as a point of reference during childbirth to indicate the progress of the presenting part (usually the baby's head)

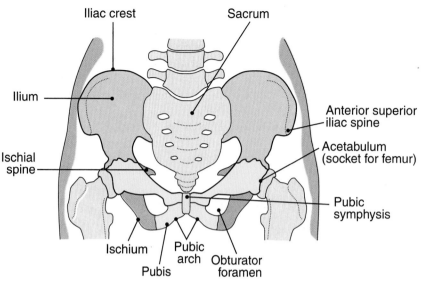

A Anterior view

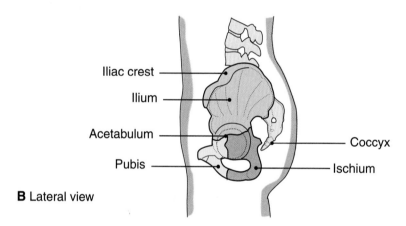

B Lateral view

FIGURE **7•15** The pelvic bones. **(A)** Anterior view. **(B)** Lateral view, shows joining of the three bones to form acetabulum.

down the birth canal. Just below this spine is the large *ischial tuberosity*, which helps support the weight of the trunk when one sits down.

- The *pubis* (PU-bis), which forms the anterior part. The joint formed by the union of the two hip bones anteriorly is called the *pubic symphysis* (SIM-fih-sis).

Portions of all three bones contribute to the formation of the *acetabulum* (as-eh-TAB-u-lum), the deep socket that holds the head of the femur (thigh bone) to form the hip joint.

The largest foramina in the entire body are found near the front of each hip bone, one on each side of the pubic symphysis. These openings are partially covered by a membrane and are called the *obturator* (OB-tu-ra-tor) *foramina* (see Fig. 7-15B).

The two ossa coxae join in forming the pelvis, a strong bony girdle completed by the sacrum and coccyx of the spine at the back (posteriorly). The pelvis supports the trunk and the organs in the lower abdomen, or pelvic cavity, including the urinary bladder, the internal reproductive organs, and parts of the intestine. The female pelvis is adapted for pregnancy and childbirth; it is broader and lighter than the male pelvis (Fig. 7-16).

The Lower Extremity

Also referred to as the lower limb, or simply the leg, the lower extremity consists of the following bones:

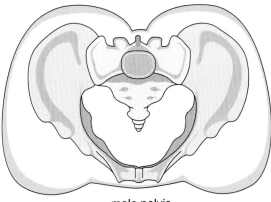

male pelvis

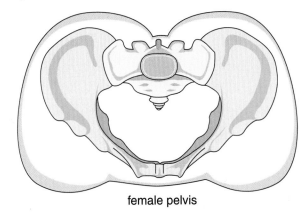

female pelvis

FIGURE **7•16** Comparison of the male pelvis and female pelvis seen from above.

- The thigh bone, called the *femur* (FE-mer), is the longest and strongest bone in the body. Proximally, it has a large ball-shaped head that joins the os coxae (Fig. 7-17). The large lateral projection at the top of the femur is the *greater trochanter* (tro-KAN-ter), used as a surface landmark. The *lesser trochanter,* a smaller elevation, is located on the medial side.
- The *patella* (pah-TEL-lah), or kneecap, is embedded in the tendon of the large anterior thigh muscle, the quadriceps femoris, where it crosses the knee joint. It is an example of a *sesamoid* (SES-ah-moyd) *bone,* a type of bone that develops within a tendon or a joint capsule.
- There are two bones in the lower leg. Medially (on the great toe side), the *tibia,* or shin bone, is the longer, weight-bearing

bone. It has a sharp anterior ridge that can be felt at the surface of the leg. Laterally, the slender *fibula* (FIB-u-lah) does not reach the knee joint; thus, it is not a weight-bearing bone. The *medial malleolus* (mal-LE-o-lus) is a downward projection at the lower end of the tibia; it forms the prominence on the inner aspect of the ankle (Fig. 7-18). The *lateral malleolus,* at the lower end of the fibula, forms the prominence on the outer aspect of the ankle.

- The structure of the foot is similar to that of the hand. However, the foot supports the weight of the body, so it is stronger and less mobile than the hand. There are seven *tarsal bones* associated with the ankle and foot. These are named and illustrated in Figure 7-18. The largest of these is the *calcaneus* (kal-KA-ne-us), or heel bone.
- Five *metatarsal bones* form the framework of the instep, and the heads of these bones form the ball of the foot.
- The *phalanges* of the toes are counterparts of those in the fingers. There are three of these in each toe except for the great toe, which has only two.

✔ CHECKPOINT **6**:

What division of the skeleton consists of the bones of the shoulder girdle, hip, and extremities?

DISORDERS OF BONE

Metabolic Disorders

Osteoporosis (os-te-o-po-RO-sis) is a disorder of bone formation in which there is a lack of normal calcium salt deposits and a decrease in bone protein. There is an increased breakdown of bone tissue without increase in the deposit of new bone by osteoblasts. The bones thus become fragile and break easily; most often involving the spine, pelvis, and long bones. Although everyone loses bone tissue with age, this condition is most apparent in postmenopausal women as a result of a decrease in hormone levels. Several treatment choices are available, including hormonal

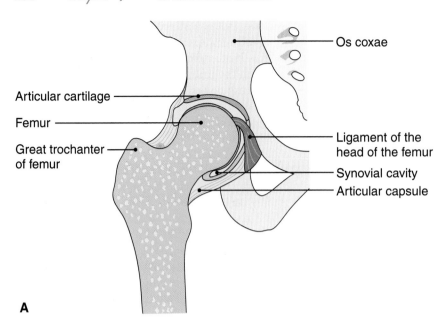

Os coxae

Articular cartilage

Femur

Great trochanter
of femur

Ligament of the
head of the femur

Synovial cavity

Articular capsule

A

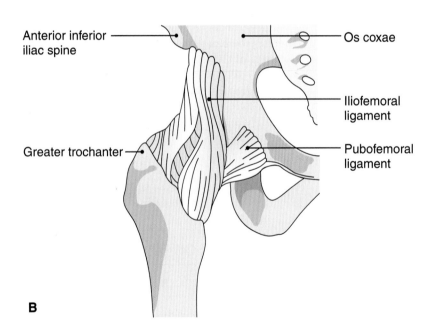

Anterior inferior
iliac spine

Os coxae

Iliofemoral
ligament

Pubofemoral
ligament

Greater trochanter

B

FIGURE **7•17** Hip joint. **(A)** Frontal section through right hip joint. **(B)** Anterior view showing ligaments.

and nonhormonal medications to reduce bone resorption. An increase in calcium intake throughout life delays the onset and decreases the severity of this disorder. Weight-bearing exercise is also important. Changes in bone can be followed with radiographic bone density tests to determine possible loss of bone mass.

Abnormal calcium metabolism may cause various bone disorders. In one of these, called Paget's disease, or ***osteitis deformans*** (os-te-I-tis de-FOR-mans), the bones undergo periods of calcium loss followed by periods of excessive deposition of calcium salts. As a result, the bones become deformed. Cause and cure are not known at the present time. The bones also can become decalcified owing to the effect of a tumor of the parathyroid gland (see Chap. 12).

Rickets is a rare childhood disease character-

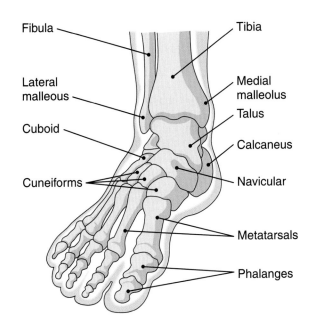

<small>FIGURE **7•18**   Bones of the right foot.</small>

ized by numerous bone deformities. Deficiency of the active form of vitamin D prevents the absorption of calcium and phosphorus salts through the intestine. These mineral salts are then not available for deposit into bone. The bones remain soft and become distorted.

Tumors

Tumors that develop in bone tissue may be benign, as is the case with certain cysts, or they may be malignant, as are osteosarcomas. In the latter case, the tumor originates most often in the bone tissue of a femur or a tibia, usually in a young person. In older people, metastases from epithelial tumors or carcinomas of various organs may spread to many bones.

Infection

Osteomyelitis (os-te-o-mi-eh-LI-tis) is an inflammation of bone caused by ***pyogenic*** (pi-o-JEN-ik) (pus-producing) bacteria. It may remain localized, or it may spread through the bone to involve the marrow and the periosteum. The bacteria may reach the bone through the bloodstream or by way of an injury in which the skin has been broken.

Before the advent of antibiotics, bone infec-

tions were resistant to treatment, and the prognosis for people with such infections was poor. Now, there are fewer cases because many bloodstream infections are prevented or treated early and do not progress to affect the bones. If those bone infections that do appear are treated promptly, the chance of a cure is usually excellent.

Structural Disorders

Abnormalities of the spinal curves, known as ***curvatures of the spine*** (Fig. 7-19), include an exaggeration of the thoracic curve, or ***kyphosis*** (ki-FO-sis) (hunchback), and an excessive lumbar curve, called ***lordosis*** (lor-DO-sis) (swayback). The most common of these disorders is ***scoliosis*** (sko-le-O-sis), a lateral curvature of the vertebral column. In extreme cases, there may be compression of some of the internal organs. Scoliosis occurs in the rapid growth period of the teens, more often in girls than in boys. Early discovery and treatment produce good results.

Cleft palate is a congenital deformity in which there is an opening in the roof of the mouth owing to faulty union of the maxillary bones. An infant born with this defect has diffi-

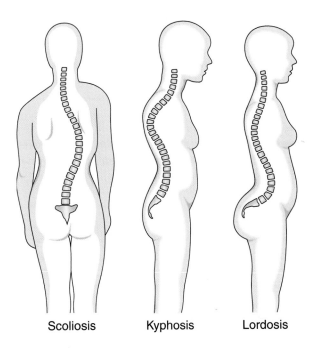

Scoliosis   Kyphosis   Lordosis

<small>FIGURE **7•19**   Abnormalities of the spinal curves.</small>

culty nursing because the mouth communicates with the nasal cavity above, and the baby therefore sucks in air rather than milk. Surgery is usually performed to correct the condition.

Flatfoot is a common disorder in which the tendons and ligaments that support the long arch of the foot are weakened and the curve of the arch flattens (see Fig. 7-18). This arch normally helps to absorb shock and distribute body weight and aids in walking. Flatfoot may be brought on by excess weight or poor posture and may also be due to a hereditary failure of the arch to form. It may cause difficulty or pain in walking. An arch support may be helpful in treating flatfoot.

Skeletal Changes in the Aging

The aging process includes significant changes in all connective tissues including bone. There is a loss of calcium salts and a decrease in the amount of protein formed in bone tissue. The reduction of collagen in bone and in tendons, ligaments, and skin contributes to the stiffness so often found in older people. Muscle tissue is also lost throughout adult life. Thus, there is a tendency to decrease the exercise that is so important to the maintenance of bone tissue.

Changes in the vertebral column with age lead to a loss in height. About 1.2 cm (about 0.5 inches) are lost each 20 years beginning at 40 years of age, owing primarily to a thinning of the intervertebral disks (between the bodies of the vertebrae). Even the vertebral bodies themselves may lose height in later years. The costal (rib) cartilages become calcified and less flexible, and the chest may decrease in diameter by 2 to 3 cm (about 1 inch), mostly in the lower part. To learn about how to keep bones strong, see Healthy Bones.

Fractures

Severe force is capable of causing a **fracture** in almost any bone (Fig. 7-20). The word **fracture** means "a break or rupture in a bone." Such injuries may be classified as follows:

- **Closed fracture,** which is a simple fracture of the bone with no open wound
- **Open fracture,** in which a broken bone

A Strong and Healthy Skeleton

The development of strong, healthy bones throughout the skeleton must begin early in childhood. The maintenance of a healthy skeleton is a lifelong effort. The process of building sound bone tissue requires certain dietary components along with consistent, periodic exercise.

The physical strength of bone tissue is derived from the presence of calcium phosphate in the bone's matrix or anatomic scaffolding. The higher the calcium phosphate content, the stronger and healthier the bone is. For calcium phosphate to be deposited in the bones' matrix, it must first be absorbed into the bloodstream from the foods we eat. The presence of calcium in the blood stream is needed not only for bone growth and development but also for blood clotting, nerve and muscle signaling, and other processes. Typically, blood calcium is used for these processes before it is stored in the bones. Because many of us do not take in enough dietary calcium, the bones generally do not receive enough calcium for storage. In fact, if not enough dietary calcium is available, the body pulls stored calcium out of the bones to ensure muscle, nerve, and clotting functions.

Overall, the amount of calcium in the bloodstream and the amount available to the bones for storage is dependent upon complex hormonal mechanisms, as well as the presence of adequate blood levels of vitamins A and D. However, the storage of calcium in bone tissue is also directly affected by exercise. Physical stress on the bones as occurs during strenuous exercise, especially during periods of growth, causes a direct increase in deposition of calcium at points where the bone is under stress. The long bones of the arms and legs build lines of strength along the direction force simply through everyday exercise. All bones respond to exercise by increasing in size and strength.

The health and strength of an individual's bones is dependent on both good nutrition and exercise, beginning in early childhood and continuing throughout life.

protrudes through the skin or an external wound leads to a broken bone
- **Greenstick fracture,** in which one side of the bone is broken and the other is bent. These are most common in children.

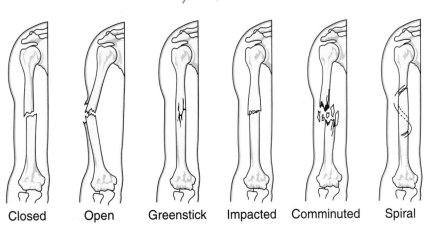

Figure **7•20** Types of fractures.   Closed   Open   Greenstick   Impacted   Comminuted   Spiral

- **Impacted fracture,** in which the broken ends of the bone are jammed into each other
- **Comminuted** (KOM-ih-nu-ted) **fracture,** in which there is more than one fracture line and the bone is splintered or crushed
- **Spiral fracture,** in which the bone has been twisted apart. These are relatively common in skiing accidents.

The most important step in first aid care of fractures is to prevent movement of the affected parts. Protection by simple splinting after careful evaluation of the situation, leaving as much as possible "as is," and a call for expert help are usually the safest measures. People who have back injuries may be spared serious spinal cord damage if they are carefully and correctly moved on a firm board or door. If trained paramedics or rescue personnel can reach the scene, a "hands off" rule for the untrained is strongly recommended. If there is no external bleeding, covering the victim with blankets may help combat shock. First aid should always be immediately directed toward the control of hemorrhage.

THE JOINTS

An **articulation,** or **joint,** is an area of junction or union between two or more bones.

Kinds of Joints

Joints are classified into three main types on the basis of the material between the bones.

They may also be classified according to the degree of movement permitted (Table 7-2):

- **Fibrous joint.** The bones in this type of joint are held together by fibrous connective tissue. An example is a **suture** (SU-chur) between bones of the skull. This type of joint is immovable and is termed a **synarthrosis** (sin-ar-THRO-sis).
- **Cartilaginous joint.** The bones in this type of joint are connected by cartilage. Examples are the joint between the pubic bones of the pelvis—the pubic symphysis—and the joints between the bodies of the vertebrae. This type of joint is slightly movable and is termed an **amphiarthrosis** (am-fe-ar-THRO-sis).
- **Synovial** (sin-O-ve-al) **joint.** The bones in this type of joint have a potential space between them called the **joint cavity,** which contains a small amount of thick, colorless fluid. This lubricant, **synovial fluid,** resembles uncooked egg white (*ov* is the root meaning "egg") and is secreted by the membrane that lines the joint cavity. The synovial joint is freely movable and is termed a **diarthrosis** (di-ar-THRO-sis). Most joints are synovial joints; they are described in more detail next.

 CHECKPOINT **7**:

What are the three types of joints classified according to the type of material between the bones?

Table 7•2   Types of Joints

Name	Movement	Material between the bones	Examples
Fibrous	Immovable (Synarthrosis)	No joint cavity; fibrous connective tissue between bones	Sutures between bones of skull

fibrous joint
(suture)

Cartilaginous	Slightly movable (Amphiarthrosis)	No joint cavity; cartilage between bones	Pubic symphysis; joints between bodies of vertebrae

cartilaginous joint
(symphysis)

Synovial	Freely movable (Diarthrosis)	Joint cavity containing synovial fluid	Gliding, hinge, pivot, condyloid, saddle, ball-and-socket joints

synovial joint

More About Synovial Joints

Structure of Synovial Joints

The bones in freely movable joints are held together by *ligaments,* bands of fibrous connective tissue. Additional ligaments reinforce and help stabilize the joints at various points (see Fig. 7-17). Also, for strength and protection, there is a *joint capsule* of connective tissue that encloses each joint and is continuous with the periosteum of the bones. The bone surfaces in freely movable joints are protected by a smooth layer of hyaline cartilage called the *articular* (ar-TIK-u-lar) *cartilage.*

Near some joints are small sacs called *bursae* (BER-se), which are filled with synovial fluid. These lie in areas subject to stress and help ease movement over and around the joints. Inflammation of a bursa, as a result of injury or irritation, is called *bursitis.*

Types of Synovial Joints

Synovial joints may be classified according to the types of movement they allow (Table 7-3).

The knee is illustrated as an example of a synovial joint in Figure 7-21. Although basically a hinge joint, the knee is complex and has some of the properties of a gliding joint as well. An x-ray picture of the knee is shown in Figure 7-22.

Movement at Synovial Joints

The chief function of the freely movable joints is to allow for changes of position and so provide for motion. These movements are named to describe changes in the positions of body parts (Fig. 7-23). For example, there are four kinds of angular movement, or movement that changes the angle between bones, as listed below:

- *Flexion* (FLEK-shun) is a bending motion that decreases the angle between bones, as in bending the fingers to close the hand.
- *Extension* is a straightening motion that increases the angle between bones, as in straightening the fingers to open the hand.
- *Abduction* (ab-DUK-shun) is movement away from the midline of the body, as in moving the arms straight out to the sides.
- *Adduction* is movement toward the midline of the body, as in bringing the arms

back to their original position beside the body.

A combination of these angular movements enables one to execute a movement referred to as *circumduction* (ser-kum-DUK-shun). To perform this movement, stand with your arm outstretched and draw a large imaginary circle in the air. Note the smooth combination of flexion, abduction, extension, and adduction that makes circumduction possible.

Rotation refers to a twisting or turning of a bone on its own axis, as in turning the head from side to side to say "no," or rotating the forearm to turn the palm up and down.

There are special movements that are characteristic of the forearm and the ankle:

- *Supination* (su-pin-A-shun) is the act of turning the palm up or forward; *pronation* (pro-NA-shun) turns the palm down or backward.
- *Inversion* (in-VER-zhun) is the act of turning the sole inward, so that it faces the opposite foot; *eversion* (e-VER-zhun) turns the sole outward, away from the body.
- In *dorsiflexion* (dor-sih-FLEK-shun), the foot is bent upward at the ankle, narrowing the angle between the leg and the top of the foot; in *plantar flexion*, the toes point downward, as in toe dancing, flexing the arch of the foot.

> ✔ CHECKPOINT **8**:
>
>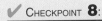
> What is the most freely movable type of joint?

Disorders of Joints

Joints are subject to certain disorders of a mechanical nature, examples of which are *dislocations* and *sprains*. A dislocation is a derangement of the parts of the joint. Ball-and-socket joints, which have the widest range of motion, also have the greatest tendency to dislocate. The shoulder joint is the most frequently dislocated joint in the body. A sprain is the wrenching of a joint with rupture or tearing of the ligaments. Injuries may cause abnormal accumulation of fluid in the joint cav-

Type of joint	Description	Examples
Gliding joint	Bone surfaces slide over one another	Joints in the wrist and ankles. (See Figs. 7-14 and 7-18) 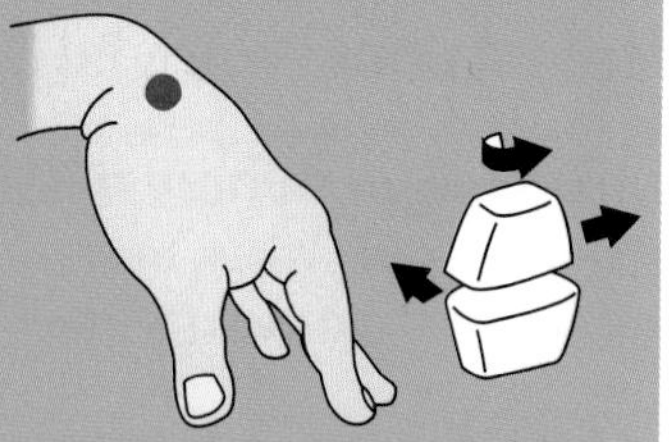
Hinge joint	Allows movement in one direction, changing the angle of the bones at the joint.	Elbow joint, joints between phalanges of fingers and toes. (See Figs. 7-13, 7-14 and 7-18) 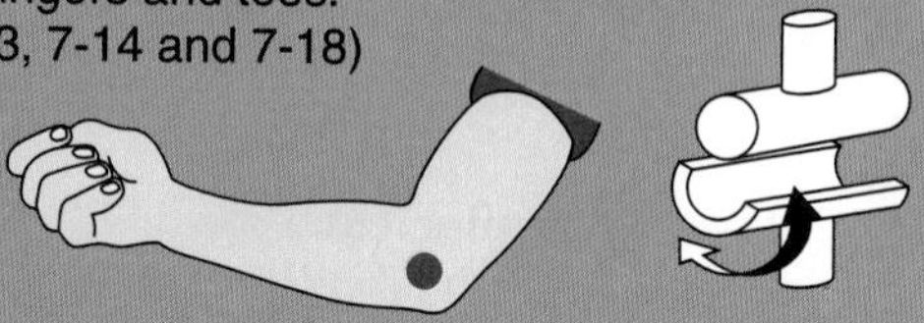
Pivot joint	Allows rotation around the length of the bone.	Joint between first and second cervical vertebrae, joint at proximal ends of the radius and ulna. (See Figs. 7-8 and 7-13) 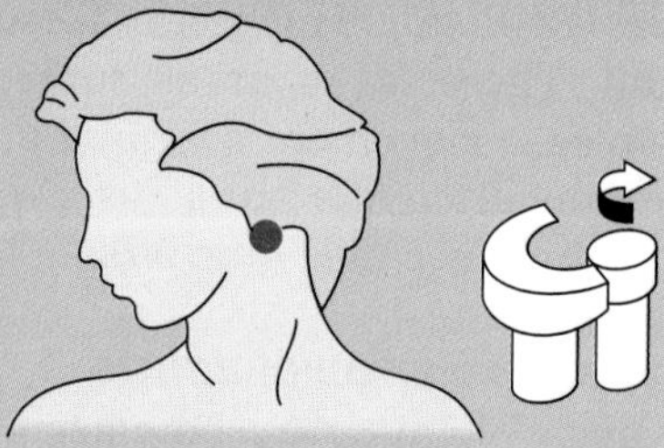
Condyloid joint	Allows movement in two directions	Joint between the metacarpal and the first phalanx of the finger (knuckle) (See Fig. 7-14); joint between the occipital bone of the skull and the first cervical vertebra (Atlas) (See Fig. 7-8) 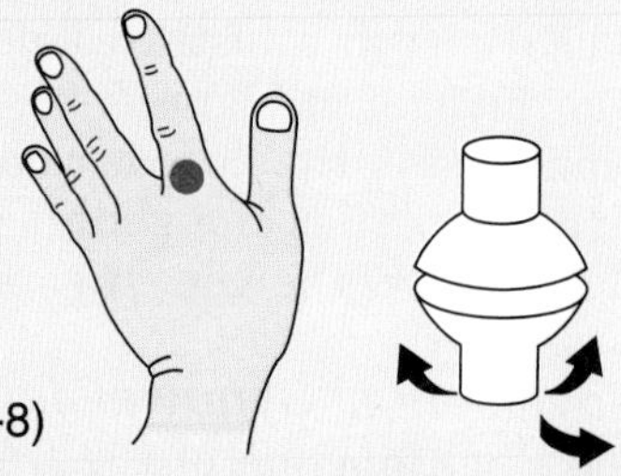
Saddle joint	Like a condyloid joint, but with deeper articulating surfaces	Joint between the wrist and the metacarpal bone of the thumb. (See Fig. 7-14) 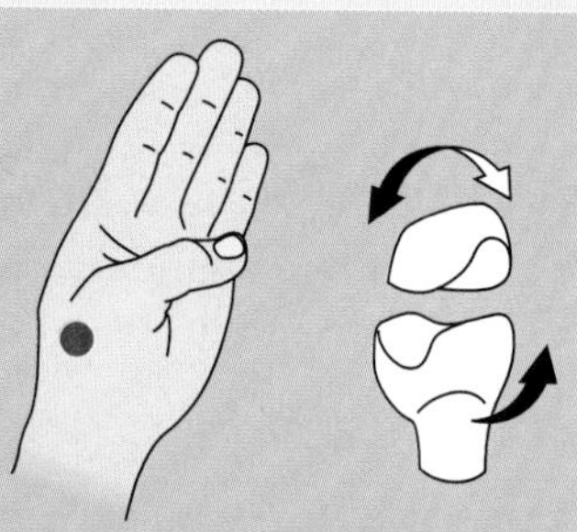
Ball-and-socket joint	Allows movement in many directions around a central point. Gives the greatest freedom of movement	Shoulder joint and hip joint (See Figs. 7-12a and 7-17) 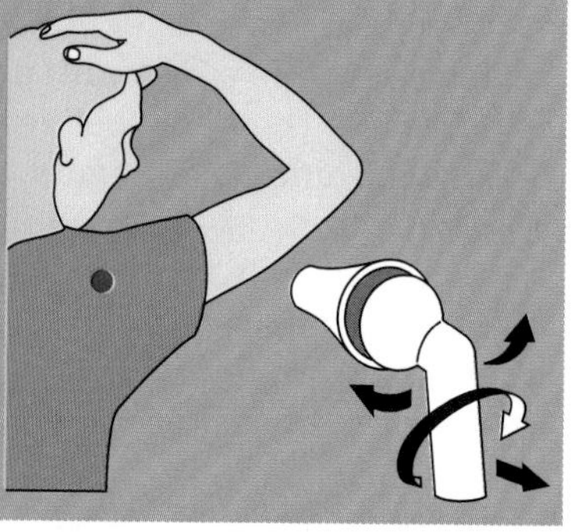

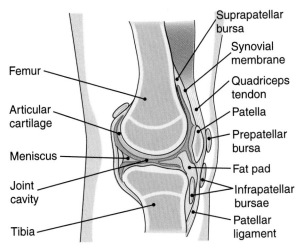

FIGURE **7•21** The knee joint (sagittal section).

ity. This fluid can be drained by a procedure called ***arthrocentesis*** (ar-thro-sen-TE-sis).

Arthritis

The most common type of joint disorder is termed ***arthritis,*** which means "inflammation of the joints." There are different kinds of arthritis, including the following:

- ***Osteoarthritis*** (os-te-o-arth-RI-tis) is a degenerative joint disease (DJD) that usually occurs in elderly people as a result of normal wear and tear. Although it appears to be a natural result of aging, such factors as obesity and repeated trauma can help bring it about. Osteoarthritis occurs mostly in joints used in weight bearing, such as the hips, knees, and spinal column. It involves degeneration of the joint cartilage, with growth of new bone at the edges of the joints. Degenerative changes include the formation of spurs at the edges of the articular surfaces, thickening of the synovial membrane, atrophy of the cartilage, and calcification of the ligaments (see Joint Replacement).
- ***Rheumatoid arthritis*** is a crippling condition characterized by swelling of the joints of the hands, the feet, and other parts of the body as a result of inflammation and overgrowth of the synovial membranes and other joint tissues. The articular cartilage is gradually destroyed, and the joint cavity develops adhesions—that is, the surfaces tend

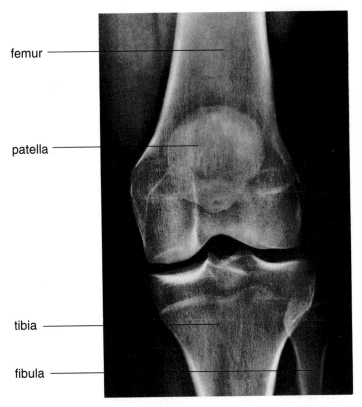

FIGURE **7•22** X-ray (radiograph) of the knee joint showing the articulating bones. (Greenspan A: Orthopedic Radiology, p. 6.2. New York, Gower, 1988)

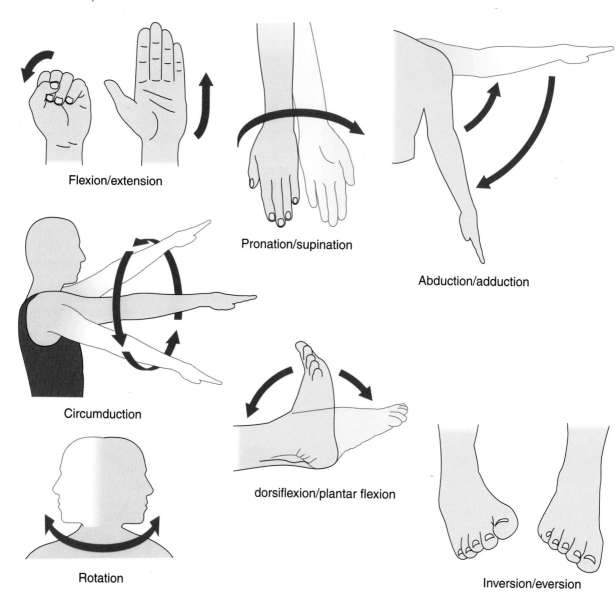

Flexion/extension

Pronation/supination

Abduction/adduction

Circumduction

dorsiflexion/plantar flexion

Rotation

Inversion/eversion

FIGURE **7•23** Movements at synovial joints.

to stick together—so that the joints stiffen and ultimately become useless. The exact cause of rheumatoid arthritis is uncertain. However, the disease shares many characteristics of disorders in which there is production of antibodies that attack normal body tissues. The role of inherited susceptibility is clear. The administration of drugs to suppress the abnormal antibody production has been successful.

• *Septic (infectious) arthritis* arises when bacteria spread to involve joint tissue, usually by way of the bloodstream. Bacteria introduced during invasive medical procedures, injections of illegal drugs, or by other means can settle in joints. A variety of organisms are commonly involved, including *Streptococcus, Staphylococcus,* and *Neisseria* species.

The joints and the bones themselves are subject to attack by the tuberculosis organism, and the result may be gradual destruction of parts of the bone near the joint.

• *Gout* is a kind of arthritis caused by a disturbance of metabolism. One of the products of metabolism is uric acid, which nor-

Joint Replacement

Since the first total hip replacement in the early 1960s, many thousands of joint replacements have been performed successfully. Joint replacements are needed when chronic arthritis or various injuries have caused serious damage, for example, in the elderly or in young athletes. The hip (the head of the femur in the acetabulum) and the knee joint are the joints that have been most commonly and most effectively restored, but shoulder, elbow, wrist, and hand joints have also been repaired.

In joint replacement surgery, the damaged ends of the articulating bones are removed or reshaped. Prosthetic heads made of synthetic material are attached, and the joint is reassembled. Special materials are available for the artificial joints that are strong and long lasting and do not corrode under the effects of body fluids. Manufacturing time and cost have been reduced by using computers to design these joints.

mally is excreted in the urine. If there happens to be an overproduction of uric acid, or for some reason not enough is excreted, the accumulated uric acid forms crystals, which are deposited as masses around the joints and other parts of the body. As a result, the joints become inflamed and extremely painful. Any joint can be involved, but the one most commonly affected is the big toe. Most victims of gout are men past middle life.

Backache

Backache is another common complaint. Some of its causes are listed below:

- Diseases of the vertebrae, such as infections or tumors, and in older people, osteoarthritis or atrophy (wasting away) of bone following long illnesses and lack of exercise
- Disorders of the intervertebral disks, especially those in the lower lumbar region. Pain may be very severe, with muscle spasms and the extension of symptoms along the course of the sciatic nerve (back of the thigh to the toes)
- Abnormalities of the lower vertebrae or of the ligaments and other supporting structures
- Disorders involving abdominopelvic organs or those in the space behind the peritoneum (such as the kidney). Variations in the position of the uterus are seldom a cause.
- Strains on the lumbosacral joint (where the lumbar region joins the sacrum) or strains on the sacroiliac joint (where the sacrum joins the ilium of the pelvis)

Backache can be prevented by attention to proper movement, good posture, and exercise. It is most important that the back itself not be used for lifting. Weight should be brought close to the body and the legs allowed to do the actual lifting. An adequate exercise program is also important.

Summary

I. Bones
- **A.** Main functions of bones—serve as body framework; protect organs; serve as levers; store calcium salts; form blood cells
- **B.** Bone structure
  1. Long bone
     a. Diaphysis—shaft
     b. Epiphysis—end
  2. Bone tissue
     a. Compact—shaft of long bones; outside of other bones
     b. Spongy—end of long bones; center of other bones
  3. Bone marrow
     a. Red—in spongy bone
     b. Yellow—in central cavity of long bones
  4. Membranes—contain bone-forming cells

a. Periosteum—covers bone

b. Endosteum—lines marrow cavity

C. Bone growth and repair

1. Cells

a. Osteoblasts—bone-forming cells

b. Osteocytes—mature bone cells that maintain bone

c. Osteoclasts—bone cells that break down (resorb) bone

2. Formation of a long bone—begins in center of shaft and continues at ends of bone; growing area forms line across epiphysis

D. Bone markings

1. Projections—head, process, crest, spine

2. Depressions and holes—foramen, sinus, fossa, meatus

II. **Divisions of the skeleton**

A. Bones of the axial skeleton

1. Skull

a. Cranial—frontal, parietal, temporal, ethmoid, sphenoid, occipital

b. Facial—mandible, maxilla, zygomatic, nasal, lacrimal, vomer, palatine, inferior nasal conchae

c. Other—ossicles (of ear), hyoid

d. Infant skull—fontanels (soft spots)

2. Trunk

a. Vertebral column—divisions: cervical, thoracic, lumbar, sacral, coccygeal

b. Thorax

(1) Sternum—manubrium, body, xiphoid process

(2) Ribs

(a) True—first seven pairs

(b) False—remaining five pairs, including two floating ribs

B. Bones of the appendicular skeleton

1. Shoulder girdle—clavicle, scapula

2. Upper extremity—humerus, ulna, radius, carpals, metacarpals, phalanges

3. Pelvic bones—os coxae (hip bone): ilium, ischium, pubis

4. Lower extremity—femur, patella, tibia, fibula, tarsals, metatarsals, phalanges

III. **Disorders of bone**

A. Metabolic—osteoporosis, osteitis deformans, rickets

B. Tumors

C. Infection—osteomyelitis

D. Structural disorders—curvature of the spine, cleft palate, flat foot

E. Changes in aging—loss of calcium salts, decreased production of collagen, thinning of intervertebral disks, loss of flexibility

F. Fractures—closed, open, greenstick, impacted, comminuted, spiral

IV. **Joints** (articulations)

A. Kinds of joints

1. Fibrous—immovable (synarthrosis)

2. Cartilaginous—slightly movable (amphiarthrosis)

3. Synovial—freely movable (diarthrosis)

B. More about synovial joints

1. Structure of synovial joints

a. Joint cavity—contains synovial fluid

b. Ligaments—hold joint together

c. Joint capsule—strengthens and protects joint

d. Articular cartilage—covers ends of bones

e. Bursae—fluid-filled sacs near joints; cushion and protect joints and surrounding tissue

2. Types of synovial joints—gliding, hinge, pivot, condyloid, saddle, ball-and-socket

3. Movement at synovial joints—flexion, extension, abduction, adduction, circumduction, rotation, supination, pronation, inversion, eversion, dorsiflexion, plantar flexion

C. Disorders of Joints

1. Dislocations and sprains

2. Arthritis—osteoarthritis, rheumatoid arthritis, infectious arthritis, gout

3. Backache

Questions for Study and Review

1. List five functions of bones.
2. Explain the difference between the terms in each of the following pairs:
   a. *osteoblast* and *osteoclast*
   b. *red marrow* and *yellow marrow*
   c. *periosteum* and *endosteum*
   d. *compact bone* and *spongy bone*
   e. *epiphysis* and *diaphysis*
3. What is an osteocyte and where are osteocytes located?
4. Define *resorption* as it applies to bone.
5. Name the two divisions of the skeleton. What parts of the skeleton are in each?
6. Name the main cranial and facial bones.
7. What is a sinus? Name several bones in which there are sinuses.
8. Define *fontanel* and name the largest fontanel.
9. What are the main divisions of the vertebral column? the ribs?
10. Name the bones of the upper and lower appendicular skeleton.
11. Name the bones on which you would find the following bone markings: mastoid process, acromion, olecranon, iliac crest, trochanter, medial malleolus, lateral malleolus, trochlea, ischial tuberosity, acetabulum, glenoid cavity, xiphoid process.
12. What is a foramen? Give at least two examples of foramina.
13. Describe osteoporosis, osteomyelitis, and rickets.
14. Name and describe three abnormal curves of the spine.
15. Describe six types of fractures.
16. Name three effects of aging on the skeletal system.
17. List three types of joints. Describe the amount of movement that occurs at each type. Find an example of each type in the chapter illustrations.
18. Describe where each of the following is found in a synovial joint: joint capsule, articular cartilage, and synovial fluid.
19. Name six types of synovial joints and give one example of the location of each. Find one example of each in the chapter illustrations.
20. Differentiate between the terms in each of the following pairs:
    a. *flexion* and *extension*
    b. *abduction* and *adduction*
    c. *supination* and *pronation*
    d. *inversion* and *eversion*
    e. *circumduction* and *rotation*
    f. *dorsiflexion* and *plantar flexion*
21. Describe four joint diseases.

✔ Answers to Checkpoints

1. Compact bone makes up the main shaft of long bones and the outer layer of other bones; spongy bone makes up the ends of the long bones and the center of other bones.
2. The shaft of the long bone is the diaphysis; the end of a long bone is the epiphysis.
3. Calcium compounds are deposited in the matrix of bone to harden it.
4. The markings on bones help to form joints, serve as points for muscle attachments, and allow passage of nerves and blood vessels.
5. The axial skeleton consists of bones of the skull and trunk.
6. The appendicular skeleton consists of bones of the shoulder girdle, hip, and extremities.
7. The three types of joints classified according to the material between the bones are fibrous, cartilaginous, and synovial.
8. The most freely movable type of joint is a synovial joint or diarthrosis.

The Muscular System

SELECTED KEY TERMS

The following terms are defined in the Glossary:

acetylcholine

actin

antagonist

aponeurosis

bursitis

fascicle

glycogen

insertion

lactic acid

myalgia

myoglobin

myosin

neuromuscular junction

neurotransmitter

origin

oxygen debt

prime mover

synapse

tendinitis

tendon

tonus

BEHAVIORAL OBJECTIVES

After careful study of this chapter, you should be able to:

1. Compare the three types of muscle tissue
2. Describe three functions of skeletal muscle
3. Briefly describe how skeletal muscles contract
4. List the substances needed in muscle contraction and describe the function of each
5. Define the term *oxygen debt*
6. List several compounds that delay the onset of oxygen debt
7. Cite the effects of exercise on muscles
8. Compare isotonic and isometric contractions
9. Explain how muscles work in pairs to produce movement
10. Compare the workings of muscles and bones to lever systems
11. Explain how muscles are named
12. Name some of the major muscles in each muscle group and describe the main function of each
13. Describe how muscles change with age
14. List the major muscular disorders

TYPES OF MUSCLE

There are three kinds of muscle tissue: smooth, cardiac, and skeletal muscle, as introduced in Chapter 4. After a brief description of all three types (Table 8-1), this chapter concentrates on skeletal muscle, which has been studied the most.

Smooth Muscle

Smooth muscle makes up the walls of the hollow body organs as well as those of the blood vessels and respiratory passageways. It moves involuntarily, producing the wavelike motions of peristalsis that move substances through a system. Smooth muscle fibers (cells) are tapered at each end and have a single, central nucleus. The cells appear smooth under the microscope because they do not contain the visible bands, or *striations*, that are seen in the other types of muscle cells. Smooth muscle may contract in response to a nerve impulse, hormonal stimulation, stretching, and other stimuli. The muscle contracts and relaxes slowly and can remain contracted for a long time.

Cardiac Muscle

Cardiac muscle, also involuntary, makes up the wall of the heart and creates the pulsing action of that organ. The cells of cardiac muscle are striated, like those of skeletal muscle. They dif-fer in having one nucleus per cell and branching interconnections. The electrical impulse that produces contraction of cardiac muscle is generated within the muscle but can be modified by nervous stimuli and hormones.

Skeletal Muscle

When viewed under the microscope, skeletal muscle cells appear heavily striated (Fig. 8-1). The arrangement of protein threads within the cell that produces these striations is described later. The cells are very long and cylindrical and have multiple nuclei per cell. Skeletal muscle is stimulated to contract by the nervous system, and it usMually contracts and relaxes rapidly. Because it is under conscious control, skeletal muscle is described as voluntary.

Skeletal muscle is attached to bones and produces movement at the joints. These muscles constitute the largest amount of muscle tissue of the body, making up about 40% of the total body weight. This muscular system is composed of almost 700 individual skeletal muscles. Although each one is a distinct structure, muscles usually act in groups to execute body movements.

✔ CHECKPOINT **1**:

What are the three types of muscle?

Table 8•1	Comparison of the Different Types of Muscle		
	SMOOTH	**CARDIAC**	**SKELETAL**
Location	Wall of hollow organs, vessels, respiratory passageways	Wall of heart	Attached to bones
Cell characteristics	Tapered at each end, single nucleus, nonstriated	Branching networks, single nucleus, lightly striated	Long and cylindrical; multinucleated; heavily striated
Control Action	Involuntary. Produces peristalsis; contracts and relaxes slowly; may sustain contraction	Involuntary. Pumps blood out of heart; self-excitatory but influenced by nervous system and hormones	Voluntary. Produces movement at joints; stimulated by nervous system; contracts and relaxes rapidly

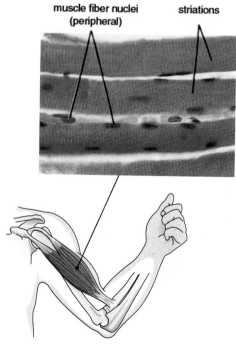

muscle fiber nuclei (peripheral)   striations

FIGURE **8•1**   Microscopic view of skeletal muscle fibers (cells) showing multiple nuclei and striations. (Cormack DH: Essential Histology. Philadelphia, JB Lippincott, 1993)

MUSCULAR SYSTEM

Functions

The three primary functions of skeletal muscles are:

- Movement of the skeleton. Muscles are attached to bones and contract to change the position of the bones at a joint.
- Maintenance of posture. A steady partial contraction of muscle, known as *muscle tone*, keeps the body in position. Some of the muscles involved in maintaining posture are the large muscles of the thighs, back, neck, and shoulders as well as the abdominal muscles.
- Generation of heat. Most of the heat needed to keep the body at 37°C (98.6°F) is generated by muscles. Heat is a natural byproduct of muscle cell metabolism. When we are cold, muscles can boost their heat output by the rapid small contractions we know of as *shivering*.

Structure of a Muscle

In forming whole muscles, individual muscle fibers are arranged in bundles, or *fascicles* (FAS-ih-kls), held together by connective tissue (Fig. 8-2). Deeper layers of connective tissue surround each individual fiber in the bundle. The entire muscle is then encased in a tough connective tissue sheath that is part of the *deep fascia.* All these supporting tissues merge to form the tendon that attaches the muscle to a bone. Each muscle also has a rich supply of blood vessels and nerves.

Muscle Cells in Action

Skeletal muscle fibers are stimulated by nerve impulses coming from the brain and the spinal cord (see Chap. 9). Nerve cell fibers (axons) carry impulses to the muscles, each fiber branching to supply from a few to more than 100 individual muscle cells.

The Neuromuscular Junction

The point at which a nerve fiber contacts a muscle cell is called the *neuromuscular junction* (Fig. 8-3). It is here that a chemical classified as a *neurotransmitter* is released from the neuron to stimulate the muscle fiber. The specific neurotransmitter released here is *acetylcholine* (as-e-til-KO-lene), which is found elsewhere in the body as well. A great deal is known about the events that occur at this junction, and this information is important in understanding muscle action.

The neuromuscular junction is an example of a *synapse* (SIN-aps), a point of communication between cells. Between the cells there is a tiny space, the *synaptic cleft,* across which the neurotransmitter must travel. Until its release, the neurotransmitter is stored in tiny bubbles, called *vesicles,* in the endings of the nerve fiber. Once released, the neurotransmitter crosses the synaptic cleft and attaches to receptors, which are proteins imbedded in the muscle cell membrane. The membrane is folded at this point to increase surface area and hold a maximum number of receptors. The receiving membrane of the muscle cell is known as the *motor end plate*.

Muscle fibers, like nerve cells, show the property of *excitability;* that is, they are able to transmit electrical current along the cell membrane. When the muscle is stimulated at the neuromuscular junction, an electrical impulse is generated that spreads rapidly along the muscle cell membrane. This spreading wave of electrical current is called the *action potential* because it calls the muscle cell into action. Chapter 9 provides more information on synapses and the action potential.

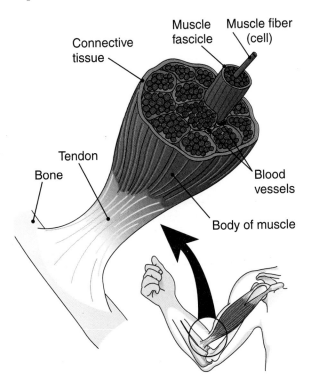

FIGURE **8•2** Structure of a skeletal muscle showing connective tissue coverings.

Connective tissue · Muscle fascicle · Muscle fiber (cell) · Tendon · Bone · Blood vessels · Body of muscle

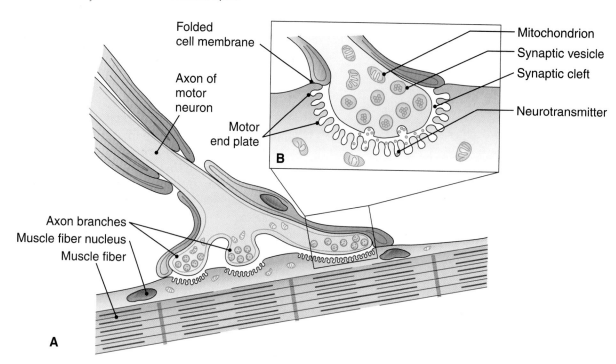

FIGURE **8•3**   Neuromuscular junction. **(A)** The branched end of a motor neuron makes contact with the membrane of a muscle fiber (cell). **(B)** Enlarged view.

Contraction

Another important property of muscle tissue is **contractility.** This is the capacity of a muscle fiber to undergo shortening and to change its shape, becoming thicker. Studies of muscle chemistry and observation of cells under the powerful electron microscope have given a concept of how muscle cells work.

These studies reveal that each skeletal muscle fiber contains many threads, or filaments, made of two kinds of proteins, called *actin* (AK-tin) and *myosin* (MI-o-sin). Filaments made of actin are thin and light; those made of myosin are heavy and dark. The filaments are present in alternating bundles within the muscle cell (Fig. 8-4). It is the alternating bands of light actin and heavy myosin filaments that give skeletal muscle its striated appearance. They also give a view of what occurs when muscles contract.

In movement, the myosin filaments "latch on" to the actin filaments by means of many paddle-like extensions. These attachments are described as *cross-bridges* between the two types of filaments. Using the energy of ATP for repeated movements, the cross-bridges, like the oars of a boat, pull all the actin strands closer together. As the overlapping filaments slide together, the muscle fiber contracts, becoming

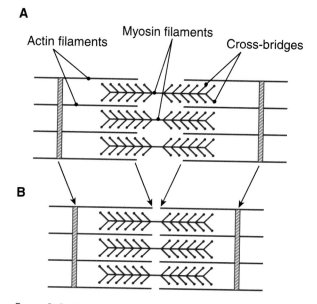

FIGURE **8•4**   The sliding filament mechanism of skeletal muscle contraction. **(A)** Muscle is in a relaxed state. **(B)** Muscle has contracted and the myosin cross bridges have moved to new sites to prepare for another "pull."

shorter and thicker. Figure 8-4 shows a section of muscle in the relaxed and contracted state. Note that the filaments overlap increasingly as the cell contracts. (In reality, not all the cross-bridges are moving at the same time. About one half are forward at any time, and the rest are preparing for another swing.)

✔ CHECKPOINT **4**:

What are two properties of muscle cells that are needed for response to a stimulus?

The Role of Calcium

It is well known that the mineral calcium is needed for muscle contraction. Calcium uncovers points on the actin where cross-bridges can form between the filaments so that the sliding action can begin. The calcium needed for contraction is stored within the endoplasmic reticulum (ER) of the muscle cell and is released into the cytoplasm when the cell is stimulated by a nerve fiber. Muscles relax when nerve stimulation stops and the calcium is pumped back into the ER (see Rigor Mortis).

Muscles and Energy

As noted earlier, all muscle contraction requires energy in the form of ATP. The source of this energy is the oxidation (commonly called "burning") of nutrients within the cells.

Rigor Mortis

After death, muscles enter a stage of rigidity known as *rigor mortis.* The calcium that triggers contraction escapes from its storage areas and causes the muscle filaments to slide together. Because all metabolism has ceased, however, there is no ATP to power further movement of the cross-bridges, and the filaments remain in a contracted position. This stiffness lasts for about 24 hours, then gradually fades as body tissues begin to decay. The rate at which these changes occur varies with the individual and the environment.

To produce ATP, muscle cells must have an adequate supply of oxygen and glucose or other usable nutrient. These substances are constantly brought to the cells by the circulation, but muscle cells also store a small reserve supply of each. Additional oxygen is stored in the form of a compound similar to the blood's hemoglobin but located specifically in muscle cells, as indicated by the prefix *myo-* in its name, ***myoglobin*** (mi-o-GLO-bin). Additional glucose is stored as a compound that is built from glucose molecules and is called ***glycogen*** (GLI-ko-jen). Glycogen can be broken down into glucose when needed by the muscle cells, for example, during vigorous exercise.

✔ CHECKPOINT **5**:

Muscle cells obtain energy for contraction from the oxidation of nutrients. What compound is formed in oxidation that supplies the energy for contraction?

Oxygen Debt

Oxygen plays an important role in preventing the accumulation of ***lactic acid,*** a waste product of metabolism that causes muscle fatigue. During strenuous activity, a person may not be able to breathe in oxygen rapidly enough to meet the needs of the hard-working muscles. The increased demands are met at first by the energy-rich compounds that are stored in the tissues. However, continual exercise depletes these stores.

For a short time, glucose may be used without the benefit of oxygen. In this case, lactic acid is formed in the cells by an alternate pathway of metabolism. This anaerobic process (occurring without oxygen) permits greater magnitude of activity than would otherwise be possible, as, for example, allowing sprinting instead of jogging.

Anaerobic metabolism can continue until buildup of lactic acid causes the muscle to fatigue. As lactic acid accumulates, the person is said to develop an ***oxygen debt***. After stopping exercise, he or she must continue to take in more oxygen by continued rapid breathing (panting) until the debt is paid in full. That is, enough oxygen must be taken in to convert the lactic acid to other substances that can be metabolized further. In addition, the energy-rich compounds that are stored in the cells must be replenished.

✔ CHECKPOINT **6**:

When muscles work without oxygen, a compound is produced that causes muscle fatigue. What is the name of this compound?

Effects of Exercise

Changes that occur as muscle metabolism increases during exercise cause *vasodilation* (vas-o-di-LA-shun)—an increase in the diameter of blood vessels—thereby allowing blood to flow more easily to these tissues. As muscles work, more blood is pumped back to the heart. The temporarily increased load on the heart acts to strengthen the heart muscle and to improve its circulation. The chambers of the heart gradually enlarge to accommodate more blood.

Regular exercise also improves breathing and respiratory efficiency. Circulation in the capillaries surrounding the alveoli (air sacs) is increased, and this brings about enhanced gas exchange. Athletic training leads to more efficient distribution and use of oxygen so that the onset of oxygen debt is delayed. Even moderate regular exercise has the additional benefits of weight control, strengthening of the bones, decreased blood pressure, and decreased risk of heart attacks. The effects of exercise on the body are studied in the fields of sports medicine and exercise physiology (see Exercise for Health).

Types of Muscle Contractions

Muscle *tone* refers to a partially contracted state of the muscles that is normal even when the muscles are not in use. The maintenance of this tone, or *tonus* (TO-nus), is due to the action of the nervous system in keeping the muscles in a constant state of readiness for action. Muscles that are little used soon become flabby, weak, and lacking in tone.

The Benefits of Regular Exercise

A well-balanced program of regular exercise can produce benefits to the muscular, cardiovascular, respiratory systems, and other systems, helping to build and maintain overall good health. Exercise can not only help you feel good, but look good as well. In order for an exercise program to produce maximum benefits, it must contain the following three components: stretching, aerobic exercise, and strength training.

Stretching helps to keep a muscle at its optimal length. Under the stress of repeated contractions, a muscle tends to shorten as each individual muscle fiber becomes stronger. Within groups of opposing or antagonistic muscles, one group of muscles or muscle fibers usually becomes stronger than the rest. This leads to muscle shortening on the side with the stronger fibers. Stretching promotes all fibers in the muscle relaxing to optimal length. A stretched muscle fiber is stronger because it contracts over a greater length. Stretching also helps to promote balance and keeps joints limber. Gentle stretching should be done both before and after a round of aerobic exercise or strength training.

Aerobic exercise is the heart of any program. Aerobic exercise should begin with a warm-up of about 5 minutes after stretching. The warm-up allows the cardiovascular and respiratory systems to gear up for increased oxygen demand. The aerobic cycle then involves a period of between 20 and 30 minutes of muscle work in which the muscles undergo a repetitive cycle of contraction and relaxation. This cycle increases the muscle stamina and, with consistency, can greatly increase endurance. Aerobic exercise prepares the muscle for the challenge of strength training.

Strength training uses resistance against active contraction to build muscle mass. This is known as the *primary principle;* all muscle tissue must work against a load to become stronger and larger. A muscle used repetitively against little or no load will not increase in strength, although some increase in size may occur. To increase strength, a muscle must be consistently contracted to at least 50% of its maximum length. This cycle should be repeated as 3 sets of 6 contractions, 3 times a
continued

week. At this level, the muscle achieves maximum strength while avoiding fatigue.

Any cycle of aerobic or strength training should be followed by a cooldown period. This involves reducing a muscle group's workload gradually over at least 10 minutes. A cooldown helps keep the blood from returning to the heart too quickly. It lets the heart and lungs readjust to a resting level and allows the circulatory system adequate time to flush out waste products built up during exercise.

A consistent regimen of appropriate exercise 3 times a week increases muscle size and strength and strengthens the cardiovascular and respiratory systems. The immune system is also stimulated by exercise. The road to good health is indeed best walked or biked instead of driven.

In addition to the partial contractions that are responsible for muscle tone, there are two other types of contractions on which the body depends:

- *Isotonic* (i-so-TON-ik) *contractions* are those in which the tone or tension within the muscle remains the same but the muscle as a whole shortens, producing movement; that is, work is accomplished. Lifting weights, walking, running, or any other activity in which the muscles become shorter and thicker (forming bulges) are isotonic contractions.
- *Isometric* (i-so-MET-rik) *contractions* are those in which there is no change in muscle length but there is a great increase in muscle tension. Pushing against an immovable force produces an isometric contraction. For example, if you push the palms of your hands hard against each other, there is no movement, but you can feel the increased tension in your arm muscles.

Most movements of the body involve a combination of both isotonic and isometric contractions. When walking, for example, some muscles contract isotonically to propel the body forward, but at the same time, other muscles are contracting isometrically to keep your body in position.

THE MECHANICS OF MUSCLE MOVEMENT

Attachments of Skeletal Muscles

Most muscles have two or more points of attachment to the skeleton. The muscle is attached to a bone at each end by means of a cordlike extension called a *tendon* (Fig. 8-5). All of the connective tissue within and around the muscle merges to form the tendon, which then attaches directly to the periosteum of the bone (see Fig. 8-2). In some instances, a broad sheet called an *aponeurosis* (ap-o-nu-RO-sis) may attach muscles to bones or to other muscles, as in the abdomen (Fig. 8-7) or across the top of the skull (Fig. 8-9).

In moving the bones, one end of a muscle is attached to a more freely movable part of the skeleton, and the other end is attached to a relatively stable part. The less movable (more fixed) attachment is called the *origin;* the attachment to the part of the body that the muscle puts into action is called the *insertion.* When a muscle contracts, it pulls on both points of attachment, bringing the more movable insertion closer to the origin and thereby causing movement of the body part. Figure 8-5 shows the action of the biceps brachii (in the upper arm) in flexing the arm at the elbow. The insertion on the radius of the forearm is brought to-

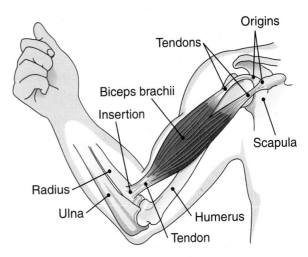

FIGURE **8•5** Diagram of a muscle showing three attachments to bones—two origins and one insertion.

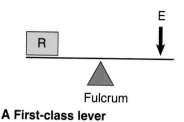

E

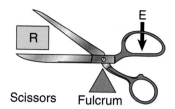

A First-class lever

Scissors   Fulcrum

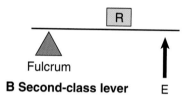

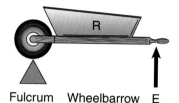

B Second-class lever   E

Fulcrum   Wheelbarrow   E

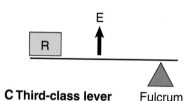

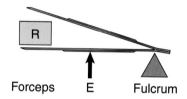

C Third-class lever   Fulcrum

Forceps   E   Fulcrum

FIGURE **8•6**   Levers. Three types of levers and tools that illustrate each. R = resistance (weight). E = effort (force).

ward the origin at the scapula of the shoulder girdle.

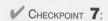

> ✔ CHECKPOINT **7**:
>
> Muscles are attached to bones by means of tendons: one attached to a less movable part of the skeleton, and one attached to a movable part. What are the names of these two attachment points?

Muscles Work Together

Many of the skeletal muscles function in pairs. A movement is performed by muscle called the ***prime mover;*** the muscle that produces an opposite movement is known as the ***antagonist.*** Clearly, for any given movement, the antagonist must relax when the prime mover contracts. For example, when the biceps brachii at the front of the arm contracts to flex the arm, the triceps brachii at the back must relax; when the triceps brachii contracts to extend the arm, the biceps brachii must relax. In addition to prime movers and antagonists, there are also

muscles that serve to steady body parts or to assist prime movers.

As the muscles work together, body movements are coordinated, and a large number of complicated movements can be carried out. At first, however, the nervous system must learn to coordinate any new, complicated movement. Think of a child learning to walk or to write, and consider the number of muscles she or he uses unnecessarily or forgets to use when the situation calls for them.

> ✔ CHECKPOINT **8**:
>
> Muscles work together to produce movement. What is the name of the muscle that produces a movement as compared with the muscle that produces an opposite movement?

Levers and Body Mechanics

Proper body mechanics help conserve energy and ensure freedom from strain and fatigue; conversely, such ailments as lower back pain—a

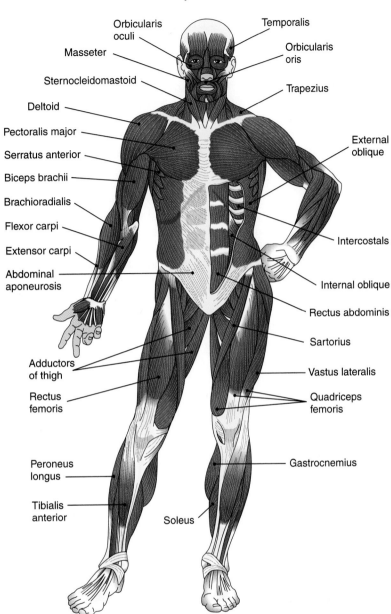

Orbicularis oculi

Temporalis

Masseter

Orbicularis oris

Sternocleidomastoid

Trapezius

Deltoid

Pectoralis major

External oblique

Serratus anterior

Biceps brachii

Brachioradialis

Flexor carpi

Extensor carpi

Intercostals

Abdominal aponeurosis

Internal oblique

Rectus abdominis

Sartorius

Adductors of thigh

Vastus lateralis

Rectus femoris

Quadriceps femoris

Gastrocnemius

Peroneus longus

Tibialis anterior

Soleus

FIGURE **8•7** Superficial muscles, anterior (front) view.

common complaint—can be traced to poor body mechanics. Body mechanics have special significance to health workers, who are frequently called on to move patients and handle cumbersome equipment. Maintaining the body segments in correct relation to one another has a direct effect on the working capacity of the vital organs that are supported by the skeleton.

If you have had a course in physics, recall your study of levers. A lever is simply a rigid bar that moves about a fixed pivot point, the fulcrum.

There are three classes of levers, which differ only in the location of the fulcrum, the effort (force), and the resistance (weight) (see Fig. 8-6). In a first-class lever, the fulcrum is located between the resistance and the effort; a see-saw or a scissors is an example of this class. The second-class lever has the resistance located between the fulcrum and the effort; a wheelbarrow or a mattress lifted at one end is an illustration of this class. In the third-class lever, the effort is between the resistance and the fulcrum. A forceps or a tweezers is an example of this type of lever. The effort is applied in the center of the tool, between the fulcrum where the pieces join and the resistance at the tip.

The musculoskeletal system can be considered a system of levers, in which the bone is the lever, the joint is the fulcrum, and the force is applied by a muscle. Most lever systems in the body are of the third-class type. A muscle usually inserts over a joint and exerts force between the fulcrum and the resistance. That is, the fulcrum is behind both the point of effort and the weight. In Figure 8-5, the resistance is in the forearm and hand, the force is exerted at the muscle insertion on the forearm, and the fulcrum is the elbow joint. By understanding and applying knowledge of levers to body mechanics, the health care worker can improve his or her skill in carrying out numerous clinical maneuvers and procedures.

✔ CHECKPOINT **9**:

Muscles and bones work together as lever systems. Of the three classes of levers, which one represents the action of most muscles?

Anabolic Steroids

Anabolic steroids are hormones that promote metabolism and stimulate growth. They are sometimes used medically to promote muscle regeneration, for example, to prevent atrophy from disuse after surgery.

Anabolic steroids have been used illegally by athletes to boost the effects of training. These steroids, which function like the male sex hormone testosterone, are taken to increase muscle size and strength and to improve endurance. The doses needed to produce significant results are large enough to have serious side effects. These drugs are known to produce liver damage, heart disease, and abnormalities of the sex organs. They can cause infertility in both men and women. Mood swings and aggressive behavior are also observed.

To learn about the effects of steroids on muscles, see Anabolic Steroids.

SKELETAL MUSCLE GROUPS

The study of muscles is made simpler by grouping them according to body regions. Knowing how muscles are named can also help in remembering them.

Naming of Muscles

A number of different characteristics are used in naming muscles, including the following:

- Location, named for a nearby bone, for example, or for position, such as lateral, medial, internal, or external
- Size, using terms such as maximus, major, minor, longus, brevis
- Shape, such as circular (orbicularis), triangular (deltoid), trapezoid (trapezius)
- Direction of fibers, including straight (rectus) or angled (oblique)
- Number of heads (attachment points) as indicated by the suffix -*ceps*, as in biceps, triceps, quadriceps
- Action, as in flexor, extensor, adductor, abductor, levator

Often, more than one feature is used in naming. Refer to Figures 8-7 and 8-8 as you study the locations and functions of some of the skeletal muscles and try to figure out why each has the name that it does. Although they are described in the singular, most of the muscles are present on both sides of the body. The information is summarized in Table 8-2.

Muscles of the Head

The principal muscles of the head are those of facial expression and of mastication (chewing) (see Fig. 8-9).

The muscles of facial expression include ring-shaped ones around the eyes and the lips, called the ***orbicularis*** (or-bik-u-LAH-ris) ***muscles*** because of their shape (think of "orbit"). The muscle surrounding each eye is called the ***orbicu-***

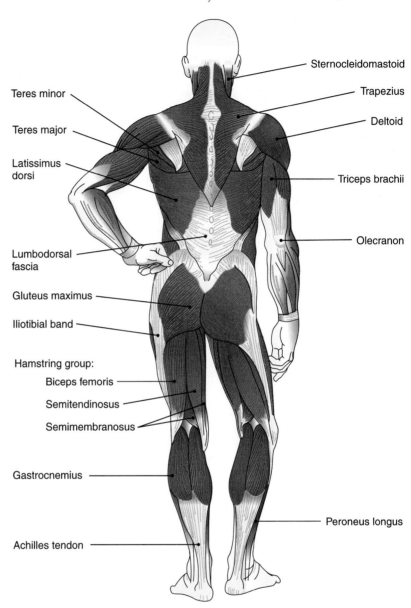

FIGURE **8•8** Superficial muscles, posterior (back) view.

Labels (clockwise from top):
- Sternocleidomastoid
- Trapezius
- Deltoid
- Triceps brachii
- Olecranon
- Peroneus longus
- Teres minor
- Teres major
- Latissimus dorsi
- Lumbodorsal fascia
- Gluteus maximus
- Iliotibial band
- Hamstring group:
  - Biceps femoris
  - Semitendinosus
  - Semimembranosus
- Gastrocnemius
- Achilles tendon

8

laris oculi (OK-u-li), whereas the muscle of the lips is the **orbicularis oris.** These muscles, of course, all have antagonists. For example, the **levator palpebrae** (PAL-pe-bre) **superioris,** or lifter of the upper eyelid, is the antagonist for the orbicularis oculi.

One of the largest muscles of expression forms the fleshy part of the cheek and is called the **buccinator** (BUK-se-na-tor). Used in whistling or blowing, it is sometimes referred to as the *trumpeter's muscle.* You can readily think of other muscles of facial expression: for in-

stance, the antagonists of the orbicularis oris can produce a smile, a sneer, or a grimace. There are a number of scalp muscles by means of which the eyebrows are lifted or drawn together into a frown.

There are four pairs of muscles of mastication, all of which insert on the mandible and move it. The largest are the **temporal** (TEM-po-ral), located above and near the ear, and the **masseter** (mas-SE-ter) at the angle of the jaw.

The tongue has two groups of muscles. The first group, called the **intrinsic muscles,** is lo-

Table 8•2 Review of Muscles

NAME	LOCATION	FUNCTION
Muscles of the Head and Neck		
Orbicularis oculi	Encircles eyelid	Closes eye
Levator palpebrae superioris	Back of orbit to upper eyelid	Opens eye
Orbicularis oris	Encircles mouth	Closes lips
Buccinator	Fleshy part of cheek	Flattens cheek; helps in eating, whistling, and blowing wind instruments
Temporal	Above and near ear	Closes jaw
Masseter	At angle of jaw	Closes jaw
Sternocleidomastoid	Along side of neck, to mastoid process	Flexes head; rotates head toward opposite side from muscle
Muscles of the Upper Extremities		
Trapezius	Back of neck and upper back, to clavicle and scapula	Raises shoulder and pulls it back; extends head
Latissimus dorsi	Middle and lower back, to humerus	Extends and adducts arm behind back
Pectoralis major	Upper, anterior chest, to humerus	Flexes and adducts arm across chest; pulls shoulder forward and downward
Serratus anterior	Below axilla on side of chest to scapula	Moves scapula forward; aids in raising arm
Deltoid	Covers shoulder joint, to lateral humerus	Abducts arm
Biceps brachii	Anterior arm, to radius	Flexes forearm and supinates hand
Triceps brachii	Posterior arm, to ulna	Extends forearm
Flexor and extensor carpi groups	Anterior and posterior forearm, to hand	Flex and extend hand
Flexor and extensor digitorum groups	Anterior and posterior forearm, to fingers	Flex and extend fingers
Muscles of the Trunk		
Diaphragm	Dome-shaped partition between thoracic and abdominal cavities	Dome descends to enlarge thoracic cavity from top to bottom
Intercostals	Between ribs	Elevate ribs and enlarge thoracic cavity
External and internal oblique; transversus and rectus abdominis	Anterolateral abdominal wall	Compress abdominal cavity and expel substances from body; flex spinal column
Levator ani	Pelvic floor	Aids defecation
Sacrospinalis	Deep in back, vertical mass	Extends vertebral column to produce erect posture
Muscles of the Lower Extremities		
Gluteus maximus	Superficial buttock, to femur	Extends thigh
Gluteus medius	Deep buttock, to femur	Abducts thigh
Iliopsoas	Crosses front of hip joint, to femur	Flexes thigh
Adductor group	Medial thigh, to femur	Adduct thigh
Sartorius	Winds down thigh, ilium to tibia	Flexes thigh and leg (to sit cross-legged)
Quadriceps femoris	Anterior thigh, to tibia	Extends leg
Hamstring group	Posterior thigh, to tibia and fibula	Flexes leg
Gastrocnemius	Calf of leg, to calcaneus	Extends foot (as in tiptoeing)
Tibialis anterior	Anterior and lateral shin, to foot	Dorsiflexes foot (as in walking on heels); inverts foot (sole inward)
Peroneus longus	Lateral leg, to foot	Everts foot (sole outward)
Flexor and extensor digitorum groups	Posterior and anterior leg, to toes	Flex and extend toes

cated entirely within the tongue. The second group, the ***extrinsic muscles,*** originate outside the tongue. It is because of these many muscles that the tongue has such remarkable flexibility and can perform so many different functions. Consider the intricate tongue motions involved in speaking, chewing, and swallowing.

Muscles of the Neck

The neck muscles tend to be ribbonlike and extend up and down or obliquely in several layers and in a complex manner. The one you will hear of most frequently is the ***sternocleidomastoid*** (ster-no-kli-do-MAS-toyd), sometimes referred

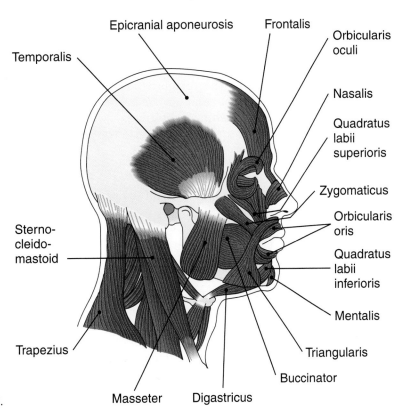

FIGURE **8•9** Muscles of the head.

to simply as the *sternomastoid*. There are two of these strong muscles, which extend from the sternum upward, across either side of the neck, to the mastoid process. Working together, they bring the head forward on the chest (flexion). Working alone, each muscle tilts and rotates the head so as to orient the face toward the side opposite that muscle. If the head is abnormally fixed in this position, the person is said to have **torticollis** (tor-tih-KOL-is), or *wryneck;* this condition may be due to injury or spasm of the muscle.

A portion of the trapezius muscle (described later) is located in the back of the neck, where it helps hold the head up (extension). Other larger deep muscles are the chief extensors of the head and neck.

Muscles of the Upper Extremities

Movement of the Shoulder and Arm
The Posterior Muscles
The position of the shoulder depends to a large extent on the degree of contraction of the **trapezius** (trah-PE-ze-us), a triangular muscle that covers the back of the neck and extends across the back of the shoulder to insert on the clavicle and scapula. The trapezius muscles enable one to raise the shoulders and pull them back. The upper portion of each trapezius can also extend the head and turn it from side to side.

The **latissimus** (lah-TIS-ih-mus) **dorsi** originates from the vertebral spine in the middle and lower back and covers the lower half of the thoracic region. The fibers of each muscle converge to a tendon that inserts on the humerus. The latissimus dorsi powerfully extends the arm, bringing it down forcibly as, for example, in swimming.

The Anterior Muscles
A large **pectoralis** (pek-to-RAL-is) **major** is located on either side of the upper part of the chest at the front of the body. This muscle arises from the sternum, the upper ribs, and the clavicle and forms the anterior "wall" of the armpit, or axilla; it inserts on the upper part of the humerus. The pectoralis major flexes and adducts the arm, pulling it across the chest.

Below the axilla, on the side of the chest, is the ***serratus*** (ser-RA-tus) ***anterior.*** It originates on the upper eight or nine ribs on the side and the front of the thorax and inserts in the scapula on the side toward the vertebrae. The serratus anterior moves the scapula forward when, for example, one is pushing something. It also aids in raising the arm above the horizontal level.

The Shoulder Muscles

The ***deltoid*** covers the shoulder joint and is responsible for the roundness of the upper part of the arm just below the shoulder. This area is often used as an injection site. Arising from the shoulder girdle (clavicle and scapula), the deltoid fibers converge to insert on the lateral side of the humerus. Contraction of this muscle abducts the arm, raising it laterally to the horizontal position.

The shoulder joint allows for a very wide range of movement. This freedom of movement is possible because the humerus fits into a shallow socket, the glenoid cavity of the scapula. This joint requires the support of four deep muscles and their tendons. In certain activities, such as swinging a golf club, playing tennis, or pitching a baseball, these four muscles, which compose the ***rotator cuff,*** may be injured, and even torn. Surgery is often required for repair of the rotator cuff.

Movement of the Forearm and Hand

The ***biceps brachii*** (BRA-ke-i), located on the front of the arm, is the muscle you usually display when you want to "flex your muscles" to show your strength. It inserts on the radius and serves to flex the forearm. It is a supinator of the hand (see Fig. 8-5).

The ***triceps brachii,*** located on the back of the arm, inserts on the olecranon of the ulna. The triceps has been called the *boxer's muscle* because it straightens the elbow when a blow is delivered. It is also important in pushing because it converts the arm and forearm into a sturdy rod.

Muscles That Move the Hand

Most of the muscles that move the hand and fingers originate from the radius and the ulna. Some of them insert on the carpal bones of the wrist, whereas others have long tendons that cross the wrist and insert on bones of the hand and the fingers.

The ***flexor carpi*** and the ***extensor carpi muscles*** are responsible for many movements of the hand. Muscles that produce finger movements are the several ***flexor digitorum*** (dij-e-TO-rum) and the ***extensor digitorum muscles.***

Special groups of muscles in the fleshy parts of the hand are responsible for the intricate movements that can be performed with the thumb and the fingers. The freedom of movement of the thumb has been one of the most useful capacities of humans.

Muscles of the Trunk

Muscles of Respiration

The most important muscle involved in the act of breathing is the ***diaphragm.*** This dome-shaped muscle forms the partition between the thoracic cavity above and the abdominal cavity below (Fig. 8-10). When the diaphragm contracts, the central dome-shaped portion is pulled downward, thus enlarging the thoracic cavity from top to bottom.

The ***intercostal muscles*** are attached to and fill the spaces between the ribs. The external and internal intercostals run at angles in opposite directions. Contraction of the intercostal muscles serves to elevate the ribs, thus enlarging the thoracic cavity from side to side and from front to back. The mechanics of breathing are described in Chapter 18.

✔ CHECKPOINT **10:**

What muscle is most important in breathing?

Muscles of the Abdomen and Pelvis

The wall of the abdomen has three layers of muscle that extend from the back (dorsally) and around the sides (laterally) to the front (ventrally). They are the ***external abdominal oblique*** on the outside, the ***internal abdominal oblique*** in the middle, and the ***transversus abdominis,*** the innermost. The connective tissue from these muscles extends forward and

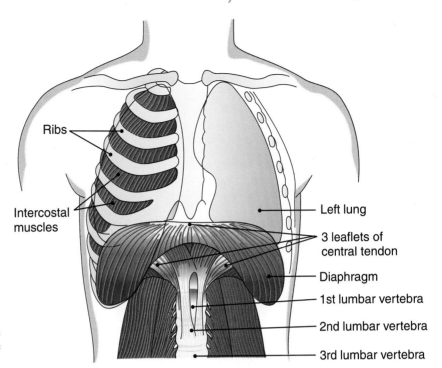

Ribs

Intercostal
muscles

Left lung

3 leaflets of
central tendon

Diaphragm

1st lumbar vertebra

2nd lumbar vertebra

3rd lumbar vertebra

FIGURE **8•10** The diaphragm forms
the partition between the thoracic
cavity and the abdominal cavity.

encloses the vertical ***rectus abdominis*** of the
anterior abdominal wall. The fibers of these
muscles, as well as their connective tissue extensions (aponeuroses), run in different directions, resembling the layers in plywood and resulting in a strong abdominal wall. The midline
meeting of the aponeuroses forms a whitish
area called the ***linea alba*** (LIN-e-ah Al-ba),
which is an important landmark on the abdomen. It extends from the tip of the sternum to
the pubic joint (see Fig. 8-7).

These four pairs of abdominal muscles act
together to protect the internal organs and compress the abdominal cavity, as in coughing,
emptying the bladder (urination) and bowel
(defecation), sneezing, vomiting, and childbirth
(labor). The two oblique muscles and the rectus
abdominis help bend the trunk forward and
sideways.

The pelvic floor, or ***perineum*** (per-ih-NE-
um), has its own form of diaphragm, shaped
somewhat like a shallow dish. One of the principal muscles of this pelvic diaphragm is the ***levator ani*** (le-VA-tor A-ni), which acts on the rectum and thus aids in defecation. The superficial
and deep muscles of the female perineum are
shown in Figure 8-11.

✔ CHECKPOINT **11**:

What structural feature gives strength to the muscles of the abdominal wall?

Deep Muscles of the Back
The deep muscles of the back, which act on
the vertebral column itself, are thick vertical
masses that lie under the trapezius and latissimus dorsi. The longest muscle is the
sacrospinalis (sa-kro-spin-A-lis), which helps
maintain the vertebral column in an erect posture.

Muscles of the Lower Extremities

The muscles in the lower extremities, among
the longest and strongest muscles in the body,
are specialized for locomotion and balance.

Movement of the Thigh and Leg
The ***gluteus maximus*** (GLU-te-us MAK-sim-
us), which forms much of the fleshy part of the
buttock, is relatively large in humans because
of its support function when a person is standing in the erect position. This muscle extends

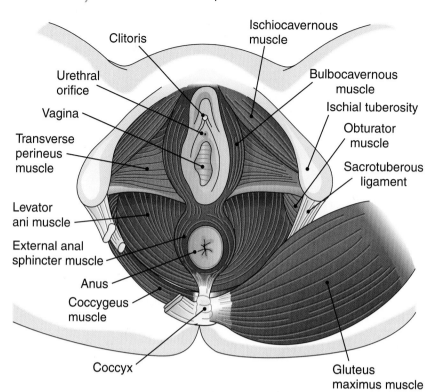

FIGURE **8•11**   Muscles of the female perineum (pelvic floor).

the thigh and is important in walking and running. The **gluteus medius,** which is partially covered by the gluteus maximus, serves to abduct the thigh, and is one of the sites used for intramuscular injections.

The **iliopsoas** (il-e-o-SO-as) arises from the ilium and the bodies of the lumbar vertebrae; it crosses the front of the hip joint to insert on the femur. It is a powerful flexor of the thigh and helps keep the trunk from falling backward when one is standing erect.

The **adductor muscles** are located on the medial part of the thigh. They arise from the pubis and ischium and insert on the femur. These strong muscles press the thighs together, as in grasping a saddle between the knees when riding a horse.

The **sartorius** (sar-TO-re-us) is a long, narrow muscle that begins at the iliac spine, winds downward and inward across the entire thigh, and ends on the upper medial surface of the tibia. It is called the *tailor's muscle* because it is used in crossing the legs in the manner of tailors, who in days gone by sat cross-legged on the floor.

The front and sides of the femur are covered by the **quadriceps femoris** (KWOD-re-seps FEM-or-is), a large muscle that has four heads of origin. The individual parts are as follows: in the center, covering the anterior thigh, the **rectus femoris**; on either side, the **vastus medialis** and **vastus lateralis**; deeper in the center, the **vastus intermedius.** One of these muscles (rectus femoris) originates from the ilium, and the other three are from the femur, but all four have a common tendon of insertion on the tibia. You may remember that this is the tendon that encloses the knee cap, or patella. This muscle extends the leg, as in kicking a ball. The vastus lateralis is also a site for intramuscular injections.

The **hamstring muscles** are located in the posterior part of the thigh. Their tendons can be felt behind the knee as they descend to insert on the tibia and fibula. The hamstrings flex the leg on the thigh, as in kneeling. Individually, moving from lateral to medial position, they are the **biceps femoris,** the **semimembranosus,** and the **semitendinosus.**

Movement of the Foot

The ***gastrocnemius*** (gas-trok-NE-me-us) is the chief muscle of the calf of the leg. It has been called the *toe dancer's muscle* because it is used in standing on tiptoe. It ends near the heel in a prominent cord called the **Achilles tendon,** which attaches to the calcaneus (heel bone). The Achilles tendon is the largest tendon in the body.

Another leg muscle that acts on the foot is the ***tibialis*** (tib-e-A-lis) ***anterior,*** located on the front of the leg. This muscle performs the opposite function of the gastrocnemius. Walking on the heels uses the tibialis anterior to raise the rest of the foot off the ground (dorsiflexion). This muscle is also responsible for inversion of the foot. The muscle for eversion of the foot is the ***peroneus*** (per-o-NE-us) ***longus,*** located on the lateral part of the leg. The long tendon of this muscle crosses under the foot, forming a sling that supports the transverse (metatarsal) arch.

The toes, like the fingers, are provided with flexor and extensor muscles. The tendons of the extensor muscles are located in the top of the foot and insert on the superior surface of the toe bones (phalanges). The flexor digitorum tendons cross the sole of the foot and insert on the undersurface of the toe bones.

EFFECTS OF AGING ON MUSCLES

Beginning at about 40 years of age, there is a gradual loss of muscle cells with a resulting decrease in the size of each individual muscle. There is also a loss of power, notably in the extensor muscles, such as the large sacrospinalis near the vertebral column. This causes the "bent over" appearance of a hunchback (kyphosis), which in women is often referred to as the *dowager's hump.* Sometimes, there is a tendency to bend (flex) the hips and knees. In addition to causing the previously noted changes in the vertebral column (see Chap. 7), these effects on the extensor muscles result in a further decrease in the elderly person's height. Activity and exercise throughout life delay and decrease these undesirable effects of aging. Even among the elderly, resistance exercise, such as weight lifting, increases muscle strength and function.

MUSCULAR DISORDERS

Spasms and Injuries

A ***spasm*** is a sudden and involuntary muscular contraction, which is always painful. A spasm of the visceral muscles is called **colic,** a good example of which is the spasm of the intestinal muscles often referred to as a *bellyache.* Spasms also occur also in the skeletal muscles. If the spasms occur in a series, the condition may be called a **seizure** or **convulsion.**

Cramps are strong, painful contractions of muscles, especially of the leg and foot. They are most likely to follow unusually strenuous activity. Cramps that occur during sleep or rest are called *recumbency cramps.*

Strains and **sprains** are common muscle injuries caused by overuse or overstretching. *Charley horse* is soreness and stiffness in a muscle caused by strain; the term usually refers to strain of the quadriceps muscle of the thigh. Sprains are more severe and can involve detachment of muscles from bones or tearing of muscle cells as well as damage to other structures, such as ligaments, blood vessels, and nerves. Much of the pain and swelling accompanying a sprain can be prevented by the immediate application of ice packs, which constrict some of the smaller blood vessels and reduce internal bleeding.

Atrophy (AT-ro-fe) is a wasting or decrease in the size of a muscle when it cannot be used, such as when an extremity must be placed in a cast after a fracture.

Diseases

Muscular dystrophy (DIS-tro-fe) is a group of disorders in which there is deterioration of muscles that still have intact nerve function. These disorders all progress at different rates. The most common type, which is found most frequently in male children, causes weakness and paralysis. Death is due to weakness of the cardiac muscle or paralysis of the respiratory muscles. Life expectancy is about 20 years for the most common type of muscular dystrophy, and about 40 years for the other types. Progress toward definitive treatment for some forms of the disease may be possible now that the genetic defects that cause them have been identified.

Myasthenia gravis (mi-as-THE-ne-ah GRA-vis) is characterized by chronic muscular fatigue brought on by the slightest exertion. It affects adults and begins with the muscles of the head. Drooping of the eyelids (ptosis) is a common early symptom. This disease is caused by a defect in transmission at the neuromuscular junction.

Myalgia (mi-AL-je-ah) means "muscular pain"; *myositis* (mi-o-SI-tis) is a term that indicates actual inflammation of muscle tissue. *Fibrositis* (fi-bro-SI-tis) means "inflammation of connective tissues" and refers particularly to those tissues associated with muscles and joints. Usually, these disorders appear in combination as *fibromyositis,* which may be acute, with severe pain on motion, or may be chronic. Sometimes, the application of heat, together with massage and rest, relieves the symptoms.

Disorders of Associated Structures

Bursitis is inflammation of a bursa, a fluid-filled sac that minimizes friction between tissues and bone. Some bursae communicate with joints; others are closely related to muscles. Sometimes, bursae develop spontaneously in response to prolonged friction. Bursitis can be very painful, with swelling and limitation of motion. Some examples of bursitis are listed below:

* *Student's elbow,* in which the bursa over the point of the elbow (olecranon) is inflamed due to long hours of leaning on the elbow while studying

* *Ischial bursitis,* which is said to be common among people who must sit a great deal, such as taxicab drivers and truckers
* *Housemaid's knee,* in which the bursa in front of the patella is inflamed. This form of bursitis is found in people who must often kneel
* *Subdeltoid bursitis* in the shoulder region, a fairly common form

In some cases a local anesthetic, corticosteroids, or both may be injected to relieve the pain of bursitis.

Bunions are enlargements commonly found at the base and medial side of the great toe. Usually, prolonged pressure has caused the development of a bursa, which has then become inflamed. Special shoes may be necessary if surgery is not performed.

Tendinitis (ten-din-I-tis), an inflammation of muscle tendons and their attachments, occurs most often in athletes who overexert themselves. It frequently involves the shoulder, the hamstring muscle tendons at the knee, and the Achilles tendon near the heel. *Tenosynovitis* (ten-o-sin-o-VI-tis), which involves the synovial sheath that encloses tendons, is found most often in women in their 40s after an injury or surgery. It may involve swelling and severe pain with activity.

Carpal tunnel syndrome involves the tendons of the flexor muscles of the fingers as well as the nerves supplying the hand and fingers. Numbness and weakness of the hand is caused by pressure on the median nerve as it passes through a tunnel formed by the carpal bones of the wrist. Carpal tunnel syndrome is one of the most common of the repetitive-use disorders. It affects many workers who use their hands and fingers strenuously, such as factory workers, keyboard operators, and musicians.

Summary

I. Types of muscle
   A. Smooth muscle
      1. In walls of hollow organs, vessels, and respiratory passageways
      2. Cells tapered, single nucleus, nonstriated
      3. Involuntary; produces peristalsis; contracts and relaxes slowly
   B. Cardiac muscle
      1. Muscle of heart wall
      2. Cells branch; single nucleus; lightly striated
      3. Involuntary; self-excitatory
   C. Skeletal muscle
      1. Attached to bones and moves skeleton
      2. Cells long, cylindrical; multiple nuclei; heavily striated
      3. Voluntary; contracts and relaxes rapidly

II. Muscular system
   A. Functions
      1. Movement of skeleton
      2. Maintenance of posture
      3. Generation of heat
   B. Structure of a muscle
      1. Held by connective tissue around individual fibers, fascicles (bundles), whole muscle
   C. Muscle cells in action
      1. Neuromuscular junction—point where nerve fiber stimulates muscle cell
      2. Contraction—sliding together of filaments to shorten muscle
         a. Actin—thin and light
         b. Myosin—heavy and dark
      3. Calcium—allows cross-bridges to form between actin and myosin
   D. Muscles and energy
      1. ATP—supplies energy
      2. Myoglobin—stores energy
      3. Glycogen—stores glucose
      4. Oxygen debt—develops during strenuous exercise
         a. Anaerobic metabolism
         b. Yields lactic acid
   E. Effects of exercise
      1. Vasodilation to bring blood to tissues
      2. Improved breathing
   F. Types of muscle contractions
      1. Tonus—partially contracted state
      2. Isotonic contractions—muscle shortens to produce movement
      3. Isometric contractions—tension increases, but muscle does not shorten

III. Mechanics of muscle movement
   A. Attachments of skeletal muscles
      1. Tendon—cord of connective tissue that attaches muscle to bone
         a. Origin—attached to more fixed part
         b. Insertion—attached to moving part
      2. Aponeurosis—broad band of connective tissue that attaches muscle to bone or other muscle
   B. Muscles work together
      1. Prime mover—performs movement
      2. Antagonist—produces opposite movement
      3. Others—steady body parts and assist prime mover
   C. Levers and body mechanics—muscles function with skeleton as lever systems
      1. Lever—bone
      2. Fulcrum—joint
      3. Force—muscle contraction

IV. Skeletal muscle groups
   A. Naming of muscles—location, size, shape, direction of fibers, number of heads, action
   B. Muscles of the head
   C. Muscles of the neck
   D. Muscles of the upper extremities
   E. Muscles of the trunk
   F. Muscles of the lower extremities

V. Effects of aging on muscles
      1. Decrease in size of muscles
      2. Weakening of muscles, especially extensors

VI. Muscular disorders
   A. Spasms and injuries
      1. Spasm—colic, seizure, convulsion
      2. Strains, sprains
      3. Atrophy—wasting
   B. Diseases
      1. Muscular dystrophy—group of disorders
      2. Myasthenia gravis
      3. Myalgia, myositis, fibromyositis
   C. Disorders of associated structures—bursitis, bunions, tendinitis, carpal tunnel syndrome

Questions for Study and Review

1. Compare smooth, cardiac, and skeletal muscle with respect to location, structure, and function.
2. List the functions of skeletal muscle.
3. Describe the structure of muscles from fiber to deep fascia.
4. Explain the role of each of the following in muscle contraction: actin and myosin, calcium, ATP, myoglobin, glycogen.
5. When does oxygen debt occur? What is the role of lactic acid in oxygen debt? How is oxygen debt eliminated?
6. What are some valuable effects of exercise?
7. Differentiate between the terms in each of the following pairs:
   a. *isotonic contraction* and *isometric contraction*
   b. *tendon* and *aponeurosis*
   c. *muscle origin* and *muscle insertion*
   d. *prime mover* and *antagonist*
   e. *bursitis* and *tendinitis*
8. What are levers and how do they work? The forceps is an example of which class of lever? When muscles and bones act as lever systems, what part of the body is the fulcrum?
9. List six characteristics by which muscles are named.
10. Name and describe the functions of the principal muscles of the head and neck, upper extremities, trunk, and lower extremities.
11. Name three muscles used for intramuscular injections.
12. What effect does aging have on muscles?
13. Define *spasm* and give examples of spasms.
14. Define *atrophy* and give one cause.
15. What are muscular dystrophies, and what are some of their effects?
16. What is bursitis? Describe several forms.

✔ ANSWERS TO CHECKPOINTS

1. The three types of muscle are smooth muscle, cardiac muscle, and skeletal muscle.
2. The three main functions of skeletal muscle are movement of the skeleton, maintenance of posture, and generation of heat.
3. The special synapse where a nerve cell makes contact with a muscle cell is the neuromuscular junction.
4. Two properties of muscle cells that are needed for response to a stimulus are excitability and contractility.
5. ATP is the form of energy produced by the oxidation of nutrients that supplies the energy for contraction of muscle cells.
6. Lactic acid is produced when muscles work without oxygen, causing muscle fatigue.
7. The attachment of a muscle to a less movable part of the skeleton is the origin; the attachment of a muscle to a movable part of the skeleton is the insertion.
8. The muscle that produces a movement is called the prime mover; the muscle that produces an opposite movement is the antagonist.
9. The action of most muscles is represented by a third-class lever in which the fulcrum is behind the point of effort and the weight.
10. The diaphragm is the muscle most important in breathing.
11. The muscles of the abdominal wall are strengthened by having the fibers of these muscles run in different directions.

Of the four chapters in this unit, two describe the nervous system and some of its many parts and complex functions. The organs of special sense and other sensory receptors are allotted an additional separate chapter. The fourth chapter in this unit discusses hormones and the organs that produce them. Working with the nervous system, these hormones play an important role in coordination and control.

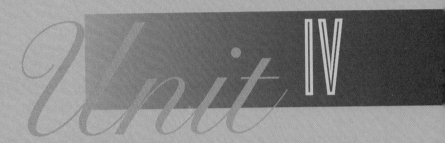

Unit IV

COORDINATION AND CONTROL

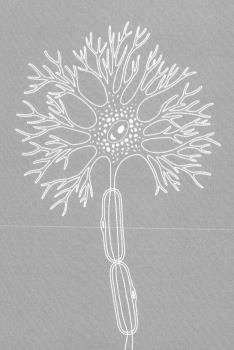

The Nervous System: The Spinal Cord and Spinal Nerves

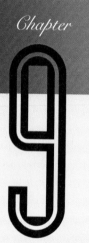

Chapter 9

BEHAVIORAL OBJECTIVES

After careful study of this chapter, you should be able to:

1. Describe the organization of the nervous system according to structure and function

2. Explain the purpose of neuroglia

3. Describe the structure of a neuron

4. Briefly describe the transmission of a nerve impulse

5. Explain the role of myelin in nerve conduction

6. Briefly describe transmission at a synapse

7. Define *neurotransmitter* and give several examples of neurotransmitters

8. Name three types of nerves and explain how they differ from each other

9. List the components of a reflex arc

10. Describe the spinal cord and name several of its functions

11. Define a reflex and give several examples

12. Describe and name the spinal nerves and three of their main plexuses

13. Compare the location and functions of the sympathetic and parasympathetic nervous systems

14. Describe several disorders of the spinal cord and of the spinal nerves

None of the body systems is capable of functioning alone. All are interdependent and work together as one unit to maintain normal conditions, termed *homeostasis*. The nervous system serves as the chief coordinating agency for all systems. Conditions both within and outside the body are constantly changing. The nervous system must detect and respond to these changes (known as *stimuli*) so that the body can adapt itself to new conditions. The nervous system has been compared to a telephone exchange, in that the brain and the spinal cord act as switching centers and the nerves act as cables for carrying messages to and from these centers.

THE NERVOUS SYSTEM AS A WHOLE

Structural Divisions

The parts of the nervous system may be grouped according to structure or function. The anatomic, or structural, divisions of the nervous system are as follows (Fig. 9-1):

- The *central nervous system* (CNS) includes the brain and spinal cord.
- The *peripheral* (per-IF-er-al) *nervous system* (PNS) is made up of all the nerves outside the CNS. It includes all the *cranial nerves* that carry impulses to and from the brain and all the *spinal nerves* that carry messages to and from the spinal cord.

The CNS and PNS together include all of the nervous tissue in the body.

Functional Divisions

Functionally, the nervous system is divided according to whether control is voluntary or involuntary and according to what type of tissue is stimulated (Table 9-1). Any tissue or organ that carries out a command from the nervous system is called an *effector*, all of which are muscles or glands.

The *somatic nervous system* is controlled voluntarily (by conscious will), and all the effectors are skeletal muscles (described in Chap. 8). The involuntary division of the nervous system is called the *autonomic nervous system* (ANS), with reference to its automatic activity, or the *visceral nervous system,* because it controls smooth muscle, cardiac muscle, and glands, much of which make up the soft body organs, the viscera.

The ANS is further subdivided into a *sympathetic nervous system* and a *parasympathetic nervous system* based on organization and how each affects specific organs. The ANS is described later in this chapter.

Although these divisions are helpful for study

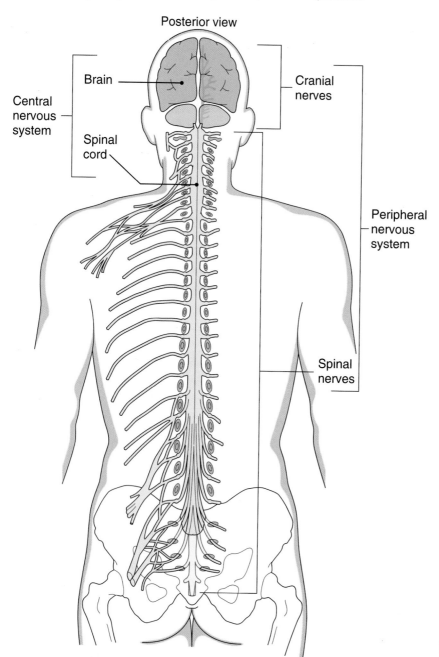

Posterior view

Brain

Central nervous system

Spinal cord

Cranial nerves

Peripheral nervous system

Spinal nerves

FIGURE **9•1** Anatomic divisions of the nervous system.

purposes, the lines that divide the nervous system according to function are not as distinct as those that classify the system structurally. For example, the diaphragm, a skeletal muscle, typically functions in breathing without conscious thought. In addition, we have certain rapid reflex responses involving skeletal muscles—drawing the hand away from a hot stove,

for example—that do not involve the brain. In contrast, people can be trained to consciously control involuntary functions, such as blood pressure, heart rate, and breathing rate, by techniques known as *biofeedback*.

To learn more about some of the effects of the nervous system on the rest of the body, see Mind Over Body: Your Own Healing Powers.

Table 9•1   **Functional Divisions of the Nervous System**

CHARAC-TERISTICS	SOMATIC NERVOUS SYSTEM	AUTONOMIC NERVOUS SYSTEM
Control Effectors	Voluntary Skeletal muscle	Involuntary Smooth muscle, cardiac muscle, and glands
Subdivisions		Sympathetic and parasympathetic systems

✔ CHECKPOINT **1**:

What are the two divisions of the nervous system based on structure?

✔ CHECKPOINT **2**:

The nervous system can be divided functionally into two divisions based on type of control and effectors. What division is voluntary and controls skeletal muscle, and what division is involuntary and controls involuntary muscles and glands?

Mind Over Body: Your Own Healing Powers

For more than 1000 years Eastern medicine has taught that the health of the body is entirely dependent upon the health of the mind. Western medicine has traditionally rejected this idea, preferring to rely upon well-documented studies of scientific fact. However, since the middle 1980s, western medical practitioners have put forth many well-founded studies to prove that our eastern colleagues have been right all along.

The earliest studies to indicate that the brain was indeed a very powerful physiological organ were undertaken in the early and middle 1960s. These studies set out to document that many "mental" illnesses such as schizophrenia and manic depression were indeed physiological disorders. In the years since, studies have continued to show that many physical symptoms are tied to what would have previously been thought of as "it's all just in your head."

"Bad" emotional stress, including feelings of depression, inability to cope, or anger, fear, loss, or rejection, causes distinct changes in the biochemistry of the brain, which may appear as physical ailments. When the body is experiencing "bad stress," the cardiovascular system works harder and less efficiently. The respiratory system has a harder time keeping up with demands for oxygen and the immune system has a more difficult time fighting off invading pathogens. The body's metabolism has trouble supplying the increased demand for energy needed to cope with the negative stress. In essence, the systems are geared more toward fighting the effects of stress than taking care of the body. As a result, people tend to get sick when they are under significant stress.

Conversely, positive or "good stress" leads to a general increase in a person's overall health. Feelings of happiness, joy, contentment, fulfillment, love, and companionship lead to positive changes in the biochemistry of the brain. The heart pumps more slowly and more efficiently, the lungs work more easily, the immune system is boosted to fight off disease.

Studies have now shown that:

- Men and women in solid, long-lasting relationships live longer than their single counterparts and experience less significant illness throughout their adult lives.
- Those who experience a significant stress are seven times more likely to become ill than the average person.
- Faith, prayer, and meditation, regardless of religious affiliation, may lead to shorter hospital stays, lower blood pressure, increased circulation, and extension of life-span by an average of 7.26 years.
- Laughter really is the best medicine, having been shown to directly stimulate the immune system.

Limiting our exposure to negative stress and exploiting the benefits of positive stress has a definite impact on our lives.

Neuroglia

In addition to conducting tissue, the nervous system contains cells that serve for support and protection. Collectively, these connective tissue cells are called *neuroglia* (nu-ROG-le-ah) or *glial* (GLI-al) *cells.* There are different types of neuroglia, each with specialized functions, some of which are the following:

- To protect nervous tissue
- To support nervous tissue and bind it to other structures
- To aid in repair of cells
- To act as phagocytes to remove pathogens and impurities
- To regulate the composition of fluids around and between cells

Unlike nerve cells, neuroglia continue to multiply throughout life. Because of their capacity to reproduce, most tumors of the nervous system are tumors of neuroglial tissue.

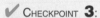

✔ CHECKPOINT **3**:

The nonconducting cells of the nervous system serve in protection and support. What are these cells called?

NEURONS AND THEIR FUNCTIONS

Structure of a Neuron

The functional cells of the nervous system are highly specialized cells called *neurons* (Fig. 9-2). The main portion of each neuron, the cell body, contains the nucleus and other organelles typically found in cells. A distinguishing feature of the neurons, however, are the long, thread-like fibers that extend out from the cell body and carry impulses across the cell. There are two kinds of fibers: dendrites and axons.

- *Dendrites* are neuron fibers that conduct impulses *to* the cell body. Most dendrites have a highly branched, treelike appearance (see Fig. 9-2). In fact, the name comes from a Greek word meaning "tree." Den-

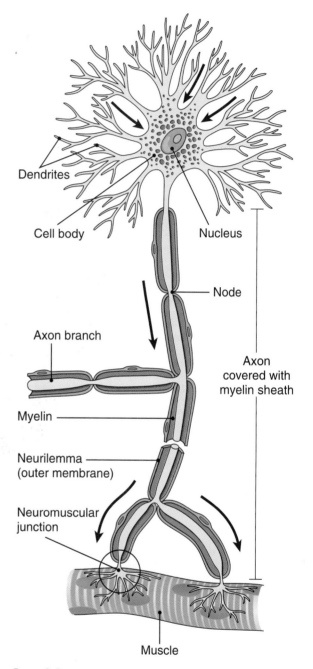

FIGURE **9•2** Diagram of a motor neuron. The break in the axon denotes length. The arrows show the direction of the nerve impulse.

drites function as *receptors* in the nervous system. That is, they receive the stimulus that begins a neural pathway. In Chapter 11, we describe how the dendrites of the sensory system may be modified to respond to a specific type of stimulus.

- ***Axons*** (AK-sons) are neuron fibers that conduct impulses *away from* the cell body. These impulses may be delivered to another neuron, to a muscle, or to a gland. An axon is a single fiber, which may be quite long and which branches at its end.

The Myelin Sheath

Some axons are covered with a fatty material called ***myelin*** that insulates and protects the fiber (Fig. 9-3). In the PNS, this covering is produced by special neuroglia called ***Schwann*** (shvahn) ***cells,*** that wrap around the axon like a jelly roll depositing layers of myelin. When the sheath is complete, small spaces remain between the individual cells. These tiny gaps, called ***nodes,*** are important in speeding the conduction of nerve impulses.

The outermost membranes of the Schwann cells form a thin coating known as the ***neurilemma*** (nu-rih-LEM-mah). This covering is a part of the mechanism by which some peripheral nerves repair themselves when injured. Under some circumstances, damaged nerve cell fibers may regenerate by growing into the sleeve formed by the neurilemma. Cells of the brain and the spinal cord are myelinated, not by Schwann cells, but by other neuroglia. As a result, they have no neurilemma. If they are injured, the damage is permanent. Even in the peripheral nerves, however, repair is a slow and uncertain process.

Myelinated axons, because of the color of the myelin, are called ***white fibers*** and are found in the ***white matter*** of the brain and spinal cord as well as in the nerve trunks in all parts of the body. The fibers and cell bodies of the ***gray matter*** are not covered with myelin.

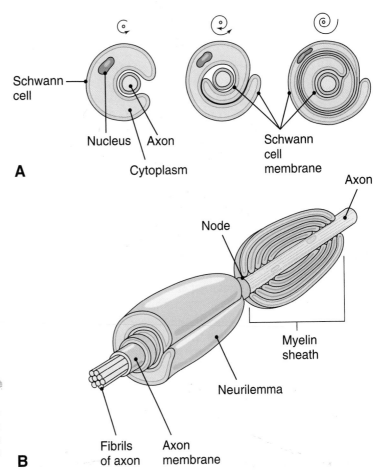

FIGURE **9•3** Formation of a myelin sheath. **(A)** Schwann cells wrap around the axon creating a myelin coating. **(B)** Outermost layer of the Schwann cell forms the neurilemma. Spaces between the cells are the nodes.

9

> ✔ CHECKPOINT **4**:
>
> The neuron, the functional unit of the nervous system, has long fibers extending from the cell body. What is the name of the fiber that carries impulses toward the cell body and what is the name of the fiber that carries impulses away from the cell body?

> ✔ CHECKPOINT **5**:
>
> Myelin is a substance that covers and protects some axons. What color describes myelinated fibers, and what color describes unmyelinated tissue of the nervous system?

Types of Neurons

The job of neurons in the PNS is to relay information constantly either to or from the CNS. Neurons that conduct impulses *to* the spinal cord and brain are described as *sensory neurons,* also *afferent neurons.* Those cells that carry impulses *from* the CNS out to muscles and glands are *motor neurons,* also *efferent neurons.* Neurons that relay information within the CNS are *interneurons,* also called *central* or *association neurons.*

Nerves and Tracts

Everywhere in the nervous system, neuron fibers are collected into bundles of varying size. A bundle of fibers located within the PNS is a *nerve.* A bundle of fibers within the CNS is a *tract.*

Tracts are located in the brain and also in the spinal cord, where they conduct impulses to and from the brain. A nerve or tract can be compared to an electric cable made up of many wires. As with muscles, the "wires," or nerve cell fibers, in a nerve or tract are bound together with connective tissue.

A few of the cranial nerves contain only sensory fibers for conducting impulses toward the brain. These are described as *sensory (afferent) nerves.* A few of the cranial nerves contain only motor fibers for conducting impulses away from the brain and are classified as *motor (ef-*

ferent) nerves. Most of the cranial nerves and *all* of the spinal nerves contain both sensory *and* motor fibers and are referred to as *mixed nerves.* Note that in a mixed nerve, impulses may be traveling in two directions (toward or away from the CNS), but each individual fiber in the nerve is carrying impulses in one direction only. Think of the nerve as a large highway. Traffic may be going north and south, for example, but each car is going forward in only one direction.

> ✔ CHECKPOINT **6**:
>
> Nerves are bundles of neuron fibers in the PNS. These nerves may be carrying impulses either toward or away from the CNS. What name is given to nerves that convey impulses toward the CNS, and what name is given to nerves that transport away from the CNS?

THE NERVOUS SYSTEM AT WORK

The Nerve Impulse

The mechanics of nerve impulse conduction are complex but can be compared to the spread of an electric current along a wire. What follows is a brief description of the electric changes that occur as a resting neuron is stimulated and transmits a nerve impulse.

The cell membrane of an unstimulated (resting) neuron carries an electric charge. This charge is maintained by ions (charged particles) concentrated on either side of the membrane. At rest, the inside of the membrane is negative as compared with the outside. In this state, the membrane is said to be *polarized.*

A *nerve impulse* starts with a local reversal in this charge, which then spreads along the membrane like a current (Fig. 9-4). This sudden electric change in the membrane is called an *action potential,* as described in Chapter 8 on the muscles. When this reversal occurs, the membrane is said to *depolarize.* The reversal occurs rapidly (in less than one thousandth of a second) and is followed at each point along the membrane by an immediate return to the original state so that the membrane can be stimu-

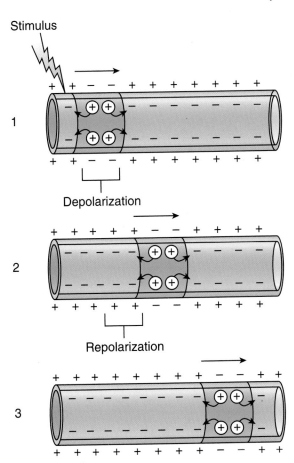

Figure **9•4**   Spread of an action potential along a neuron.

lated again. When the membrane returns to its resting state, it is said to *repolarize*. Depolarization and repolarization are brought about by rapid shifts in sodium and potassium ions across the cell membrane. A stimulus can be defined as any force (*e.g.,* electric, chemical, or mechanical) that can start an action potential, which then spreads along the membrane as a nerve impulse.

The Role of Myelin in Conduction
In an unmyelinated fiber, the action potential spreads continuously along the membrane of the cell (see Fig. 9-4). When myelin is present on an axon, however, it insulates the fiber against the spread of current. This would appear to slow or stop conduction along these fibers, but in fact, the myelin sheath speeds conduction. In this case, the action potential must "jump" like a spark from node (space) to

node along the sheath (see Fig. 9-3), and this type of conduction is actually faster than continuous conduction.

> ✔ CHECKPOINT **7**:
>
> An action potential occurs in two stages. In the first stage, the charge on the membrane reverses, and in the second stage, it returns to the resting state. What terms are used to describe the membrane in these two stages?

The Synapse

Neurons do not work alone; impulses must be transferred between neurons to convey information within the nervous system. The point of junction for transmission of the nerve impulse is the *synapse* (SIN-aps), a term that comes from a Greek word meaning "to clasp" (Fig. 9-5).

As described in Chapter 8, information must be passed from one cell to another across a tiny gap between the cells, the synaptic cleft. Within the branched endings of the axon are small vesicles (bubbles) containing a type of chemical known as a *neurotransmitter.* When a nerve impulse traveling along a neuron reaches the end of the axon, the axon releases its neurotransmitter into the narrow gap, the *synaptic cleft*, between the cells. The neurotransmitter then acts as a chemical signal to stimulate the next cell, described as the *postsynaptic cell.* The cell that releases the neurotransmitter is the *presynaptic cell.*

On the receiving membrane, usually that of a dendrite, but sometimes another part of the cell, there are special sites, or *receptors*, ready to pick up and respond to specific neurotransmitters. Receptors in the postsynaptic cell membrane influence how or if that cell will respond to a given neurotransmitter.

Neurotransmitters
Although there are many known neurotransmitters, the main ones are *epinephrine* (ep-ih-NEF-rin), also called *adrenaline;* a related compound, *norepinephrine* (nor-ep-ih-NEF-rin), or *noradrenaline;* and *acetylcholine* (as-e-til-KO-lene). Acetylcholine (ACh) is the neurotransmitter released at the neuromuscu-

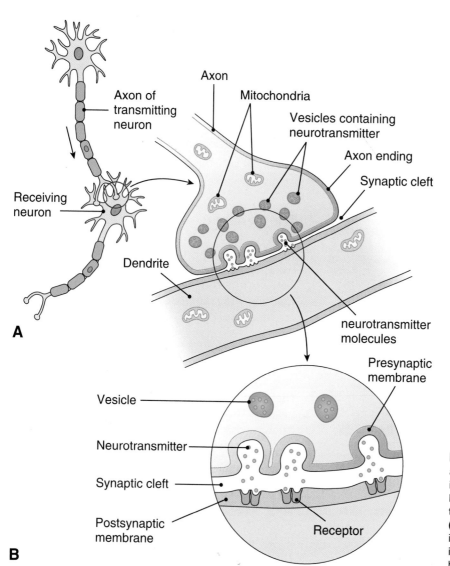

Axon

Axon of transmitting neuron

Mitochondria

Vesicles containing neurotransmitter

Axon ending

Synaptic cleft

Receiving neuron

Dendrite

neurotransmitter molecules

A

Presynaptic membrane

Vesicle

Neurotransmitter

Synaptic cleft

Postsynaptic membrane

Receptor

B

FIGURE **9•5** **(A)** A synapse. The axon ending has vesicles containing neurotransmitter, which is released across the synaptic cleft to the membrane of the next cell. **(B)** Close-up of a synapse showing receptors for neurotransmitter in the postsynaptic cell membrane.

lar junction, the synapse between a neuron and a muscle cell. All three of the above neurotransmitters function in the ANS. It is common to think of neurotransmitters as stimulating the cells they reach; in fact, they have been described as such in this discussion. Note, however, that some of these chemicals act to inhibit the postsynaptic cell and keep it from reacting.

The connections between neurons can be quite complex. One cell can branch to stimulate many receiving cells, or a single cell may be stimulated by a number of different axons (Fig. 9-6). The cell's response is based on the total effects of all the neurotransmitters it receives at any one time.

After its release into the synaptic cleft, the neurotransmitter may follow several paths for removal:

- It may slowly diffuse away from the synapse.
- It may be destroyed rapidly by enzymes in the synaptic cleft.
- It may be taken back into the presynaptic cell to be used again.

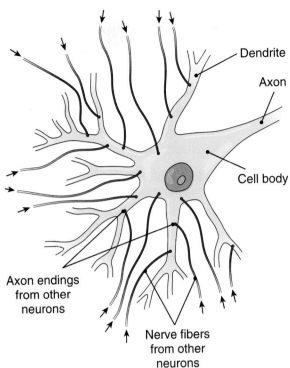

FIGURE **9•6**   A single neuron is stimulated by axons of many other neurons.

Dendrite

Axon

Cell body

Axon endings from other neurons

Nerve fibers from other neurons

The method of removal is a factor in determining how long a neurotransmitter will act.

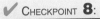

✔ CHECKPOINT **8**:

Chemicals are needed to carry information across the synaptic cleft at a synapse. As a group, what are all these chemicals called?

The Reflex Arc

As the nervous system functions, both external and internal stimuli are received, interpreted, and acted on. A complete pathway through the nervous system from stimulus to response is termed a *reflex arc* (Fig. 9-7). This is the basic functional pathway of the nervous system. The basic parts of a reflex arc are the following:

- *Receptor*—the end of a dendrite or some specialized receptor cell, as in a special sense organ, that detects a stimulus
- *Sensory neuron,* or afferent neuron—a cell that transmits impulses *toward* the CNS

9

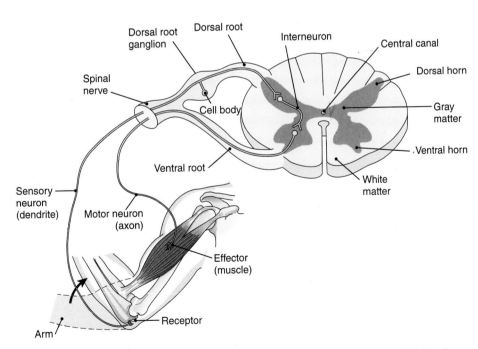

Dorsal root ganglion

Dorsal root

Spinal nerve

Cell body

Sensory neuron (dendrite)

Motor neuron (axon)

Ventral root

Effector (muscle)

Arm

Receptor

Interneuron

Central canal

Dorsal horn

Gray matter

Ventral horn

White matter

FIGURE **9•7**   Reflex arc showing the pathway of impulses and a cross section of the spinal cord.

- **Central nervous system**—where impulses are coordinated and a response is organized. One or more interneurons may carry impulses to and from the brain, may function within the brain, or may distribute impulses to different regions of the spinal cord. Almost every response involves connecting neurons in the CNS.
- **Motor neuron,** or efferent neuron—a cell that carries impulses *away from* the CNS
- **Effector**—a muscle or a gland outside the CNS that carries out a response

At its simplest, a reflex arc can involve just two neurons, one sensory and one motor, with a synapse in the CNS. There are few reflex arcs that require only this minimal number of neurons. The knee-jerk reflex described later is one of the few examples in humans. Most reflex arcs involve many more, even hundreds, of connecting neurons within the CNS. The many intricate patterns that make the nervous system so responsive and adaptable also make it difficult to study, and investigation of the nervous system is one of the most active areas of research today.

✔ CHECKPOINT **9**:

What name is given to a pathway through the nervous system from a stimulus to an effector?

THE SPINAL CORD

Location of the Spinal Cord

The spinal cord is contained in and protected by the vertebrae, which fit together to form a continuous tube extending from the occipital bone to the coccyx (Fig. 9-8). In the embryo, the spinal cord occupies the entire spinal canal, extending down into the tail portion of the vertebral column. The column of bone grows much more rapidly than the nerve tissue of the cord, however, and eventually, the end of the cord no longer reaches the lower part of the spinal canal. This disparity in growth continues to increase, so that in adults, the cord ends in the region just below the area to which the last rib attaches (between the first and second lumbar vertebrae).

Structure of the Spinal Cord

The spinal cord (see Fig. 9-7) has a small, irregularly shaped internal section that consists of gray matter (nerve cell bodies) and a larger area surrounding this gray part that consists of white matter (nerve cell fibers). The gray matter is so arranged that a column of cells extends up and down dorsally, one on each side; another column is found in the ventral region on each side. These two pairs of columns, called the **dorsal** and **ventral horns,** give the gray matter an H-shaped appearance in cross-section. In the center of the gray matter is a small channel, the **central canal**, that contains cerebrospinal fluid, the liquid that circulates around the brain and spinal cord. The white matter consists of thousands of myelinated axons arranged in three areas external to the gray matter on each side.

✔ CHECKPOINT **10**:

The spinal cord contains both gray and white matter. How is this tissue arranged in the spinal cord?

Functions of the Spinal Cord

Linking the Spinal Nerves to the Brain
The white matter of the spinal cord is divided into tracts that convey impulses to and from the brain. As shown in Figure 9-7, sensory impulses from peripheral receptors enter the dorsal horn of the spinal cord. They are then transmitted upward toward the brain in *ascending tracts* of the white matter.

Motor impulses traveling down from the brain are carried in *descending tracts* until they exit through the ventral horn of the gray matter to reach an effector.

Reflex Activities
A **reflex** is a rapid, simple, and automatic response involving very few neurons. Reflexes are

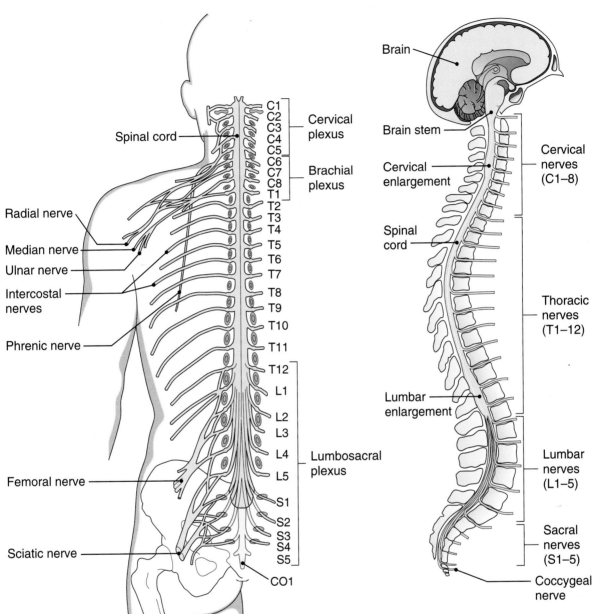

FIGURE **9•8** Spinal cord and spinal nerves showing plexuses. **(A)** Posterior view. **(B)** Lateral view.

specific; a given stimulus always produces the same response.

When you fling out an arm or leg to catch your balance, withdraw from a painful stimulus, or blink to avoid an object approaching your eyes, you are experiencing reflex behavior. A simple reflex arc that passes through the spinal cord alone and does not involve the brain is termed a ***spinal reflex.***

The ***stretch reflex,*** in which a muscle is stretched and responds by contracting, is one example. If you tap the tendon below the kneecap (the patellar tendon), the muscle of the anterior thigh (quadriceps femoris) contracts, eliciting the knee-jerk reflex (Fig. 9-9).

Such stretch reflexes may be evoked by appropriate tapping of most large muscles (such as the triceps brachii in the arm and the gas-

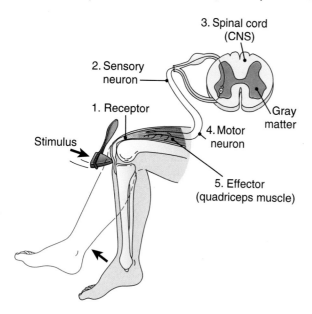

3. Spinal cord
(CNS)

2. Sensory
neuron

1. Receptor

Stimulus

Gray
matter

4. Motor
neuron

5. Effector
(quadriceps muscle)

FIGURE 9•9   The patellar (knee-jerk) reflex.

trocnemius in the calf of the leg). Because reflexes are simple and predictable, they are used in physical examinations to test the condition of the nervous system.

✔ CHECKPOINT **11**:

What are the two main functions of the spinal cord?

Medical Procedures Involving the Spinal Cord

Lumbar Puncture

It is sometimes necessary to remove a small amount of cerebrospinal fluid (CSF) from the nervous system for testing. CSF is the fluid that circulates in and around the brain and spinal cord. This fluid is taken from the space below the spinal cord to avoid damage to nervous tissue. Because the spinal cord is only about 18 inches long and ends some distance above the level of the hip line, a lumbar puncture or spinal tap is usually done between the third and fourth lumbar vertebrae, at about the level of the top of the hipbone. The sample that is removed can then be studied in the laboratory for evidence of disease or injury.

Administration of Drugs

Anesthetics or medications are sometimes injected into the space below the cord. The anesthetic agent temporarily blocks all sensation from the lower part of the body. This method of giving anesthesia has an advantage for certain types of procedures or surgery; the patient is awake but feels nothing in his or her lower body.

The spinal route also can be used to administer pain medication.

Disorders Involving the Spinal Cord

Diseases

Multiple sclerosis (MS) is a disease in which the myelin sheath around axons is damaged and the neuron fibers themselves degenerate. Both the spinal cord and the brain are affected. Although the cause of MS is not completely understood, there is strong evidence that it involves an attack on the myelin sheath by a person's own immune system, a situation described as *autoimmunity*. Genetic makeup, in combination with environmental factors, may trigger MS. Some research suggests that a prior viral or bacterial infection, even one that occurred many years before, may set off the disease.

MS progresses at different rates depending on the individual, and it may be marked by episodes of relapse and remission. At this point, no cure has been found for MS, but drugs that stop the autoimmune response and drugs that relieve MS symptoms are currently under study.

Amyotrophic (ah-mi-o-TROF-ik) *lateral sclerosis* is a disorder of the nervous system in which motor neurons are destroyed. The progressive destruction causes muscle atrophy and loss of motor control until finally the affected person is unable to swallow or talk.

Poliomyelitis (po-le-o-mi-eh-LI-tis) ("polio") is a viral disease of the nervous system that occurs most commonly in children. Polio is spread by ingestion of water contaminated with feces containing the virus. Infection of the gastrointestinal tract leads to passage of the virus into the blood, from which it spreads to the CNS. Poliovirus tends to multiply in motor neurons in the spinal cord, leading to paralysis, including paralysis of the breathing muscles.

Polio has been virtually eliminated in many countries through the use of vaccines against the disease—first the injected Salk vaccine developed in 1954, followed by the Sabin oral vaccine. A goal of the World Health Organization (WHO) is the total eradication of polio by worldwide vaccination programs.

Tumors

Tumors that affect the spinal cord commonly arise in the support tissue in and around the cord. They are frequently tumors of the nerve sheaths, the meninges, or neuroglia. Symptoms are caused by pressure on the cord and the roots of the spinal nerves. These include pain, numbness, weakness, and loss of function. Spinal cord tumors are diagnosed by magnetic resonance imaging (MRI) or other imaging techniques, and treatment is by surgery and radiation.

Injuries

Injuries to the spinal cord occur when bones of the spinal column are broken or dislocated, such as in motor vehicle crashes and swimming and diving accidents. Gunshot or shrapnel wounds may also damage the cord to varying degrees. Because the nervous tissue of the brain and cord cannot repair itself, severing of the cord causes paralysis of all the muscles supplied by nerves below the level of the injury. Loss of sensation and motion in the lower part of the body is called *paraplegia* (par-ah-PLE-je-ah).

SPINAL NERVES

Location and Structure of the Spinal Nerves

There are 31 pairs of spinal nerves, each pair numbered according to the level of the spinal cord from which it arises (see Fig. 9-8). Each nerve is attached to the spinal cord by two roots: the *dorsal root* and the *ventral root* (see Fig. 9-7). On each dorsal root is a marked swelling of gray matter called the *dorsal root ganglion,* which contains the cell bodies of the

sensory neurons. A *ganglion* (GANG-le-on) is any collection of nerve cell bodies located outside the CNS. Fibers from sensory receptors throughout the body lead to these dorsal root ganglia.

The ventral roots of the spinal nerves are a combination of motor (efferent) fibers that supply muscles and glands (effectors). The cell bodies of these neurons are located in the ventral gray matter (ventral horns) of the cord. Because the dorsal (sensory) and ventral (motor) roots are combined to form the spinal nerve, all spinal nerves are mixed nerves.

Branches of the Spinal Nerves

Each spinal nerve continues only a short distance away from the spinal cord and then branches into small posterior divisions and larger anterior divisions. The larger anterior branches interlace to form networks called *plexuses* (PLEK-sus-eze), which then distribute branches to the body parts (see Fig. 9-8). The three main plexuses are described as follows:

- The *cervical plexus* supplies motor impulses to the muscles of the neck and receives sensory impulses from the neck and the back of the head. The phrenic nerve, which activates the diaphragm, arises from this plexus.
- The *brachial* (BRA-ke-al) *plexus* sends numerous branches to the shoulder, arm, forearm, wrist, and hand. The radial nerve emerges from the brachial plexus.
- The *lumbosacral* (lum-bo-SA-kral) *plexus* supplies nerves to the pelvis and legs. The largest branch in this plexus is the *sciatic* (si-AT-ik) *nerve,* which leaves the dorsal part of the pelvis, passes beneath the gluteus maximus muscle, and extends down the back of the thigh. At its beginning, it is nearly 1 inch thick, but it soon branches to the thigh muscles; near the knee, it forms two subdivisions that supply the leg and the foot.

To learn about how the organization of the spinal nerves affects skin sensations, see Dermatomes.

Dermatomes

Sensory neurons from all over the skin, except for the skin of the face and scalp, feed information into the spinal cord through the spinal nerves. The skin surface can be mapped into distinct regions that are supplied by a single spinal nerve. Each of these regions is called a *dermatome* (DER-mah-tome) (see illustration on page 157.).

Stimulation of the skin within a given dermatome is carried over the corresponding spinal nerve. This information can be used to identify the spinal nerve or spinal segment that is involved in an injury. In some areas, the dermatomes are not absolutely distinct. Some dermatomes may share a nerve supply with neighboring regions. For this reason, it is necessary to numb several adjacent dermatomes to achieve successful anesthesia.

✔ CHECKPOINT **12**:

How many pairs of spinal nerves are there?

Disorders of the Spinal Nerves

Peripheral neuritis (nu-RI-tis), or peripheral neuropathy, is the degeneration of nerves supplying the distal areas of the extremities. It affects both sensory and motor function, causing symptoms of pain and paralysis. Causes include chronic intoxication (alcohol, lead, drugs), infectious diseases (meningitis), metabolic diseases (diabetes, gout), or nutritional diseases (vitamin deficiency, starvation). Identification and treatment of the underlying disorder is most important. Because peripheral neuritis is a symptom rather than a disease, a complete physical examination may be needed to establish its cause.

Sciatica (si-AT-ih-kah) is a form of peripheral neuritis characterized by severe pain along the sciatic nerve and its branches. The most common causes of this disorder are rupture of a disk between the lower lumbar vertebrae and arthritis of the lower part of the spinal column.

Herpes zoster, commonly known as *shingles,* is characterized by numerous blisters along the course of certain nerves, most commonly the intercostal nerves, which are branches of the thoracic spinal nerves in the waist area. It is caused by a reactivation of a prior infection by the chickenpox virus and involves an attack on the sensory cell bodies inside the spinal ganglia. Initial symptoms include fever and pain, followed in 2 to 4 weeks by the appearance of vesicles (fluid-filled skin lesions). The drainage from these vesicles contains highly contagious liquid. The neuralgic pains may persist for years and can be distressing. This infection may also involve the first branch of the fifth cranial nerve and cause pain in the eyeball and surrounding tissues. Early treatment of a recurrent attack with antiviral drugs may reduce the neuralgia.

THE AUTONOMIC NERVOUS SYSTEM

Characteristics of the Autonomic Nervous System

The autonomic (visceral) nervous system regulates the action of the glands, the smooth muscles of hollow organs and vessels, and the heart muscle. These actions are carried on automatically; whenever a change occurs that calls for a regulatory adjustment, it is made without conscious awareness.

The sensory neurons in this system are grouped with those that come from the skin and voluntary muscles. In contrast, the *efferent* neurons, which supply the glands and the involuntary muscles, are arranged in a distinct pattern, which has led to their separation for study purposes into **sympathetic** and **parasympathetic** divisions (Fig. 9-10).

All autonomic pathways contain two motor neurons connecting the spinal cord with the effector organ. The two neurons synapse in ganglia that serve as relay stations along the way. The first neuron, the **preganglionic neuron**, extends from the spinal cord to the ganglion. The second neuron, the **postganglionic neuron**, travels from the ganglion to the effector. This differs from the voluntary (somatic) nervous system, in which each motor nerve fiber

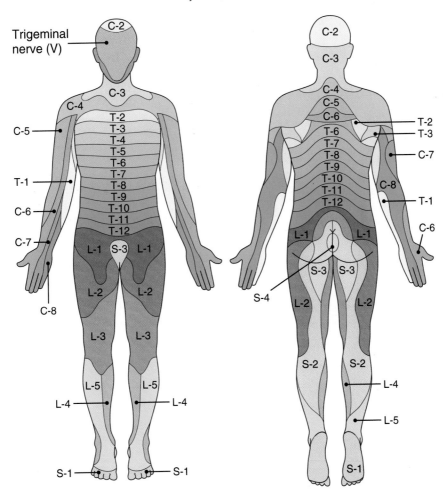

extends all the way from the spinal cord to the skeletal muscle with no intervening synapse. Some of the autonomic fibers are within the spinal nerves; some are within the cranial nerves (see Chap. 10).

✔ CHECKPOINT **13**:

How many neurons are there in each motor pathway of the ANS?

Divisions of the Autonomic Nervous System

The characteristics of the two divisions of the ANS are described below. The information is summarized in Table 9-2.

Sympathetic Nervous System

The sympathetic motor neurons originate in the spinal cord with cell bodies in the thoracic and lumbar regions, the ***thoracolumbar*** (tho-rah-ko-LUM-bar) area. These fibers arise from the spinal cord at the level of the first thoracic nerve down to the level of the second lumbar spinal nerve. From this part of the cord, nerve fibers extend to ganglia where they synapse with second neurons, the fibers of which extend to the glands and involuntary muscle tissues.

Many of the sympathetic ganglia form the ***sympathetic chains,*** two cordlike strands of ganglia that extend along either side of the spinal column from the lower neck to the upper abdominal region.

In addition, the nerves that supply the organs of the abdominal and pelvic cavities synapse in

SYMPATHETIC SYSTEM   **PARASYMPATHETIC SYSTEM**

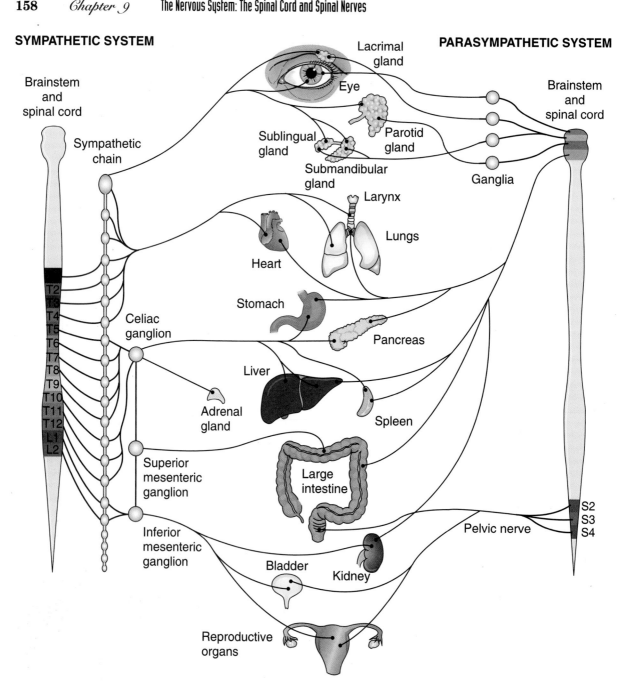

Figure **9•10** Autonomic nervous system (only one side is shown).

three single **collateral ganglia** farther from the spinal cord.

The postganglionic neurons of the sympathetic system, with few exceptions, act on their effectors by releasing the neurotransmitter epinephrine (adrenaline) and the related compound norepinephrine (noradrenaline). This system is therefore described as **adrenergic,** which means "activated by adrenaline."

Parasympathetic Nervous System
The parasympathetic motor pathways begin in the **craniosacral** (kra-ne-o-SAK-ral) areas, with fibers arising from cell bodies in the brain-

Table 9•2	Divisions of the Autonomic Nervous System	
CHARACTERISTICS	SYMPATHETIC NERVOUS SYSTEM	PARASYMPATHETIC NERVOUS SYSTEM
Origin of fibers	Thoracic and lumbar regions of the spinal cord; thoracolumbar	Brain stem and sacral regions of the spinal cord; craniosacral
Location of ganglia	Sympathetic chain and three single collateral ganglia	Terminal ganglia in or near the effector organ
Neurotransmitter	Adrenaline and noradrenaline; adrenergic	Acetylcholine; cholinergic
Effects (see Table 9-3)	Response to stress; fight-or-flight response	Reverses stress response; stimulates some activities

stem (midbrain and medulla) and the lower (sacral) part of the spinal cord. From these centers, the first fibers extend to autonomic ganglia that are usually located near or within the walls of the effector organs and are called **terminal ganglia**. The pathways then continue along postganglionic neurons that stimulate the involuntary tissues.

The neurons of the parasympathetic system release the neurotransmitter acetylcholine, leading to the description of this system as **cholinergic** (activated by acetylcholine).

Functions of the Autonomic Nervous System

Most organs are supplied by both sympathetic and parasympathetic fibers, and the two systems generally have opposite effects. The sympathetic part of the ANS tends to act as an accelerator for those organs needed to meet a stressful situation. It promotes what is called the **fight-or-flight response** because in the most primitive terms, the person must decide to stay and "fight it out" with the enemy or to run away from danger. If you think of what happens to a person who is frightened or angry, you can easily remember the effects of impulses from the sympathetic nervous system:

- Increase in the rate and force of heart contractions
- Increase in blood pressure due partly to the more effective heartbeat and partly to constriction of small arteries in the skin and the internal organs
- Dilation of blood vessels to skeletal

muscles, bringing more blood to these tissues
- Dilation of the bronchial tubes to allow more oxygen to enter
- Stimulation of the central portion of the adrenal gland. This produces hormones, including epinephrine, that prepare the body to meet emergency situations in many ways (see Chap. 12). The sympathetic nerves and hormones from the adrenal gland reinforce each other
- Increase in metabolism
- Dilation of the pupil and decrease in focusing ability (for near objects)

The sympathetic system also acts as a brake on those systems not directly involved in the response to stress, such as the urinary and digestive systems. If you try to eat while you are angry, you may note that your saliva is thick and so small in amount that you can swallow only with difficulty. Under these circumstances, when food does reach the stomach, it seems to stay there longer than usual.

The parasympathetic part of the ANS normally acts as a balance for the sympathetic system once a crisis has passed. The parasympathetic system brings about constriction of the pupils, slowing of the heart rate, and constriction of the bronchial tubes. It also stimulates the formation and release of urine and activity of the digestive tract. Saliva, for example, flows more easily and profusely, and its quantity and fluidity increase.

Most organs of the body receive both sympathetic and parasympathetic stimulation, the effects of the two systems on a given organ generally being opposite. Table 9-3 shows some of the actions of these two systems.

Table 9•3   Effects of the Sympathetic and Parasympathetic Systems on Selected Organs

EFFECTOR	SYMPATHETIC SYSTEM	PARASYMPATHETIC SYSTEM
Pupils of eye	Dilation	Constriction
Sweat glands	Stimulation	None
Digestive glands	Inhibition	Stimulation
Heart	Increased rate and strength of beat	Decreased rate and strength of beat
Bronchi of lungs	Dilation	Constriction
Muscles of digestive system	Decreased contraction (peristalsis)	Increased contraction
Kidneys	Decreased activity	None
Urinary bladder	Relaxation	Contraction and emptying
Liver	Increased release of glucose	None
Penis	Ejaculation	Erection
Adrenal medulla	Stimulation	None
Blood vessels to		
Skeletal muscles	Dilation	Constriction
Skin	Constriction	None
Respiratory system	Dilation	Constriction
Digestive organs	Constriction	Dilation

✔ CHECKPOINT **14**:

Which division of the ANS stimulates a stress response, and which division reverses the stress response?

See Cell Receptors—Getting the Message.

Disorders of the Autonomic Nervous System

Injuries due to wounds by penetrating objects or to tumors, hemorrhage, or spinal column dislocations or fractures may cause damage to the sympathetic chain. In addition to these rather obvious kinds of disorders, there are a great number of conditions in which symptoms, such as heart palpitations, increased blood pressure, and stomach aches, suggest autonomic malfunctions but in which the cause is not well understood. These disorders are related to psychological factors involved in the functioning of the viscera and may arise from the close interrelations of the brain, brain stem, and spinal cord and the ANS.

The ANS, together with the endocrine system, regulates our responses to stress. This interrelation and the effects of prolonged stress are discussed in more detail in Chapter 12.

Cell Receptors— Getting the Message

The nervous system functions by means of neurotransmitters, chemicals that carry information from cell to cell across the synapse. Just as important as the neurotransmitters are the "docking sites" for these chemicals, the receptors on the receiving (postsynaptic) cell membranes. The same neurotransmitter may have different effects, depending on the nature of the receptor.

Acetylcholine (ACh) stimulates muscle contraction at the neuromuscular junction, the point where an axon contacts a skeletal muscle. When functioning in the parasympathetic nervous system, however, ACh stimulates some tissues, such as the digestive organs, but inhibits others, such as the heart. These differences depend on the receptors on the postsynaptic cell membrane.

Some drugs work by blocking receptors for specific neurotransmitters. For example, the beta-blocking agents used to regulate the heart in cardiac disease inhibit the receptors for adrenaline, a neurotransmitter that increases the rate and strength of heart contractions.

Summary

I. **The nervous system as a whole**
   A. Structural divisions—anatomic
      1. Central nervous system (CNS)—brain and spinal cord
      2. Peripheral nervous system (PNS)—spinal and cranial nerves
   B. Functional divisions—physiologic
      1. Somatic nervous system—voluntary; supplies skeletal muscles
      2. Autonomic (visceral) nervous system—involuntary; supplies smooth muscle, cardiac muscle, glands
   C. Neuroglia
      1. Nonconducting cells
      2. Protect and support nervous tissue

II. **Neurons and their functions**
   A. Structure of a neuron
      1. Cell body
      2. Cell fibers
         a. Dendrite—carries impulses to cell body
         b. Axon—carries impulses away from cell body
      3. Myelin sheath
         a. Covers and protects some axons
         b. Speeds conduction
         c. Made by Schwann cells in PNS; neuroglia in CNS
         d. Neurilemma—outermost layer of Schwann cell; aids axon repair
         e. White matter—myelinated tissue; gray matter—unmyelinated tissue
   B. Types of neurons
      1. Sensory (afferent)—carry impulses toward CNS
      2. Motor (efferent)—carry impulses away from CNS
   C. Nerves and tracts—bundles of neuron fibers
      1. Nerve—in peripheral nervous system
         a. Sensory (afferent) nerve—contains only fibers that carry impulses toward the CNS (from a receptor)
         b. Motor (efferent) nerve—contains only fibers that carry impulses away from the CNS (to an effector)
         c. Mixed nerve—contains both sensory and motor fibers
      2. Tract—in central nervous system

III. **The nervous system at work**
   A. Nerve impulse (action potential)—electric current that spreads along nerve fiber
   B. Synapse—junction between neurons where a nerve impulse is transmitted from one neuron to the next
      1. Neurotransmitter—carries impulse across synapse
      2. Receptors—in postsynaptic membrane; pick up neurotransmitters
      3. Neurotransmitter removed by diffusion, destruction by enzyme, return to presynaptic cell
   C. Reflex arc—pathway through the nervous system
      1. Receptor—detects stimulus
      2. Sensory neuron—receptor to CNS
      3. Central neuron—in CNS
      4. Motor neuron—CNS to effector
      5. Effector—muscle or gland that responds

IV. **Spinal cord**
   A. Location of the spinal cord—in vertebral column; ends between first and second lumbar vertebrae
   B. Structure of the spinal cord—H-shaped area of gray matter surrounded by white matter
   C. Functions of the spinal cord
      1. Links spinal nerves to brain
      2. Reflex activities
         a. Reflex—simple, rapid, automatic response using few neurons
         b. Examples—stretch reflex, eye blink, withdrawal reflex
         c. Spinal reflex—coordinated in spinal cord

D. Medical procedures involving the spinal cord
  a. Lumbar puncture
  b. Administration of drugs
E. Disorders involving the spinal cord
  1. Diseases—poliomyelitis, multiple sclerosis, amyotrophic lateral sclerosis
  2. Tumors
  3. Injuries

V. Spinal nerves—31 pairs
A. Location and structure of the spinal nerves
  1. Roots
    a. Sensory (dorsal)
    b. Motor (ventral)
B. Branches of the spinal nerves—plexuses: networks formed by anterior branches
  1. Cervical plexus
  2. Brachial plexus
  3. Lumbosacral plexus
C. Disorders of the spinal nerves—peripheral neuritis, sciatica, herpes zoster

VI. Autonomic nervous system—motor (efferent) division of the visceral (involuntary) nervous system
A. Characteristics of the autonomic nervous system
  1. Involuntary
  2. Controls glands, smooth muscle, heart (cardiac) muscle
B. Divisions of the autonomic nervous system
  1. Sympathetic nervous system
    a. Thoracolumbar
    b. Adrenergic—uses adrenaline
  2. Parasympathetic system
    a. Craniosacral
    b. Cholinergic—uses acetylcholine
C. Functions of the autonomic nervous system
  1. Sympathetic—stimulates fight-or-flight (stress) response
  2. Parasympathetic—returns body to normal
  3. Usually have opposite effects on an organ
D. Disorders of the autonomic nervous system

Questions for Study and Review

1. What is the main function of the nervous system?
2. Name the two structural divisions of the nervous system.
3. Name the organs or structures controlled by the somatic nervous system; by the visceral nervous system.
4. Define the following terms: *neuron, myelin, synapse, ganglion, Schwann cell.*
5. What are neuroglia? Give some examples of their functions.
6. Differentiate between the terms in each of the following pairs:
   a. *axon* and *dendrite*
   b. *gray matter* and *white matter*
   c. *receptor* and *effector*
   d. *afferent* and *efferent*
   e. *sensory* and *motor*
   f. *nerve* and *tract*
7. Without the label, how would you know that the neuron in Figure 9-2 is a motor neuron? Is this neuron a part of the somatic or visceral nervous system?
8. What is a mixed nerve? Give several examples.
9. Describe a nerve impulse. How does conduction along a myelinated fiber differ from conduction along an unmyelinated fiber?
10. What is a synapse? Briefly describe what occurs at a synapse.

11. What are neurotransmitters? Give several examples of neurotransmitters.
12. Name the components of a reflex arc.
13. Locate and describe the spinal cord. Name two of its functions.
14. Describe a reflex. Give several examples of reflexes.
15. Name and describe two spinal cord disorders.
16. Define a spinal nerve. How many pairs of spinal nerves are there?
17. Differentiate between the dorsal and ventral roots of a spinal nerve.
18. Define a *plexus.* Name the three main plexuses of the spinal nerves.
19. Name two disorders of the spinal nerves.
20. What are the functions of the sympathetic part of the ANS, and how do these compare with those of the parasympathetic nervous system?

✔ ANSWERS TO CHECKPOINTS

1. Structurally, the nervous system can be divided into a central and a peripheral nervous system.
2. The somatic nervous system is voluntary and controls skeletal muscle; the autonomic (visceral) nervous system is involuntary and controls involuntary muscles and glands.
3. The nonconducting cells of the nervous system that serve in protection and support are the neuroglia (glial cells).
4. The fiber of the neuron that carries impulses toward the cell body is the dendrite; the fiber that carries impulses away from the cell body is the axon.
5. Myelinated fibers are white, and unmyelinated tissues are gray.
6. Nerves that convey impulses toward the CNS are sensory (afferent) nerves; nerves that convey impulses away from the CNS are motor (efferent) nerves.
7. In the first stage of an action potential, the charge on the membrane reverses and the membrane is described as being depolarized. In the second stage of an action potential, the membrane returns to the resting state and is described as repolarized.
8. All the chemicals used to carry information across the synaptic cleft are neurotransmitters.
9. A reflex arc is a pathway through the nervous system from a stimulus to an effector.
10. In the spinal cord, an H-shaped section of gray matter is located internally, and the white matter is located around it. The gray matter extends in two pairs of columns called dorsal and ventral horns.
11. The spinal cord links the spinal nerves to the brain and coordinates reflexes.
12. There are 31 pairs of spinal nerves.
13. There are two neurons in each motor pathway of the autonomic nervous system.
14. The sympathetic system stimulates a stress response, and the parasympathetic system reverses it.

9

The Nervous System: The Brain and Cranial Nerves

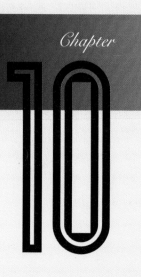

Chapter

10

BEHAVIORAL OBJECTIVES

After careful study of this chapter, you should be able to:

1. Give the location and functions of the four main divisions of the brain

2. Name and locate the three subdivisions of the brain stem

3. Name and describe the three meninges

4. Cite the function of cerebrospinal fluid and describe where and how this fluid is formed

5. Cite one function of the cerebral cortex in each lobe of the cerebrum

6. Cite the names and functions of the 12 cranial nerves

7. Describe several methods used to image the brain

8. List some disorders that involve the brain or the cranial nerves

THE BRAIN AND ITS PROTECTIVE STRUCTURES

Main Parts of the Brain

The brain occupies the cranial cavity and is covered by membranes, fluid, and the bones of the skull. Although the various regions of the brain are in communication and function together, the brain may be divided into distinct areas for ease of study (Fig. 10-1):

- The *cerebrum* (SER-e-brum) is the largest part of the brain. It is divided into right and left *cerebral* (SER-e-bral) *hemispheres* by a deep groove called the *longitudinal fissure.*
- The *diencephalon* (di-en-SEF-ah-lon) is the area between the cerebral hemispheres and the brain stem. It includes the thalamus and the hypothalamus.
- The *brain stem* connects the cerebrum and diencephalon with the spinal cord. The upper portion of the brain stem is the *midbrain.* Below that, and plainly visible from the inferior view of the brain, are the *pons* (ponz) and the *medulla oblongata* (meh-DUL-lah ob-long-GAH-tah). The pons connects the midbrain with the medulla, whereas the medulla connects the brain with the spinal cord through a large opening in the base of the skull (foramen magnum).
- The *cerebellum* (ser-eh-BEL-um) is lo-cated immediately below the back part of the cerebral hemispheres and is connected with the cerebrum, brain stem, and spinal cord by means of the pons. The word *cerebellum* means "little brain."

Each of these divisions is described in greater detail later in this chapter.

✔ CHECKPOINT **1**:

What are the main divisions of the brain?

Coverings of the Brain and Spinal Cord

The *meninges* (men-IN-jez) are three layers of connective tissue that surround both the brain and spinal cord to form a complete enclosure. The outermost of these membranes, the *dura mater* (DU-rah MA-ter), is the thickest and toughest of the meninges. (*Mater* is from the Latin meaning "mother," referring to the protective function of the meninges; *dura* means "hard"). Inside the skull, the dura mater splits in certain places to provide venous channels, called *dural sinuses,* for the drainage of blood coming from the brain tissue.

The middle layer of the meninges is the *arachnoid* (ah-RAK-noyd). This membrane is loosely attached to the deepest of the meninges by web-

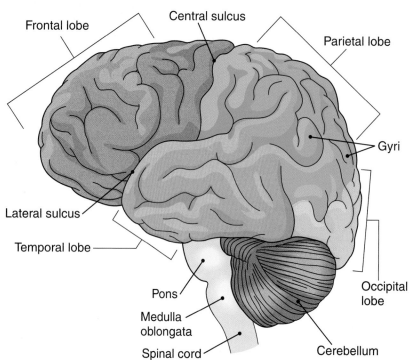

Frontal lobe
Central sulcus
Parietal lobe
Gyri
Lateral sulcus
Temporal lobe
Pons
Medulla oblongata
Spinal cord
Cerebellum
Occipital lobe

FIGURE **10•1** External surface of the brain showing the main parts and some of the lobes and sulci of the cerebrum.

like fibers, allowing a space for the movement of cerebrospinal fluid (CSF) between the two membranes. (*Arachnoid* is from the Latin word for spider because of its weblike appearance).

The innermost layer around the brain, the ***pia mater*** (PI-ah MA-ter), is attached to the nervous tissue of the brain and spinal cord and follows all the contours of these structures (Fig. 10-2). It is made of a delicate connective tissue in which there are many blood vessels (*pia* meaning "tender" or "soft"). The blood supply to the brain is carried, to a large extent, by the pia mater.

Disorders of the Meninges

Meningitis (men-in-JI-tis) is an inflammation of the brain and spinal cord coverings. It may be caused by viruses or by bacteria, including *Neisseria meningitidis, Haemophilus influenzae, Streptococcus pneumoniae,* and *Escherichia coli.* In many cases, an injury, invasive procedure, septicemia, or adjoining infection allows the entry of pathogenic organisms. Diagnosis is by lumbar puncture and examination of the CSF removed. Early treatment with antibiotics can have good results. Untreated cases have a

high death rate. Vaccines are available against some of the bacteria that cause meningitis.

Trauma to the head may cause bleeding between the skull and the brain. Arterial bleeding outside the dura causes an ***epidural hematoma,*** with rapidly progressing symptoms, including coma and dilated pupils. A tear in the wall of a dural sinus causes a ***subdural hematoma,*** with a slow leak and less dramatic symptoms. Frequent observations of level of consciousness, pupil response, and extremity reflexes are important in the patient with a head injury.

✔ CHECKPOINT **2**:
_____

The meninges are protective membranes around the brain and spinal cord. What are the names of the three layers of the meninges from the outermost to the innermost?

Cerebrospinal Fluid

Cerebrospinal (ser-e-bro-SPI-nal) ***fluid*** is a clear liquid that circulates in and around the brain and spinal cord (Fig. 10-3). The function

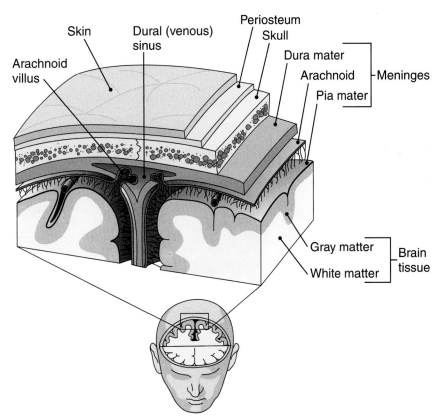

FIGURE **10•2** Frontal (coronal) section of the top of the head showing meninges and related parts.

of the CSF is to support nervous tissue and to cushion shocks that would otherwise injure these delicate structures. This fluid also carries nutrients to the cells and transports waste products from the cells.

CSF flows freely through the brain and spinal cord and finally flows out into the subarachnoid space of the meninges. Much of the fluid is then returned to the blood through projections called *arachnoid villi* in the dural sinuses.

Ventricles

CSF is formed in four spaces within the brain called *ventricles* (VEN-trih-klz) (Fig. 10-4). A vascular network in each ventricle, the *choroid* (KOR-oyd) *plexus,* forms CSF by filtration of the blood and by cellular secretion.

The four ventricles that produce CSF extend somewhat irregularly into the various parts of the brain. The largest are the lateral ventricles in the two cerebral hemispheres. Their extensions into the lobes of the cerebrum are called *horns.* These paired ventricles communicate with a midline space, the third ventricle, by

means of openings called *foramina* (fo-RAM-in-ah). The third ventricle is surrounded by the diencephalon. Continuing down from the third ventricle, a small canal, called the *cerebral aqueduct,* extends through the midbrain into the fourth ventricle, which is located between the brain stem and the cerebellum. This ventricle is continuous with the central canal of the spinal cord. In the roof of the fourth ventricle are three openings that allow the escape of CSF to the area that surrounds the brain and spinal cord.

> 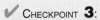 CHECKPOINT **3**:
>
> In addition to the meninges, CSF helps to support and protect the brain and spinal cord. Where is CSF produced?

Hydrocephalus

Any obstruction to the flow of CSF, for example, in injury to the membranes around the three exit openings, may cause the condition called *hydrocephalus* (hi-dro-SEF-ah-lus). As the fluid accu-

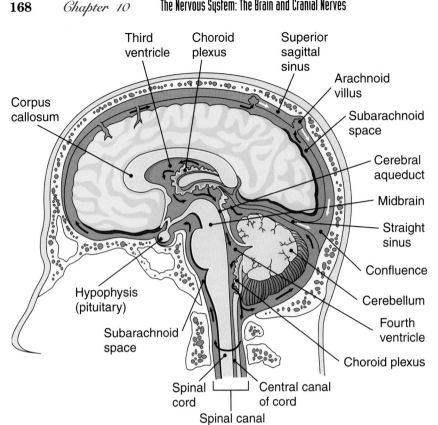

Figure **10•3** Flow of CSF from choroid plexuses back to the blood in dural sinuses is shown by the black arrows; flow of blood is shown by the white arrows.

mulates, the mounting pressure can squeeze the brain against the skull and destroy brain tissue.

Hydrocephalus is more common in infants than in adults. Because the fontanels of the skull have not closed in the infant, the cranium itself can become greatly enlarged. In contrast, in the adult, cranial enlargement cannot occur, so that even a slight increase in fluid results in symptoms of increased pressure within the skull and damage to brain tissue. Treatment of hydrocephalus involves the creation of a shunt to drain excess CSF from the brain.

DIVISIONS OF THE BRAIN

Cerebral Hemispheres

Each cerebral hemisphere is divided into four visible *lobes* named for the overlying cranial bones. These are the frontal, parietal, temporal, and occipital lobes (see Fig. 10-1). In addition, there is a small fifth lobe deep within each hemisphere that cannot be seen from the surface. Not much is known about this lobe, which is called the *insula.*

The outer nervous tissue of the cerebral hemispheres is gray matter that makes up the *cerebral cortex.* This thin layer of gray matter is the most highly evolved portion of the brain and is responsible for conscious thought, reasoning, and abstract mental functions. Specific functions are localized in the cortex of the different lobes, as described in greater detail later.

The cortex is arranged in folds forming elevated portions known as *gyri* (JI-ri), which are separated by shallow grooves called *sulci* (SUL-si) (see Fig. 10-1). Although there are many sulci, the following two are especially important landmarks:

- The *central sulcus,* which lies between the frontal and parietal lobes of each hemisphere at right angles to the longitudinal fissure
- The *lateral sulcus,* which curves along

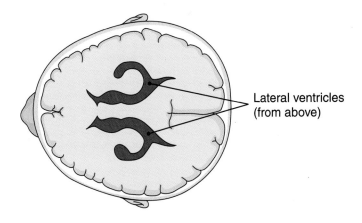

Lateral ventricles
(from above)

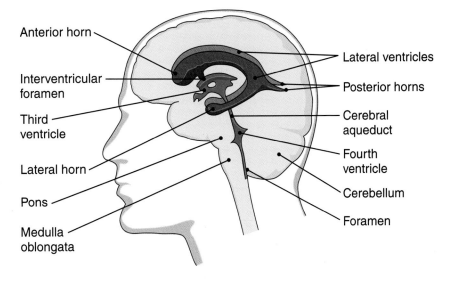

Anterior horn

Interventricular
foramen

Third
ventricle

Lateral horn

Pons

Medulla
oblongata

Lateral ventricles

Posterior horns

Cerebral
aqueduct

Fourth
ventricle

Cerebellum

Foramen

10

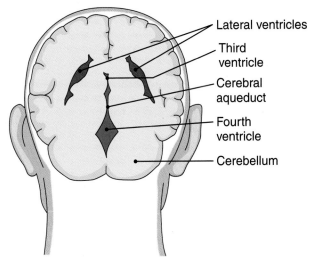

Lateral ventricles

Third
ventricle

Cerebral
aqueduct

Fourth
ventricle

Cerebellum

Figure **10•4**   Ventricles of the
brain seen from three views.

the side of each hemisphere and separates the temporal lobe from the frontal and parietal lobes (see Fig. 10-1)

Internally, the cerebral hemispheres are made largely of white matter and a few islands of gray matter. The white matter consists of myelinated fibers that connect the cortical areas with each other and with other parts of the nervous system.

An important band of white matter is the **corpus callosum** located at the bottom of the longitudinal fissure (see Fig. 10-3). This band acts as a bridge between the right and left hemispheres, permitting impulses to cross from one side of the brain to the other.

The **internal capsule** is a crowded strip of white matter composed of many myelinated fibers (forming tracts).

Basal ganglia are masses of gray matter located deep within each cerebral hemisphere. These groups of neurons help regulate body movement and facial expressions communicated from the cerebral cortex. The neurotransmitter **dopamine** (DO-pah-mene) is secreted by the neurons of the basal ganglia.

Functions of the Cerebral Cortex

It is within the cerebral cortex, the layer of gray matter that forms the surface of each cerebral hemisphere, that impulses are received and analyzed. These activities form the basis of knowledge. The brain "stores" information, much of which can be recalled on demand by means of the phenomenon called *memory*. It is in the cerebral cortex that thought processes such as association, judgment, and discrimination take place. Conscious deliberation and voluntary actions also arise from the cerebral cortex.

Although the various areas of the brain act in coordination to produce behavior, particular functions are localized in the cortex of each lobe. Some of these are described below:

- The **frontal lobe,** which is relatively larger in humans than in any other organism, lies in front of the central sulcus. This lobe contains the motor area, which directs movement (Fig. 10-5). Because of the way in which motor fibers cross to opposite sides in the central nervous system, the left

side of the brain governs the right side of the body, and the right side of the brain governs the left side of the body. The frontal lobe also contains two areas important in speech (the speech centers are discussed later).

- The **parietal lobe** occupies the upper part of each hemisphere and lies just behind the central sulcus. This lobe contains the **sensory area,** in which impulses from the skin, such as touch, pain, and temperature, are interpreted. The estimation of distances, sizes, and shapes also take place here.

- The **temporal lobe** lies below the lateral sulcus and folds under the hemisphere on each side. This lobe contains the **auditory area** for receiving and interpreting impulses from the ear. The **olfactory area,** concerned with the sense of smell, is located in the medial part of the temporal lobe; it is stimulated by impulses arising from receptors in the nose.

- The **occipital lobe** lies behind the parietal lobe and extends over the cerebellum. This lobe contains the **visual area** for interpreting impulses arising from the retina of the eye.

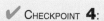

✔ CHECKPOINT **4**:

Higher functions of the brain occur in a thin layer of gray matter on the surface of the cerebral hemispheres. What is the name of this outer layer of gray matter?

Communication Areas

The ability to communicate by written and verbal means is an interesting example of the way in which areas of the cerebral cortex are interrelated (Fig. 10-6). The development and use of these areas are closely connected with the process of learning.

- The **auditory areas** are located in the temporal lobe. In one of these areas, sound impulses transmitted from the environment are detected, whereas in the surrounding area (auditory association area), the sounds are interpreted and understood. The beginnings of language are learned by

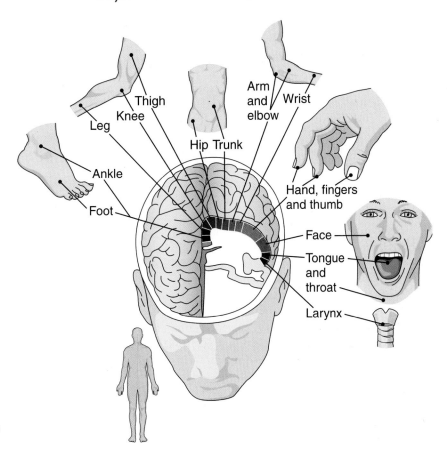

FIGURE **10•5** Motor areas of the cerebral cortex (frontal lobe).

10

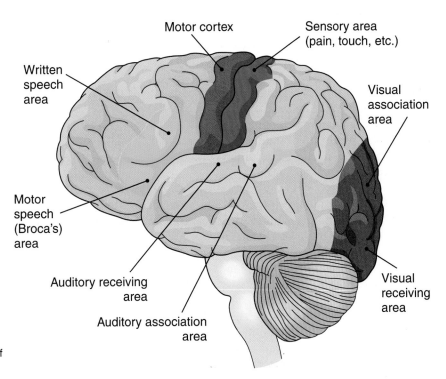

FIGURE **10•6** Functional areas of the cerebral cortex.

auditory means; thus, the auditory area for understanding sounds is near the auditory receiving area of the cortex. Babies often appear to understand what is being said long before they do any talking themselves. It is usually several years before children learn to read or write words.

- The **motor areas** for communication by speech and writing are located in front of the lowest part of the motor cortex in the frontal lobe. Because the lower part of the motor cortex controls the muscles of the head and neck, it seems logical to think of the motor speech center as an extension forward in this area. The muscles of speech (in the tongue, the soft palate, and the larynx) are controlled here, in a region named **Broca's** (bro-KAHZ) **area**, after its discoverer. A person who suffers damage to this area, as by a stroke, may have difficulty in producing speech (motor aphasia). Similarly, the written speech center is located in front of the cortical area that controls the muscles of the arm and hand. The ability to write words is usually one of the last phases in the development of learning words and their meanings.

- The **visual areas** of the cortex in the occipital lobe are also involved in communication. Here, visual images of language are received. These visual impulses are then interpreted as words in the visual area that lies in front of the receiving cortex. The ability to read with understanding is also developed in this area. You might *see* writing in the Japanese language, for example, but this would involve only the visual receiving area in the occipital lobe unless you could also *read* the words.

There is a functional relation among areas of the brain. Many neurons must work together to enable a person to receive, interpret, and respond to verbal and written messages as well as to touch (tactile stimulus) and other sensory stimuli.

Memory and the Learning Process

Memory is the mental faculty for recalling ideas. In the initial stage of the memory process, sensory signals (*e.g.,* visual, auditory)

are retained for a very short time, perhaps only fractions of a second. Nevertheless, they can be used for further processing. **Short-term memory** refers to the retention of bits of information for a few seconds or perhaps a few minutes, after which the information is lost unless reinforced. **Long-term memory** refers to the storage of information that can be recalled at a later time. There is a tendency for a memory to become more fixed the more often a person repeats the remembered experience; thus, short-term memory signals can lead to long-term memories. Furthermore, the more often a memory is recalled, the more indelible it becomes; such a memory can be so deeply fixed in the brain that it can be recalled immediately.

Careful anatomic studies have shown that tiny extensions called *fibrils* form at the synapses in the cerebral cortex, so that impulses can travel more easily from one neuron to another. The number of these fibrils increases with age. Physiologic studies show that rehearsal (repetition) of the same information again and again accelerates and potentiates the degree of transfer of short-term memory into long-term memory. A person who is wide awake memorizes far better than does a person who is in a state of mental fatigue. It has also been noted that the brain is able to organize information so that new ideas are stored in the same areas in which similar ones had been stored before.

To learn about preventing damage to the brain and loss of memory, read about preventing concussion in Watch Your Head!

The Diencephalon

The **diencephalon,** or interbrain, is located between the cerebral hemispheres and the brain stem. It can be seen by cutting into the central section of the brain. The **thalamus** (THAL-ahmus) and the **hypothalamus** are included in the diencephalon (Fig. 10-7).

The two parts of the thalamus form the lateral walls of the third ventricle. Nearly all sensory impulses travel through the masses of gray matter that form the thalamus. The role of the thalamus is to sort out the impulses and direct them to particular areas of the cerebral cortex.

The hypothalamus is located in the midline

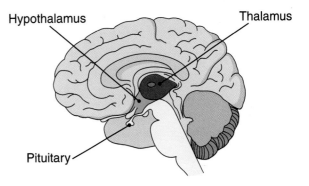

Hypothalamus Thalamus

Pituitary

FIGURE **10•7** Diagram showing the relationship among the thalamus, hypothalamus, and pituitary (hypophysis).

Watch Your Head!

Closed head injury (CHI) is the leading cause of death due to neurologic illness or injury for people under 50 years of age. Damage to brain tissues occurs either from penetrating trauma of the head or from acceleration–deceleration events where a head in motion suddenly comes to a stop. Nervous tissue, blood vessels, and possibly the meninges may be bruised, torn, lacerated, or ruptured. Depending upon the degree and type of tissue damage, the patient may be said to have suffered a concussion, cerebral contusion, or cerebral laceration along with edema. Recovery from a concussion is usually complete, with no longstanding effects. However, recovery from a significant contusion or a laceration with edema is a serious challenge. Mortality rates in these more severe injuries approach 50%; treatment is usually supportive in nature and may do little to change the outcome. The most unfortunate fact regarding CHIs is that they are largely preventable.

Any head injury may be lessened, if not prevented, by taking a few precautions.

- Whenever riding in a moving vehicle, wear both the lap and shoulder belts, and adjust the headrest to sit directly behind the back of your skull.
- Whenever you participate in outside sports or activities, wear a safety helmet. Young children are especially vulnerable since their skulls may not be completely fused and calcified at the time of injury.
- Children should never be swung around to play "airplane" nor should they ever be vigorously bounced or shaken.

Although treatment of CHIs has advanced in recent years, prevention is still the best weapon we have against these potentially serious and fatal injuries.

pothalamus, as is the pituitary gland. The hypothalamus thus influences the heartbeat, the contraction and relaxation of the walls of blood vessels, hormone secretion, and other vital body functions.

To learn more about the function of sleep, see Sleep.

✔ CHECKPOINT **5**:

What are the two main portions of the diencephalon and what do they do?

The Limbic System

Along the border between the cerebrum and the diencephalon is a region known as the *limbic system.* This system is involved in emotional states and behavior. It includes the *hippocampus* (shaped like a sea horse), located under the lateral ventricles, which functions in learning and the formation of long-term memory. It also includes regions that stimulate the *reticular formation,* a network that extends along the brain stem and governs wakefulness and sleep. The limbic system thus links the conscious functions of the cerebral cortex and the automatic functions of the brain stem.

The Brain Stem

The brain stem is composed of the midbrain, the pons, and the medulla oblongata. These structures connect the cerebrum and diencephalon with the spinal cord.

area below the thalamus and forms the floor of the third ventricle. It helps to maintain homeostasis by controlling body temperature, water balance, sleep, appetite, and some emotions, such as fear and pleasure. Both the sympathetic and parasympathetic divisions of the autonomic nervous system are under the control of the hy-

Sleep

Although everybody does it, there are still many mysteries about how, why, and when we sleep. Study of brain waves with the electroencephalograph has shown that sleep occurs in two phases. One of these, rapid-eye-movement (REM) sleep, is associated with dreaming.

As we descend from drowsiness into deep sleep, we progress through a non–rapid-eye-movement (NREM) phase. Although all the triggers for falling asleep are not known, a major factor is the amount of light received through the eyes. This signals the hypothalamus to regulate sleep–wake cycles. About 1 to 1½ hours after falling asleep, short periods of REM sleep with dreaming occur. These then alternate with NREM sleep at intervals of about 90 minutes. Extreme fatigue and sedatives decrease the amount of REM sleep in favor of deep NREM sleep. Also, infants have a much greater percentage of REM sleep; this declines with age.

Sleep rests the body, improves learning, and strengthens the immune system. There is also evidence that REM sleep helps the brain to sort memories.

The Midbrain

The **midbrain,** located below the center of the cerebrum, forms the forward part of the brain stem. Four rounded masses of gray matter that are hidden by the cerebral hemispheres form the upper part of the midbrain; these four bodies act as relay centers for certain eye and ear reflexes. The white matter at the front of the midbrain conducts impulses between the higher centers of the cerebrum and the lower centers of the pons, medulla, cerebellum, and spinal cord. Cranial nerves III and IV originate from the midbrain.

The Pons

The **pons** lies between the midbrain and the medulla, in front of the cerebellum (see Fig. 10-1). It is composed largely of myelinated nerve fibers, which serve to connect the two halves of the cerebellum with the brain stem as well as with the cerebrum above and the spinal cord below.

The pons is an important connecting link between the cerebellum and the rest of the nervous system, and it contains nerve fibers that carry impulses to and from the centers located above and below it. Certain reflex (involuntary) actions, such as some of those regulating respiration, are integrated in the pons. Cranial nerves V through VIII originate from the pons.

The Medulla Oblongata

The **medulla oblongata** of the brain is located between the pons and the spinal cord (see Fig. 10-1). It appears white externally because, like the pons, it contains many myelinated nerve fibers. Internally, it contains collections of cell bodies (gray matter) called **nuclei,** or *centers.* Among these are vital centers, such as the following:

- The **respiratory center** controls the muscles of respiration in response to chemical and other stimuli.
- The **cardiac center** helps regulate the rate and force of the heartbeat.
- The **vasomotor** (vas-o-MO-tor) **center** regulates the contraction of smooth muscle in the blood vessel walls and thus controls blood flow and blood pressure.

The ascending sensory fibers that carry messages through the spinal cord up to the brain travel through the medulla, as do descending motor fibers. These groups of fibers form tracts (bundles) and are grouped together according to function.

The motor fibers from the motor cortex of the cerebral hemispheres extend down through the medulla, and most of them cross from one side to the other (decussate) while going through this part of the brain. It is the crossing of motor fibers in the medulla that causes the right cerebral hemisphere to control muscles in the left side of the body and the left cerebral hemisphere to control muscles in the right side of the body, a characteristic termed *contralateral* (opposite side) *control.*

The medulla is an important reflex center; here, certain neurons end, and impulses are relayed to other neurons. The last four pairs of cranial nerves (IX through XII) are connected with the medulla.

✔ CHECKPOINT **6**:

What are the three subdivisions of the brain stem?

✔ CHECKPOINT **7**:

What are some functions of the cerebellum?

The Cerebellum

The *cerebellum* is made up of three parts: the middle portion (vermis) and two lateral hemispheres. Like the cerebral hemispheres, the cerebellum has an outer area of gray matter and an inner portion that is largely white matter. The functions of the cerebellum are as follows:

- To aid in the *coordination of voluntary muscles* so that they will function smoothly and in an orderly fashion. Disease of the cerebellum causes muscular jerkiness and tremors.
- To aid in the *maintenance of balance* in standing, walking, and sitting as well as during more strenuous activities. Messages from the internal ear and from sensory receptors in tendons and muscles aid the cerebellum.
- To aid in the *maintenance of muscle tone* so that all muscle fibers are slightly tensed and ready to produce necessary changes in position as quickly as may be necessary.

BRAIN STUDIES

Imaging the Brain

A major tool for clinical study of the brain is the *CT* (computed tomography) *scan,* which provides multiple x-ray pictures taken from different angles simultaneously. By means of a computer, the information is organized and displayed as photographs of the bone, soft tissue, and cavities of the brain (Fig. 10-8). Anatomic lesions, such as tumors or scar tissue accumulations, are readily seen.

MRI (magnetic resonance imaging) gives even clearer pictures of the brain without the use of dyes or x-rays. The method is based on computerized interpretation of the movements of atomic nuclei following their exposure to radio waves within a powerful magnetic field. Although MRI is more expensive and takes longer than CT imaging, it gives more views of the brain and may reveal tumors, scar tissue, and hemorrhaging not shown by CT.

With *PET* (positron emission tomography) one

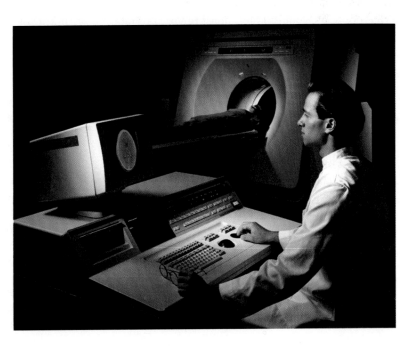

FIGURE **10•8** CT scanner. (Photograph courtesy of Philips Medical Systems)

can actually visualize the brain in action. With this method, a radioactively labeled substance (*e.g.,* glucose) is followed as it moves through the brain. As tasks are performed, regions of the cortex that are involved become "hot."

The Electroencephalograph

The interactions of the billions of nerve cells in the brain give rise to measurable electric currents. These may be recorded by an instrument called the ***electroencephalograph*** (e-lek-tro-en-SEF-ah-lo-graf). The recorded tracings or brain waves produce an electroencephalogram (EEG).

DISORDERS OF THE BRAIN

Stroke, or ***cerebrovascular*** (ser-e-bro-VAS-ku-lar) ***accident*** (CVA), is by far the most common kind of brain disorder. The most common cause of stroke is a blood clot that blocks the flow of blood to an area of brain tissue. Another frequent cause is the rupture of a blood vessel resulting in ***cerebral hemorrhage*** and destruction of brain tissue. Stroke is most common among people older than 40 years of age and those with arterial wall damage, diabetes, or high blood pressure. Restoring blood flow to the affected area can reduce long-term damage. This can be done surgically or by administration of clot-dissolving medication, usually followed by medication to reduce brain swelling and minimize further damage.

The effect of a stroke depends on the location of the artery and the extent of the involvement. Damage of the white matter of the internal capsule in the lower part of the cerebrum may cause extensive paralysis of the side opposite the affected area. Such a paralysis is called ***hemiplegia*** (hem-e-PLE-je-ah), and the paralyzed person is described as ***hemiplegic*** (hem-e-PLE-jik).

One possible aftereffect of stroke or other injury to the brain is ***aphasia*** (ah-FA-ze-ah), a loss or defect in language communication. There may be a loss of the ability to speak or write (expressive aphasia) or a loss of understanding of written or spoken language (receptive aphasia). The type of aphasia present depends on what part of the brain is affected. The lesion that causes aphasia in the right-handed person is likely to be in the left cerebral hemisphere.

Often, much can be done for stroke victims by patient retraining and much understanding. The brain has tremendous reserves for adapting itself to different conditions. In many cases, some means of communication can be found even though speech areas are damaged.

Cerebral palsy (PAWL-ze) is a disorder caused by brain damage occurring before or during the birth process. It is characterized by diverse muscular disorders varying in degree: it may consist of only slight weakness of the lower extremity muscles or, at the other extreme, of paralysis of all four extremities as well as the speech muscles. With muscle and speech training and other therapeutic approaches, children with cerebral palsy can be helped.

Epilepsy is a chronic disorder involving an abnormality of the electric activity of the brain with or without apparent changes in the nervous tissues. One manifestation of epilepsy is seizure activity, which may be so mild that it is hardly noticeable or so severe that it results in loss of consciousness. In most cases, the cause is not known. The study of brain waves on an EEG usually shows abnormalities and is helpful in both diagnosis and treatment. Many people with epilepsy can lead normal, active lives with appropriate medical treatment.

Tumors of the brain may develop in people of any age but are somewhat more common in young and middle-aged adults than in other groups. Most brain tumors originate from the neuroglia (connective tissue of the brain) and are called ***gliomas.*** The symptoms produced depend on the type of tumor, its location, its destructiveness, and the degree to which it compresses the brain tissue. Involvement of the frontal portion of the cerebrum often causes mental symptoms, such as changes in personality and in levels of consciousness. Early surgery, chemotherapy, and radiation therapy offer hope of cure in some cases.

Inflammation of the brain is termed ***encephalitis*** (en-sef-ah-LI-tis), based on the scientific name for the brain, which is *encephalon*. There are many causes of such disease, including viruses transmitted by insects or ticks. The

Prozac and Other Psychoactive Drugs

Prozac (chemical name, fluoxetine) and related compounds are among the newest in a long line of chemicals that have an effect on the brain. Many of the psychoactive drugs in use today operate by affecting the levels and activities of neurotransmitters. Specifically, Prozac increases the activity of serotonin in the brain by blocking the membrane transporters that carry the neurotransmitter back into the presynaptic cell at the synapse. Like other "reuptake" inhibitors, Prozac causes the neurotransmitter to remain active at the synapse for a longer period, and this translates into a mood-elevating effect.

Prozac is widely used to treat depression, but because of its minimal side effects, it is also used to treat much less serious disorders, such as anxiety attacks, feelings of inadequacy, and the repetitive behavior of obsessive-compulsive disorder.

Why these drugs have the effects that they do is still in question. Also unknown is why they require 2 to 4 weeks to take effect. They may, however, shed some light on the chemical nature of psychiatric problems and their biologic basis.

invasion of brain tissue by lymphocytes (white blood cells) is accompanied by swelling of the brain and diffuse nerve cell destruction. Typical symptoms include fever, vomiting, and coma.

Degenerative Diseases

Alzheimer's (ALZ-hi-merz) *disease* is a disorder of the brain resulting from an unexplained degeneration of the cerebral cortex and hippocampus. The disorder develops gradually and eventually causes severe intellectual impairment with mood changes and confusion. Memory loss, especially for recent events, is a common early symptom. Changes in the brain occur many years before noticeable signs of the disease appear. These changes include the development of amyloid, an abnormal protein, and a tangling of neuron fibers that prevents communication between cells. At present, there is no cure, but a number of drugs have been developed that can delay the progression of early disease. It has been shown that in some groups, the hormone estrogen, vitamin E, and anti-inflammatory drugs have shown some promise of delaying the onset of Alzheimer's disease.

Multi-infarct dementia represents the accumulation of brain damage due to chronic ischemia (lack of blood supply), such as would be caused by a series of small strokes. There is a stepwise deterioration of function. People with multi-infarct dementia are troubled by progressive loss of memory, judgment, and cognitive function. Many people older than 80 years of age have some evidence of this disorder.

Parkinson's disease is a progressive neurologic condition characterized by tremors, rigidity of limbs and joints, slow movement, and impaired balance. The disease arises from cell death in a part of the brain (substantia nigra) that produces the neurotransmitter dopamine. The average age of onset is 55 years.

The main therapy for Parkinson's disease is administration of L-dopa, a substance that is capable of entering the brain and converting to dopamine. Drugs are now available that mimic the effects of dopamine or increase the effectiveness of L-dopa. Other approaches to treatment include implanting fetal cells that can do the job of the missing cells and implanting a device that electrically stimulates the brain to control symptoms of Parkinson's disease.

To learn more about psychoactive medications, see Prozac and Other Psychoactive Drugs.

✔ CHECKPOINT **8**:

Aphasia is a possible result of stroke or other injury to the brain. What is aphasia?

CRANIAL NERVES

Location of the Cranial Nerves

There are 12 pairs of cranial nerves (in this discussion, when a cranial nerve is identified, a pair is meant). They are numbered, usually in Roman numerals, according to their connection with the brain, beginning at the front and proceeding back (Fig. 10-9). Except for the first two

10

10

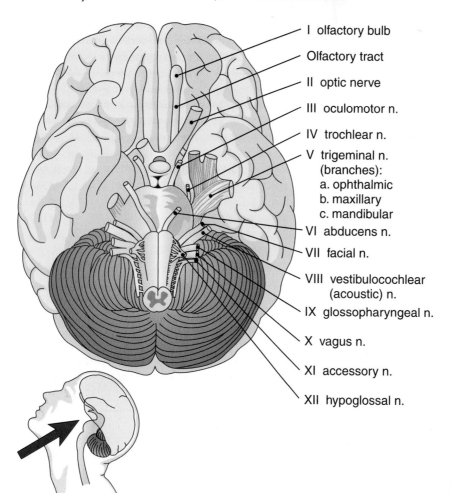

I olfactory bulb

Olfactory tract

II optic nerve

III oculomotor n.

IV trochlear n.

V trigeminal n.
(branches):
a. ophthalmic
b. maxillary
c. mandibular

VI abducens n.

VII facial n.

VIII vestibulocochlear
(acoustic) n.

IX glossopharyngeal n.

X vagus n.

XI accessory n.

XII hypoglossal n.

FIGURE **10•9** Base of the brain showing cranial nerves.

pairs, all the cranial nerves arise from the brain stem. The first 9 pairs and the 12th pair supply structures in the head.

General Functions of the Cranial Nerves

From a functional point of view, we may think of the kinds of messages the cranial nerves handle as belonging to one of four categories:

- *Special sensory impulses,* such as those for smell, taste, vision, and hearing
- *General sensory impulses,* such as those for pain, touch, temperature, deep muscle sense, pressure, and vibrations
- *Somatic motor impulses* resulting in voluntary control of skeletal muscles
- *Visceral motor impulses* producing invol-

untary control of glands and involuntary muscles (cardiac muscle and smooth muscle). These motor pathways are part of the autonomic nervous system, parasympathetic division.

Names and Functions of the Cranial Nerves

A few of the cranial nerves (I, II, and VIII) contain only sensory fibers; some (III, IV, VI, XI, and XII) contain all or mostly motor fibers. The remainder (V, VII, IX, and X) contain both sensory and motor fibers; they are known as *mixed nerves.* All 12 nerves are listed below:

I. The *olfactory nerve* carries smell impulses from receptors in the nasal mucosa to the brain.

II. The ***optic nerve*** carries visual impulses from the eye to the brain.

III. The ***oculomotor nerve*** is concerned with the contraction of most of the eye muscles.

IV. The ***trochlear*** (TROK-le-ar) ***nerve*** supplies one eyeball muscle.

V. The ***trigeminal*** (tri-JEM-in-al) ***nerve*** is the great sensory nerve of the face and head. It has three branches that transport general sense impulses (*e.g.,* pain, touch, temperature) from the eye, the upper jaw, and the lower jaw. The third branch is joined by motor fibers to the muscles of mastication (chewing).

VI. The ***abducens*** (ab-DU-senz) ***nerve*** is another nerve sending controlling impulses to an eyeball muscle.

VII. The ***facial nerve*** is largely motor. The muscles of facial expression are all supplied by branches from the facial nerve. This nerve also includes special sensory fibers for taste (anterior two thirds of the tongue), and it contains secretory fibers to the smaller salivary glands (the submandibular and sublingual) and to the lacrimal (tear) gland.

VIII. The ***vestibulocochlear*** (ves-tib-u-lo-KOK-le-ar) ***nerve*** carries sensory impulses for hearing and for equilibrium from the inner ear. This nerve was formerly called the *auditory* or *acoustic nerve.*

IX. The ***glossopharyngeal*** (glos-o-fah-RIN-ge-al) ***nerve*** contains general sensory fibers from the back of the tongue and the pharynx (throat). This nerve also contains sensory fibers for taste from the posterior third of the tongue, secretory fibers that supply the largest salivary gland (parotid), and motor nerve fibers to control the swallowing muscles in the pharynx.

X. The ***vagus*** (VA-gus) ***nerve*** is the longest cranial nerve. (Its name means "wanderer.") It supplies most of the organs in the thoracic and abdominal cavities. This nerve also contains motor fibers to the larynx (voice box) and pharynx and to glands that produce digestive juices and other secretions.

XI. The ***accessory nerve*** (formerly called the *spinal accessory nerve*) is a motor nerve with two branches. One branch controls two muscles of the neck, the trapezius and sternocleidomastoid; the other supplies muscles of the larynx.

XII. The ***hypoglossal nerve,*** the last of the 12 cranial nerves, carries impulses controlling the muscles of the tongue.

✔ CHECKPOINT **9**: _____

How many pairs of cranial nerves are there?

✔ CHECKPOINT **10**: _____

The cranial nerves are classified as being sensory, motor, or mixed. What is a mixed nerve?

Disorders Involving the Cranial Nerves

Destruction of optic nerve (II) fibers may result from increased pressure of the eye fluid on the nerves, as occurs in glaucoma, from the effect of poisons, and from some infections. Certain medications, when used in high doses for a long period of time, can damage the branch of the vestibulocochlear nerve responsible for hearing.

Injury to a nerve that contains motor fibers causes paralysis of the muscles supplied by these fibers. The oculomotor nerve (III) may be damaged by certain infections or various poisonous substances. Because this nerve supplies so many muscles connected with the eye, including the levator, which raises the eyelid, injury to it causes a paralysis that usually interferes with eye function.

Bell's palsy is a facial paralysis caused by damage to the facial nerve (VII), usually on one side of the face. This injury results in distortion of the face because of one-sided paralysis of the muscles of facial expression.

Neuralgia (nu-RAL-je-ah) in general means "nerve pain." A severe spasmodic pain affecting the fifth cranial nerve is known as ***trigeminal neuralgia*** or ***tic douloureux*** (tik du-lu-RU). At first, the pain comes at relatively long intervals, but as time goes on, it is likely to appear at shorter intervals and to be of longer duration. Treatments include microsurgery and high-frequency current.

10

AGING OF THE NERVOUS SYSTEM

The nervous system is one of the first systems to develop in the embryo. By the beginning of the third week of development, the rudiments of the central nervous system have appeared.

Beginning with maturity, the nervous system begins to undergo changes. The brain begins to decrease in size and weight due to a loss of cells, especially in the cerebral cortex. These losses are accompanied by a decrease in synapses and in neurotransmitters. The speed of processing information decreases, and movements are slowed. Memory diminishes, especially for recent events. Changes in the vascular system throughout the body with a narrowing of the arteries (atherosclerosis) reduce blood flow to the brain. Degeneration of vessels increases the likelihood of stroke.

Despite this depressing news, the nervous system, like other body systems, has vast reserves. Changes vary from person to person in location and severity, and most elderly people are able to cope with life's demands.

10

Summary

I. **The brain and its protective structures**
  A. Main parts of the brain—cerebrum, diencephalon, brain stem, cerebellum
  B. Coverings of the brain and spinal cord
    1. Meninges
      a. Dura mater—tough outermost layer
      b. Arachnoid—weblike middle layer
      c. Pia mater—vascular innermost layer
    2. Meningitis—inflammation of the meninges
  C. Cerebrospinal fluid (CSF)
    1. Circulates around and within brain and spinal cord
    2. Cushions and protects
    3. Ventricles—four spaces within brain where CSF is produced
      a. Choroid plexus—vascular network in ventricle that produces CSF
    4. Hydrocephalus—accumulation of CSF

II. **Divisions of the brain**
  A. Cerebral hemispheres
    1. Lobes—frontal, parietal, temporal, occipital, insula
    2. Cortex—outer layer of gray matter
      a. Functions—interpretation, memory, conscious thought, judgment, voluntary actions
    3. Corpus callosum—connecting band of white matter
  B. Diencephalon—area between cerebral hemispheres and brain stem
    1. Thalamus—directs sensory impulses to cortex
    2. Hypothalamus—maintains homeostasis, controls pituitary
    3. Limbic system
      a. Contains parts of cerebrum and diencephalon
      b. Controls emotion and behavior
  C. Brain stem
    1. Midbrain—involved in eye and ear reflexes
    2. Pons—connecting link for other divisions
    3. Medulla oblongata
      a. Connects with spinal cord
      b. Contains vital centers for respiration, heart rate, vasomotor activity
  D. The cerebellum—regulates coordination, balance, muscle tone

III. **Brain studies**
  A. Imaging the brain
    1. Computed tomography (CT)
    2. Magnetic resonance imaging (MRI)

3. Positron emission tomography (PET)

B. Electroencephalograph (EEG)

IV. Disorders of the brain

1. Cerebrovascular accident (CVA); stroke
   a. Causes—cerebral hemorrhage, blood clot
   b. Effects—paralysis, aphasia
2. Cerebral palsy, epilepsy
3. Tumors
4. Encephalitis—inflammation of the brain

A. Degenerative diseases
1. Alzheimer's disease, multi-infarct dementia, Parkinson's disease

V. Cranial nerves—12 pairs

A. Location of the cranial nerves

B. General functions of the cranial nerves
1. Carry special and general sensory impulses
2. Carry somatic and visceral motor impulses

C. Names and functions of the cranial nerves
1. Sensory (I, II, VIII)
2. Motor (III, IV, VI, XI, XII)
3. Mixed (V, VII, IX, X)

D. Disorders—Bell's palsy, trigeminal neuralgia

VI. Aging of the nervous system

Questions for Study and Review

1. Name and locate the main parts of the brain and briefly describe the main functions of each.
2. Name the covering of the brain and the spinal cord. Name and describe its three layers. What is an infection of this covering called?
3. What is the purpose of the CSF? Where and how is CSF formed? Describe hydrocephalus.
4. Name the four surface lobes of the cerebral hemispheres and describe functions of the cortex in each.
5. Name and describe the communication areas.
6. What are the differences between short-term and long-term memory, and how is each attained?
7. Describe the thalamus. Where is it located? What are its functions?
8. What activities does the hypothalamus regulate?
9. What is the limbic system and what are its functions?
10. Name and locate three divisions of the brain stem.
11. Name and describe six brain disorders.
12. Name four general functions of the cranial nerves.
13. Name and describe the functions of the 12 cranial nerves. What are some disorders of the cranial nerves?

✔ ANSWERS TO CHECKPOINTS

1. The main divisions of the brain are the cerebrum, the diencephalon, the brain stem, and the cerebellum.
2. The three layers of the meninges are the dura mater, the arachnoid, and the pia mater.
3. CSF is produced in the ventricles of the brain. The two lateral ventricles are in the cerebral hemispheres, the third ventricle is in the diencephalon, and the fourth is between the brain stem and the cerebellum.
4. The outer layer of gray matter of the cerebral hemispheres where higher functions occur is the cerebral cortex.
5. The thalamus of the diencephalon directs sensory input to the cerebral cortex; the hypothalamus helps to maintain homeostasis.
6. The three subdivisions of the brain stem are the midbrain, the pons, and the medulla oblongata.
7. The cerebellum aids in coordination of voluntary muscles, maintenance of balance, and maintenance of muscle tone.
8. Aphasia is loss or defect in language communication.
9. There are 12 pairs of cranial nerves.
10. A mixed nerve has both sensory and motor fibers.

The Sensory System

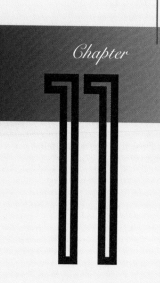

SELECTED KEY TERMS

The following terms are defined in the Glossary:

accommodation

cataract

choroid

cochlea

conjunctiva

convergence

cornea

glaucoma

lacrimal

lens (crystalline lens)

organ of Corti

ossicle

proprioceptor

refraction

retina

sclera

semicircular canal

tympanic membrane

vestibule

vitreous body

BEHAVIORAL OBJECTIVES

After careful study of this chapter, you should be able to:

1. Describe the function of the sensory system

2. Differentiate between the special and general senses and give examples of each

3. Describe the structure of the eye

4. Define *refraction* and list the refractive media of the eye

5. Differentiate between the rods and the cones of the eye

6. Compare the functions of the extrinsic and intrinsic muscles of the eye

7. Describe the nerve supply to the eye

8. List several disorders of the eye

9. Describe the three divisions of the ear

10. Describe the receptors for hearing and for equilibrium with respect to location and function

11. List several disorders of the ear and hearing

THE SENSES

The sensory system serves to protect the individual by detecting changes in the environment. An environmental change becomes a *stimulus* when it initiates a nerve impulse, which then travels to the central nervous system (CNS) by way of a sensory (afferent) neuron. Many stimuli arrive from the external environment and are detected at or near the surface of the body. Others, such as the stimuli from the viscera, originate internally and help to maintain homeostasis.

Receptors

The part of the nervous system that detects a stimulus is the **receptor,** which may be one of the following:

- The free dendrite of a sensory neuron, such as the receptors for pain
- A modified ending, or **end-organ,** on the dendrite of an afferent neuron, such as those for touch and temperature
- A special cell associated with an afferent neuron, such as the rods and cones of the retina of the eye and the receptors in the other special sense organs.

Regardless of the type of stimulus or the type of receptor involved, a stimulus becomes a sensation—something we experience—only when the nerve impulse it generates is interpreted by a specialized area of the cerebral cortex to which it travels.

Special and General Senses

One way of classifying the senses is according to the distribution of the receptors. A **special sense** is localized in a special sense organ; a **general sense** is widely distributed throughout the body.

- *Special senses*
  - *Vision* from receptors in the eye
  - *Hearing* from receptors in the internal ear
  - *Equilibrium* from receptors in the internal ear
  - *Taste* from the tongue receptors
  - *Smell* from receptors in the upper nasal cavities
- *General senses*
  - *Pressure, heat, cold, pain,* and *touch* from the skin and internal organs
  - Sense of *position* from the muscles, tendons, and joints

For more information, see Mechanoreceptors.

Mechanoreceptors

Sensory receptors can be classified according to the stimulus to which they respond. Thermoreceptors, such as those in the skin, detect change in temperature; photoreceptors in the retina of the eye respond to light; and chemoreceptors, such as those for taste and smell, detect chemicals.

Mechanoreceptors respond to movement, such as stretch, pressure, or vibration. The receptors that provide awareness of body position are examples, as are those that monitor stretch and tone of muscle fibers. Pressure and touch receptors in the skin are also mechanoreceptors.

In the ear, the receptors for hearing and equilibrium are mechanoreceptors. Both these receptors function by means of ciliated cells that respond to movement. In the vestibular apparatus, movements of the head trigger impulses that help to regulate balance. In the cochlea, sound waves cause movement of cilia and generate the impulses involved in hearing.

THE EYE AND VISION

Protection of the Eyeball

In the embryo, the eye develops as an outpocketing of the brain. The eye is a delicate organ, and nature has carefully protected it by means of the following structures:

- The skull bones form the walls of the eye orbit (cavity) and serve to protect more than half of the dorsal part of the eyeball.
- The eyelid aids in protecting the front of the eye. The eyelid can be closed to keep harmful materials out of the eye, and blinking helps to lubricate the eye. A muscle, the levator palpebrae, is attached to the upper eyelid. When this muscle contracts, it keeps the eye open. If the muscle becomes weaker with age, the eyelids may droop and interfere with vision, a condition called *ptosis.*
- The eyelashes and eyebrow help to keep foreign matter out of the eye.

- A thin membrane, the ***conjunctiva*** (kon-junk-TI-vah), lines the eyelid and covers the anterior portion of the eyeball.
- Tears, produced by the ***lacrimal*** (LAK-rih-mal) ***glands,*** lubricate the eye, wash away small foreign objects that enter the eye, and contain an enzyme that protects against infection.

The Conjunctiva

The conjunctiva is a thin membrane that lines the inner surface of the eyelid and covers the anterior part of the eyeball up to the edge of the cornea at the center. Cells within the conjunctiva produce mucus that aids in lubricating the eye. As the conjunctiva extends from the eyelid to the front of the eye, a sac is formed. The lower portion of the conjunctival sac can be used to instill drops of medication.

With age, there is often a thinning and drying of the conjunctiva, resulting in inflammation and enlarged blood vessels.

The Lacrimal Apparatus

Tears, produced by the ***lacrimal*** (LAK-rih-mal) ***gland*** (Fig. 11-1), serve to keep the conjunctiva moist. As tears flow across the eye from the lacrimal gland, located in the upper lateral part of the orbit, the fluid carries away small particles that have entered the conjunctival sacs. The tears are then carried into ducts near the nasal corner of the eye where they drain into the nose by way of the ***nasolacrimal*** (na-zo-LAK-rih-mal) ***duct*** (see Fig. 11-1). Any excess

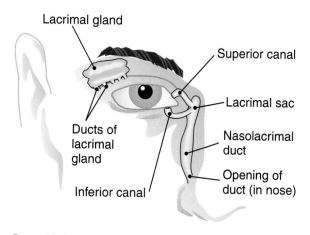

FIGURE **11•1**   Lacrimal apparatus.

of tears causes a "runny nose"; a greater over-production of them results in the spilling of tears onto the cheeks.

With age, the lacrimal gland produces less secretion, but those tears that are produced may overflow to the cheek because of plugging of the nasolacrimal ducts, which would normally carry the tears away from the eye.

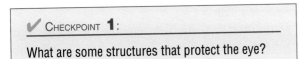

✔ CHECKPOINT **1**:

What are some structures that protect the eye?

Coats of the Eyeball

The eyeball has three separate coats, or tunics (Fig. 11-2). The outermost tunic, called the **sclera** (SKLE-rah), is made of tough connective tissue. It is commonly referred to as the *white of the eye.*

The second tunic of the eyeball is the **choroid** (KO-royd). Composed of a delicate network of connective tissue interlaced with many blood vessels, this coat contains much dark brown pigment. The choroid may be compared to the dull black lining of a camera in that it prevents incoming light rays from scattering and reflecting off the inner surface of the eye. The blood vessels at the back of the eye can reveal signs of disease, and visualization of these vessels with an *ophthalmoscope* (of-THAL-mo-skope) is an important part of a medical examination.

The innermost tunic, the **retina** (RET-ih-nah), is the actual receptor layer of the eye. It contains the light-sensitive cells known as **rods** and **cones,** which generate the nerve impulses associated with the sense of vision.

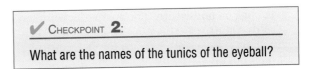

✔ CHECKPOINT **2**:

What are the names of the tunics of the eyeball?

Pathway of Light Rays and Refraction

As light rays pass through the eye toward the retina, they travel through a series of transparent, colorless parts (see Fig. 11-2). On the way, they undergo a process known as **refraction,**

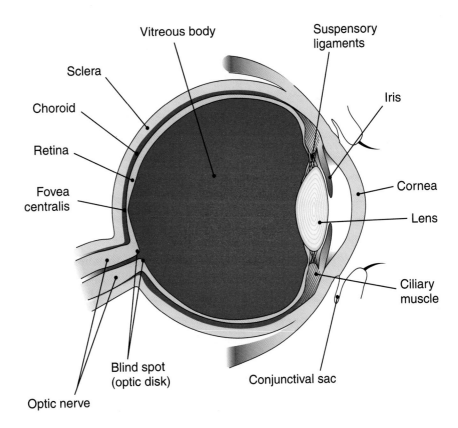

FIGURE **11•2** The eye.

which is the bending of light rays as they pass from one substance to another substance of different density. This refraction of the light rays makes it possible for light from a very large area to be focused on a very small surface, the retina, where the receptors are located. The following are, in order from the outside to the inside, the transparent refracting parts, or *media,* of the eye:

- The *cornea* (KOR-ne-ah) is a forward continuation of the sclera, but it is transparent and colorless, whereas the rest of the sclera is opaque and white. The cornea is referred to frequently as the *window* of the eye. It bulges forward slightly and is the main refracting structure of the eye. The cornea has no blood vessels; it is nourished by the fluids that constantly wash over it.
- The *aqueous* (A-kwe-us) *humor,* a watery fluid that fills much of the eyeball in front of the lens, helps maintain the slight forward curve of the cornea.
- The *lens,* technically called the *crystalline lens,* is a clear, circular structure made of a firm, elastic material. The lens has two bulging surfaces and is thus described as biconvex. The lens is important in light refraction because it is elastic and its thickness can be adjusted to focus light for near or distance vision.
- The *vitreous* (VIT-re-us) *body* is a soft jellylike substance that fills the entire space behind the lens. Like the aqueous humor, it is important in maintaining the shape of the eyeball as well as in aiding in refraction.

Note that the light rays passing through the eye are actually overrefracted so that an image falls on the retina upside down and backward. It is the job of the visual centers of the brain to reverse the images.

✔ CHECKPOINT **3:**

What are the structures that refract light as it passes through the eye?

Function of the Retina

The retina has a complex structure with multiple layers of cells (Fig. 11-3). The deepest layer is a pigmented layer just anterior to the choroid. Next are the rods and cones, the receptor cells of the eye, named for their shape. Details on how these two types of cells differ are presented Table 11-1.

The rods are highly sensitive to light and thus function in dim light, but they do not provide a sharp image. They are more numerous than the cones and are distributed more toward the front of the retina. When you enter into dim light, such as a darkened movie theater, you cannot see for a short period. It is during this time that the rods are beginning to function, a change that is described as *dark adaptation.* When you are able to see again, images are blurred and appear only in shades of gray because the rods are unable to differentiate colors.

The cones function in bright light, are sensitive to color, and give sharp images. The cones are localized at the center of the retina, especially at a point near the optic nerve called the *fovea centralis* (FO-ve-ah sen-TRA-lis). There are three types of cones, each sensitive to either red, green, or blue light. Color blindness results from a lack of cones in the retina. People who completely lack cones are totally color blind; those who lack one type of cone are partially color blind. This disorder, because of its pattern of inheritance, occurs almost exclusively in males.

The rods and cones function by means of pigments that are sensitive to light. The rod pigment is *rhodopsin* (ro-DOP-sin) or visual purple. Manufacture of these pigments requires vitamin A. If vitamin A is lacking in the diet, a person may have difficulty seeing in dim light because there is too little light to activate the rods, a condition termed *night blindness.*

Nerve impulses from the rods and cones flow into sensory neurons that eventually merge to form the optic nerve (cranial nerve II), which connects with the retina at the back of the eye (see Fig. 11-2). The impulses travel to the visual center in the occipital cortex of the brain.

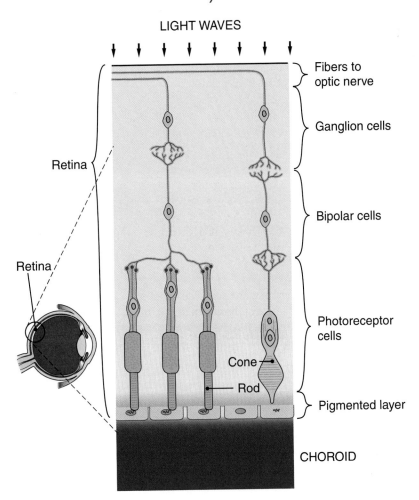

LIGHT WAVES

Fibers to optic nerve

Ganglion cells

Bipolar cells

Photoreceptor cells

Cone

Rod

Pigmented layer

Retina

Retina

CHOROID

FIGURE **11•3** Structure of the retina.

Table 11•1	Comparison of the Rods and Cones of the Retina	
CHARACTERISTIC	RODS	CONES
Shape	Cylindrical	Flask shaped
Number	About 120 million in each retina	About 6 million in each retina
Distribution	Toward the periphery (front) of the retina	Concentrated at the center of the retina
Stimulus	Dim light	Bright light
Visual acuity (sharpness)	Low	High
Pigments	Rhodopsin (visual purple)	Pigments sensitive to red, green, or blue
Color perception	None; shades of gray	Respond to color

The coordinated actions needed for vision are summarized in Table 11-2.

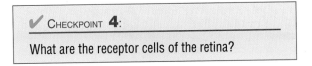

✔ CHECKPOINT **4**:

What are the receptor cells of the retina?

Muscles of the Eye

There are two groups of muscles associated with the eye:

* The voluntary muscles attached to the outer surface of the eyeball are the ***extrinsic*** (eks-TRIN-sik) ***muscles***.
* The involuntary muscles located within the

Table 11•2	Events Needed for Vision

Refraction of light
Adjustment of the pupil by muscles of the iris
Adjustment of the lens by the ciliary muscle (accommodation)
Convergence of the eyes by extrinsic eye muscles
Stimulation of receptor cells (rods and cones) in retina
Transmission of impulses to the brain by means of the optic nerve
Interpretation of impulses in cortex of occipital lobe

eyeball are the ***intrinsic*** (in-TRIN-sik) ***muscles.***

The Extrinsic Muscles

The six ribbonlike extrinsic muscles connected with each eye originate on the bones of the orbit and insert on the surface of the sclera (Fig. 11-4). They are named for their location and the direction of the muscle fibers. These muscles pull on the eyeball in a coordinated fashion so that both eyes center on one visual field. This process of ***convergence*** is necessary to formation of a clear image on the retina. Having the image come from a slightly different angle from each retina is believed to be important for three-dimensional (stereoscopic) vision, a characteristic of primates.

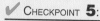
✔ CHECKPOINT **5**:

What is the function of the extrinsic muscles of the eye?

The Intrinsic Muscles

The intrinsic muscles are found in two circular structures within the eye (see Fig. 11-2):

* The ***iris,*** the colored or pigmented part of the eye, is composed of two types of muscles. The size of the central opening of the iris, called the ***pupil,*** is governed by the action of these two sets of muscles, one of which is arranged in a circular fashion, and the other of which extends in a radial manner like the spokes of a wheel.
* The ***ciliary muscle*** is shaped somewhat like a flattened ring with a hole the size of the outer edge of the iris. This muscle alters the shape of the lens during the process of accommodation (described later).

The purpose of the iris is to regulate the amount of light entering the eye. In the presence of bright light, the circular muscle fibers of the iris contract, reducing the size of the pupil. This narrowing is termed *constriction.* In contrast, if the light is dim, the radial muscles contract, and the opening is pulled outward and enlarged. This enlargement of the pupil is known as *dilation.*

The pupil changes size, too, according to whether one is looking at a near object or a distant one. Viewing a near object causes the pupil to become smaller; viewing a distant object causes it to enlarge.

The muscle of the ciliary body is similar in direction and method of action to the radial muscle of the iris. When the ciliary muscle contracts, it draws forward and removes the tension on the ***suspensory ligaments,*** which hold the lens in place (see Fig. 11-2). The elastic lens then recoils and becomes thicker in much the same way that a rubber band thickens when the pull on it is released. When the ciliary

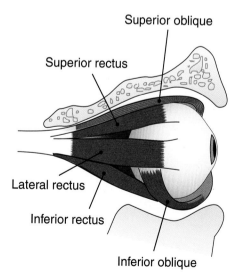

Superior oblique

Superior rectus

Lateral rectus

Inferior rectus

Inferior oblique

FIGURE **11•4** Extrinsic muscles of the eye (medial rectus not shown)

body relaxes, the lens becomes flattened. These actions change the refractive ability of the lens.

The process of ***accommodation*** involves co-ordinated eye changes to enable a person to focus on near objects. The ciliary body contracts, thereby thickening the lens, and the circular muscle fibers of the iris contract to decrease the size of the opening of the pupil. In young people, the lens is elastic, and therefore its thickness can be readily adjusted according to the need for near or distance vision. With aging, the lens loses its elasticity and therefore its ability to adjust to near vision by thickening, making it difficult to focus clearly on close objects. This condition is called ***presbyopia*** (pres-be-O-pe-ah), which literally means "old eye."

✔ CHECKPOINT **6**:

What is the function of the iris?

✔ CHECKPOINT **7**:

What is the function of the ciliary muscle?

Nerve Supply to the Eye

Two sensory nerves supply the eye (Fig. 11-5):

- The ***optic nerve*** (cranial nerve II) carries visual impulses from the retinal rods and cones to the brain.
- The ***ophthalmic*** (of-THAL-mik) ***branch of the trigeminal nerve*** (cranial nerve V) carries impulses of pain, touch, and temperature from the eye and surrounding parts to the brain.

The optic nerve arises from the retina a little toward the medial or nasal side of the eye. There are no retinal rods and cones in the area of the optic nerve. Consequently, no image can form on the retina at this point, which is known as the blind spot or ***optic disk.***

Near the optic disk is the tiny depressed area in the retina known as the fovea centralis, which contains the highest concentration of cones and is the point of sharpest vision (see Fig. 11-2). The fovea is contained within a yellowish spot, the macula. This area may show degenerative changes with age.

There are three nerves that carry motor im-

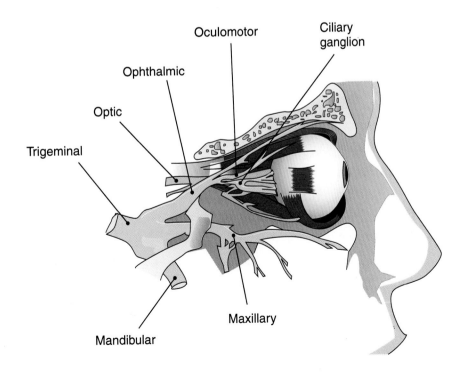

FIGURE **11•5** Nerves of the eye.

pulses to the muscles of the eyeball. The largest is the oculomotor nerve (cranial nerve III), which supplies voluntary and involuntary motor impulses to all the muscles but two. The other two nerves, the trochlear (cranial nerve IV) and the abducens (cranial nerve VI), each supply one voluntary muscle.

✔ CHECKPOINT **8**:

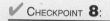

What is cranial nerve II and what does it do?

Eye Disorders

Errors of Refraction

Hyperopia (hi-per-O-pe-ah), or farsightedness, is usually due to an abnormally short eyeball (Fig. 11-6). In this situation, the focal point is behind the retina because light rays cannot bend sharply enough to focus on the retina. Objects must be moved away from the eye to be seen clearly. Farsightedness is normal in the infant but usually corrects itself by the time the child uses the eyes more for near vision. To a certain extent, the ciliary muscle can thicken the lens (accommodate) and thereby enable a

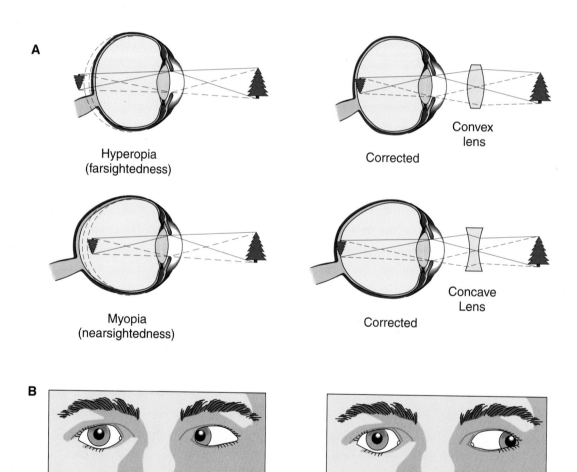

A

Hyperopia
(farsightedness)

Convex
lens

Corrected

Myopia
(nearsightedness)

Concave
Lens

Corrected

B

Convergent strabismus

Divergent strabismus

FIGURE **11•6** Errors of refraction. **(A)** Hyperopia (farsightedness) and myopia (nearsightedness) **(B)** Strabismus.

person to focus objects on the too-near retina. Glasses with convex lenses that increase the refraction of light rays can correct for the visual disturbance.

Myopia (mi-O-pe-ah), or nearsightedness, is another defect of the eye also related to development. In this case, the eyeball is too long or the cornea bends the light rays too sharply, so that the focal point is in front of the retina (see Fig. 11-6). Distant objects appear blurred and may appear clear only if brought near the eye. A concave lens is used to correct for myopia. This alters the angle of refraction so that the focal point is moved backward. Nearsightedness in a young person becomes worse each year until the person reaches his or her 20s.

Another common visual defect, **astigmatism** (ah-STIG-mah-tism), is due to irregularity in the curvature of the cornea or the lens. As a result, light rays are incorrectly bent, causing blurred vision. Astigmatism is often found in combination with hyperopia or myopia, so that a careful eye examination is needed to obtain the correct prescription for corrective lenses. Surgical techniques are now available to correct some visual defects and eliminate the need for eyeglasses or contact lenses. Such refractive surgery can be used to correct nearsightedness, farsightedness, and astigmatism. In these procedures, the cornea is reshaped to change the refractive angle of light as it passes through.

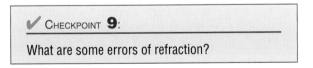

✔ CHECKPOINT **9**:

What are some errors of refraction?

Strabismus

Strabismus (strah-BIZ-mus) is a deviation of the eye that results from lack of coordination of the eyeball muscles. That is, the two eyes do not work together. In **convergent strabismus,** the eye deviates toward the nasal side, or medially. This disorder gives an appearance of being cross-eyed. In **divergent strabismus,** the affected eye deviates laterally.

If these disorders are not corrected early, the transmission and interpretation of visual impulses from the affected eye to the brain is decreased. The brain does not develop ways to "see" images from the eye. Care by an ophthal-

mologist as soon as the condition is detected may result in restoration of muscle balance. In some cases, glasses and patching of one eye correct the defect, whereas in others, surgery may be required.

Infections

Inflammation of the membrane that lines the eyelid and covers the front of the eyeball is called **conjunctivitis** (kon-junk-tih-VI-tis). It may be acute or chronic and may be caused by a variety of irritants and pathogens. "Pinkeye" is a highly contagious acute conjunctivitis that is usually caused by cocci or bacilli. Sometimes, irritants such as wind and excessive glare cause an inflammation, which may in turn lead to susceptibility to bacterial infection.

Inclusion conjunctivitis is an acute eye infection caused by **Chlamydia trachomatis** (klah-MID-e-ah trah-KO-mah-tis). This same organism causes a sexually transmitted disease of the reproductive tract. In underdeveloped countries where this infection appears in chronic form, it is known as **trachoma**. If not treated, scarring of the conjunctiva and cornea can cause blindness. The use of antibiotics and proper hygiene to prevent reinfection has reduced the incidence of blindness from this disorder in many parts of the world.

An acute infection of the eye of the newborn, caused by organisms acquired during passage through the birth canal, is called **ophthalmia neonatorum** (of-THAL-me-ah ne-o-na-TO-rum). The usual cause is gonococcus, chlamydia, or some other sexually transmitted organism. Preventive doses of an appropriate antiseptic or antibiotic solution are routinely administered into the conjunctiva of newborns just after birth.

The iris, choroid coat, ciliary body, and other parts of the eyeball may become infected by various organisms. Such disorders are likely to be serious; fortunately, they are not common. Syphilis spirochetes, tubercle bacilli, and a variety of cocci may cause these painful infections. They may follow a sinus infection, tonsillitis, conjunctivitis, or other disorder in which the infecting agent can spread from nearby structures. The care of these conditions usually should be in the hands of an **ophthalmologist** (of-thal-MOL-o-jist), a physician who specializes in the diagnosis and treatment of disorders of the eye.

Injuries

The most common eye injury is a laceration or scratch of the cornea caused by a foreign body. Injuries caused by foreign objects or by infection may result in scar formation in the cornea, leaving an area of opacity through which light rays cannot pass. If such an injury involves the central area in front of the pupil, blindness may result.

Because the cornea lacks blood vessels, a person can receive a corneal transplant without danger of rejection. Eye banks store corneas obtained from donors, and corneal transplantation is a fairly common procedure.

Severe traumatic injuries to the eye, such as penetration of deeper structures, may not be subject to surgical repair. In such cases, an operation to remove the eyeball, a procedure called **enucleation** (e-nu-kle-A-shun), is performed.

It is important to prevent infection in cases of injury to the eye. Even a tiny scratch can become so seriously infected that blindness may result. Injuries by pieces of glass and other sharp objects are a frequent cause of eye damage. The incidence of accidents involving the eye has been greatly reduced by the use of protective goggles.

Cataracts

A *cataract* is an opacity of the lens or the outer covering of the lens. An early cataract causes a gradual loss of visual acuity (sharpness). An untreated cataract leads to complete loss of vision. Surgical removal of the lens with the implantation of an artificial lens is a highly successful procedure for restoring vision. Although the cause of cataracts is not known, age is a factor, as is excess exposure to ultraviolet rays. Diseases such as diabetes, as well as certain medications, are known to accelerate the development of cataracts.

Glaucoma

Glaucoma is a condition characterized by excess pressure of the aqueous humor. This fluid is produced constantly from the blood, and after circulation in the eye, it is reabsorbed into the bloodstream. Interference with the normal reentry of this fluid to the bloodstream leads to an increase in pressure inside the eyeball.

The most common type of glaucoma usually progresses rather slowly, with vague visual disturbances being the only symptom. In most cases, the high pressure of the aqueous humor causes destruction of some optic nerve fibers before the person is aware of visual change. Many cases of glaucoma are diagnosed by the measurement of pressure in the eye. This measurement is part of a routine eye examination for people older than 35 years or for those with a family history of glaucoma. Early diagnosis and continuous treatment with medications to reduce pressure frequently results in the preservation of vision.

Disorders Involving the Retina

Diabetes as a cause of blindness is increasing in the United States. In **diabetic retinopathy** (ret-in-OP-ah-the), the retina is damaged by blood vessel hemorrhages and growth of new vessels. Other disorders of the eye directly related to diabetes include optic atrophy, in which the optic nerve fibers die; cataracts, which occur earlier and with greater frequency among diabetics than among nondiabetics; and retinal detachment.

In cases of **retinal detachment,** the retina becomes separated from the underlying layer of the eye as a result of trauma or an accumulation of fluid or tissue between the layers. This disorder may develop slowly or may occur suddenly. If it is left untreated, complete detachment can occur, resulting in blindness. Surgical treatment includes a sort of "spot welding" with an electric current or a weak laser beam. A series of pinpoint scars (connective tissue) develops to reattach the retina.

Macular degeneration is another leading cause of blindness. This name refers to the macula, the yellow area of the retina that contains the fovea centralis, the point of sharpest vision. Changes in this area distort the center of the visual field. In one form of macular degeneration, material accumulates on the retina, causing gradual loss of vision. In another form, abnormal blood vessels grow under the retina, caus-

- The *outer ear* includes an outer projection and a canal.
- The *middle ear* is an air space containing three small bones.
- The *inner ear* is the most complex and contains the sensory receptors for hearing and equilibrium.

The Outer Ear

The external portion of the ear consists of a visible projecting portion, the *pinna* (PIN-nah), or the *auricle* (AW-rih-kl), and a canal that leads into the deeper parts of the ear. The purpose of the pinna is to direct sound waves into the ear, but it is probably of little importance in humans. Leading in from the pinna is an opening, the *external auditory canal,* or *meatus* (me-A-tus), which extends medially for about 2.5 cm or more, depending on which wall of the canal is measured. The skin lining this tube is thin and, in the first part of the canal, contains many *ceruminous* (seh-RU-mih-nus) *glands.* The *cerumen* (seh-RU-men), or wax, may become dried and impacted in the canal and must then be removed. The same kinds of disorders that involve the skin elsewhere—atopic dermatitis, boils, and other infections—may also affect the skin of the external auditory canal.

At the end of the auditory canal is the *tympanic* (tim-PAN-ik) *membrane,* or eardrum, which serves as a boundary between the external auditory canal and the middle ear cavity. It vibrates freely as sound waves enter the ear.

The Middle Ear

The Ossicles

The middle ear cavity is a small, flattened space that contains three small bones, or *ossicles* (OS-ih-klz). The three ossicles are joined in such a way that they amplify the sound waves received by the tympanic membrane and then transmit the sounds to the fluid in the inner ear. The handlelike part of the first bone, or *malleus* (MAL-e-us), is attached to the tympanic membrane, whereas the headlike portion is connected with the second bone, called the *incus* (ING-kus). The innermost of the ossicles

---

ing it to detach. Laser surgery may stop the growth of these vessels and delay vision loss. Factors contributing to macular degeneration are smoking, exposure to sunlight, and a high cholesterol diet. Some forms are known to be hereditary (see Protecting the Eye).

THE EAR

The ear is the sense organ for both hearing and equilibrium (Fig. 11-7). It may be divided into three main sections:

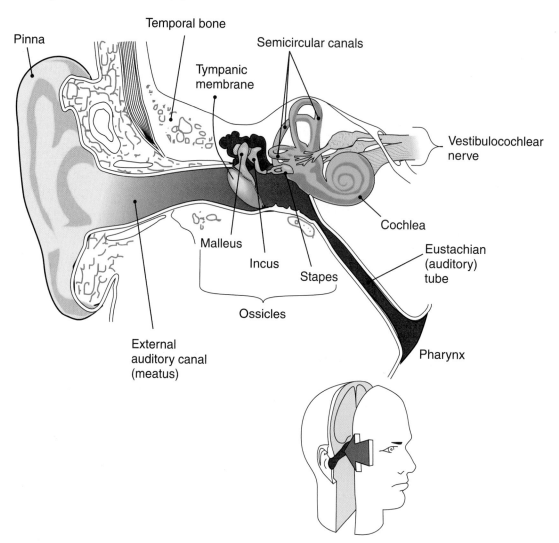

FIGURE **11•7** The ear, showing the outer, middle, and inner divisions.

is shaped somewhat like a stirrup and is called the **stapes** (STA-peze). The base of the stapes is in contact with a membrane covering the **oval window** of the inner ear. This membrane in turn vibrates and transmits the sound waves to the fluid of the inner ear.

✔ CHECKPOINT **10**:

What are the ossicles of the ear and what do they do?

The Eustachian Tube

The **eustachian** (u-STA-shun) **tube** (auditory tube) connects the middle ear cavity with the throat, or **pharynx** (FAR-inks) (see Fig. 11-7). This tube opens to allow pressure to equalize on the two sides of the tympanic membrane. The valve that closes the tube can be forced open by swallowing hard, yawning, or blowing with the nose and mouth sealed, as is done when one is experiencing pain from pressure changes in an airplane.

The mucous membrane of the pharynx is continuous through the eustachian tube into the middle ear cavity, and organisms may travel along the membrane, causing infection of the middle ear.

At the back of the middle ear cavity is an opening into the mastoid air cells, which are spaces inside the mastoid process of the temporal bone.

The Inner Ear

The most complicated and important part of the ear is the internal portion, which is described as a *labyrinth* (LAB-ih-rinth) because it has a complex mazelike construction. It consists of three separate areas hollowed out inside the temporal bone (see Fig. 11-7). The skeleton of the inner ear is called the **bony labyrinth**. Its three divisions are as follows:

- The **vestibule,** which is next to the oval window and is composed of two chambers (the utricle and saccule)
- The **semicircular canals,** three projecting bony tubes located toward the back
- The **cochlea** (KOK-le-ah), coiled like a snail shell and located toward the front

All three divisions of the bony labyrinth contain a fluid called **perilymph** (PER-e-limf).

Within the bony labyrinth is an exact replica of this bony shell made of membrane, much like an inner tube within a tire. The tubes and chambers of this **membranous labyrinth** are filled with a fluid called **endolymph** (EN-do-limf). The endolymph is within the membranous labyrinth, and the perilymph is all around it. These fluids are important to the sensory functions of the inner ear.

Hearing

The organ of hearing, called the **organ of Corti** (KOR-te), consists of ciliated receptor cells located inside the membranous cochlea, or **cochlear duct** (Fig. 11-8). Sound waves enter the external auditory canal and cause the tympanic membrane to vibrate. These vibrations are amplified by the ossicles and transmitted by them to the perilymph of the inner ear. The sound waves enter the upper chamber of the cochlea (the vestibular duct), travel to the top of the cochlea, and then continue through the lower chamber of the cochlea (the tympanic duct). As the sound waves move through the fluids in these chambers, they set up vibrations in the endolymph of the cochlear duct. These vibrations stimulate the tiny, hairlike cilia on the receptor cells, setting up nerve impulses that travel to the brain in the **cochlear nerve,** a branch of the eighth cranial nerve (formerly called the *auditory* or *acoustic nerve*).

Sound waves ultimately leave the ear through another membrane-covered space in the bony labyrinth, the **round window.**

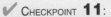

✔ CHECKPOINT **11**:

What is the name of the organ of hearing and where is it located?

Equilibrium

The other sensory receptors in the inner ear are those related to equilibrium (Fig. 11-9). They are located in the vestibule and the semicircular canals, which together make up the vestibular apparatus.

Receptors located in the two small sacs of the vestibule function to sense the position of the head or the position of the body when moving in a straight line, as in a moving vehicle. This aspect of equilibrium is termed **static equilibrium.**

The receptors for **dynamic equilibrium,** which function when the body is spinning or moving in a different direction, are located at the bases of the semicircular canals.

Receptors for the sense of equilibrium are also ciliated cells. As the head moves, a shift in the position of the cilia within their surrounding fluid generates a nerve impulse. Nerve fibers from the vestibule and from the semicircular canals form the **vestibular** (ves-TIB-u-lar) **nerve,** which joins the cochlear nerve to form the vestibulocochlear nerve, the eighth cranial nerve.

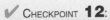

✔ CHECKPOINT **12**:

Where are the receptors for equilibrium located?

Disorders of the Ear

Otitis Media

Infection of the middle ear cavity, **otitis media** (o-TI-tis ME-de-ah), is relatively common. A variety of bacteria and viruses may cause otitis

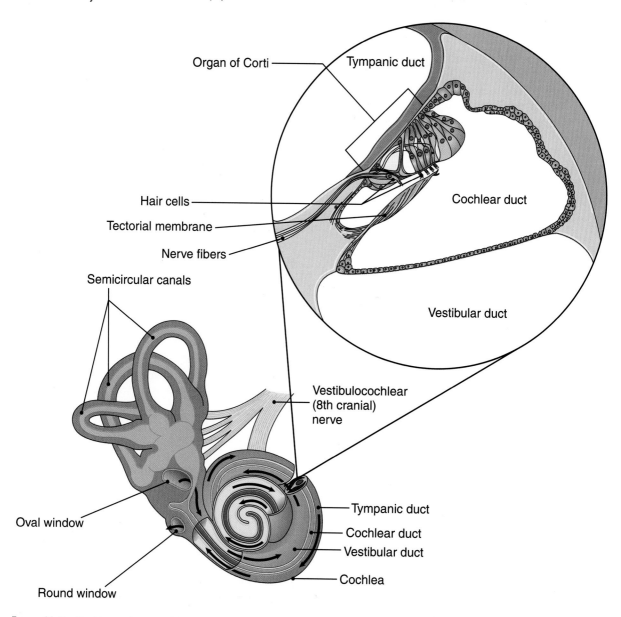

FIGURE **11•8** Cochlea and organ of Corti. The arrows show the direction of sound waves in the cochlea.

media, and it is a frequent complication of measles, influenza, and other infections, especially those of the pharynx. Transmission of pathogens from the pharynx to the middle ear happens most often in children, partly because the eustachian tube is relatively short and horizontal in the child; in the adult, the tube is longer and tends to slant down toward the pharynx. Antibiotic drugs have reduced complications and have caused a marked reduction in the amount of surgery done to drain middle ear infections. In some cases, however, pressure from pus or exudate in the middle ear can be relieved only by cutting the tympanic membrane, a procedure called a *myringotomy* (mir-in-GOT-o-me). Placement of a **tympanostomy**

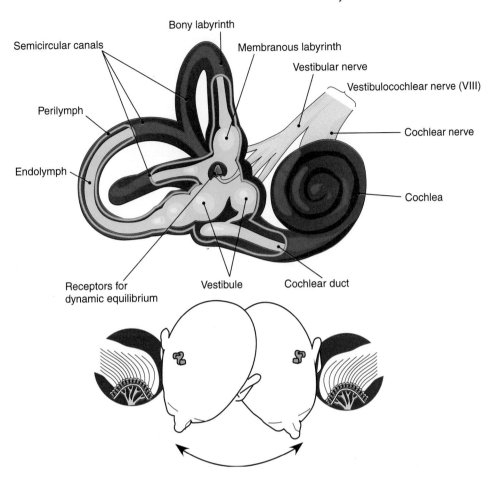

FIGURE **11•9**   Inner ear showing action of receptors for dynamic equilibrium.

(tim-pan-OS-to-me) **tube** in the eardrum allows pressure to equalize and prevents further damage to the eardrum.

Hearing Loss

Another disorder of the ear is hearing loss, which may be partial or complete. When the loss is complete, the condition is called ***deafness.*** The two main types of hearing loss are ***conductive hearing loss*** and ***sensorineural hearing loss.***

Conductive hearing loss is due to interference with the passage of sound waves from the outside to the inner ear. In this condition, there may be obstruction of the external canal by wax or a foreign body. Blockage of the eustachian tube prevents the equalization of air pressure on both sides of the tympanic membrane, thereby decreasing the ability of the membrane to vibrate. Another cause of conductive hearing loss is damage to the tympanic membrane and ossicles resulting from chronic otitis media or from ***otosclerosis*** (o-to-skle-RO-sis), a hereditary disease that causes bone changes in the stapes that prevent its normal vibration. Surgical removal of the diseased stapes and its replacement with an artificial device allows conduction of sound from the ossicles to the oval window and the cochlea.

Sensorineural hearing loss may involve the cochlea, the vestibulocochlear nerve, or the brain areas concerned with hearing. It may result from prolonged exposure to loud noises, from the use of certain drugs for long periods, or from exposure to various infections and toxins.

Presbycusis (pres-be-KU-sis) is a slowly progressive hearing loss that often accompanies aging. The condition involves gradual atrophy of the sensory receptors and the nerve fibers in the cochlear nerves. As a result, the affected person may experience a sense of isolation and depression, so that psychological help may be desirable. Because the ability to hear high-pitched sounds is usually lost first, it is important to address elderly people in clear, low-pitched tones.

OTHER SPECIAL SENSE ORGANS

The sense organs of taste and smell are designed to respond to chemical stimuli.

Sense of Taste

The sense of taste involves receptors in the tongue and two different nerves that carry taste impulses to the brain (Fig. 11-10). The taste receptors, known as *taste buds,* are located along the edges of small, depressed areas called *fis-*

sures. Taste buds are stimulated only if the substance to be tasted is in solution or dissolves in the fluids of the mouth. Receptors for four basic tastes are localized in different regions, forming a "taste map" of the tongue:

- *Sweet* tastes are most acutely experienced at the tip of the tongue (hence the popularity of lollipops and ice cream cones).
- *Sour* tastes are most effectively detected by the taste buds located at the sides of the tongue.
- *Salty* tastes are most acute at the anterior sides of the tongue.
- *Bitter* tastes are detected at the back part of the tongue.

The nerves of taste include the facial and the glossopharyngeal cranial nerves (VII and IX). The interpretation of taste impulses is probably accomplished by the lower front portion of the brain, although there may be no sharply

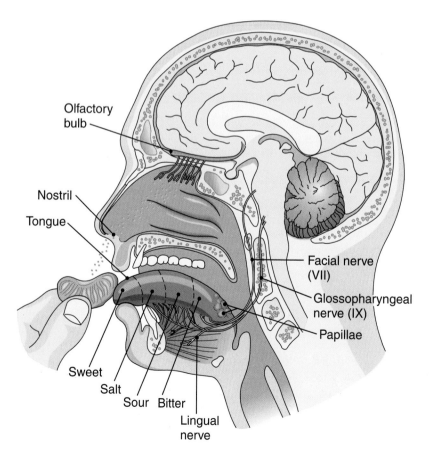

FIGURE **11•10**   Organs of taste and smell.

separate taste, or **gustatory** (GUS-tah-to-re) **center**.

Sense of Smell

The importance of the sense of smell is often underestimated. This sense helps to detect gases and other harmful substances in the environment and helps to warn of spoiled food. Smells can trigger memories and other psychological responses. Smell is also important in sexual behavior.

The receptors for smell are located in the **olfactory** (ol-FAK-to-re) **epithelium** of the upper part of the nasal cavity (see Fig. 11-10). Again, the chemicals detected must be in solution in the fluids that line the nose. Because these receptors are high in the nasal cavity, one must "sniff" to bring odors upward in the nose.

The impulses from the receptors for smell are carried by the olfactory nerve (I), which leads directly to the olfactory center in the temporal cortex of the brain. The interpretation of smell is closely related to the sense of taste, but a greater variety of dissolved chemicals can be detected by smell than by taste. The smell of foods is just as important in stimulating appetite and the flow of digestive juices as is the sense of taste.

The olfactory receptors deteriorate with age, with the result that food becomes less appealing. It is important when presenting food to elderly people that the food look inviting so as to stimulate their appetites.

✔ CHECKPOINT **13**:

What are the special senses that respond to chemical stimuli?

THE GENERAL SENSES

Unlike the *special* sensory receptors, which are localized within specific sense organs, limited to a relatively small area, the *general* sensory receptors are scattered throughout the body. These include receptors for touch, pressure, heat, cold, position, and pain (Fig. 11-11).

Sense of Touch

The touch receptors, **tactile** (TAK-til) **corpuscles,** are found mostly in the dermis of the skin and around hair follicles. Sensitivity to touch varies with the number of touch receptors in different areas. They are especially numerous and close together in the tips of the fingers and the toes. The lips and the tip of the tongue also contain many of these receptors and are very sensitive to touch. Other areas, such as the back of the hand and the back of the neck, have fewer receptors and are less sensitive to touch.

Sense of Pressure

It has been found that even when the skin is anesthetized, there is still consciousness of pressure. These sensory end-organs for deep sensibility are located in the subcutaneous tissues beneath the skin and also near joints, muscles, and other deep tissues. They are sometimes referred to as *receptors for deep touch.*

Sense of Temperature

The temperature receptors are free nerve endings. They are widely distributed in the skin. There are separate receptors for heat and cold, and they vary in distribution. A warm object stimulates only the heat receptors, and a cool object affects only the cold receptors. Internally, there are temperature receptors in the hypothalamus of the brain, which help to adjust body temperature according to the temperature of the blood passing through.

Sense of Position

Receptors located in muscles, tendons, and joints relay impulses that aid in judging one's position and changes in the locations of body parts in relation to each other. They also inform the brain of the amount of muscle contraction and tendon tension. These rather widespread receptors, known as **propriocep-**

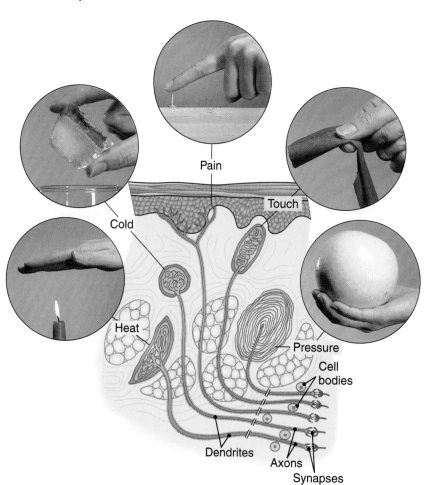

Pain

Touch

Cold

Heat

Pressure

Cell bodies

Dendrites

Axons

Synapses

tors (pro-pre-o-SEP-tors), are aided in this function by the equilibrium receptors of the internal ear.

Information received by these receptors is needed for the coordination of muscles and is important in such activities as walking, running, and many more complicated skills, such as playing a musical instrument. These muscle receptors also play an important part in maintaining muscle tone and good posture as well as allowing for the adjustment of the muscles for the particular kind of work to be done. The nerve fibers that carry impulses from these receptors enter the spinal cord and ascend to the brain in the posterior part of the cord. The cerebellum is a main coordinating center for these impulses.

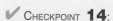

✔ CHECKPOINT **14**:

What are proprioceptors and where are they located?

Sense of Pain

Pain is the most important protective sense. The receptors for pain are widely distributed. They are found in the skin, muscles, and joints and to a lesser extent in most internal organs (including the blood vessels and viscera). Pain receptors are not enclosed in capsules as are the sensory end-organs; rather, they are merely branchings of the nerve fiber, called ***free nerve endings.***

There are two pathways for the transmission

of pain to the CNS, one for acute, sharp pain, and the other for slow, chronic pain. Thus, a single strong stimulus produces the immediate sharp pain, followed in a second or so by the slow, diffuse, burning pain that increases in severity with the passage of time.

Sometimes, the cause of pain cannot be remedied quickly, and occasionally it cannot be remedied at all. In the latter case, it is desirable to relieve the pain. Some pain relief methods that have been found to be effective include the following:

1. *Analgesic drugs.* An analgesic (an-al-JE-zik) is a drug that relieves pain. There are two main categories of such agents:
   a. *Nonnarcotic analgesics* act locally to reduce inflammation and are effective for mild to moderate pain. Most of these drugs are commonly known as nonsteroidal anti-inflammatory drugs (NSAIDs). Examples are ibuprofen (i-bu-PRO-fen) and naproxen (na-PROK-sen).
   b. *Narcotics* act on the CNS to alter the perception and response to pain. Effective for severe pain, narcotics are administered by varied methods, including orally and by intramuscular injection. They are also effectively administered into the space surrounding the spinal cord. An example of a narcotic drug is morphine.
2. *Anesthetics.* Although most commonly used to prevent pain during surgery, anesthetic injections are also used to relieve certain types of chronic pain.
3. *Endorphins* (en-DOR-fins) are released naturally from certain regions of the brain and are associated with the control of pain. Massage, acupressure, and electric stimulation are among the techniques that are thought to activate this system of natural pain relief.
4. Applications of *heat* or *cold* can be a simple but effective means of pain relief, either alone or in combination with medications. Care must be taken to avoid injury caused by excessive heat or cold.
5. *Relaxation* or *distraction techniques* in-

Referred Pain

Referred pain is a term used to describe pain that is felt in an outer part of the body—particularly the skin—but actually originates in an internal organ located near that particular area of skin. Liver and gallbladder disease often cause referred pain in the skin over the right shoulder. Spasm of the coronary arteries that supply the heart may cause pain in the left shoulder and the left arm.

The reason for this referral of pain is that some neurons have the twofold duty of conducting impulses from visceral pain receptors and from pain receptors in neighboring areas of the skin. The brain cannot differentiate between these two possible sources, but because most pain sensations originate in the skin, the brain automatically assigns the pain to this more likely place of origin.

clude several methods that reduce perception of pain in the CNS. Relaxation techniques counteract the fight-or-flight response to pain and complement other pain-control methods.

To learn more about pain, see Referred Pain.

SENSORY ADAPTATION

When sensory receptors are exposed to a continuous stimulus, receptors often adjust themselves so that the sensation becomes less acute. The term for this phenomenon is *sensory adaptation.* For example, if you immerse your hand in very warm water, it may be uncomfortable; however, if you leave your hand there, soon the water will feel less hot (even if it has not cooled appreciably).

Receptors adapt at different rates. Those for warmth, cold, and light pressure adapt rapidly. In contrast, those for pain do not adapt. In fact, the sensations from the slow pain fibers tend to increase over time. This variation in receptors allows us to save energy by not responding to unimportant stimuli while always heeding the warnings of pain.

Summary

I. **The senses**—protect by detecting changes (stimuli) in the environment
   A. Special and general senses
      1. Special senses—vision, hearing, equilibrium, taste, smell
      2. General senses—pain, touch, temperature, pressure, position

II. **The eye and vision**
   A. Protection of the eyeball—bony orbit, eyelid, eyelashes, conjunctiva, tears (lacrimal apparatus)
   B. Coats of the eyeball
      1. Sclera—white of the eye
         a. Cornea—anterior
      2. Choroid—pigmented; contains blood vessels
      3. Retina—receptor layer
   C. Pathway of light rays and refraction
      1. Refraction—bending of light rays as they pass through substances of different density
      2. Refracting parts (media)—cornea, aqueous humor, lens, vitreous body
   D. Function of the retina
      1. Cells
         a. Rods—cannot detect color; function in dim light
         b. Cones—detect color; function in bright light
      2. Pigments—sensitive to light; rod pigment is rhodopsin
   E. Muscles of the eye
      1. Extrinsic muscles—six move each eyeball
      2. Intrinsic muscles
         a. Iris—colored ring around pupil; regulates the amount of light entering the eye
         b. Ciliary body—regulates the thickness of the lens for accommodation
   F. Nerve supply to the eye
      1. Sensory nerves
         a. Optic nerve (II)—carries impulses from retina to brain
         b. Ophthalmic branch of trigeminal (V)
      2. Motor nerves—move eyeball
         a. Oculomotor (III), trochlear (IV), abducens (VI)
   G. Eye disorders
      1. Errors of refraction—hyperopia (farsightedness), myopia (nearsightedness), astigmatism
      2. Strabismus
      3. Infections—conjunctivitis, ophthalmia neonatorum
      4. Injuries
      5. Cataracts
      6. Glaucoma
      7. Retinal disorders

III. **The ear**
   A. Outer ear—pinna, auditory canal (meatus), tympanic membrane (eardrum)
   B. Middle ear
      1. Ossicles—malleus, incus, stapes
      2. Eustachian tube—connects middle ear with pharynx to equalize pressure
   C. Inner ear—bony labyrinth and membranous labyrinth
      1. Vestibule—contains receptors for static equilibrium
      2. Semicircular canals—contain receptors for dynamic equilibrium
      3. Cochlea—contains receptors for hearing (organ of Corti)
      4. Nerve—vestibulocochlear (auditory) nerve (VIII)
   D. Disorders of the ear
      1. Otitis media—infection
      2. Hearing loss

IV. **Other special sense organs**
   A. Sense of taste—gustatory sense
      1. Receptors—taste buds
      2. Tastes—sweet, sour, salty, bitter
      3. Nerves—facial (VII) and glossopharyngeal (IX)
   B. Sense of smell—olfactory sense
      1. Receptors—in upper part of nasal cavity
      2. Nerve—olfactory nerve (I)

V. General senses
  A. Sense of touch
  B. Sense of pressure
  C. Sense of temperature
  D. Sense of position—receptors are proprioceptors in muscles, tendons, joints
  E. Sense of pain—receptors are free nerve endings

  1. Relief—analgesic drugs, anesthetics, endorphins, heat, cold, relaxation and distraction techniques

VI. Sensory adaptation—adjustment of receptors so that sensation becomes less acute

Questions for Study and Review

1. What is the function of the senses?
2. Define *sensory receptor* and give several examples.
3. List the five special senses.
4. List six general senses.
5. List five protective devices for the eye
6. Name the three coats (tunics) of the eye.
7. Trace the path of a light ray from the outside of the eye to the retina.
8. What happens to light when it is refracted and what causes refraction?
9. How does the retina function in vision?
10. List the extrinsic muscles of the eye. What is their function?
11. List the intrinsic muscles of the eye. What is their function?
12. What is near accommodation? What structures of the eye are necessary for near accommodation?
13. List five cranial nerves associated with the eye and give the function of each.
14. What are some possible causes of blindness?
15. Describe the structures that sound waves pass through in traveling through the ear to the receptors for hearing.
16. What parts of the ear function in equilibrium?
17. What cranial nerve carries impulses from the ear? Name the two branches.
18. List some causes of hearing loss.
19. Name the four basic tastes. Where are the taste receptors?
20. Describe the olfactory apparatus.
21. Where are the receptors for the sense of position located?
22. Name several types of pain-relieving drugs. Describe several methods for relieving pain that do not involve drugs.
23. What does *adaptation* mean with respect to the senses? How does sensory adaptation differ among the senses?
24. Differentiate between the terms in each of the following pairs:
    a. *special sense* and *general sense*
    b. *hyperopia* and *myopia*
    c. *presbyopia* and *presbycusis*
    d. *rods* and *cones*
    e. *static* and *dynamic equilibrium*
    f. *endolymph* and *perilymph*
    g. *gustatory* and *olfactory*

11

1. Structures that protect the eye include the skull bones, eyelid, eyelashes, eyebrow, conjunctiva, and lacrimal gland.
2. The tunics (coats) of the eyeball are the sclera, choroid, and retina.
3. The structures that refract light as it passes through the eye to the retina are the cornea, aqueous humor, lens, and vitreous body.
4. The receptor cells of the retina are the rods and cones.
5. The extrinsic eye muscles pull on the eyeball so that both eyes center on one visual field, a process known as convergence.
6. The iris adjusts the size of the pupil to regulate the amount of light that enters the eye.
7. The ciliary muscle adjusts the thickness of the lens to allow for accommodation for near vision.
8. Cranial nerve II is the optic nerve. It carries impulses from the retinal rods and cones to the brain.
9. Hyperopia, myopia, and astigmatism are some errors of refraction.
10. The ossicles of the middle ear are three small bones, the malleus, incus, and stapes, that transmit sound waves from the tympanic membrane to the inner ear.
11. The organ of hearing is the organ of Corti located in the cochlear duct within the cochlea.
12. The receptors for equilibrium are located in the vestibular apparatus, which consists of the vestibule and the semicircular canals.
13. The senses of taste and smell are the special senses that respond to chemical stimuli.
14. Proprioceptors are the receptors that respond to change in position. They are located in muscles, tendons, and joints.

11

The Endocrine System: Glands and Hormones

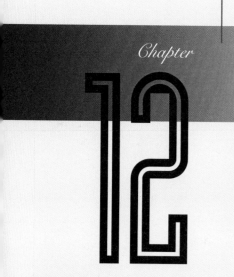
SELECTED KEY TERMS

The following terms are defined in the Glossary:

endocrine

hormone

hypothalamus

pituitary (hypophysis)

prostaglandin

receptor

steroid

target tissue

BEHAVIORAL OBJECTIVES

After careful study of this chapter, you should be able to:

1. Compare the effects of the nervous system and the endocrine system in controlling the body
2. Describe the functions of hormones
3. Explain how hormones are regulated
4. Identify the glands of the endocrine system on a diagram
5. List the hormones produced by each endocrine gland and describe the effects of each on the body
6. Describe how the hypothalamus controls the anterior and posterior pituitary
7. Describe the effects of hyposecretion and hypersecretion of the various hormones
8. List tissues other than the endocrine glands that produce hormones
9. List some medical uses of hormones
10. Explain how the endocrine system responds to stress

The endocrine system consists of a group of glands that produces regulatory chemicals called **hormones.** The endocrine system and the nervous system work together to control and coordinate all other systems of the body. The nervous system and the endocrine system are the two main controlling and coordinating systems of the body. The nervous system controls such rapid activity as muscle movement and intestinal activity by means of electrical and chemical stimuli. The effects of the endocrine system occur more slowly and over a longer period and involve chemical stimuli only. The effects of these chemical messengers are widespread.

Although the nervous and endocrine systems differ in some respects, the two systems are closely related. The activity of the pituitary gland, which in turn regulates other glands, is controlled by a part of the brain. The connections between the nervous system and the endocrine system enable endocrine function to adjust to the demands of a changing environment.

HORMONES

Functions of Hormones

Hormones are chemical messengers that have specific regulatory effects on certain cells or organs in the body. Hormones are released directly into the bloodstream, by which they are carried to all parts of the body. They regulate growth, metabolism, reproduction, and behavior. Some hormones affect many tissues, for example, growth hormone, thyroid hormone, and insulin. Others affect only specific tissues. One pituitary hormone, thyroid-stimulating hormone (TSH), acts only on the thyroid gland; another (ACTH) stimulates only the outer portion of the adrenal gland.

The specific tissue acted on by each hormone is the *target tissue.* The cells that make up these tissues have *receptors* in the plasma membrane or within the cytoplasm to which the hormone attaches. Once attached to the cell, the hormone affects cell activities, regulating the manufacture of proteins, changing the permeability of the membrane, or affecting metabolic reactions.

Chemistry

Chemically, hormones fall into two main categories:

- *Amino acid compounds.* Most hormones are proteins or related compounds also made of amino acids. All hormones except those of the adrenal cortex and the sex glands fall into this category.
- *Steroids* are hormones derived from lipids.

They are produced by the adrenal cortex and the sex glands.

> ✔ CHECKPOINT **1**:
>
> What are hormones and what are some effects of hormones?

Regulation of Hormones

The amount of each hormone that is secreted is normally kept within a specific range. Negative feedback is the method used to regulate these levels. That is, the concentration of the hormone itself acts as a brake on further secretion of that hormone. Each endocrine gland tends to oversecrete its hormone, exerting more effect on the target tissue. When the target tissue becomes too active, there is a negative effect on the endocrine gland, which then decreases its secretory action.

The release of hormones may fall into a rhythmic pattern. Hormones of the adrenal cortex follow a 24-hour cycle related to a person's sleeping pattern, with the level of secretion greatest just before arising and least at bedtime. Hormones of the female menstrual cycle follow a monthly pattern.

The remainder of this chapter deals with hormones and the tissues that produce them. Refer to Figure 12-1 to locate each of the endocrine glands as you study. The information on the endocrine glands and their hormones is summarized in Table 12-1. Each section also includes information on the effects of oversecretion or undersecretion of a hormone. This information is summarized in Table 12-2.

> ✔ CHECKPOINT **2**:
>
> Hormone levels are normally kept within a specific range. What method is used to regulate secretion of hormones?

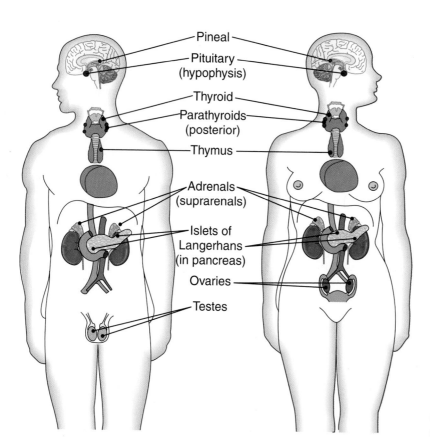

Pineal
Pituitary (hypophysis)
Thyroid
Parathyroids (posterior)
Thymus
Adrenals (suprarenals)
Islets of Langerhans (in pancreas)
Ovaries
Testes

FIGURE **12•1** The endocrine glands.

Table 12•1   The Endocrine Glands and Their Hormones

GLAND	HORMONE	PRINCIPAL FUNCTIONS
Anterior pituitary	GH (growth hormone)	Promotes growth of all body tissues
	TSH (thyroid-stimulating hormone)	Stimulates thyroid gland to produce thyroid hormones
	ACTH (adrenocorticotropic hormone)	Stimulates adrenal cortex to produce cortical hormones; aids in protecting body in stress situations (injury, pain)
	PRL (prolactin)	Stimulates secretion of milk by mammary glands
	FSH (follicle-stimulating hormone)	Stimulates growth and hormone activity of ovarian follicles; stimulates growth of testes; promotes development of sperm cells
	LH (luteinizing hormone); ICSH (interstitial cell–stimulating hormone) in males	Causes development of corpus luteum at site of ruptured ovarian follicle in female; stimulates secretion of testosterone in male
Posterior pituitary	ADH (antidiuretic hormone; vasopressin)	Promotes reabsorption of water in kidney tubules; stimulates smooth muscle tissue of blood vessels to constrict
	Oxytocin	Causes contraction of uterine muscle; causes ejection of milk from mammary glands
Thyroid	Thyroxine (T_4) and triiodothyronine (T_3)	Increases metabolic rate, influencing both physical and mental activities; required for normal growth
	Calcitonin	Decreases calcium level in blood
Parathyroids	Parathyroid hormone	Regulates exchange of calcium between blood and bones; increases calcium level in blood
Adrenal medulla	Epinephrine and norephinephrine	Increases blood pressure and heart rate; activates cells influenced by sympathetic nervous system plus many not affected by sympathetic nerves
Adrenal cortex	Cortisol (95% of glucocorticoids)	Aids in metabolism of carbohydrates, proteins, and fats; active during stress
	Aldosterone (95% of mineralcorticoids)	Aids in regulating electrolytes and water balance
	Sex hormones	May influence secondary sexual characteristics
Pancreatic islets	Insulin	Aids transport of glucose into cells; required for cellular metabolism of foods, especially glucose; decreases blood sugar levels
	Glucagon	Stimulates liver to release glucose, thereby increasing blood sugar levels
Testes	Testosterone	Stimulates growth and development of sexual organs (testes, penis) plus development of secondary sexual characteristics, such as hair growth on body and face and deepening of voice; stimulates maturation of sperm cells
Ovaries	Estrogens (*e.g.*, estradiol)	Stimulates growth of primary sexual organs (uterus, tubes) and development of secondary sexual organs, such as breasts, plus changes in pelvis to ovoid, broader shape
	Progesterone	Stimulates development of secretory parts of mammary glands; prepares uterine lining for implantation of fertilized ovum; aids in maintaining pregnancy
Thymus	Thymosin	Promotes growth of T cells active in immunity
Pineal	Melatonin	Regulates mood, sexual development, and daily cycles in response to the amount of light in the environment

12

Table 12•2   Disorders Associated with Endocrine Dysfunction

HORMONE	HYPERSECRETION	HYPOSECRETION
Growth hormone	Gigantism (children), acromegaly (adults)	Dwarfism (children)
Antidiuretic hormone	Syndrome of inappropriate antidiuretic hormone (SIADH)	Diabetes insipidus
Aldosterone	Aldosteronism	Addison's disease
Cortisol	Cushing's syndrome	Addison's disease
Thyroid hormone	Graves' disease, thyrotoxicosis	Cretinism (children), myxedema (adults)
Insulin	Hypoglycemia	Diabetes mellitus
Parathyroid hormone	Bone degeneration	Tetany (muscle spasms)

THE ENDOCRINE GLANDS AND THEIR HORMONES

The Pituitary

The *pituitary* (pih-TU-ih-tar-e), or *hypophysis* (hi-POF-ih-sis), is a small gland about the size of a cherry. It is located in a saddlelike depression of the sphenoid bone just behind the point at which the optic nerves cross. It is surrounded by bone except where it connects with the brain by a stalk called the *infundibulum* (in-fun-DIB-u-lum). The gland is divided into two parts, the *anterior lobe* and the *posterior lobe.* The hormones released from each lobe are shown in Figure 12-2.

The pituitary is often called the *master gland* because it releases hormones that affect the working of other glands, such as the thyroid, gonads (gonads), and adrenal glands. (Hormones

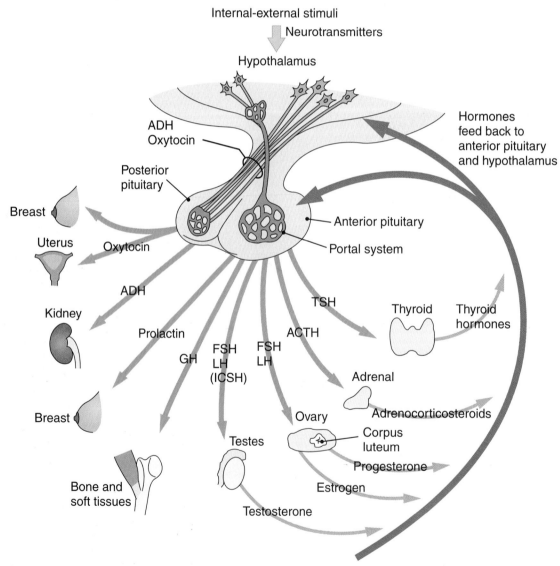

Figure **12•2** Pituitary gland and its relations to the brain and target tissues. Hypothalamic-releasing hormones influence the anterior pituitary through a portal system. Tropic hormones from the anterior pituitary affect the working of various other glands. The hypothalamus communicates with the posterior pituitary through tracts.

that stimulate other glands may be recognized by the ending *-tropin*, as in *thyrotropin*, which means "acting on the thyroid gland.") However, the pituitary itself is controlled by the **hypothalamus** of the brain, to which it is connected by the infundibulum (stalk) (see Fig. 12-2). The infundibulum carries secretions and nerve impulses from the hypothalamus to the pituitary.

The hormones produced in the anterior pituitary are not released from the gland until chemical messengers called **releasing hormones** arrive from the hypothalamus. These releasing hormones are sent to the anterior pituitary by way of a special type of circulatory pathway called a **portal system.** By this circulatory "detour," some of the blood that leaves the hypothalamus travels to capillaries in the anterior pituitary before returning to the heart. As the blood circulates through the capillaries, it delivers the hormones that stimulate the release of anterior pituitary secretions.

The two hormones of the posterior pituitary (antidiuretic hormone, or ADH, and oxytocin) are actually produced in the hypothalamus and stored in the posterior pituitary. Their release is controlled by nerve impulses that travel over pathways (tracts) between the hypothalamus and the posterior pituitary.

✔ CHECKPOINT **3**:
_____

What part of the brain controls the pituitary?

Hormones of the Anterior Lobe

- **Growth hormone (GH)**, or **somatotropin** (so-mah-to-TRO-pin), acts directly on most body tissues, promoting protein manufacture that is essential for growth. Produced throughout life, GH causes increase in size and height to occur in youth, before the closure of the epiphyses of long bones. A young person with a deficiency of GH will remain small, though well proportioned, unless treated with adequate hormone (see Growth Hormone).
- **Thyroid-stimulating hormone (TSH),** or **thyrotropin** (thi-ro-TRO-pin), stimulates the thyroid gland to produce thyroid hormones.

- **Adrenocorticotropic** (ad-re-no-kor-te-ko-TRO-pik) **hormone (ACTH)** stimulates the cortex of the adrenal glands.
- **Prolactin** (pro-LAK-tin) **(PRL)** stimulates the production of milk in the female.
- **Gonadotropins** (gon-ah-do-TRO-pinz), acting on the gonads, regulate the growth, development, and functioning of the reproductive systems in both males and females. The two gonadotropins are the following:
  - **Follicle-stimulating hormone (FSH)** stimulates the development of eggs in the ovaries and sperm cells in the testes.
  - **Luteinizing** (LU-te-in-i-zing) **hormone (LH)** causes ovulation in females and sex hormone secretion in both males and females; in males, the hormone is called *interstitial cell–stimulating hormone (ICSH).*

Growth Hormone

Growth hormone, also called **somatotropin,** is produced by the anterior pituitary gland. Its release is regulated by growth hormone–releasing hormone (GHRH) and growth hormone–inhibiting hormone (GHIH), also called **somatostatin,** from the hypothalamus.

Although growth hormone mainly affects the development of bones and muscles, it has a general effect on most other tissues as well, stimulating an increase in protein synthesis. It also stimulates the liver to release fatty acids for energy when the level of blood glucose drops. In this capacity, it is released during times of stress. The production of growth hormone is controlled by its concentration in the blood; by the level of other hormones, including those from the adrenal, thyroid, and sex glands; and by the level of nutrients in the blood.

Insufficient growth hormone results in pituitary dwarfism. This condition can be prevented by administering growth hormone to children who lack it. Growth hormone is now produced by genetic engineering. The gene for the hormone is introduced into harmless bacteria, which then produce large quantities in laboratory cultures.

Hormones of the Posterior Lobe

- *Antidiuretic* (an-ti-di-u-RET-ik) *hormone (ADH)* promotes the reabsorption of water from the kidney tubules and thus decreases the excretion of water. Large amounts of this hormone cause contraction of the smooth muscle of blood vessels and raise blood pressure. Inadequate amounts of ADH cause excessive loss of water and result in a disorder called *diabetes insipidus*. This type of diabetes should not be confused with diabetes mellitus, which is due to inadequate amounts of insulin.
- *Oxytocin* (ok-se-TO-sin) causes contraction of the muscle of the uterus and milk ejection from the breasts. Under certain circumstances, commercial preparations of this hormone are administered during or after childbirth to cause the uterus to contract.

✔ CHECKPOINT **4**:

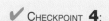

Some of the anterior pituitary hormones end with the suffix *-tropin*. What does this suffix mean?

Tumors of the Pituitary

The effects of pituitary tumors depend on the types of cells in the excess tissue (see Table 12-2). Some of these tumors contain an excessive number of the cells that produce growth hormone. A person who develops such a tumor in childhood will grow to an abnormally tall stature, a condition called *gigantism* (ji-GAN-tizm). Although people with this condition are large, they are usually very weak.

If the GH-producing cells become overactive in the adult, a disorder known as *acromegaly* (ak-ro-MEG-ah-le) develops. In acromegaly, the bones of the face, hands, and feet widen. The fingers resemble a spatula, and the face takes on a grotesque appearance: the nose widens, the lower jaw protrudes, and the forehead bones may bulge. Often, these pituitary tumors involve the optic nerves and cause blindness.

Tumors may destroy the secreting tissues of the pituitary so that signs of underactivity develop. Patients with this condition often become obese and sluggish and may exhibit signs of underactivity of other endocrine glands that are controlled by the pituitary, such as the ovaries, testes, or thyroid.

Evidence of tumor formation in the pituitary gland may be obtained by radiographic examinations of the skull; the pressure of the tumor distorts the saddlelike space for the pituitary. Computed tomography (CT) and magnetic resonance imaging (MRI) scans are also used to diagnose pituitary abnormalities.

The Thyroid Gland

The largest of the endocrine glands is the *thyroid*, which is located in the neck (Fig. 12-3). The thyroid has two oval parts called the *lateral lobes*, one on either side of the larynx (voice box). A narrow band called the *isthmus* (IS-mus) connects these two lobes. A connective tissue capsule encloses the entire gland.

Hormones of the Thyroid Gland

The thyroid produces two hormones that regulate metabolism. The principal hormone is *thyroxine* (thi-ROK-sin), which is symbolized as T_4, based on the iodine content. The other hormone, triiodothyronine (tri-i-o-do-THI-ro-nin), is T_3. These hormones function to increase the rate of metabolism in body cells. In particular, they increase energy metabolism and protein metabolism. Thyroid hormones are necessary along with growth hormones for normal growth to occur.

The thyroid gland needs an adequate supply of iodine in the blood to produce these hormones. Iodine deficiency is rare now due to widespread

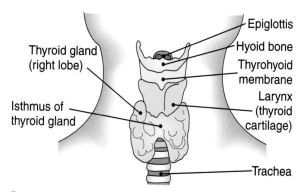

FIGURE **12•3** Thyroid gland (anterior view) in relation to the larynx and trachea.

availability of this mineral in vegetables, seafood, dairy products, and processed foods.

Another hormone produced by the thyroid gland is **calcitonin** (kal-sih-TO-nin), which is active in calcium metabolism. This hormone is discussed later in connection with the parathyroid gland.

Disorders of the Thyroid Gland

A **goiter** is an enlargement of the thyroid gland, which may or may not be associated with overproduction of hormone. A **simple goiter** is the uniform overgrowth of the thyroid gland, with a smooth appearance. An **adenomatous** (ad-eh-NO-mah-tus), or **nodular, goiter** is an irregular-appearing goiter accompanied by tumor formation.

For various reasons, the thyroid gland may become either underactive or overactive. Underactivity of the thyroid, known as **hypothyroidism** (hi-po-THI-royd-izm), shows up as two characteristic states related to age:

- **Cretinism** (KRE-tin-izm), a condition resulting from hypothyroidism in infants and children. The usual cause is a failure of the thyroid gland to form during fetal development. The infant suffers lack of physical growth and lack of mental development. Early and continuous treatment with replacement hormone can alter the outlook of this disease. Most states require newborns to have a blood test to detect this disorder.
- **Myxedema** (mik-seh-DE-mah), the result of atrophy (wasting) of the thyroid in the adult. The patient becomes sluggish both mentally and physically. The skin and the hair become dry, and a peculiar swelling of the tissues of the face develops. Because thyroid hormone can be administered orally, the patient with myxedema can be restored to health easily, although treatment must be maintained throughout life.

Hyperthyroidism is the opposite of hypothyroidism, that is, overactivity of the thyroid gland with excessive secretion of hormone. A common form of hyperthyroidism is **exophthalmic** (ek-sof-THAL-mik) **goiter,** or **Graves' disease,** which is characterized by a goiter, bulging of the eyes, a strained appearance of the face, intense nervousness, weight loss, a rapid pulse, sweating, tremors, and an abnormally quick metabolism. Treatment of hyperthyroidism may take the the following forms:

- Suppression of hormone production with medication
- Destruction of thyroid tissue with radioactive iodine
- Surgical removal of part of the thyroid gland

An exaggerated form of hyperthyroidism with a sudden onset is called a **thyroid storm.** Untreated, it is usually fatal, but with appropriate care, most affected people can be saved.

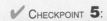

> ✔ CHECKPOINT **5**:
>
> What is the effect of thyroxine on cells?

Tests of Thyroid Function

The most frequently used tests of thyroid function are blood tests in which the uptake of radioactive iodine added to a blood sample is measured. These very sensitive tests are used to detect abnormal thyroid function and to monitor response to drug therapy. A test for the level of thyroid-stimulating hormone (from the pituitary) is frequently done at the same time. Further testing involves giving a person radioactive iodine orally. The amount and distribution of the rays emitted from the radioactive iodine accumulated by the thyroid gland are then measured.

The Parathyroid Glands

Behind the thyroid gland, and embedded in its capsule, are four tiny **parathyroid glands** (Fig. 12-4). The secretion of these glands, **parathyroid hormone (PTH),** is one of three substances that regulate calcium metabolism. The other two hormones are **calcitonin** and **hydroxycholecalciferol** (hi-drok-se-ko-le-kal-SIF-eh-rol)

Calcium Metabolism

PTH promotes the release of calcium from bone tissue, thus increasing the amount of calcium circulating in the bloodstream. PTH also causes

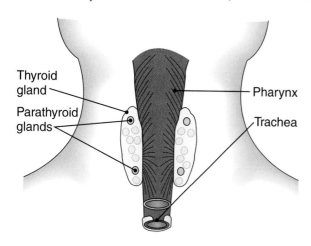

FIGURE **12•4** Posterior view of the thyroid gland showing the parathyroid glands embedded in its surface.

the kidney to retain calcium. Calcitonin, produced by the thyroid gland, lowers the amount of calcium circulating in the blood. Calcitonin does this by promoting the deposit of calcium in bone tissue. Hydroxycholecalciferol, the active form of vitamin D, is produced by modification of the vitamin in the liver and then the kidney. Hydroxycholecalciferol increases absorption of calcium by the intestine to raise blood calcium levels. These three substances work together to regulate the amount of calcium in the blood and provide calcium for bone maintenance and other functions.

Disorders of the Parathyroid Glands

Inadequate production of parathyroid hormone, as a result of removal or damage to the parathyroid glands, for example, causes a series of muscle contractions involving particularly the hands and face. These spasms are due to a low concentration of blood calcium, and the condition is called *tetany* (TET-ah-ne). This low calcium tetany should not be confused with the infection called *tetanus* (lockjaw).

In contrast, if there is excess production of PTH, as may happen in tumors of the parathyroid glands, calcium is removed from its normal storage place in the bones and released into the bloodstream. The loss of calcium from the bones leads to fragile bones that fracture easily. Because the kidneys ultimately excrete the calcium, the formation of kidney stones is common in such cases.

✔ CHECKPOINT **6**:

What mineral is regulated by parathyroid hormone?

The Adrenal Glands

The *adrenals,* or *suprarenals,* are two small glands located above the kidneys. Each adrenal gland has two parts that act as separate glands. The inner area is called the *medulla,* and the outer portion is called the *cortex.*

Hormones From the Adrenal Medulla

The hormones of the adrenal medulla are released in response to stimulation by the sympathetic nervous system. The principal hormone produced by the medulla is *epinephrine,* also called *adrenaline.* Another hormone released from the adrenal medulla, *norepinephrine,* is closely related chemically and is similar in its actions to epinephrine. These two hormones are referred to as the *fight-or-flight hormones* because of their effects during emergency situations. We have already learned about these hormones in studying the autonomic nervous system. When released from nerve endings instead of being released directly into the bloodstream, they function as neurotransmitters.

Some of their effects are as follows:

* Stimulation of the involuntary muscle in the walls of the arterioles, causing these

muscles to contract and blood pressure to rise accordingly

- Conversion of the glycogen stored in the liver into glucose. The glucose is poured into the blood and brought to the voluntary muscles, permitting them to do an extraordinary amount of work
- Increase in the heart rate
- Increase in the metabolic rate of body cells
- Dilation of the bronchioles, through relaxation of the smooth muscle of their walls

---

✔ CHECKPOINT **7**:

The main hormone from the adrenal medulla also functions as a neurotransmitter in the sympathetic nervous system. What is the name of this hormone?

Hormones From the Adrenal Cortex

There are three main groups of hormones secreted by the adrenal cortex:

- *Glucocorticoids* (glu-ko-KOR-tih-koyds) maintain the carbohydrate reserve of the body by promoting the conversion of amino acids into glucose (sugar) instead of protein. The production of these hormones increases in times of stress to aid the body in responding to unfavorable conditions. Glucocorticoids also have the ability to suppress the inflammatory response and are often administered as medication for this purpose. The major hormone of this group is *cortisol,* which is also called *hydrocortisone.*
- *Mineralocorticoids* (min-er-al-o-KOR-tih-koyds) are important in the regulation of electrolyte balance. They control the reabsorption of sodium and the secretion of potassium by the kidney tubules. The major hormone of this group is *aldosterone* (al-DOS-ter-one).
- *Sex hormones* are normally secreted, but in small amounts; their effects in the body are slight.

Disorders of the Adrenal Cortex

Hypofunction of the adrenal cortex gives rise to a condition known as *Addison's disease,* a disease characterized chiefly by muscle atrophy

(loss of tissue), weakness, skin pigmentation, and disturbances in salt and water balance.

Hypersecretion of cortisol results in a condition known as *Cushing's syndrome,* the symptoms of which include obesity with a round face, thin skin that bruises easily, muscle weakness, bone loss, and elevated blood sugar. Use of steroid drugs also may produce these symptoms. If aldosterone is secreted in excess, as a result of hyperfunction of the adrenal cortex, the condition is termed aldosteronism.

Adrenal gland tumors give rise to a wide range of symptoms resulting from an excess or a deficiency of the hormones secreted.

✔ CHECKPOINT **8**:

What effect does cortisol have on glucose levels in the blood?

The Pancreas

Hormones of the Pancreas

Scattered throughout the *pancreas* are small groups of specialized cells called *islets* (I-lets), also known as the *islets of Langerhans* (LAHNG-er-hanz). A microscopic view of the pancreas showing the islet cells is presented in Figure 12-5. These cells make up the endocrine portion of the pancreas and function independently from the exocrine part of the pancreas, which produces digestive juices and releases them through ducts. The most important hormone secreted by these islets is *insulin.*

Insulin is active in the transport of glucose across plasma membranes. Once inside a cell, glucose is metabolized for energy. Insulin also increases the rate at which the liver changes excess glucose into fatty acids, which can then be converted to fats and stored in adipose tissue. Through these actions, insulin has the effect of lowering the level of sugar in the blood. Insulin has other metabolic effects as well. It promotes the uptake of amino acids into cells and improves the manufacture of these amino acids into proteins.

A second hormone produced by the islet cells is *glucagon* (GLU-kah-gon), which works with insulin to regulate blood sugar levels. Glucagon

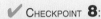

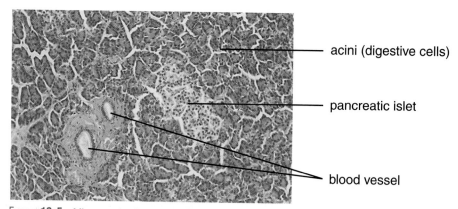

FIGURE **12•5** Microscopic view of pancreatic cells. Light staining islet cells are seen among the cell clusters (acini) that produce digestive juices. (Courtesy of Dana Morse Bittus and B. J. Cohen)

causes the liver to release stored glucose into the bloodstream. Glucagon also increases the rate at which glucose is made from proteins in the liver. In these two ways, glucagon increases blood sugar.

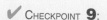

> ✔ CHECKPOINT **9**:
>
> What two hormones produced by the islets of the pancreas act to regulate glucose levels in the blood?

Disorders of the Pancreatic Islets

When the pancreatic islet cells fail to produce enough insulin, glucose is not available to the cells to be oxidized (burned) for energy. Instead, the sugar remains in the blood and then must be removed by the kidneys and excreted in the urine. This condition, called ***diabetes mellitus*** (di-ah-BE-teze mel-LI-tus), is the most common endocrine disorder.

Diabetes is divided into two types:

* Insulin-dependent diabetes mellitus (IDDM) is less common but more severe. It is also known as *type I diabetes* (formerly known as *juvenile diabetes*). This disease usually appears by age 30 years and is brought on by an autoimmune (self) destruction of the insulin-producing cells in the islets. People with IDDM need close monitoring of blood sugar levels and injections of insulin.
* Non–insulin-dependent diabetes mellitus

(NIDDM), or *type II diabetes,* characteristically occurs in overweight adults. These people retain the ability to secrete varying amounts of insulin, depending on the severity of the disease. However, the ability of their body cells to respond to the hormone is diminished. This disease can be controlled with diet, oral medication to improve insulin production and increase its effectiveness, and, for the obese patient, weight reduction. Treatment with injectable insulin may be necessary during illness or other stress.

Diabetic patients can control their disease by following their prescribed diet consistently, taking medication as ordered, eating at regular times, and following a regular program of exercise. The advent of the pocket-sized blood glucose test meter has enabled the diabetic patient to achieve closer control of his or her disease. People taking insulin injections are subject to episodes of low blood sugar and should carry notification of their disease.

Diabetes is associated with many long-term complications, including the following:

* Abnormal fat metabolism. Low insulin levels result in the release of more fatty acids from adipose cells. The liver converts the fatty acids into phospholipids and cholesterol. The result is a high level of fats in the bloodstream and the accelerated development of atherosclerosis (arterial degeneration).

- Damage to arteries, including those of the retina and heart. Capillaries, such as those in the kidney, are often damaged as well.
- Damage to peripheral nerves, with accompanying pain and loss of sensation. Damage to the autonomic nervous system can result in poor stomach emptying.
- Decreased transport of amino acids, the building blocks of proteins. This may explain the weakness and poor tissue repair seen in people that have been diabetic for many years. It may also explain the reduced resistance to infection noted in diabetic patients.

Tight control of blood sugar in cases of diabetes can reduce the severity of long-term complications. Control is achieved by testing the blood sugar four times a day and injecting insulin twice a day. An alternate method for administration of insulin is by means of a pump that provides an around-the-clock supply. The insulin is placed in a device that then injects it into the subcutaneous tissues of the abdomen.

Most insulin in use today is a "human" type that is produced by bacteria through genetic engineering. The insulin obtained from animal pancreases is now modified so that it causes fewer adverse reactions.

✔ CHECKPOINT **10**:

What hormone is low or ineffective in cases of diabetes mellitus?

The Sex Glands

The sex glands, the ovaries of the female and the testes of the male, not only produce the sex cells but also are important endocrine organs. The hormones produced by these organs are needed in the development of the sexual characteristics, which usually appear in the early teens, and for the maintenance of the reproductive organs once full development has been attained. Those features that typify a male or female other than the structures directly concerned with reproduction are termed ***secondary sex characteristics***. They include a deep voice and facial and body hair in males, and wider hips and a greater ratio of fat to muscle in females.

Hormones of the Sex Glands

The main male sex hormone or ***androgen*** (AN-dro-jen) produced by the male sex glands is ***testosterone*** (tes-TOS-ter-one).

In the female, the hormones that most nearly parallel testosterone in their actions are the ***estrogens*** (ES-tro-jens). Estrogens contribute to the development of the female secondary sex characteristics and stimulate the development of the mammary glands, the onset of menstruation, and the development and functioning of the reproductive organs.

The other hormone produced by the female sex glands, called ***progesterone*** (pro-JES-ter-one), assists in the normal development of pregnancy. All the sex hormones are discussed in more detail in Chapter 23.

✔ CHECKPOINT **11**:

In addition to controlling reproduction, sex hormones confer certain features associated with male and female gender. What are these features called as a group?

The Thymus Gland

The ***thymus gland*** is a mass of lymphoid tissue that lies in the upper part of the chest above the heart. This gland is important in the development of immunity. Its hormone, ***thymosin*** (THI-mo-sin), assists in the maturation of certain white blood cells known as T cells (T lymphocytes) after they have left the thymus gland and taken up residence in lymph nodes throughout the body.

The Pineal Gland

The ***pineal*** (PIN-e-al) ***gland*** is a small, flattened, cone-shaped structure located posterior to the midbrain and connected to the roof of the third ventricle. The pineal produces the hormone ***melatonin*** (mel-ah-TO-nin) during the

12

Seasonal Affective Disorder

We all sense that long dark days make us blue and sap our motivation. Are these learned responses or is there a physical basis for them? Studies have shown that the amount of light in the environment truly does have a physical effect on behavior.

Evidence that light alters mood comes from people who are intensely affected by the dark days of winter—people who suffer from *seasonal affective disorder,* aptly abbreviated SAD. When days shorten, these people feel sleepy, depressed, and anxious. They tend to overeat, especially carbohydrates.

Daily exposure to bright lights has been found to improve the mood of most people with SAD. Exposure for 15 minutes after rising in the morning may be enough, but some people require longer sessions both morning and evening. Light exerts its effects on the pineal gland of the brain. As it strikes the retina of the eye, it sets up impulses that decrease the amount of melatonin produced by the pineal. Because melatonin is known to depress mood, the final effect of light is to act as a mood elevator. Other aids incude aerobic exercise, stress management techniques, and antidepressant medications.

- The stomach secretes a hormone that stimulates its digestive activity.
- The small intestine secretes hormones that stimulate the production of digestive juices and help regulate the process of digestion.
- The kidneys produce a hormone called *erythropoietin* (e-rith-ro-POY-eh-tin), which stimulates red blood cell production in the bone marrow. This hormone is produced when there is a decreased supply of oxygen in the blood.
- The atria of the heart produce a substance called *atrial natriuretic* (na-tre-u-RET-ik) *peptide (ANP)* in response to increased filling of the atria. ANP increases loss of sodium by the kidneys and lowers blood pressure.
- The *placenta* (plah-SEN-tah) produces several hormones during pregnancy. These cause changes in the uterine lining and, later in pregnancy, help to prepare the breasts for lactation. Pregnancy tests are based on the presence of placental hormones.

dark period of each day. Little hormone is produced during daylight hours. This pattern of hormone secretion influences the regulation of sleep–wake cycles (see Seasonal Affective Disorder). Melatonin also appears to delay the onset of puberty.

OTHER HORMONE-PRODUCING TISSUES

Originally, the word *hormone* applied to the secretions of the endocrine glands only. The term now includes various substances produced in the body that have regulatory actions, either locally or at a distance from where they are produced. Many body tissues produce substances that have strong effects in regulating the local environment. Some of these other hormone-producing organs are the following:

Prostaglandins

Prostaglandins (pros-tah-GLAN-dins) are a group of local hormones made by most body tissues. They are produced, act, and are rapidly inactivated in or close to the sites of origin. A bewildering array of functions has been ascribed to these substances. Some prostaglandins cause constriction of blood vessels, of bronchial tubes, and of the intestine, whereas others cause dilation of these same structures. Prostaglandins are active in promoting inflammation; certain anti-inflammatory drugs, such as aspirin, act by blocking the production of prostaglandins. Some of the prostaglandins have been used to induce labor or abortion and have been recommended as possible contraceptive agents.

Overproduction of prostaglandins by the uterine lining (endometrium) can cause painful cramps of the muscle of the uterus. Treatment with drugs that are prostaglandin inhibitors has been successful in some cases. Much has been written about these substances, and extensive research on them continues.

HORMONES AND TREATMENT

Hormones used for medical treatment are obtained from several different sources. Some hormones are extracted from animal tissues for use as medication. Some hormones and hormone-like substances are available in synthetic form, meaning that they are manufactured in commercial laboratories. A few hormones are produced by the genetic engineering technique of recombinant DNA. In this method, a gene for the cellular manufacture of a given product is introduced in the laboratory into the common bacterium, *Escherichia coli.* The organisms are then grown in quantity, and the desired substance is harvested and purified.

A few examples of the use of natural and synthetic hormones in treatment are noted here:

- *Growth hormone* is used for the treatment of children with a deficiency of this hormone. Adequate supplies are available from recombinant DNA techniques.
- *Insulin* is used in the treatment of diabetes mellitus. Types of insulin available include "human" insulin produced by recombinant DNA methods and hormone obtained from animal pancreases.
- *Adrenal steroids,* primarily the glucocorticoids, are used for the relief of inflammation in such diseases as rheumatoid arthritis, lupus erythematosus, asthma, and cerebral edema; for immunosuppression after organ transplantation; and for the relief of the stress symptoms of shock.
- *Epinephrine* (adrenaline) has many uses, including stimulation of the heart muscle when rapid response is required, treatment of asthmatic attacks by relaxation of the muscles of the small bronchial tubes, and treatment of the acute allergic reaction called *anaphylaxis* (an-ah-fi-LAK-sis).
- *Thyroid hormones* are used in the treatment of hypothyroid conditions (cretinism and myxedema) and as replacement therapy after surgical removal of the thyroid gland.
- *Oxytocin* is used to contract the uterine muscle.

- *Androgens,* including testosterone and androsterone, are used in severe chronic illness to aid tissue building and promote healing.
- *Estrogen and progesterone* as purified synthetic drugs are used as oral contraceptives (birth control pills; "the pill"). They are highly effective in preventing pregnancy. Occasionally, they give rise to unpleasant side effects, such as nausea. More rarely, they cause serious complications, such as thrombosis (blood clots) or hypertension (high blood pressure). Any woman taking birth control pills should have a medical examination every 6 months. Preparations of estrogen and progesterone also are used to treat symptoms associated with menopause.

HORMONES AND STRESS

Stress in the form of physical injury, disease, emotional anxiety, and even pleasure calls forth a specific response from the body that involves both the nervous system and the endocrine system. The nervous system response, the "fight-or-flight" response, is mediated by parts of the brain, especially the hypothalamus, and by the autonomic nervous system. The hypothalamus also triggers the release of ACTH from the anterior pituitary. The hormones released from the adrenal cortex as a result of stimulation by ACTH raise the levels of glucose and other nutrients in the blood and inhibit inflammation. Growth hormone, thyroid hormones, sex hormones, and insulin may also be released.

These hormones help the body meet stressful situations. Unchecked, however, they are harmful to the body and may lead to such stress-related disorders as high blood pressure, heart disease, ulcers, back pain, and headaches. Cortisones decrease the immune response, leaving the body more open to infection.

Although no one would enjoy a life totally free of stress in the form of stimulation and challenge, unmanaged stress, or "distress," has negative effects on the body. For this reason, techniques such as biofeedback and meditation to control stress are useful. The simple measures of setting priorities, getting adequate periods of relaxation, and getting regular physical exercise are important in maintaining total health. See Learning to Control Stress Reactions.

✔ CHECKPOINT **12**:

What are some hormones released in time of stress?

AGING AND THE ENDOCRINE SYSTEM

Some of the changes associated with aging, such as loss of muscle and bone tissue, can be linked to changes in the endocrine system. The main clinical conditions associated with the endocrine system involve the pancreas and the thyroid.

Many elderly people develop adult-onset diabetes mellitus as a result of decreased secretion of insulin, which is made worse by poor diet, inactivity, and increased body fat. Some elderly people also show the effects of decreased thyroid hormone secretion.

Decline in the sex hormones during the middle-aged years occurs in both males and females. These changes come from decreased activity of the gonads but also involve the more basic level of the pituitary gland and the secretion of gonadotropic hormones. Decrease in bone mass leading to osteoporosis is one result of these declines. With age, there is also a decrease in levels of growth hormone and diminished activity of the adrenal cortex.

Thus far, the only commonly applied treatment for endocrine failure associated with age has been sex hormone replacement therapy for women at menopause. This supplementation has shown beneficial effects on mucous membranes, the cardiovascular system, bone mass, and mental function.

Taking Control of the Stress in Your Life

In today's complicated world, everyday stress is a part of our normal routine. Every now and then the pressures build until we are "stressed out." Research has conclusively shown that this feeling is not simply in your mind but is a physiologic reaction to stress.

When we encounter a stressful event, our nervous system signals the adrenal medulla to secrete the hormones epinephrine and norepinephrine directly into the bloodstream. This results in similar effects as when these hormones are released from nerve endings upon stimulation of the sympathetic nervous system. The difference is, when the hormones are secreted directly into the bloodstream, their effects are as much as 3 to 5 times stronger, and last up to 10 times longer than when they are released from nerve endings. When we encounter excessive stress, both hormones build up in the bloodstream and cause adverse effects such as restlessness, feeling jittery, inability to concentrate, inability to eat or sleep, and ultimately significant fatigue and possibly depression. Most of these effects can be reduced or eliminated by techniques of stress reduction, for example:

- Biofeedback focuses on an unconscious process to bring it into conscious perception; with structured, focused thought, the process can often be changed.
- Transcendental meditation uses a repetition of a "mantra," a specific word closely associated with a process to control or change that process.
- Guided imagery uses pleasing music, natural sounds, and visual images to steal focus away from unpleasant stimuli.
- Repetitive physical modalities use a physical action (exercise) rather than a mantra to focus attention.
- Coordinated relaxation exercises such as slow, deep breathing or repetitive contraction and relaxation of muscles also focus the mind's control.

Summary

I. Hormones

A. Functions of hormones
  1. Affect other cells or organs—target tissue
  2. Widespread effects on growth, metabolism, reproduction
  3. Local effects

B. Chemistry—chemical types
  1. Amino acid compounds—proteins and related compounds
  2. Steroids
     a. Derived from lipids
     b. Produced by adrenal cortex and sex glands

C. Regulation of hormones—negative feedback

II. Endocrine glands and their hormones

A. Pituitary
  1. Regulated by hypothalamus
     a. Anterior pituitary—releasing hormones sent through portal system
     b. Posterior pituitary—stores hormones; released by nervous stimulation
  2. Anterior lobe hormones
     a. Growth hormone (GH)
     b. Thyroid-stimulating hormone (TSH)
     c. Adrenocorticotropic hormone (ACTH)
     d. Prolactin (PRL)
     e. Follicle-stimulating hormone (FSH)
     f. Luteinizing hormone (LH)
  3. Posterior lobe hormones
     a. Antidiuretic hormone (ADH)
     b. Oxytocin
  4. Pituitary tumors—may cause underactivity or overactivity of pituitary

B. Thyroid gland
  1. Hormones
     a. Thyroxine—influences cell metabolism
     b. Calcitonin—decreases blood calcium levels
  2. Abnormalities
     a. Goiter—enlarged thyroid
     b. Hypothyroidism—causes cretinism or myxedema
     c. Hyperthyroidism—Graves' disease (exophthalmic goiter), a common example
  3. Thyroid function tests—radioactive iodine used

C. Parathyroid glands—secrete parathyroid hormone (PTH), which increases blood calcium levels

D. Adrenal glands
  1. Hormones of adrenal medulla (inner region)
     a. Epinephrine and norepinephrine—act as neurotransmitters
  2. Hormones of adrenal cortex (outer region)
     a. Glucocorticoids—released during stress; e.g., cortisol
     b. Mineralocorticoids—regulate water and electrolyte balance; e.g., aldosterone
     c. Sex hormones—produced in small amounts

E. Pancreas—islet cells of pancreas secrete hormones
  1. Insulin
     a. Lowers blood glucose
     b. Lack causes diabetes mellitus
  2. Glucagon
     a. Raises blood glucose

F. Sex glands—needed for reproduction and development of secondary sex characteristics
  1. Testes—secrete testosterone
  2. Ovaries—secrete estrogen and progesterone

G. Thymus gland—secretes thymosin, which aids in development of T lymphocytes

H. Pineal gland—secretes melatonin
  1. Regulates sexual development and sleep–wake cycles
  2. Controlled by environmental light

III. Other hormone-producing tissues
  1. Stomach and small intestine—se-

crete hormones that regulate digestion

2. Kidneys—secrete erythropoietin, which increases production of red blood cells

3. Atria of heart—ANP causes loss of sodium by kidney and lowers blood pressure

4. Placenta—secretes hormones that maintain pregnancy and prepare breasts for lactation

A. Prostaglandins—other cells throughout body produce prostaglandins, which have varied effects

IV. Hormones and treatment
1. Growth hormone—treatment of deficiency in children
2. Insulin—treatment of diabetes mellitus
3. Steroids—reduction of inflammation, suppression of immunity
4. Epinephrine—treatment of asthma, anaphylaxis, shock
5. Thyroid hormone—treatment of hypothyroidism
6. Oxytocin—contraction of uterine muscle
7. Androgens—promote healing
8. Estrogen and progesterone—contraception, symptoms of menopause

V. Hormones and stress

VI. Aging and the endocrine system

Questions for Study and Review

1. Compare the actions of the nervous system and the endocrine system.
2. Define *hormone.* Describe some general functions of hormones.
3. Give three examples of amino acid hormones; of steroid hormones.
4. Define *target tissue.*
5. Name the two divisions of the pituitary gland. Name the hormones released from each division and describe the effects of each.
6. What type of system connects the anterior pituitary with the hypothalamus? What is carried to the pituitary by this system?
7. Where is the thyroid gland located? What is its main hormone, and what does it do?
8. Describe the effects of hypothyroidism and hyperthyroidism.
9. How is thyroid function measured?
10. What is the main purpose of PTH? What are the effects of removal of the parathyroid glands? of excess secretion of PTH?
11. Name the two divisions of the adrenal glands and describe the effects of the hormones from each.
12. What are the results of hypofunction of the adrenal cortex?
13. What are the results of hyperfunction of the adrenal cortex? What common therapy produces similar symptoms?
14. What are the main purposes of insulin in the body? Name and describe the condition characterized by insufficient production of insulin.
15. Name the male and female sex hormones and briefly describe what each does.
16. Name the hormone produced by the thymus gland; by the pineal body. What are the effects of each?
17. Name five organs other than the endocrine glands that secrete hormones.
18. What are some of the various functions that have been ascribed to prostaglandins?
19. List several hormones that are released during stress.

✔ ANSWERS TO CHECKPOINTS

1. Hormones are chemicals that have specific regulatory effects on certain cells or organs in the body. Some of their effects are to regulate growth, metabolism, reproduction, and behavior.
2. Negative feedback is used to regulate the secretion of hormones.
3. The hypothalamus controls the pituitary.
4. The ending *-tropin* means a hormone that acts on another gland.
5. Thyroxine increases metabolism in cells.
6. The mineral calcium is regulated by PTH.
7. The main hormone from the adrenal medulla is epinephrine (adrenaline).
8. Cortisol raises the level of glucose in the blood.
9. The two hormones produced by the pancreatic islets that regulate glucose levels are insulin and glucagon.
10. Insulin is low or ineffective in cases of diabetes mellitus.
11. Secondary sex characteristics are features associated with gender other than reproductive activity.
12. Some hormones released in time of stress are epinephrine, norepinephrine, ACTH, cortisol, growth hormone, thyroid hormones, sex hormones, and insulin.

12

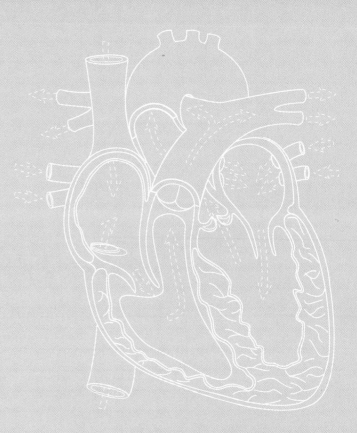

The chapters of this unit discuss the blood, the heart, the blood vessels, and the lymphatic system as well as body defenses, immunity, and vaccines. It is the purpose of this unit to emphasize the importance of transportation and immune systems in maintaining normal body functions.

Unit V

CIRCULATION AND BODY DEFENSE

The Blood

Chapter

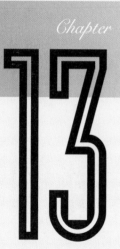

13

SELECTED KEY TERMS

The following terms are defined in the Glossary:

agglutination

anemia

antiserum

centrifuge

coagulation

erythrocyte

fibrin

hematocrit

hemoglobin

hemolysis

hemorrhage

hemostasis

leukemia

leukocyte

plasma

platelet (thrombocyte)

serum

thrombocytopenia

BEHAVIORAL OBJECTIVES

After careful study of this chapter, you should be able to:

1. List the functions of the blood
2. List the main ingredients in plasma
3. Name the three types of formed elements in the blood and give the function of each
4. Describe five types of leukocytes
5. Describe the formation of blood cells
6. Define hemostasis and cite three steps in hemostasis
7. Briefly describe the steps in blood clotting
8. Define *blood type* and explain the relation between blood type and transfusions
9. List the possible reasons for transfusions of whole blood and blood components
10. Define *anemia* and list the causes of anemia
11. Define *leukemia* and name the two types of leukemia
12. Describe several forms of clotting disorders
13. Describe the tests used to study blood

The circulating blood is of fundamental importance in maintaining homeostasis. This life-giving fluid brings nutrients and oxygen to the cells and carries away waste. Blood is pumped continuously by the heart through a closed system of vessels. The heart and blood vessels are described in Chapters 14 and 15.

Blood is classified as a connective tissue because nearly half of it is made up of cells. Blood cells share many characteristics of origination and development with other connective tissues. However, blood differs from other connective tissues in that its cells are not fixed in position; instead, they move freely in the liquid portion of the blood.

Blood is a viscous (thick) fluid that varies in color from bright scarlet to dark red, depending on how much oxygen it is carrying. The quantity of circulating blood differs with the size of the person; the average adult male, weighing 70 kg (154 pounds), has about 5 liters (5.2 quarts) of blood. This volume accounts for about 8% of total body weight.

FUNCTIONS OF THE BLOOD

The circulating blood serves the body in three ways: transportation, regulation, and protection.

Transportation

- Oxygen from inhaled air diffuses into the blood through the thin lung membranes and is carried to all the tissues of the body. Carbon dioxide, a waste product of cell metabolism, is carried from the tissues to the lungs, where it is breathed out.
- The blood transports nutrients and other needed substances, such as electrolytes (salts) and vitamins, to the cells. These materials may enter the blood from the digestive system or may be released into the blood from body stores.
- The blood transports the waste products from the cells to the sites from which they are released. For example, the kidney removes excess water, acid, electrolytes, and urea (a nitrogen-containing waste). The liver removes blood pigments, hormones, and drugs, and the lungs eliminate carbon dioxide.
- The blood carries hormones from their sites of origin to the organs they affect.

Regulation

- Buffers in the blood help keep the pH of body fluids at about 7.4. (The pH is a measure of the acidity of a solution.)

- The blood serves to regulate the amount of fluid in the tissues by means of substances (mainly proteins) that maintain the proper osmotic pressure.
- The blood transports heat that is generated in the muscles to other parts of the body, thus aiding in the regulation of body temperature.

Protection

- The blood is important in defense against disease. It carries the cells and antibodies of the immune system that protect against pathogens.
- The blood contains factors that protect against blood loss from the site of an injury.

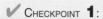

CHECKPOINT **1**:

What are some substances transported in the blood?

BLOOD CONSTITUENTS

The blood is divided into two main components. The liquid portion is the *plasma.* The *formed elements,* which include cells and cell fragments, fall into three categories, as follows:

- *Erythrocytes* (eh-RITH-ro-sites), from *erythro,* meaning "red," are the red blood cells, which transport oxygen.
- *Leukocytes* (LU-ko-sites), from *leuko,* meaning "white," are the several types of white blood cells, which protect against infection.
- *Platelets,* also called *thrombocytes* (THROM-bo-sites), are cell fragments that participate in blood clotting.

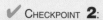

CHECKPOINT **2**:

What are the two main components of blood?

Blood Plasma

More than half of the total volume of blood is plasma. The plasma itself is 90% water. Many different substances, dissolved or suspended in the water, make up the other 10%. The plasma content may vary somewhat because substances are removed and added as the blood circulates to and from the tissues. However, the body tends to maintain a fairly constant level of most substances. For example, the level of glucose, a simple sugar, is maintained at a remarkably constant level of about one tenth of one percent (0.1%) in solution.

After water, the next largest percentage of material in the plasma is *protein.* Proteins are the principal constituents of cytoplasm and are essential to the growth and the rebuilding of body tissues. The plasma proteins include the following:

- *Albumin* (al-BU-min), the most abundant protein in plasma, is important for maintaining the osmotic pressure of the blood. This protein is manufactured in the liver.
- *Clotting factors,* necessary for blood coagulation, are also manufactured in the liver.
- *Antibodies* combat infection.
- A system of enzymes made of several proteins, collectively known as *complement,* helps antibodies in their fight against pathogens (see Chap. 17).

Nutrients are also found in the plasma. The principal carbohydrate found in the plasma is *glucose,* which is absorbed by the capillaries of the intestine after digestion. Glucose is stored mainly in the liver as glycogen and is released as needed to supply energy.

Amino acids, the products of protein digestion, are also found in the plasma. These are also absorbed into the blood through the intestinal capillaries.

Lipids constitute a small percentage of blood plasma. Lipid components include fats, cholesterol, and lipoproteins, which are proteins bound to cholesterol.

The *electrolytes* in the plasma appear primarily as chloride, carbonate, or phosphate salts of sodium, potassium, calcium, and magnesium. These salts have a variety of functions, including the formation of bone (calcium and phosphorus), the production of certain hormones (such as iodine for the production of thyroid hormones), and the maintenance of the acid–base balance (sodium and potassium carbonates and phosphates).

Other materials, such as vitamins, hormones, waste products, and drugs, also are transported in the plasma.

> ✔ CHECKPOINT **3**:
>
> Next to water, what is the most abundant type of substance in plasma?

The Formed Elements

Erythrocytes

Erythrocytes, the red blood cells (RBCs, or red cells), are tiny, disk-shaped bodies with a central area that is thinner than the edges (Fig. 13-1). They are different from other cells in that the mature form found in the circulating blood is lacking a nucleus and most of the other organelles commonly found in cells. As red cells mature, these components are lost to provide more space for the cells to carry oxygen. This vital gas is bound in the red cells to *hemoglobin* (he-mo-GLO-bin), a protein that contains iron (see Hemoglobin). Hemoglobin, combined with oxygen, gives the blood its characteristic red color. The more oxygen carried by the hemoglobin, the brighter is the red color of the blood. Therefore, the blood that goes from the lungs to the tissues is a bright red because it carries a great supply of oxygen; in contrast, the blood that returns to the lungs is a much darker red because it has given up much of its oxygen to the tissues.

Hemoglobin has two lesser functions in addition to the transport of oxygen. Hemoglobin that has given up its oxygen is able to carry hydrogen ions. In this way, hemoglobin acts as a buffer and plays an important role in acid–base balance (see Chap. 21). Hemoglobin also carries some carbon dioxide from the tissues to the

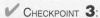

Hemoglobin

The hemoglobin molecule is a protein made of four chains of amino acids (the "globin" part of the molecule), each of which holds an iron-containing "heme" unit. It is the heme portion that binds oxygen.

Hemoglobin allows the blood to carry much more oxygen than it could carry simply dissolved in the plasma. Hemoglobin picks up oxygen in the lungs and releases it in the body tissues. When cells are active, they need more oxygen. At the same time, they generate heat and acidity. These changing conditions promote the release of oxygen from hemoglobin.

Hemoglobin is produced by red cells in the red bone marrow. It is constantly broken down as the red cells die and disintegrate. Some of its components are recycled, but dietary protein, and iron are still essential to maintain supplies.

lungs for elimination. The carbon dioxide is bound to a different part of the molecule than the part that holds oxygen, so that it does not interfere with oxygen transport.

The ability of hemoglobin to carry oxygen can be blocked by carbon monoxide. This harmful gas combines with hemoglobin to form a stable compound that can severely restrict the ability of the erythrocytes to carry oxygen. Carbon monoxide is a byproduct of the incomplete burning of fuels, such as gasoline and other petroleum products and coal, wood, and other carbon-containing materials. It also occurs in cigarette smoke and automobile exhaust.

The erythrocytes are by far the most numerous of the blood cells, averaging from 4.5 to 5 million per cubic millimeter (mm^3) of blood. (A cubic millimeter is the same as a microliter [uL], one millionth of a liter, another way of expressing the concentration of blood cells.) Because mature red cells have no nucleus and cannot divide, they must be replaced constantly. The production of red cells is stimulated by the hormone *erythropoietin* (eh-rith-ro-POY-eh-tin). This hormone is released from the kidney in response to a decrease in oxygen supply.

13

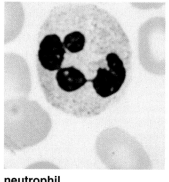
neutrophil

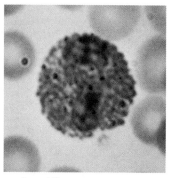
eosinophil

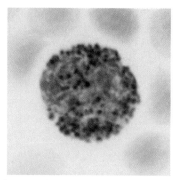
basophil

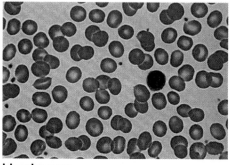
blood smear

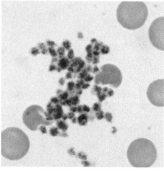
red blood cells and platelets

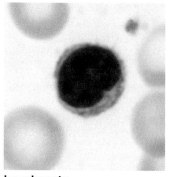
lymphocyte
A

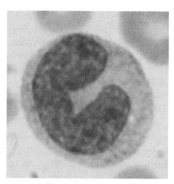
monocyte

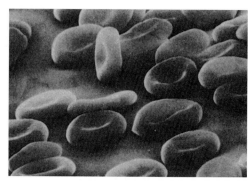
B

FIGURE **13•1** **(A)** Normal blood smear and close-up view of individual blood cells. **(B)** Red blood cells as seen by scanning electron microscopy.

> ✔ CHECKPOINT **4**:
>
> Red cells are modified to carry a maximum amount of hemoglobin. What is the function of hemoglobin?

Leukocytes

The **leukocytes,** or white blood cells (WBCs, or white cells), are different from the erythrocytes in appearance, quantity, and function (see Fig. 13-1). The cells themselves are round, but they contain prominent nuclei of varying shapes and sizes. Occurring at a concentration of 5,000 to 10,000 per cubic millimeter of blood, leukocytes are outnumbered by red cells by about 700 to 1. Although the red cells have a definite color, the leukocytes tend to be colorless.

The different types of white cells are identified by their size, the shape of the nucleus, and

Table 13•1	Leukocytes (White Blood Cells)		
TYPE OF CELL	RELATIVE PERCENTAGE (ADULT)		FUNCTION
Granulocytes			
Neutrophils (NU-tro-fils)	54%–62%		Phagocytosis
Eosinophils (e-o-SIN-o-fils)	1%–3%		Allergic reactions: defense against parasites
Basophils (BA-so-fils)	< 1%		Allergic reactions; inflammatory reactions
Agranulocytes			
Lymphocytes (LIM-fo-sites)	25%–38%		Immunity (T cells and B cells)
Monocytes (MON-o-sites)	3%–7%		Phagocytosis

the appearance of granules in the cytoplasm when the cells are stained (Table 13-1). The stain commonly used for blood is Wright's stain. This is a mixture of dyes that differentiates the various cells in blood. The relative percentage of the different types of leukocytes is a valuable clue in arriving at a medical diagnosis.

The granular leukocytes, or **granulocytes** (GRAN-u-lo-sites), are so named because they show visible granules in the cytoplasm when stained. They include the following:

- **Neutrophils** (NU-tro-fils), which show lavender granules
- **Eosinophils** (e-o-SIN-o-fils), which have beadlike, bright pink granules
- **Basophils** (BA-so-fils), which have large, dark blue granules that often obscure the nucleus

The neutrophils, which are active in fighting infections, are the most numerous of the white cells, constituting up to 60% of all leukocytes. The eosinophils and basophils make up a small percentage of the white cells but increase in number during allergic reactions.

Because the nuclei of the neutrophils are of various shapes, they are also called **polymorphs** (meaning "many forms") or simply *polys*. Other nicknames are *segs*, referring to the segmented nucleus, and *PMNs*, an abbrevi-

ation of *polymorphonuclear neutrophils*. Before reaching full maturity and becoming segmented, the nucleus of the neutrophil looks like a thick, curved band. An increase in the number of these **band cells** (also called *stab* or *staff cells*) is a sign of infection and active production of neutrophils.

The agranular leukocytes, or **agranulocytes,** are so named because they lack easily visible granules. There are two types:

- **Lymphocytes** (LIM-fo-sites) are the second most numerous of the white cells and are active in immunity.
- **Monocytes** (MON-o-sites) are the largest in size. They function as phagocytes.

Function of Leukocytes

The most important function of leukocytes is to destroy pathogens. Whenever pathogens enter the tissues, as through a wound, certain white cells (neutrophils and monocytes) are attracted to that area. They leave the blood vessels and proceed by ameboid (ah-ME-boyd), or amebalike, motion to the area of infection. There, they engulf the invaders by the process of **phagocytosis** (fag-o-si-TO-sis) (Fig. 13-2). In battling pathogens, leukocytes may be destroyed. A mixture of dead and living bacteria, together with dead and living leukocytes, forms **pus**. A collection of pus localized in one area is known as an **abscess**.

Some monocytes enter the tissues, enlarge, and mature into **macrophages** (MAK-ro-faj-ez), which are highly active in disposing of invaders or foreign material. Some lymphocytes become **plasma cells,** active in the production of circulating antibodies needed for immunity. The activities of the various white cells are further discussed in Chapter 17.

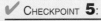

✔ CHECKPOINT **5**:

What is the most important function of leukocytes?

Platelets

Of all the formed elements, the blood **platelets** (thrombocytes) are the smallest (see Fig. 13-1). These tiny structures are not cells in them-

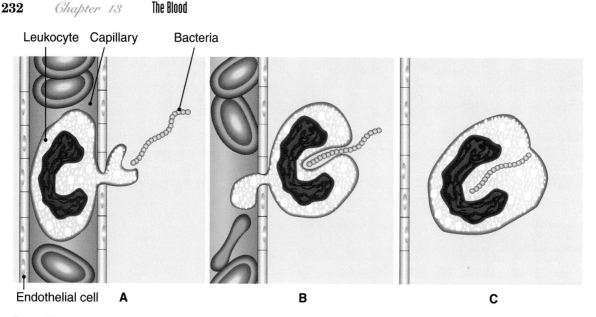

Leukocyte   Capillary   Bacteria

Endothelial cell   **A**   **B**   **C**

FIGURE **13•2**   Phagocytosis. **(A)** White blood cell squeezes through a capillary wall in the region of an infection. **(B, C)** White cells engulf the bacteria.

selves but rather fragments of cells. The number of platelets in the circulating blood has been estimated to range from 150,000 to 450,000 per cubic millimeter.

Platelets are essential to blood ***coagulation*** (clotting). When, as a result of injury, blood comes in contact with any tissue other than the innermost lining of the blood vessels, the platelets stick together and form a plug that seals the wound. The platelets then release chemicals that participate in the formation of a clot to stop blood loss. More details on these reactions are given later.

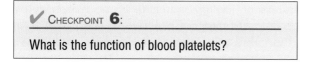

✔ CHECKPOINT **6**:

What is the function of blood platelets?

Origin of the Formed Elements

All of the formed elements of the blood are produced in red marrow, which is located in the ends of long bones and in the inner mass of all other bones. The ancestors of the blood cells are called ***stem cells***. Each kind of stem cell develops into one of the blood cell types found within the red marrow.

One group of white cells, the lymphocytes, develops to maturity in lymphoid tissue and can multiply in this tissue as well (see Chap. 16). When an invader enters the tissues, the bone marrow and lymphoid tissue go into emergency production of white cells, and their number increases enormously as a result. Detection in a blood examination of an abnormally large number of white cells is an indication of infection.

The platelets are believed to originate in the red marrow as fragments of certain giant cells called ***megakaryocytes*** (meg-ah-KAR-e-o-sites), which are formed in the red marrow. Platelets do not have nuclei or DNA, but they do contain active enzymes and mitochondria.

Life-Span of the Blood Cells

The life-span of the different types of blood cells varies considerably. For example, after leaving the bone marrow, erythrocytes circulate in the bloodstream for about 120 days. Leukocytes may appear in the circulating blood for only 6 to 8 hours. They may then enter the tissues, where they survive for longer periods—days, months, or even years. Blood platelets have a life-span of about 10 days.

In comparison with other tissue cells, most of those in the blood are short lived. The need for constant replacement of blood cells means that normal activity of the red bone marrow is absolutely essential to life.

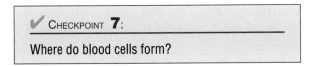

CHECKPOINT **7**:

Where do blood cells form?

HEMOSTASIS

Hemostasis (he-mo-STA-sis) is the process that prevents the loss of blood from the circulation when a blood vessel is ruptured by an injury. Events in hemostasis include the following:

- ***Contraction*** of the smooth muscles in the wall of the blood vessel. This reduces the flow of blood and loss from the defect in the vessel wall. The term for this reduction in the diameter of a vessel is *vasoconstriction*.
- Formation of a ***platelet plug***. Activated platelets become sticky and adhere to the defect to form a temporary plug.
- Formation of a ***blood clot***.

Blood Clotting

The many substances necessary for blood clotting, or coagulation, are normally inactive in the bloodstream. A balance is maintained between compounds that promote clotting, known as ***procoagulants,*** and those that prevent clotting, known as ***anticoagulants.*** In addition, there are chemicals in the circulation that act to dissolve any clots that may form. Under normal conditions, the substances that prevent clotting prevail. When an injury occurs, however, the procoagulants are activated, and a clot is formed.

The clotting process is a well-controlled series of separate events involving 12 different factors. The final step in these reactions is the conversion of a plasma protein called ***fibrinogen*** (fi-BRIN-o-jen) into solid threads of ***fibrin,*** which form the clot.

A few of the final steps involved in the forma-

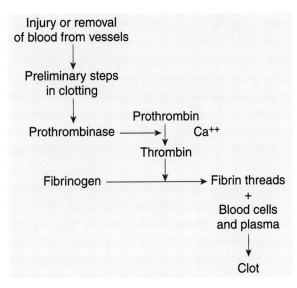

FIGURE **13•3**   Final steps in the formation of a blood clot.

tion of a blood clot are described below and diagrammed in Figure 13-3:

- Substances released from damaged tissues result in the formation of ***prothrombinase*** (pro-THROM-bih-nase), a substance that triggers the final clotting mechanism.
- Prothrombinase converts prothrombin in the blood to ***thrombin.*** Calcium is needed for this step.
- Thrombin, in turn, converts soluble fibrinogen into insoluble fibrin. ***Fibrin*** forms a network of threads that entraps plasma and blood cells to form a clot.

Blood clotting occurs in response to injury. Blood also clots when it comes into contact with some surface other than the innermost lining of a blood vessel, such as a glass or plastic tube used for a blood specimen. In this case, the preliminary steps of clotting are somewhat different and require more time. The fluid that remains after clotting has occurred is called ***serum*** (plural, *sera*). Serum contains all the components of blood plasma *except* the clotting factors.

Several methods used to measure the body's ability to coagulate blood are described later in this chapter.

BLOOD TYPES

If for some reason the amount of blood in the body is severely reduced, through **hemorrhage** (HEM-eh-rij) (excessive bleeding) or disease, the body cells suffer from lack of oxygen and nutrients. One possible measure to take in such an emergency is to administer blood from another person into the veins of the patient, a procedure called **transfusion.**

Care must be taken in transferring blood from one person to another, however, because the patient's plasma may contain substances, called *antibodies* or *agglutinins*, that can cause the red cells of the donor's blood to rupture and release their hemoglobin. Such cells are said to be **hemolyzed** (HE-mo-lized), and the resulting condition can be dangerous.

Certain proteins, called *antigens* (AN-ti-jens) or *agglutinogens,* on the surface of the red cells cause these incompatibility reactions. There are many types of these proteins on blood cells, but only two groups are particularly likely to cause a transfusion reaction, the so-called A and B antigens and the Rh factor.

The ABO Blood Type Group

Four blood types involving the A and B antigens have been recognized: A, B, AB, and O (Table 13-2). These letters indicate the type of antigen present on the red cells. If only the A antigen is present on the red cells, the person has type A blood; if only the B antigen is present, he or she has type B blood. Type AB red cells have both antigens, and type O have neither. Of course no one has antibodies to his or her own blood type antigens, or their plasma would destroy their own cells. Each person does, however, develop antibodies that react with the AB antigens he or she is lacking. It is these antibodies in the patient's plasma that can react with antigens on the donor's red cells to cause a transfusion reaction.

Testing for Blood Type

Blood sera containing antibodies to the A or B antigens are used to test for blood type. These antisera are prepared in animals using either the A or the B antigens to induce a response. Blood serum containing antibodies that can agglutinate and destroy red cells with A antigen on the surface is called **anti-A serum;** blood serum containing antibodies that can destroy red cells with B antigen on the surface is called **anti-B serum.** When combined with a blood sample in the laboratory, each antiserum causes the corresponding red cells to clump together in a process known as **agglutination** (ah-glu-tih-NA-shun). The blood's pattern of agglutination, when mixed *separately* with these two sera, reveals its blood type (Fig. 13-4). Type A reacts with anti-A serum only; type B reacts with anti-B serum only. Type AB agglutinates with both, and type O agglutinates with neither A nor B.

A blood specimen from any person who has had a prior blood transfusion or a pregnancy is tested further for the presence of any less common antibodies. Both the red cells and the serum are tested separately for any possible cross-reactions with donor blood.

Blood Compatibility

A person's blood type is determined by heredity, and the percentage of people with each of the different blood types varies in different popula-

Table 13•2	**The ABO Blood Group System**				
BLOOD TYPE	RED BLOOD CELL ANTIGEN	REACTS WITH ANTISERUM	PLASMA ANTIBODIES	CAN TAKE FROM	CAN DONATE TO
A	A	Anti-A	Anti-B	A, O	A, AB
B	B	Anti-B	Anti-A	B, O	B, AB
AB	A, B	Anti-A, Anti-B	None	AB, A, B, O	AB
O	None	None	Anti-A, anti-B	O	O, A, B, AB

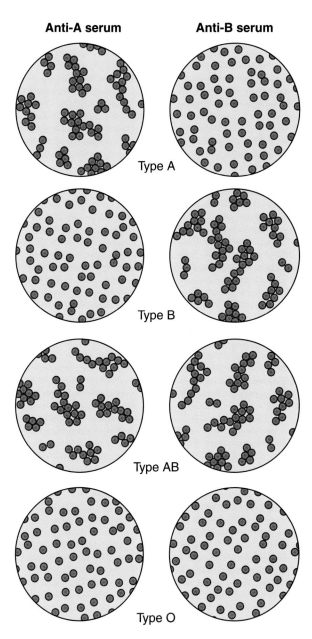

Anti-A serum **Anti-B serum**

Type A

Type B

Type AB

Type O

FIGURE **13•4** Blood typing. Red cells in type A blood are ag-glutinated (clumped) by anti-A serum; those in type B blood are agglutinated by anti-B serum. Type AB blood cells are ag-glutinated by both sera, and type O blood is not agglutinated by either serum.

tions. About 45% of the white population of the United States has type O blood.

In an emergency, type O blood can be given to any ABO type because the cells lack both A and B antigens and will not react with either A or B antibodies. Conversely, type AB blood contains no antibodies to agglutinate red cells, and peo-ple with this blood type can therefore receive blood from any ABO type donor (see Table 13-2). Under normal circumstances, it is safest to give blood of the same type.

The Rh Factor

More than 85% of the population of the United States has another red cell antigen group called the **Rh factor,** named for *Rh*esus monkeys, in which it was first found. Rh is also known as the *D antigen*. People with this antigen are said to be **Rh positive;** those who lack this protein are said to be **Rh negative.** If Rh-positive blood is given to an Rh-negative person, he or she may produce antibodies to the "foreign" Rh anti-gens. The blood of this "Rh-sensitized" person will then destroy any Rh-positive cells received in a later transfusion.

Rh incompatibility is a potential problem in certain pregnancies. A mother who is Rh nega-tive may develop antibodies to the Rh protein of an Rh-positive fetus (the fetus having inherited this factor from the father). Red cells from the fetus that enter the mother's circulation during pregnancy and childbirth evoke the response. In a subsequent pregnancy with an Rh-positive fetus, some of the anti-Rh antibodies may pass from the mother's blood into the blood of her fetus and destroy the fetus's red cells. This con-dition is called **hemolytic disease of the new-born** (HDN). HDN is now prevented by admin-istration of immune globulin $Rh_o(D)$, trade name Rho-GAM, to the mother during preg-nancy and shortly after delivery. These pre-formed antibodies clear the mother's circulation of Rh antigens and prevent stimulation of an immune response. In many cases, a baby born with HDN could be saved by a transfusion dur-ing which much of the baby's blood is replaced with Rh-negative blood.

✔ CHECKPOINT **8**:

What are the blood antigens most often involved in incompatibility reactions?

USES OF BLOOD AND BLOOD COMPONENTS

Blood Banks

Blood can be packaged and kept in blood banks for emergencies. To keep the blood from clotting, a solution such as citrate-phosphate-dextrose-adenine (CPDA-1) is added. The blood may then be stored for up to 35 days. The supplies of blood in the bank are dated with an expiration date so that blood in which red cells may have disintegrated is not used. Blood banks usually have all types of blood and blood products available. It is important that there be an extra supply of type O, Rh-negative blood because in an emergency this type can be used for any patient. It is normal procedure to test the recipient and give blood of the same type.

A person can donate his or her own blood before undergoing elective (planned) surgery to be used during surgery if needed. This practice eliminates the possibility of incompatibility and of disease transfer as well. Such *autologous* (aw-TOL-o-gus) (self-originating) blood is stored in a blood bank until after the surgery is completed.

Whole Blood Transfusions

The transfer of whole human blood from a healthy person to a patient is often a life-saving process. Whole blood transfusions may be used for any condition in which there is loss of a large volume of blood, for example:

- In the treatment of massive hemorrhage from serious mechanical injuries
- For blood loss during internal bleeding, as from bleeding ulcers
- During or after an operation that causes considerable blood loss
- For blood replacement in the treatment of hemolytic disease of the newborn

Caution and careful evaluation of the need for a blood transfusion is the rule, however, because of the risk for transfusion reactions and the transmission of viral diseases, particularly hepatitis.

Use of Blood Components

Most often, when some ingredient of the blood is needed, it is not whole blood but a blood component that is given. Blood can be broken down into its various parts, which may be used for different purposes.

A common method for separating the blood plasma from the formed elements is by use of a *centrifuge* (SEN-trih-fuje), a machine that spins in a circle at high speed to separate components of a mixture according to density. When a container of blood is spun rapidly, all the formed elements of the blood are pulled into a clump at the bottom of the container. They are thus separated from the plasma, which is less dense. The formed elements may be further separated and used for specific purposes, for example, packed red cells alone or platelets alone.

Blood losses to the donor can be minimized by removal of the blood, separation of the desired components, and return of the remainder to the donor. The general term for this procedure is *hemapheresis* (hem-ah-fer-E-sis). If the plasma is removed and the formed elements returned to the donor, the procedure is called *plasmapheresis* (plas-mah-fer-E-sis).

Use of Plasma
Blood plasma is a very useful substance; it may be given as an emergency measure to combat shock and replace blood volume. Plasma is especially useful in situations in which blood typing and the use of whole blood are not possible, such as in natural disasters or in emergency rescues. Because the red cells have been removed from the plasma, there are no incompatibility problems; plasma can be given to anyone. Plasma separated from the cellular elements is usually further separated by chemical means into various components, such as plasma protein fraction, serum albumin, immune serum, and clotting factors.

The packaged plasma that is currently available is actually plasma protein fraction. Further separation yields serum albumin that is available in solutions of 5% or 25% concentration. In addition to use in treatment of shock, these solutions are given in cases in which plasma proteins are deficient; they increase the osmotic pressure of the blood and thus draw fluids back into circulation. The use of plasma proteins and serum albumin has increased because these blood components can be treated with heat to prevent transmission of viral diseases.

Fresh plasma may be frozen and saved. When frozen plasma is thawed, a white precipitate called ***cryoprecipitate*** (kri-o-pre-SIP-ih-tate) forms in the bottom of the container. Plasma frozen when it is less than 6 hours old and cryoprecipitate contain most of the factors needed for clotting and may be given when there is a special need for these factors.

Gamma globulin is the fraction of the plasma that contains the antibodies produced by lymphocytes when they come in contact with foreign agents, such as bacteria and viruses. Antibodies play an important role in the immune system (see Chap. 17). Commercially prepared immune sera are available for administration to patients in immediate need of antibodies, such as infants born to mothers with active hepatitis.

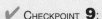

✔ CHECKPOINT **9**:

How is blood commonly separated into its component parts?

BLOOD DISORDERS

Abnormalities involving the blood may be divided into three groups:

- ***Anemia*** (ah-NE-me-ah), a disorder in which there is an abnormally low level of hemoglobin or red cells in the blood and thus impaired delivery of oxygen to the tissues. Anemia may result from the following:
  - ***Excessive loss or destruction of red cells.*** This may occur with hemorrhage or with conditions that cause hemolysis (rupture) of red cells.
  - ***Impaired production of red cells or hemoglobin.*** Both nutritional deficiencies and suppression of bone marrow may cause anemia.
- ***Leukemia*** (lu-KE-me-ah), a neoplastic disease of the blood characterized by an increase in the number of white cells.
- ***Clotting disorders.*** These disorders are characterized by an abnormal tendency to bleed due to a breakdown in the body's clotting mechanism.

Anemia

Anemia Due to Excessive Loss or Destruction of Red Cells

Excessive loss of red cells occurs with hemorrhage, which may be sudden and acute or gradual and chronic.

The average adult has about 5 liters of blood. If a person loses as much as 2 liters suddenly, death usually results. If the loss is gradual, however, over a period of weeks, or months, the body can compensate and withstand the loss of as much as 4 or 5 liters. If the cause of the chronic blood loss, such as bleeding ulcers, excessive menstrual flow, and bleeding hemorrhoids (piles), can be corrected, the body is usually able to restore the blood to normal. This process can take as long as 6 months, and until the blood returns to normal, the affected person may have anemia.

Anemia caused by the excessive destruction of red cells is called ***hemolytic*** (he-mo-LIH-tik) ***anemia.*** The spleen, along with the liver, normally destroys old red cells. Occasionally, an overactive spleen destroys the cells too rapidly, causing anemia. Infections may also cause the loss of red cells. For example, the malarial parasite multiplies in red cells and destroys them, and certain bacteria, particularly streptococci, produce a toxin that causes hemolysis.

Certain inherited diseases that cause the production of abnormal hemoglobin may also result in hemolytic anemia. The hemoglobin in normal adult cells is of the A type and is designated *HbA*. In the inherited disease **sickle cell anemia,** the hemoglobin in many of the red cells is abnormal. When these cells give up their oxygen to the tissues, they are transformed from the normal disk shape into a sickle shape (Fig. 13-5). These sickle cells are fragile and tend to break easily. Because of their odd shape, they also tend to become tangled in masses that can block smaller blood vessels. When obstruction

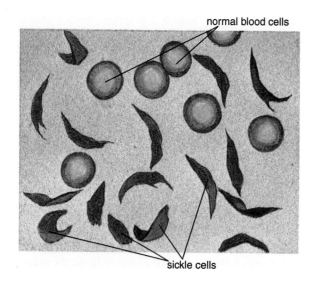

normal blood cells

sickle cells

FIGURE **13•5** Sickling of red blood cells in sickle cell anemia.

occurs, there may be severe joint swelling and pain, especially in the fingers and toes, as well as abdominal pain. This aspect of sickle cell anemia is referred to as *painful crisis.*

Sickle cell anemia occurs almost exclusively in black people. About 8% of African Americans have one of the genes for the abnormal hemoglobin and are said to have the **sickle cell trait.** It is only when the involved gene is transmitted from both parents that the clinical disease appears. About 1% of African Americans have two of these genes and thus have **sickle cell disease.** One drug has been found to reduce the frequency of painful crisis in certain adults. Hydroxyurea causes the body to make some hemoglobin of an alternate form (fetal hemoglobin) so that the red cells are not as susceptible to sickling. People taking hydroxyurea require blood tests every 2 weeks to assess for bone marrow suppression due to this drug.

Anemia Due to Impaired Production of Red Cells or Hemoglobin

Many factors can interfere with normal red cell production. Anemia that results from a deficiency of some nutrient is referred to as *nutritional anemia.* These conditions may arise from a deficiency of the specific nutrient in the diet, from an inability to absorb the nutrient, or from

drugs that interfere with the body's use of the nutrient.

Deficiency Anemia

The most common nutritional anemia is **iron-deficiency anemia.** Iron is an essential constituent of hemoglobin. The average diet usually provides enough iron to meet the needs of the adult male, but this diet often is inadequate to meet the needs of growing children and women of childbearing age.

A diet deficient in proteins or vitamins can also result in anemia. Folic acid, one of the B complex vitamins, is necessary for the production of blood cells. Folic acid deficiency anemia occurs in people with alcoholism, in elderly people on poor diets, and in infants or others suffering from intestinal disorders that interfere with the absorption of this water-soluble vitamin.

Pernicious (per-NISH-us) **anemia** is characterized by a deficiency of vitamin B_{12}, a substance essential for the proper formation of red cells. The cause is a permanent deficiency of **intrinsic factor,** a secretion in the gastric juice that is responsible for the absorption of vitamin B_{12} from the intestine. Neglected pernicious anemia can bring about deterioration in the nervous system, causing difficulty in walking, weakness and stiffness in the extremities, mental changes, and permanent damage to the spinal cord. Early treatment, including the intramuscular injection of vitamin B_{12} and attention to a prescribed diet, ensures an excellent outlook. This treatment must be kept up for the rest of the patient's life if good health is to be maintained. See Preventing Nutritional Anemia.

Bone Marrow Suppression

The decreased production of red cells may also be brought about by **bone marrow suppression** or failure. One type of bone marrow failure, **aplastic** (a-PLAS-tik) **anemia,** may be caused by a variety of physical and chemical agents. Chemical substances that injure the bone marrow include certain prescribed drugs and toxic agents such as gold compounds, arsenic, and benzene. Physical agents that may

Preventing Nutritional Anemia

The term "anemia" has long been misused as a primary diagnosis. In its correct usage, the term refers to a set of complex signs and symptoms that are generally related to a decrease in numbers of red blood cells (RBC) and/or hemoglobin (Hb) in the blood. Nutritional anemias may be caused by deficiencies of iron, vitamin C, vitamin B_{12}, and folate. They are usually easily controlled through changes in dietary intake. Not recognizing and therefore not treating even mild anemias could be a serious mistake, since the presence of any type of anemia indiciates an underlying disorder. To avoid nutritional anemias:

- Make sure your diet contains ample iron. Because iron is poorly absorbed from the intestines, most individuals barely meet the recommended dietary allowance (RDA). This can be especially important in women who lose iron through menstruation, lactation, or any other blood loss. The best sources of dietary iron are red meats; although vegetables and bran also contain iron, it is not as readily absorbed as the iron in meat.
- Increase vitamin C intake if needed. Vitamin C (ascorbic acid) is known to directly effect absorption of iron from the intestinal tract. Vitamin C deficiency inevitably leads to anemia. Eating citrus fruits and green leafy vegetables will ensure enough vitamin C to have adequate iron absorption.
- Build up stores of vitamin B_{12} in your body. Vitamin B_{12} deficiency also leads to anemia. This vitamin is found in red meats (especially liver), eggs, milk, and red vegetables, such as red cabbage and beets. B_{12} can only be absorbed from a full stomach as digestive proteins and enzymes are necessary for its absorption.
- Take in plenty of folate. Both vitamin B_{12} and folate are needed for the maturation of red cells. Folate is found in many plant and animal tissues and is absorbed from the large intestine. Foods high in folate are green leafy vegetables, yeasts, liver, and mushrooms. Inadequate intake of folate is common and many medications interfere with its absorption, as does alcohol.

injure the marrow include x-rays, atomic radiation, radium, and radioactive phosphorus.

The damaged bone marrow fails to produce either red or white cells, so that the anemia is accompanied by **leukopenia** (lu-ko-PE-ne-ah), a drop in the number of white cells. Removal of the toxic agent, followed by blood transfusions until the marrow is able to resume its activity, may result in recovery. Bone marrow transplantations have also been successful.

A less severe depression of the bone marrow may develop in patients with certain chronic diseases, such as cancer, kidney or liver disorders, and rheumatoid arthritis. Some medications are now available to stimulate production of specific types of blood cells by the bone marrow.

> ✔ CHECKPOINT **10**:
>
> What is anemia?

Leukemia

Leukemia is a neoplastic blood disease characterized by an enormous increase in the number of white cells due to a cancer of the tissues that produce these cells. Although the cells are high in number, they are immature and cannot perform their normal jobs. They also crowd out the other blood cells.

As noted earlier, the white cells have two main sources: red marrow, also called *myeloid tissue,* and lymphoid tissue. If this wild proliferation of white cells stems from a tumor of the bone marrow, the condition is called **myelogenous** (mi-eh-LOJ-en-us) **leukemia.** When the cancer arises in the lymphoid tissue, so that most of the abnormal cells are lymphocytes, the condition is called **lymphocytic** (lim-fo-SIT-ik) **leukemia.**

The cause of leukemia is unknown. Both inborn factors and various environmental agents have been implicated. Among the latter are chemicals (such as benzene), x-rays, radioactive substances, and viruses.

Patients with leukemia exhibit the general symptoms of anemia because the white cells overwhelm the red cells. In addition, they have a tendency to bleed easily, owing to a lack of platelets. The spleen is greatly enlarged, and several other organs may be increased in size because of the accumulation of white cells within them. Treatment consists of x-ray therapy and chemotherapy (drug treatment), but the disease is malignant and thus may be fatal. With new methods of chemotherapy, the outlook is improving, and many patients survive for years.

✔ CHECKPOINT **11**:

What is leukemia?

Clotting Disorders

A characteristic common to all clotting disorders is a disruption of the coagulation process, which brings about abnormal bleeding.

Hemophilia (he-mo-FIL-e-ah) is a rare hereditary bleeding disorder. This disease influenced history by its occurrence in some of the royal families of Russia and Western Europe. All forms of hemophilia are characterized by a deficiency of a specific clotting factor, so that any cut or bruise may cause serious abnormal bleeding. The needed clotting factors are now available in concentrated form for treatment in cases of injury, preparation for surgery, or painful bleeding into the joints, a frequent occurrence in hemophilia.

The most common clotting disorder is a deficient number of circulating platelets (thrombocytes). The condition, called *thrombocytopenia* (throm-bo-si-to-PE-ne-ah), results in hemorrhage in the skin or mucous membranes. The decrease in the number of platelets may be due to decreased production or to increased destruction of platelets. There are several possible causes of thrombocytopenia, including diseases of the red bone marrow, liver disorders, and various drug toxicities. When a drug is the cause of the disorder, its withdrawal leads to immediate recovery.

A serious disorder of clotting involving excessive coagulation is *disseminated intravascular coagulation* (DIC). This disease occurs in cases of tissue damage due to massive burns, trauma, certain acute infections, cancer, and some disorders of childbirth. During the progress of DIC, platelets and various clotting factors are used up faster than they can be produced, and serious hemorrhaging may result.

✔ CHECKPOINT **12**:

What blood components are low in cases of thrombocytopenia?

BLOOD STUDIES

Many kinds of studies can be done on blood, and some of these have become a standard part of a routine physical examination. Machines that are able to perform several tests at the same time have largely replaced manual procedures, particularly in large institutions. Standard blood tests are listed in Tables 2 and 3 of Appendix 3.

The Hematocrit

The *hematocrit* (he-MAT-o-krit), the volume percentage of red cells in whole blood, is determined by spinning of a blood sample in a high-speed centrifuge for 3 to 5 minutes. In this way, the cellular elements are separated out from the plasma.

The hematocrit is expressed as the volume of packed red cells per unit volume (100 mL) of whole blood. For example, if a laboratory report states "hematocrit, 38%," that means that there are 38 mL red cells per 100 mL whole blood. In other words, 38% of the whole blood is red cells. For adult men, the normal range is 42 to 54 mL per 100 mL blood, whereas for adult women the range is slightly lower, 36 to 46 mL per 100 mL blood. These normal ranges, like all normal ranges for humans, may vary depending on the method used and the interpretation of the results by an individual laboratory. Hematocrit values much below or much above these figures point to an abnormality requiring further study.

Hemoglobin Tests

A sufficient amount of hemoglobin in red cells is required for adequate delivery of oxygen to the tissues. To measure its level, the hemoglobin is released from the red cells, and the color of the blood is compared with a known color scale. Hemoglobin is expressed in grams per 100 mL (dL) whole blood. Normal hemoglobin concentrations for adult males range from 14 to 17 g per 100 mL blood. Values for adult women are in a somewhat lower range, at 12 to 15 g per 100 mL blood. A decrease in hemoglobin to below normal levels signifies anemia.

Normal and abnormal types of hemoglobin can be separated and measured by the process of *electrophoresis* (e-lek-tro-fo-RE-sis). In this procedure, an electric current is passed through the liquid that contains the hemoglobin. This test is useful in the diagnosis of sickle cell anemia and other disorders caused by abnormal types of hemoglobin.

Blood Cell Counts

Most laboratories use automated methods for obtaining the data for blood counts. Visual counts are sometimes done using a *hemocytometer* (he-mo-si-TOM-eh-ter), a ruled slide used to count the cells in a given volume of blood under the microscope.

Red Cell Counts
The normal count for red cells varies from 4.5 to 5.5 million cells per cubic millimeter (µL) of blood. The leukocyte count varies from 5000 to 10,000 cells per cubic millimeter of blood.

An increase in the red cell count is called *polycythemia* (pol-e-si-THE-me-ah). This condition may be found in people who live at high altitudes and in patients with the disease *polycythemia* (pol-e-si-THE-me-ah) *vera.*

White Cell Counts
In *leukopenia*, the white count is below 5000 cells per cubic millimeter. This condition is indicative of depressed bone marrow or a neoplasm of the bone marrow. In *leukocytosis* (lu-ko-si-TO-sis), the white cell count is in excess of 10,000 cells per cubic millimeter. This condition is characteristic of most bacterial infections. It may also occur after hemorrhage, in cases of gout, and in uremia, a result of kidney disease.

Platelet Counts
It is difficult to count platelets directly because they are so small. More accurate counts can be obtained with automated methods. These counts are necessary for the evaluation of platelet loss (thrombocytopenia) such as occurs after radiation therapy or cancer chemotherapy. The normal platelet count ranges from 150,000 to 450,000 per cubic millimeter of blood, but counts may fall to 100,000 or less without causing serious bleeding problems. If a count is very low, a platelet transfusion may be given.

The Blood Slide (Smear)

In addition to the above tests, the *complete blood count* (CBC) includes the examination of a stained blood slide. In this procedure, a drop of blood is spread thinly and evenly over a glass slide, and a special stain (Wright's) is applied to differentiate the otherwise colorless white cells. The slide is then studied under the microscope. The red cells are examined for abnormalities in size, color, or shape and for variations in the percentage of immature forms, known as reticulocytes (see Reticulocytes). The number of platelets is estimated. Parasites, such as the malarial organism and others, may be found. In

Reticulocytes

As they mature, red cells go through a series of stages in which they lose their nucleus and most other organelles. In one of the last stages of development, ribosomes that are still remaining in the cell appear as a network when stained. Cells at this stage are called *reticulocytes* (reh-TIK-u-lo-sites). A small percentage of reticulocytes normally appears in the blood. Changes in these numbers can be used in diagnosis.

When red cells are lost or destroyed, as from bleeding or some form of hemolytic anemia, production of red cells is "stepped up" to compensate for the loss. Greater numbers of reticulocytes are then released into the blood before reaching full maturity, and counts increase above the average. A decrease in the number of circulating reticulocytes suggests that there is a problem with the manufacture of red cells, as in cases of deficiency anemias or suppression of bone marrow activity.

addition, a ***differential white count*** is done. This is an estimation of the percentage of each type of white cell in the smear. Because each type of white cell has a specific function, changes in their proportions can be a valuable diagnostic aid.

✔ CHECKPOINT **13**:

The hematocrit is a common blood test. What is a hematocrit?

Blood Chemistry Tests

Batteries of tests on blood serum are often done by machine. One machine, the Sequential Multiple Analyzer (SMA), provides for the running of some 20 tests per minute. Tests for electrolytes, such as sodium, potassium, chloride, and bicarbonate, as well as for blood glucose, blood urea nitrogen (BUN), and ***creatinine*** (kre-AT-in-in), another nitrogen waste product, may be performed at the same time.

Other tests check for enzymes. Increased levels of ***CPK*** (creatine phosphokinase), ***LDH*** (lactic dehydrogenase), and other enzymes indicate tissue damage, such as that which may occur in heart disease. An excess of ***alkaline phosphatase*** (FOS-fah-tase) could indicate a liver disorder or metastatic cancer involving bone (see Table 3 in Appendix 3).

Blood can be tested for amounts of lipids, such as cholesterol, triglycerides (fats), and lipoproteins, or for amounts of plasma proteins. Many of these tests help in evaluating disorders that may involve various vital organs. For example, the presence of more than the normal amount of glucose (sugar) dissolved in the blood, a condition called ***hyperglycemia*** (hi-per-gli-SE-me-ah), is found most frequently in patients with unregulated diabetes. Sometimes, several evaluations of sugar content are done after the administration of a known amount of glucose. This procedure is called the ***glucose tolerance test*** and is usually given along with another test that determines the amount of sugar in the urine. This combination of tests can indicate faulty cell metabolism. The list of blood chemistry tests is extensive and is constantly increasing. We may now obtain values for various hormones, vitamins, antibodies, and toxic or therapeutic drug levels.

Coagulation Studies

Nature prevents the excessive loss of blood from small vessels by the formation of a clot. Before surgery and under some other circumstances, it is important to know that the time required for coagulation to take place is within normal limits. Because clotting is a rather complex process involving many reactants, a delay may be due to a number of different causes, including lack of certain hormonelike substances, calcium salts, or vitamin K.

Each of the various clotting factors has been designated by a Roman numeral, ranging from I to XIII. Factor I is fibrinogen, factor II is prothrombin, factor III is tissue factor, and factor IV is assigned to calcium ions. The amounts of all these factors may be determined and evaluated on a percentage basis, aiding in the diagnosis and treatment of some bleeding disorders.

Additional tests for coagulation include tests for bleeding time, clotting time, capillary strength, and platelet function.

Bone Marrow Biopsy

A special needle is used to obtain a small sample of red marrow from the sternum, sacrum, or iliac crest in a procedure called a ***bone marrow biopsy.*** If marrow is taken from the sternum, the procedure may be referred to as a ***sternal puncture.*** Examination of the cells gives valuable information that can aid in the diagnosis of bone marrow disorders, including leukemia and certain kinds of anemia.

Summary

I. Functions of the blood
A. Transportation—of oxygen, carbon dioxide, nutrients, minerals, vitamins, hormones, waste
B. Regulation—of pH, fluid balance, body temperature
C. Protection—against foreign organisms, blood loss

II. Blood constituents
A. Plasma—liquid component
1. Water—main ingredient
2. Proteins—albumin, clotting factors, antibodies, complement
3. Nutrients—carbohydrates, lipids, amino acids
4. Electrolytes (minerals)
5. Waste products
6. Hormones and other materials
B. The formed elements
1. Erythrocytes (red cells)—carry oxygen bound to hemoglobin
2. Leukocytes (white cells)
   a. Granulocytes—neutrophils (polymorphs, segs, PMNs), eosinophils, basophils
   b. Agranulocytes—lymphocytes, monocytes
3. Platelets (thrombocytes)—necessary for blood clotting
C. Origin of formed elements—produced in red bone marrow from stem cells

III. Hemostasis—prevention of blood loss
1. Contraction of blood vessels
2. Formation of platelet plug
3. Formation of blood clot
A. Blood clotting
1. Regulators
   a. Procoagulants—promote clotting
   b. Anticoagulants—prevent clotting
2. 12 clotting factors (I–XII)
3. Final steps in blood clotting
   a. Prothrombinase converts prothrombin to thrombin
   b. Thrombin converts fibrinogen to solid threads of fibrin
   c. Threads form clot
4. Serum—fluid that remains after blood has clotted

IV. Blood types
A. ABO blood type group—types A, B, AB, and O
1. Tested by mixing blood sample with antisera to different antigens
2. Incompatible transfusions cause destruction of donor red cells
B. Rh factor—positive or negative

V. Uses of blood and blood components
A. Blood banks—store blood
1. Autologous blood—donated for a person's own use
B. Whole blood transfusions—used only to replace large blood losses
C. Use of blood components—formed elements separated by centrifugation
D. Use of plasma
1. Protein fractions
2. Cryoprecipitate—obtained by freezing; contains clotting factors
3. Gamma globulin—contains antibodies

VI. Blood disorders
A. Anemia—lack of hemoglobin or red cells
1. Loss of cells or destruction of cells
2. Impaired production of cells
   a. Deficiency anemia
   b. Pernicious anemia
   c. Bone marrow suppression
B. Leukemia—excess production of white cells
1. Myelogenous leukemia—cancer of bone marrow
2. Lymphocytic leukemia—cancer of lymphoid tissue
C. Clotting disorders
1. Hemophilia—lack of clotting factors
2. Thrombocytopenia—lack of platelets
3. Disseminated intravascular coagulation (DIC)

13

VII. Blood studies

A. Hematocrit—measures percentage of packed red cells in whole blood

B. Hemoglobin tests—color test, electrophoresis

C. Blood cell counts

D. Blood slide (smear)

E. Blood chemistry tests—electrolytes, waste products, enzymes, glucose, hormones

F. Coagulation studies—clotting factor assays, bleeding time, clotting time, capillary strength, platelet function

G. Bone marrow biopsy

Questions for Study and Review

1. How does the color of blood vary with the amount of oxygenation?
2. What is the average total quantity of circulating blood?
3. Name the three main purposes of blood.
4. Name the two main fractions of blood.
5. Name four main types of proteins in blood plasma. What are their purposes?
6. Name some substances carried in blood plasma other than proteins.
7. Name and describe the three main types of formed elements in blood.
8. Describe the structure and function of erythrocytes
9. Name and give the functions of the five types of leukocytes.
10. What are platelets and what is their function?
11. Where are blood cells formed?
12. Define *hemostasis.* Describe the three main steps in hemostasis.
13. Describe the three final steps in blood clotting.
14. Name the four blood types in the ABO system. What determines the different types?
15. What is the Rh factor? What proportion of the population of the United States possesses this factor? In what situations is this factor of medical importance? Why?
16. What are some of the conditions for which blood transfusions are useful?
17. What precautions should always be taken before a transfusion is given?
18. What is autologous blood?
19. What blood components are used in treatment and how are these components obtained?
20. Name the three general categories of blood disorders.
21. Differentiate among the types of anemia and give an example of each.
22. Name two kinds of leukemia. What are the symptoms of leukemia?
23. Name the main characteristics of clotting disorders and give several examples of clotting disorders.
24. What does the hematocrit measure? Cite normal hematocrit ranges for males and females.
25. Differentiate between leukopenia and leukocytosis. What are some of the conditions that result in abnormal white counts?
26. What can be learned by studying the blood smear? What is determined by a differential white count?
27. What are some evaluations made by blood chemistry tests?
28. What can be determined by a bone marrow biopsy?

✔ Answers to Checkpoints

1. Some substances transported in blood are oxygen, carbon dioxide, nutrients, electrolytes, vitamins, hormones, urea, and toxins.
2. The two main divisions of the blood are the liquid portion or plasma, and the formed elements, which include the cells and cell fragments.

3. Protein is the most abundant type of substance in plasma aside from water.
4. The function of hemoglobin is to carry oxygen in the blood.
5. The main function of leukocytes is to destroy pathogens.
6. The blood platelets are essential to blood coagulation (clotting).
7. Blood cells form in the red bone marrow.
8. The blood antigens most often involved in incompatibility reactions are the A antigen, the B antigen, and the Rh antigen.
9. Blood is commonly separated into its component parts by a centrifuge.
10. Anemia is an abnormally low level of red cells or hemoglobin in the blood.
11. Leukemia is a cancer of the tissues that produce white cells, resulting in an excess number of white cells in the blood.
12. Platelets are low in cases of thrombocytopenia.
13. The hematocrit is the volume percentage of red cells in whole blood.

The Heart and Heart Disease

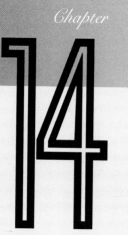

SELECTED KEY TERMS

The following terms are defined in the Glossary:

arrhythmia
atherosclerosis
atrium
coronary
diastole
echocardiograph
electrocardiograph
endocardium
epicardium
infarct
ischemia
murmur
myocardium
pacemaker
pericardium
septum
stenosis
systole
thrombosis
valve
ventricle

BEHAVIORAL OBJECTIVES

After careful study of this chapter, you should be able to:

1. Describe the three layers of the heart wall
2. Compare the functions of the right heart and left heart
3. Name the four chambers of the heart
4. Name the valves at the entrance and exit of each ventricle
5. Briefly describe blood circulation through the myocardium
6. Briefly describe the cardiac cycle
7. Name the components of the heart's conduction system
8. Explain the effects of the autonomic nervous system on the heart rate
9. List and define several terms that describe variations in heart rates
10. Explain what produces the two main heart sounds
11. Describe several common types of heart disease
12. List five actions that can be taken to minimize the risk of heart disease
13. Briefly describe four methods for studying the heart
14. Describe three approaches to the treatment of heart disease

CIRCULATION AND THE HEART

The next two chapters investigate the manner in which the blood delivers oxygen and nutrients to the cells and carries away the waste products of cell metabolism. This continuous one-way movement of the blood is known as its *circulation.* The prime mover that propels blood throughout the body is the *heart.* We shall have a look at the heart before going into the subject of the blood vessels in detail.

The heart is a muscular pump that drives the blood through the blood vessels. Slightly bigger than a fist, this organ is located between the lungs in the center and a bit to the left of the midline of the body. The strokes (contractions) of this pump average about 72 per minute and are carried on unceasingly for the whole of a lifetime.

The importance of the heart has been recognized for centuries. The fact that its rate of beating is affected by the emotions may be responsible for the frequent references to the heart in song and poetry. However, the vital functions of the heart and its disorders are of more practical importance to us.

STRUCTURE OF THE HEART

Layers of the Heart Wall

The heart is a hollow organ, the walls of which are formed of three different layers. Just as a warm coat might have a smooth lining, a thick and bulky interlining, and an outer layer of a third fabric, so the heart wall has three tissue layers (Fig. 14-1). Starting with the innermost layer, these are as follows:

- The *endocardium* (en-do-KAR-de-um) is a thin, smooth layer of cells that resembles squamous epithelium. This membrane lines the interior of the heart. Reinforced folds of this material form the valves of the heart.
- The *myocardium* (mi-o-KAR-de-um), the muscle of the heart, is the thickest layer and is responsible for pumping blood through the vessels. The unique structure of cardiac muscle is described in more detail later.
- The *epicardium* (ep-ih-KAR-de-um) forms the thin, outermost layer of the heart wall and is continuous with the serous lining of the fibrous sac that encloses the heart. These membranes together make up the *pericardium* (per-ih-KAR-de-um). The serous lining of the pericardial sac is separated from the epicardium on the heart surface by a thin film of fluid.

Special Features of the Myocardium

Cardiac muscle cells are lightly striated (striped) and have specialized partitions between the cells that appear faintly under the light microscope. These *intercalated* (in-TER-cah-la-ted) *disks* are actually modified cell membranes that allow for rapid transfer of electrical impulses between the cells. The adjective *intercalated* means "inserted between."

247

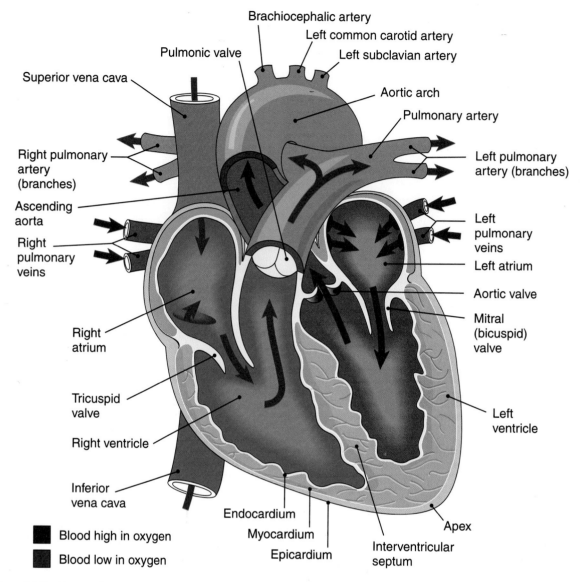

Brachiocephalic artery
Left common carotid artery
Pulmonic valve
Left subclavian artery
Superior vena cava
Aortic arch
Pulmonary artery
Right pulmonary artery (branches)
Left pulmonary artery (branches)
Ascending aorta
Left pulmonary veins
Right pulmonary veins
Left atrium
Aortic valve
Right atrium
Mitral (bicuspid) valve
Tricuspid valve
Left ventricle
Right ventricle
Inferior vena cava
Endocardium
Apex
Myocardium
Interventricular septum
Epicardium

■ Blood high in oxygen
■ Blood low in oxygen

FIGURE **14•1** Heart and great vessels.

Another feature of cardiac muscle tissue is the branching of the muscle fibers (cells). These fibers are interwoven so that the stimulation that causes the contraction of one fiber results in the contraction of a whole group. These structural features play an important role in the working of the heart muscle.

✔ CHECKPOINT **1**:

What are the names of the innermost, middle, and outermost layers of the heart?

Two Hearts and a Partition

Health care professionals often refer to the *right heart* and the *left heart*. This is because the human heart is really a double pump (Fig. 14-2). The right side pumps blood low in oxygen to the lungs through the **pulmonary circuit**. The left side pumps oxygenated blood to the remainder of the body through the **systemic circuit**. The two sides are completely separated from each other by a partition called the **septum**. The upper part of this partition is called the **interatrial** (in-ter-A-tre-al) **septum**, and

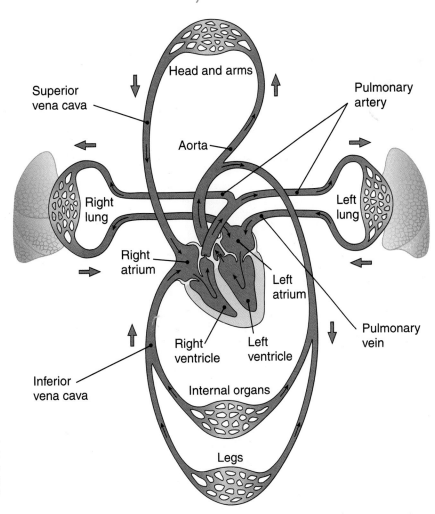

Figure **14•2** The heart is a double pump. The pulmonary circuit carries blood to the lungs to be oxygenated; the systemic circuit carries blood to all other parts of the body.

the larger, lower portion is called the ***interventricular*** (in-ter-ven-TRIK-u-lar) ***septum.*** The septum, like the heart wall, consists largely of myocardium.

Four Chambers

On either side of the heart are two chambers. The upper chamber is a receiving chamber, the ***atrium*** (A-tre-um); the lower one is a pumping chamber, the ***ventricle*** (VEN-trih-kl) (see Fig. 14-1). The chambers, listed in the order in which blood flows through them, are as follows:

1. The ***right atrium*** is a thin-walled chamber that receives the blood returning from

the body tissues. This blood, which is low in oxygen, is carried in veins, the blood vessels leading back to the heart from the body tissues. The superior vena cava brings blood from the head, chest, and arms; the inferior vena cava delivers blood from the trunk and legs.
2. The ***right ventricle*** pumps the venous blood received from the right atrium into the lungs. It pumps into a large pulmonary trunk, which then divides into right and left pulmonary arteries, which branch to the lungs. An artery is a vessel that takes blood from the heart to the tissues.
3. The ***left atrium*** receives blood high in oxygen content as it returns from the lungs in pulmonary veins.

4. The **left ventricle,** which is the chamber with the thickest wall, pumps oxygenated blood to all parts of the body. This blood goes first into the aorta (a-OR-tah), the largest artery, and then into the branching systemic arteries that take blood to the tissues. The lower pointed region of the heart, the **apex,** is formed by the left ventricle (see Fig. 14-1).

The chambers of the heart can be seen in anterior and posterior views in Figure 14-4, shown later.

✔ CHECKPOINT **2**:

The heart is divided into four chambers. What is the upper receiving chamber on each side called? What is the lower pumping chamber called?

Four Valves

One-way valves that direct the flow of blood through the heart are located at the entrance and the exit of each ventricle. The entrance valves are the **atrioventricular** (a-tre-o-ven-TRIK-u-lar) **valves;** the exit valves are the **semilunar** (sem-e-LU-nar) **valves.** (So named because each flap of these valves resembles a half-moon.) Each valve has a specific name, as follows:

- The **right atrioventricular (AV) valve** is also known as the **tricuspid** (tri-KUS-pid) **valve** because it has three cusps, or flaps, that open and close. When this valve is open, blood flows freely from the right atrium into the right ventricle. When the right ventricle begins to contract, however, the valve closes so that blood cannot return to the right atrium; this ensures forward flow into the pulmonary artery.

- The **left atrioventricular (AV) valve** is the bicuspid valve, but it is usually referred to as the **mitral** (MI-tral) **valve** (named for a miter, the pointed, two-sided hat worn by bishops). It has two heavy cusps that permit blood to flow freely from the left atrium into the left ventricle. The cusps close when the left ventricle begins to contract; this closure prevents blood from returning to the left atrium and ensures the forward flow of blood into the aorta. Both the tricuspid and mitral valves are attached by means of thin fibrous threads to muscles in the walls of the ventricles (shown in Fig. 14-6). The function of these threads, called the **chordae tendineae** (KOR-de ten-DIN-e-e), is to stabilize the valve flaps when the ventricles contract so that the force of the blood will not push them up into the atria. In this manner, they help to prevent a backflow of blood when the heart beats.

- The **pulmonic** (pul-MON-ik) **valve,** also called the *pulmonary valve,* is a semilunar valve located between the right ventricle and the pulmonary artery that leads to the lungs. As soon as the right ventricle has finished emptying itself, the valve closes to prevent blood on its way to the lungs from returning to the ventricle.

- The **aortic** (a-OR-tik) **valve** is a semilunar

Coronary arteries

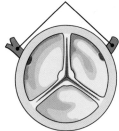

Aortic
(semilunar) valve

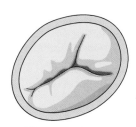

Tricuspid valve

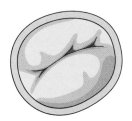

Mitral valve

FIGURE **14•3** Valves of the heart, seen from above, in the closed position.

valve located between the left ventricle and the aorta. After contraction of the left ventricle, the aortic valve closes to prevent the flow of blood back from the aorta to the ventricle.

The appearance of the heart valves in the closed position is illustrated in Figure 14-3.

> ✔ CHECKPOINT **3**:
>
> What is the purpose of valves in the heart?

Blood Supply to the Myocardium

Only the endocardium comes into contact with the blood that flows through the heart chambers. Therefore, the myocardium must have its own blood vessels to provide oxygen and nourishment and to remove waste products. Together, these blood vessels provide the *coronary circulation*. The main arteries that supply blood to the muscle of the heart are the *right* and *left coronary arteries* (Fig. 14-4).

These arteries, which are the first to branch off the aorta, arise just above the aortic semilunar valve (see Fig. 14-3). They receive blood when the heart relaxes and branch to all regions of the heart muscle. After passing through capillaries in the myocardium, blood drains into the cardiac veins and finally into the *coronary sinus* for return to the right atrium.

> ✔ CHECKPOINT **4**:
>
> The heart must have its own system of vessels to supply it with blood. What name is given to this blood supply to the heart?

FUNCTION OF THE HEART

The Work of the Heart

Although the right and left sides of the heart are separated from each other, they work together. Blood is squeezed through the chambers by a contraction of heart muscle beginning in the thin-walled upper chambers, the atria, fol-

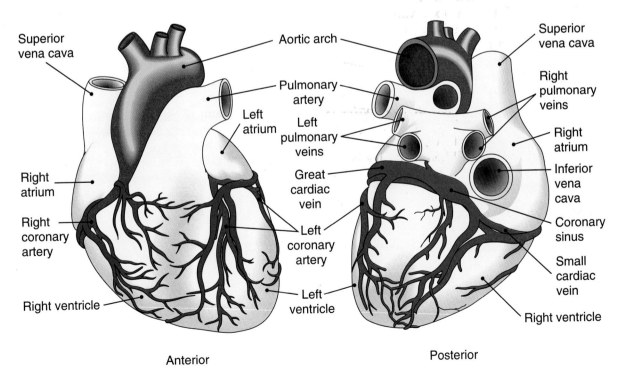

FIGURE **14•4** Coronary arteries and cardiac veins. (*left*) Anterior view, (*right*) Posterior view.

lowed by a contraction of the thick muscle of the lower chambers, the ventricles. This active phase is called **systole** (SIS-to-le), and in each case, it is followed by a resting period known as **diastole** (di-AS-to-le). The contraction of the walls of the atria is completed at the time the contraction of the ventricles begins. Thus, resting phase (diastole) begins in the atria at the same time that a contraction (systole) begins in the ventricles. After the ventricles have emptied, both chambers are relaxed for a short period as they fill with blood. Then another beat begins with contraction of the atria followed by contraction of the ventricles. This sequence of heart relaxation and contraction is called the **cardiac cycle.** At rest, each cycle takes an average of 0.8 seconds (Fig. 14-5).

Cardiac Output

A unique property of heart muscle is its ability to adjust the strength of contraction to the amount of blood received. When the heart chamber is filled and the wall stretched (within limits), the contraction is strong. As less blood enters the heart, the contraction becomes less forceful. Thus, as more blood enters the heart, as occurs during exercise, the muscle contracts

Cardiac Reserve

Like many other organs, the heart has great reserves of strength. The **cardiac reserve** is a measure of how many times more than average the heart can produce when needed. Based on a heart rate of 75 beats/minute and a stroke volume of 70 mL/beat, the average cardiac output for an adult at rest is about 5L/minute. This means that *at rest,* the heart pumps the equivalent of the total blood volume each minute.

During mild exercise, this volume might double and even double again during strenuous exercise. For most people the cardiac reserve is 4 to 5 times the resting output. In athletes exercising vigorously, the ratio may reach 6 to 7 times. In contrast, those with heart disease may have little or no cardiac reserve. They may be fine at rest but quickly become short of breath or fatigued when exercising.

with greater strength to push the larger volume of blood out into the blood vessels.

The volume of blood pumped by each ventricle in 1 minute is termed the **cardiac output.** It is the product of the **stroke volume**—the vol-

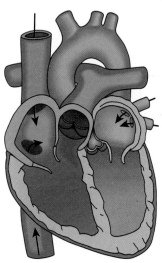

Diastole
Atria fill with blood which begins to flow into ventricles as soon as their walls relax.

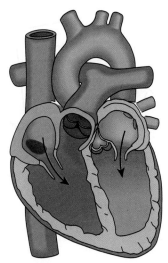

Atrial systole
Contraction of atria pumps blood into the ventricles.

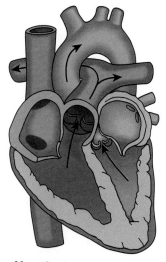

Ventricular systole
Contraction of ventricles pumps blood into aorta and pulmonary arteries.

FIGURE **14•5** Pumping cycle of the heart.

ume of blood ejected from the ventricle with each beat—and the ***heart rate***—the number of times the heart beats per minute (See Cardiac Reserve).

> ✔ CHECKPOINT **5**:
>
> The cardiac cycle consists of an alternating pattern of contraction and relaxation. What name is given to the contraction phase? to the relaxation phase?

> ✔ CHECKPOINT **6**:
>
> Cardiac output is the amount of blood pumped by each ventricle in 1 minute. What two factors determine cardiac output?

The Conduction System of the Heart

Like other muscles, the heart muscle is stimulated to contract by a wave of electrical energy that passes along the cells. This action potential is generated by specialized tissue within the heart and spreads over structures that form the heart's conduction system (Fig. 14-6). Two of these structures are tissue masses called ***nodes.*** In addition to the two nodes, there is a group of fibers called the ***atrioventricular bundle,*** which subdivides to branch through the myocardium.

The ***sinoatrial (SA) node*** is located in the upper wall of the right atrium. This node initiates the heartbeats by generating an action potential at regular intervals. Because the SA node sets the rate of heart contractions, it is called the ***pacemaker.*** The second node, lo-

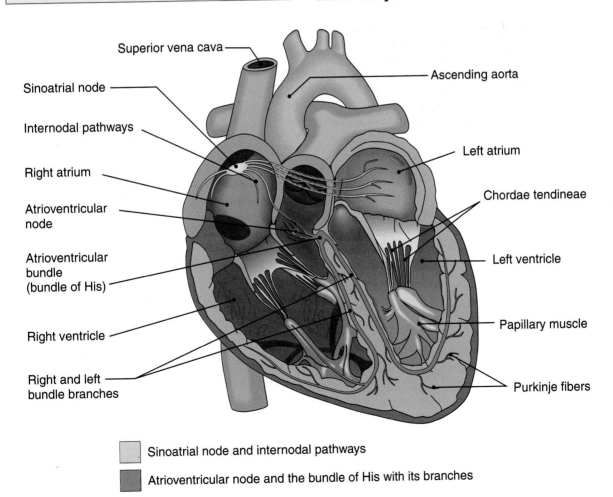

Sinoatrial node and internodal pathways

Atrioventricular node and the bundle of His with its branches

FIGURE **14•6** Conduction system of the heart.

cated in the interatrial septum at the bottom of the right atrium, is called the *atrioventricular (AV) node.*

The *atrioventricular bundle,* also known as the *bundle of His,* is located at the top of the interventricular septum; it has branches that extend to all parts of the ventricular walls. Fibers travel first down both sides of the interventricular septum in groups called the *right* and *left bundle branches.* Smaller *Purkinje* (pur-KIN-je) *fibers* then travel in a branching network throughout the myocardium of the ventricles.

The special membranes between the cells (intercalated disks) allow the rapid flow of impulses throughout the heart muscle.

The Conduction Pathway

The order in which impulses travel through the heart is as follows:

1. The sinoatrial node generates the electrical impulse that begins the heartbeat.
2. The excitation wave travels throughout the muscle of each atrium, causing the atria to contract.
3. The atrioventricular node is stimulated. The relatively slower conduction through this node allows time for the atria to contract and complete the filling of the ventricles.
4. The excitation wave travels rapidly through the bundle of His and then throughout the ventricular walls by means of the bundle branches and Purkinje fibers. The entire musculature of the ventricles contracts practically at once.

As a safety measure, a region of the conduction system other than the sinoatrial node can generate a heartbeat if the sinoatrial node fails, but it does so at a slower rate. A normal heart rhythm originating at the SA node is termed a *sinus rhythm.*

✔ CHECKPOINT **7**:

The heartbeat is started by a small mass of tissue in the upper right atrium. This is commonly called the pacemaker, but what is its scientific name?

Control of the Heart Rate

Although the fundamental beat of the heart originates within the heart itself, the heart rate can be influenced by the nervous system and by other factors in the internal environment.

The autonomic nervous system (ANS) plays a major role in modifying the heart rate according to need (Fig. 14-7). Stimulation from the sympa-

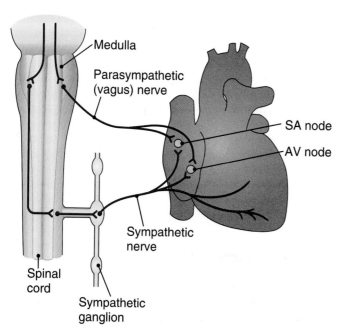

FIGURE **14•7** Nervous stimulation of the heart.

thetic nervous system increases the heart rate. During a fight-or-flight response, the sympathetic nerves can boost the cardiac output two to three times the resting value. Sympathetic fibers increase the rate of contraction by stimulating the SA and AV nodes. They also increase the force of contraction by acting directly on the fibers of the myocardium. These actions translate into increased cardiac output. Stimulation from the parasympathetic nervous system decreases the heart rate to restore homeostasis. The parasympathetic nerve that supplies the heart is the vagus nerve (cranial nerve X). It slows the heart rate by acting on the SA and AV nodes.

These ANS influences allow the heart to meet changing needs rapidly. The heart rate is also affected by substances circulating in the blood, including hormones, ions, and drugs. Regular exercise strengthens the heart and increases the amount of blood ejected with each beat. At rest, the needs of the body then can be met with a lower heart rate. Trained athletes usually have a low resting heart rate.

Variations in Heart Rates

- **Bradycardia** (brad-e-KAR-de-ah) is a relatively slow heart rate of less than 60 beats/minute. During rest and sleep, the heart may beat less than 60 beats/minute but usually does not fall below 50 beats/minute.
- **Tachycardia** (tak-e-KAR-de-ah) refers to a heart rate of more than 100 beats/minute. Tachycardia is normal during exercise or stress but may also occur under abnormal conditions.
- **Sinus arrhythmia** (ah-RITH-me-ah) is a regular variation in heart rate due to changes in the rate and depth of breathing. It is a normal phenomenon.
- **Premature beat,** also called *extrasystole,* is a beat that comes before the expected normal beat. These may occur in normal people initiated by caffeine, nicotine, or psychological stresses. They are also common in people with heart disease.

Heart Sounds

The normal heart sounds are usually described by the syllables "lubb" and "dupp." The first is a longer, lower-pitched sound that occurs at the start of ventricular systole. It is probably caused by a combination of things, mainly closure of the atrioventricular valves. The second, or "dupp," sound is shorter and sharper. It occurs at the beginning of ventricular relaxation and is due in large part to sudden closure of the semilunar valves.

Murmurs

An abnormal sound is called a **murmur** and is usually due to faulty action of a valve. For example, if a valve fails to close tightly and blood leaks back, a murmur is heard. Another condition giving rise to an abnormal sound is the narrowing (stenosis) of a valve opening.

The many conditions that can cause abnormal heart sounds include congenital defects, disease, and physiologic variations. An abnormal sound caused by any structural change in the heart or the vessels connected with the heart is called an **organic murmur.** Certain normal sounds heard while the heart is working may also be described as murmurs, such as the sound heard during rapid filling of the ventricles. To differentiate these from abnormal sounds, they are more properly called **functional murmurs.**

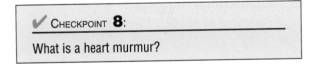

✔ CHECKPOINT **8**:

What is a heart murmur?

HEART DISEASE

Diseases of the heart and circulatory system are the most common causes of death in industrialized countries. Few escape having some damage to the heart and blood vessels in a lifetime.

Classification of Heart Disease

There are many ways of classifying heart disease. The anatomy of the heart forms the basis for one grouping of heart pathology:

- **Endocarditis** (en-do-kar-DI-tis) means "inflammation of the lining of the heart." Endocarditis may involve the lining of the chambers, but the term most commonly refers to inflammation of the endocardium of the valves and valvular disease.

- *Myocarditis* (mi-o-kar-DI-tis) is inflammation of heart muscle.
- *Pericarditis* (per-ih-kar-DI-tis) refers to disease of the serous membrane on the heart surface as well as that lining the pericardial sac.

These inflammatory diseases are often due to infection. They may also occur secondary to respiratory or other systemic diseases.

Another classification of heart disease is based on causative factors:

- *Congenital heart disease* is present at birth.
- *Rheumatic heart disease* begins with an attack of rheumatic fever in childhood or in youth.
- *Coronary* (KOR-o-na-re) *artery disease* involves the walls of the blood vessels that supply the muscle of the heart.
- *Heart failure* is due to deterioration of the heart tissues and is frequently the result of disorders of long duration such as high blood pressure.

Types of Heart Disease

Congenital Heart Disease

Congenital heart diseases are usually due to defects in the development of the fetus. The most common single defect is a hole in the septum between the two ventricles, known as *ventricular septal defect*. Two other congenital disorders represent the abnormal persistence of structures that are part of the normal fetal circulation.

Because the lungs are not used until a child is born, the fetus has some adaptations that allow blood to bypass the lungs. The ductus arteriosus (ar-te-re-O-sis) is a small blood vessel that connects the pulmonary artery and the aorta to divert blood from the lungs. This vessel normally closes of its own accord once the lungs are in use. Persistence of the vessel after birth is described as *patent* (open) *ductus arteriosus.* Also present in the fetus is a small hole, the foramen ovale (for-A-men o-VAL-e), located in

the septum between the two atria. This opening allows some blood to flow directly from the right atrium into the left atrium, bypassing the lungs. Failure of the foramen ovale to close results in an *atrial septal defect.*

In each of the above defects, part of the output of the left side of the heart goes back to the lungs instead of out to the body. A small defect remaining from the foramen ovale or a small patent ductus may cause no difficulty and is often not diagnosed until an adult is being examined for other cardiac problems. More serious defects greatly increase the work of the left ventricle and may lead to heart failure. In addition, ventricular septal defect creates high blood pressure in the lungs, which damages lung tissue.

Other congenital defects that tax the heart involve restriction of outward blood flow. *Coarctation* (ko-ark-TA-shun) *of the aorta* is a localized narrowing of the arch of the aorta. Another example is obstruction or narrowing of the pulmonary artery that prevents blood from passing in sufficient quantity from the right ventricle to the lungs.

In many cases, several congenital heart defects occur together. The most common combination is that of four specific defects known as the *tetralogy of Fallot*. The so-called "blue baby" commonly has this disorder. The blueness, or *cyanosis* (si-ah-NO-sis), of the skin and mucous membranes is caused by a relative lack of oxygen. (See Chap. 18 for other causes of cyanosis.)

In recent years, it has become possible to remedy many congenital defects by heart surgery, one of the more spectacular advances in modern medicine. A patent ductus arteriosus may also respond to drug treatment. During fetal life, prostaglandins (hormones) act to keep the ductus arteriosus open. Drugs that inhibit prostaglandins can promote closing of the duct after birth.

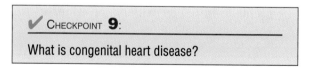

✔ CHECKPOINT **9**:

What is congenital heart disease?

Rheumatic Fever and the Heart

Certain streptococcal infections are indirectly responsible for rheumatic fever and rheumatic heart disease. The toxin produced by these streptococci causes an immune reaction that may be followed some 2 to 4 weeks later by rheumatic fever with marked swelling of the joints. The antibodies formed to combat the toxin may then attack the heart valves, producing a condition known as *rheumatic endocarditis*. The heart valves, particularly the mitral valve, become inflamed, and the normally flexible valve cusps thicken and harden so that they do not open sufficiently (mitral stenosis) or close effectively (mitral regurgitation). Either condition interferes with the flow of blood from the left atrium into the left ventricle, causing pulmonary congestion, an important characteristic of mitral heart disease. Although antibiotics are available to treat streptococcal infections, children who do not receive adequate treatment may develop rheumatic heart disease.

✔ CHECKPOINT **10**:

What types of organisms cause rheumatic fever?

Coronary Artery Disease

The coronary arteries that supply the heart muscle, like vessels elsewhere in the body, can undergo degenerative changes with time. The lumen (space) inside the vessel may gradually narrow due to progressive thickening and hardening, a process called ***atherosclerosis*** (ath-er-o-skleh-RO-sis) (Fig. 14-8*A* and *B*). Narrowing of vessels results in ***ischemia*** (is-KE-me-ah), a lack of blood supply to the areas fed by those arteries. Degenerative changes in the arterial wall also may cause the inside surface of the vessel to become roughened, promoting the formation of a blood clot (thrombus) (see Fig. 14-8*C*). In the heart, this results in a life-threatening condition known as ***coronary thrombosis***. Sudden ***occlusion*** (ok-LU-zhun), or closure, of a coronary vessel with complete obstruction of blood is commonly known as a *heart attack*. Because the area of tissue damaged in a heart attack is described as an ***infarct*** (IN-farkt), the medical term for a heart attack is ***myocardial infarction*** (MI).

The outcome of a myocardial infarction depends largely on the extent and location of the

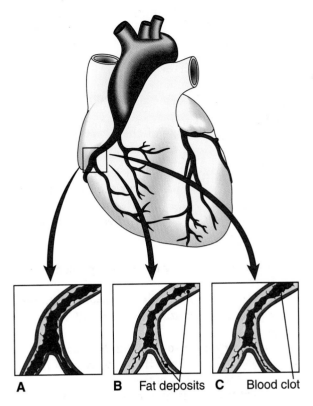

FIGURE **14•8** Coronary atherosclerosis. **(A)** Fat deposits narrow an artery leading to ischemia. **(B)** Blockage (occlusion) of a coronary artery. **(C)** Formation of a blood clot (thrombus) leading to myocardial infarction.

damage. Many people die within the first hour after onset of symptoms, but prompt, aggressive treatment can improve outcomes. Efforts are made immediately to relieve chest pain, to stabilize the heart rhythm, and to reopen the blocked vessel. Complete and prolonged lack of blood to any part of the myocardium results in necrosis (death) of tissue and weakening of the heart wall.

Angina Pectoris

Inadequate blood flow to the heart muscle results in a characteristic discomfort, called ***angina pectoris*** (an-JI-nah PEK-to-ris), felt in the region of the heart and in the left arm and the shoulder. Angina pectoris may be accompanied by a feeling of suffocation and a general sensation of forthcoming doom. Coronary artery disease is a common cause of angina pectoris, although the condition has other causes as well.

14

Abnormalities of Heart Rhythm

Coronary artery disease or myocardial infarction often results in an abnormality in the rhythm of the heartbeat, or **arrhythmia** (ah-RITH-me-ah). Extremely rapid but coordinated contractions, numbering up to 300 per minute, are described as **flutter.** Rapid, wild, and uncoordinated contractions of the heart muscle are called **fibrillation,** which may involve the atria only or both the atria and the ventricles. Ventricular fibrillation is a serious disorder because there is no effective heartbeat. It must be corrected by a **defibrillator,** a device that generates a strong electrical current that discharges all the cardiac muscle cells at once, allowing a normal rhythm to resume.

An interruption of electric impulses in the conduction system of the heart is called **heart block.** The seriousness of this condition depends on how completely the impulses are blocked. It may result in independent beating of the chambers if the ventricles respond to a second pacemaker.

Treatment of Heart Attacks

The death rate for heart attacks is high when treatment is delayed. Initial treatment involves cardiopulmonary resuscitation (CPR) and defibrillation at the scene when needed. The American Heart Association is adding training in the use of the **automated external defibrillator** (AED) to the basic course in CPR. The AED detects fatal arrhythmia and automatically delivers the correct preprogrammed shock. Work is underway to place machines in shopping centers, sports venues, and other public settings.

Prompt transport by paramedics who are equipped with cardiac monitors and who are able to give emergency drugs allows more people to arrive at the hospital emergency room alive. The next step is to restore blood flow to the ischemic areas by administering **thrombolytic** (throm-bo-LIT-ik) **drugs,** which act to dissolve the clots blocking the coronary arteries. Therapy must be given promptly to prevent permanent damage to heart muscle. In many cases, a pulmonary artery catheter (tube) is put in place to monitor cardiac function and response to medication.

Supportive care includes treatment of chest pain with intravenous (IV) morphine. Heart rhythm is monitored constantly, and medications are given to maintain a functional rhythm. Oxygen is given to improve the function of the heart muscle. Some clients require surgery, such as angioplasty or bypass graft, to preserve heart tissue; others may need a pacemaker.

Recovery from a heart attack with resumption of a normal lifestyle is possible as long as the patient follows his or her prescribed drug therapy plan, stops smoking, modifies diet, and follows a planned program to increase physical activity gradually.

✔ CHECKPOINT **11**:

Narrowing or blockage of the vessels that supply the heart muscle causes coronary artery disease. What degenerative process commonly causes narrowing of these vessels?

Heart Failure

Heart failure is a condition in which the heart is unable to pump sufficient blood to supply the tissues with oxygen and nutrients. The chambers of the heart enlarge to contain more blood than the stretched fibers are able to pump. Blood backs up into the lungs, increasing blood pressure in the lungs. The muscles of the ventricles do not get enough blood, decreasing their ability to contract. Additional mechanisms cause the retention of fluid. In an attempt to increase blood flow, the nervous system increases contraction of smooth muscle in the blood vessels, increasing blood pressure. Soon there is the accumulation of fluids in the lungs, liver, abdomen, and legs. People can live with compensated heart failure by attention to diet, drug therapy, and a balance of activity and rest.

THE HEART IN THE ELDERLY

As a person ages, the heart becomes smaller, and there is a decrease in the strength of heart muscle contraction. The valves become less flexible, and incomplete closure may produce an audible murmur. By 70 years of age, the cardiac output may decrease by as much as 35%. Damage within the conduction system can produce abnormal rhythms, including extra beats, rapid atrial beats, and slowing of ventricular rate. Temporary failure of the conduction system (heart block) can cause periodic loss of consciousness. Due to the decrease in the reserve strength of the heart, elderly people are often limited in their ability to respond to physical or emotional stress

PREVENTION OF HEART AILMENTS

Prevention of heart ailments is based on identification of cardiovascular risk factors and modification of those factors that can be changed (see Managing Cardiac Risk Factors). Risk factors that cannot be modified include the following:

- Age. The risk of heart disease increases with age.
- Gender. Males have greater risk than females. Females older than 50 years or past menopause have risk matching that of males.
- Heredity. Those with immediate family members with heart disease are at greater risk.
- Body build, in particular the hereditary tendency to deposit fat in the abdomen or on the chest surface.

Risk factors that can be changed include the following:

- Smoking, which leads to spasm and hardening of the arteries. This results in decreased blood flow and poor supply of oxygen and nutrients to heart muscle.
- Physical inactivity. Lack of exercise decreases the efficiency of the heart. It also decreases the efficiency of the skeletal muscles, which then require more work from the heart to function.
- Weight over the ideal increases risk.
- Saturated fat in the diet. Elevated fat levels in the blood lead to blockage of the coronary arteries by plaque (see What Are All Those DLs? on p. 260).

Managing Cardiac Risk Factors

Management of those risk factors for cardiac disease that we have some control over is essential to good health. Modification of these risk factors can significantly delay the onset of disease by 12 to 20 years. Each of the following modifications can have some effect by itself; however, used together the effects can be dramatic:

- Stop smoking; nicotine has been shown to increase sclerosis of the coronary arteries as well as to increase irritability of the arterial wall, leading to coronary artery spasm.
- Gain control over your weight; even marginal obesity, less than 20 pounds over your ideal weight, increases the workload on your heart by 3 times and significant obesity (more than 20 pounds) eventually leads to heart failure. If you need to lose weight, do so gradually, most physicians recommend no more than 2 to 3 pounds per week.
- Watch your diet: reduce overall intake of fats and cholesterol, paying special attention to saturated fats. Increase items that are high in monounsaturated fat (fish oils and olive oil), and vitamins A, E, and C. Increase the number of servings of grains in your diet and include plenty of vegetables while avoiding red meats.
- Exercise! A good aerobic/cardiovascular work-out, such as walking or bicycling, 3 times a week allows the heart muscle to become stronger and pump more efficiently. Remember to begin slowly and work yourself up to a regular regimen and don't forget the warm-up and cool-down parts of the routine.

The key to making any significant, lasting modifications is to do so in moderation. Drastic changes will undoubtedly be short-term and have little benefit.

- High blood pressure (hypertension) damages heart muscle.
- Diabetes and gout. Both diseases cause damage to small blood vessels.

Actions that can be taken to minimize risk factors include the following:

- Regular physical examinations, particu-

What Are All Those DLs?

Although cholesterol has received a lot of bad press in recent years, it is a necessary substance in the body. It is found in bile salts needed for digestion of fats, in hormones, and in the plasma membrane of the cell. However, high levels of cholesterol in the blood have been associated with heart disease.

It now appears that the total amount of blood cholesterol is not as important as the form in which it occurs. Cholesterol is transported in the blood in combination with other lipids and with protein, forming compounds called *lipoproteins.* These compounds are distinguished by their relative density. High-density lipoprotein (HDL) is about one-half protein, whereas low-density lipoprotein (LDL) has a higher proportion of cholesterol and less protein. VLDLs, or very-low-density lipoproteins, are substances that are converted to LDLs.

LDLs carry cholesterol from the liver to the tissues. HDLs remove cholesterol from the tissues, such as the walls of the arteries, and carry it back to the liver for reuse or disposal. Thus, high levels of HDLs indicate efficient removal of arterial plaques, whereas high levels of LDLs suggest that arteries will become clogged.

larly for middle-aged people and those with an increase in any risk factor.

- Diet to control fat intake and to keep weight close to the ideal.
- Quitting smoking. Many aids are available to assist the smoker in "kicking the habit."
- Regular exercise. Even a minimal amount of regular exercise, such as walking 30 minutes 3 times a week, has been shown to be of major benefit.
- Control of chronic illness, such as high blood pressure, diabetes, and gout. Such control can reduce the risk of cardiac involvement.

HEART STUDIES

Experienced listeners can gain much information about the heart using a *stethoscope* (STETH-o-skope). This is a relatively simple instrument used to convey sounds from within the patient's body to the ear of an examiner.

The *electrocardiograph* (*ECG* or *EKG*) is used for making records of the changes in electrical currents produced by the contracting heart muscle. It may thus reveal certain myocardial injuries. Electrical activity is picked up by electrodes placed on the surface of the skin and appears as *waves* on the ECG tracing. The P wave represents the activity of the atria; the QRS and T waves represent the activity of the ventricles (Fig. 14-9). Changes in the waves and the intervals between them are used to diagnose heart damage and arrhythmias.

Many people with heart disease undergo *catheterization* (kath-eh-ter-i-ZA-shun). In right heart catheterization, an extremely thin tube (catheter) is passed through the veins of the right arm or right groin and then into the right side of heart. A *fluoroscope* (flu-OR-o-scope), an instrument for examining deep structures with x-rays, is used to show the route taken by the catheter. The tube is passed all the way through the pulmonic valve into the large lung arteries. Blood samples are obtained along the way for testing, and pressure readings are taken.

In left heart catheterization, a catheter is

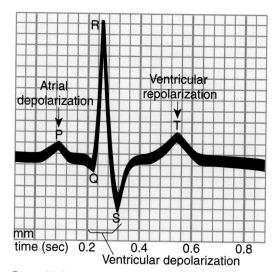

FIGURE **14•9** Normal EKG showing one cardiac cycle.

passed through an artery in the left groin or arm to the heart. Dye can then be injected into the coronary arteries to map damage to the vessels. The tube may also be passed through the aortic valve into the left ventricle for further studies.

Ultrasound consists of sound waves generated at a frequency above the range of sensitivity of the human ear. In **echocardiography** (ek-o-kar-de-OG-rah-fe), also known as *ultrasound cardiography,* high-frequency sound waves are sent to the heart from a small instrument on the surface of the chest. The ultrasound waves bounce off the heart and are recorded as they return, showing the heart in action. Movement of the echoes is traced on an electronic instrument called an *oscilloscope* and recorded on film. (The same principle is employed by submarines to detect ships.) The method is safe and painless, and it does not use x-rays. It provides information on the size and shape of heart structures, on cardiac function, and on possible heart defects.

✔ CHECKPOINT **12**:

What does ECG stand for?

TREATMENT OF HEART DISEASE

Medications

One of the oldest drugs, which is still the most important drug for many heart patients, is **digitalis** (dij-ih-TAL-is). This agent, which slows and strengthens contractions of the heart muscle, is obtained from the leaf of the foxglove, a plant originally found growing wild in many parts of Europe. Foxglove is now cultivated to ensure a steady supply of digitalis for medical purposes.

Several forms of **nitroglycerin** are used to relieve angina pectoris. This drug dilates (widens) the vessels in the coronary circulation and improves the blood supply to the heart.

Beta-adrenergic blocking agents ("betablockers") control sympathetic stimulation of the heart. They reduce the rate and strength of

heart contractions, thus reducing the heart's oxygen demand. Propanolol is one example.

Antiarrhythmic agents (*e.g.,* quinidine) are used to regulate the rate and rhythm of the heartbeat.

Slow calcium-channel blockers aid in the treatment of coronary heart disease and hypertension by several mechanisms. They may dilate vessels, control the force of heart contractions, or regulate conduction through the atrioventricular node. Their actions are based on the fact that calcium ions must enter muscle cells before contraction can occur.

Anticoagulants (an-ti-ko-AG-u-lants) are valuable drugs for heart patients. They may be used to prevent clot formation in patients with damage to heart valves or blood vessels or in patients who have had a myocardial infarction.

Artificial Pacemakers

Electric, battery-operated pacemakers that supply impulses to regulate the heartbeat have been implanted under the skin of many thousands of patients. The site of implantation is usually in the left chest area. Electrode catheters attached to the pacemaker are then passed into the heart and anchored to the chest wall. The frequency of battery pack replacement varies with the type of pacemaker. This rather simple device has saved many people whose hearts cannot beat effectively alone. In an emergency, a similar stimulus can be supplied to the heart muscle through electrodes placed externally on the chest wall.

Heart Surgery

The heart-lung machine has made possible many operations on the heart and other thoracic organs. There are several types of machines in use, all of which serve as temporary substitutes for the patient's heart and lungs. The machine siphons off the blood from the large vessels entering the heart on the right side so that no blood passes though the heart and lungs. While in the machine, the blood is oxygenated, and carbon dioxide is removed chemically. The blood is also "defoamed," or rid of air bubbles, which could fatally obstruct blood vessels. The machine then pumps the processed blood back into the general circulation by way of a large artery.

Coronary bypass surgery to relieve obstruction in the coronary arteries is a common and often successful treatment. While the damaged coronary arteries remain in place, healthy segments of blood vessels from other parts of the patient's body are grafted onto the vessels to bypass any obstructions. Usually, parts of the saphenous vein (a superficial vein in the leg) are used.

Sometimes, as many as six or seven segments are required to establish an adequate blood supply. The mortality associated with this operation is low, and most patients are able to return to a nearly normal lifestyle after recovery from the surgery. The effectiveness of this procedure diminishes over a period of years, however, owing to blockage of the replacement vessels.

Less invasive surgical procedures include the technique of ***angioplasty*** (AN-je-o-plas-te), which is used to open restricted arteries in the heart and other areas of the body. In coronary angioplasty, a catheter with a balloon is guided by fluoroscopy to the affected area. There, the balloon is inflated to break up the blockage in the coronary artery, thus restoring effective circulation to the heart muscle. To prevent repeated blockage, a small tube called a *stent* may be inserted in the vessel to keep it open.

Diseased valves may become so deformed and scarred from endocarditis that they are ineffective and often obstructive. In most cases, there is so much damage that ***valve replacement*** is the best treatment. Substitute valves made of a variety of natural and artificial materials have been used successfully.

The news media have given considerable attention to the ***surgical transplantation*** of human hearts and sometimes of lungs and hearts together. This surgery is done in specialized centers and is available to some patients with degenerative heart disease who are otherwise in good health. Tissues of the recently deceased donor and of the recipient must be as closely matched as possible to avoid rejection.

Efforts to replace a damaged heart with a completely artificial heart have not been successful so far. There are devices available, however, to assist a damaged heart in pumping during recovery from heart attack or while a patient is awaiting a donor heart.

Also in use are small defibrillators placed inside the body. These implanted automatic defibrillators are programmed to detect rapid abnormal rhythm and then deliver a direct shock to the heart. These are lifesaving devices for patients with frequent episodes of rapid ventricular arrhythmias.

Summary

I. **Circulation and the heart**—heart contractions drive blood through the blood vessels

II. **Structure of the heart**
  A. **Layers of the heart wall**
    1. Endocardium—thin inner layer
    2. Myocardium—thick muscle layer
      a. Lightly striated, intercalated disks, branching of fibers
    3. Epicardium—thin outer layer
      a. Pericardium—membrane-lined sac that encloses the heart
  B. **Two hearts and a partition**—left and right sides divided by a septum
  C. **Four chambers**
    1. Atria—left and right receiving chambers
    2. Ventricles—left and right pumping chambers
  D. **Four valves**—prevent backflow of blood

1. Tricuspid—right atrioventricular valve
2. Mitral (bicuspid)—left atrioventricular valve
3. Pulmonic (semilunar) valve—at entrance to pulmonary artery
4. Aortic (semilunar) valve—at entrance to aorta

E. Blood supply to the myocardium
   1. Coronary arteries—first branches of aorta; fill when heart relaxes
   2. Coronary sinus—collects venous blood from heart and empties into right atrium

III. **Function of the heart**
   A. The work of the heart—cardiac cycle
      1. Phases
         a. Diastole—relaxation phase
         b. Systole—contraction phase
      2. Cardiac output—volume pumped by each ventricle per minute
         a. Stroke volume—amount pumped with each beat
         b. Heart rate—number of beats per minute
   B. Conduction system of the heart
      1. Sinoatrial node (pacemaker)—at top of right atrium
      2. Atrioventricular node—between atria and ventricles
      3. Atrioventricular bundle (bundle of His)—at top of interventricular septum
         a. Bundle branches—right and left, on either side of septum
         b. Purkinje fibers—branch through myocardium of ventricles
   C. Control of the heart rate
      1. Autonomic nervous system
         a. Sympathetic system—speeds heart rate
         b. Parasympathetic system—slows heart rate through vagus nerve
      2. Others—hormones, ions, drugs
      3. Variations in heart rates
         a. Bradycardia—slower rate than normal; less than 60 beats/minute
         b. Tachycardia—faster rate than

normal; more than 100 beats/minute
      4. Sinus arrhythmia—related to breathing changes
      5. Premature beat—extrasystole
   D. Heart sounds
      1. Normal
         a. "Lubb"—occurs at closing of atrioventricular valves
         b. "Dupp"—occurs at closing of semilunar valves
      2. Abnormal—murmur

IV. **Heart disease**
   A. Classification of heart disease
      1. Anatomic classification—endocarditis, myocarditis, pericarditis
      2. Causal classification
   B. Types of heart disease
      1. Congenital heart diseases—present at birth
         a. Holes in septum
         b. Failure of fetal lung bypasses to close
         c. Narrowing of aorta or pulmonary artery
         d. Tetralogy of Fallot
      2. Rheumatic heart disease
         a. Mitral stenosis—valve cusps do not open
         b. Mitral regurgitation—valve cusps do not close
      3. Coronary artery disease
         a. Characteristics
            (1) Atherosclerosis—thickening and hardening of arteries
            (2) Ischemia—lack of blood to area fed by blocked arteries
            (3) Coronary occlusion—closure of coronary arteries, as by a thrombus (clot)
            (4) Infarct—area of damaged tissue
            (5) Angina pectoris—pain caused by lack of blood to heart muscle
            (6) Abnormal rhythm—arrhythmia
               (a) Flutter—rapid, coordinated beats
               (b) Fibrillation—rapid, unco-

14

ordinated contractions of heart muscle

    (c) Heart block—interruption of electric conduction

  b. Treatment of heart attacks—CPR, defibrillation, thrombolytic drugs, monitoring

   4. Heart failure—due to hypertension, disease, malnutrition, anemia, age

V. The heart in the elderly

VI. Prevention of heart ailments—physical examination, proper diet, quitting smoking, regular exercise, control of chronic illness

VII. Heart studies

1. Stethoscope—used to listen to heart sounds
2. Electrocardiograph (ECG, EKG)—records electrical activity as waves
3. Catheterization—thin tube inserted into heart for blood samples, pressure readings, and other tests

4. Fluoroscope—examines deep tissue with x-rays; used to guide catheter
5. Echocardiography—uses ultrasound to record pictures of heart in action

VIII. Treatment of heart disease

A. Medications—examples are digitalis, nitroglycerin, beta-adrenergic blocking agents, antiarrhythmic agents, slow channel calcium-channel blockers, anticoagulants

B. Artificial pacemakers—electronic devices implanted under skin to regulate heartbeat

C. Heart surgery
1. Bypass—vessels grafted to detour blood around blockage
2. Angioplasty—balloon catheter used to open blocked arteries
3. Valve replacement
4. Heart transplantation
5. Artificial hearts—experimental

14

Questions for Study and Review

1. What are the three layers of the heart wall?
2. Describe the characteristics of heart muscle tissue.
3. Name the sac around the heart.
4. What is a partition in the heart called? Name two such partitions.
5. Name the chambers of the heart and tell what each does.
6. Explain the purpose of valves in the heart and name the four valves in the heart.
7. Why does the myocardium need its own blood supply? Name the arteries that supply blood to the heart.
8. Explain the contraction pattern of the cardiac cycle.
9. Define *cardiac output*. What determines cardiac output?
10. What are the parts of the heart's conduction system called and where are these structures located? Outline the order in which the excitation waves travel.
11. Compare the effects of the sympathetic and parasympathetic nervous systems on the working of the heart.
12. What two syllables are used to indicate normal heart sounds and at what times in the heart cycle can they be heard?
13. Inflammation of the heart structures is the basis for a classification of heart pathology. List the three terms in this classification and explain each.
14. What is meant by *congenital heart disease*? Give some examples.
15. What part does infection play in rheumatic heart disease?

16. What is coronary artery disease?
17. What is the effect of a thrombus in an artery supplying the heart wall?
18. What are some of the effects of heart failure?
19. What changes occur in the heart with age?
20. List some risk factors for heart disease that cannot be modified. List some that can be modified.
21. What is a stethoscope?
22. What is an electrocardiograph and what is its purpose?
23. Of what value is heart catheterization and how is it carried out?
24. How is echocardiography used to study the heart?
25. How does digitalis help a person who has heart muscle damage?
26. Why are artificial pacemakers used?
27. What is the purpose of coronary bypass surgery?
28. What is coronary angioplasty and how does it benefit the heart?
29. Differentiate between the terms in each of the following pairs:
    a. *pulmonary* and *systemic circuit*
    b. *interatrial* and *interventricular*
    c. *systole* and *diastole*
    d. *stroke volume* and *heart rate*
    e. *tachycardia* and *bradycardia*
    f. *functional murmur* and *organic murmur*
    g. *flutter* and *fibrillation*

✔ ANSWERS TO CHECKPOINTS

1. The innermost layer of the heart is the endocardium, the middle is the myocardium, and the outermost is the epicardium.
2. The upper chamber on each side of the heart is the atrium; each lower chamber is the ventricle.
3. Valves direct the flow of blood through the heart.
4. The coronary circulation is the blood supply to the heart.
5. The contraction phase of the cardiac cycle is systole; the relaxation phase is diastole.
6. Cardiac output is determined by the stroke volume, the volume of blood ejected from the ventricle with each beat, and by the heart rate, the number of times the heart beats per minute.
7. The small mass of tissue that starts the heartbeat is the sinoatrial (SA) node.
8. A heart murmur is an abnormal heart sound.
9. Congenital heart disease is a defect present at birth.
10. Rheumatic fever is caused by certain streptococci.
11. Atherosclerosis commonly causes narrowing of the coronary vessels.
12. ECG stands for electrocardiography.

14

Blood Vessels and Blood Circulation

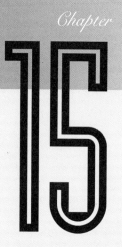

SELECTED KEY TERMS

The following terms are defined in the Glossary:

anastomosis

aorta

arteriole

artery

atherosclerosis

capillary

embolus

endothelium

hemorrhage

hypertension

hypotension

ischemia

phlebitis

pulse

shock

sinusoid

sphygmomanometer

vasoconstriction

vasodilation

vein

venule

BEHAVIORAL OBJECTIVES

After careful study of this chapter, you should be able to:

1. Differentiate among the three main types of vessels in the body with regard to structure and function
2. Compare the locations and functions of the pulmonary and systemic circuits
3. Name the four sections of the aorta and list the main branches of each section
4. Define *anastomosis*. Cite the function of anastomoses and give several examples
5. Compare superficial and deep veins and give examples of each type
6. Name the main vessels that drain into the superior and inferior venae cavae
7. Define *venous sinus* and give four examples
8. Describe the structure and function of the hepatic portal system
9. Explain how materials are exchanged across the capillary wall
10. Describe the factors that regulate blood flow
11. Define *pulse* and list factors that affect the pulse rate
12. List several factors that affect blood pressure
13. Explain how blood pressure is commonly measured
14. List some disorders that involve the blood vessels
15. List steps in first aid for hemorrhage
16. List four types of shock

The blood vessels, together with the four chambers of the heart, form a closed system in which blood is carried to and from the tissues. Although whole blood does not leave the vessels, components of the plasma and tissue fluids can be exchanged through the walls of the tiniest vessels, the capillaries.

The vascular system is easier to understand if you refer to the appropriate illustrations in this chapter as the vessels are described. When this information is added to what you already know about the blood and the heart, a picture of the cardiovascular system as a whole will emerge.

BLOOD VESSELS

Types of Blood Vessels

On the basis of function, blood vessels may be divided into three groups:

- *Arteries* carry blood away from the heart and toward the capillaries in the tissues. Blood is pumped out of the ventricles into the arteries. The smallest arteries are called *arterioles* (ar-TE-re-olz).
- *Veins* drain capillaries in the tissues and return the blood to the heart. The smallest veins are the *venules* (VEN-ulz).
- *Capillaries* allow for exchanges between

the blood and body cells, or between the blood and air in the lung tissues. The capillaries connect the arterioles and venules.

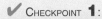
✔ CHECKPOINT **1**:

What are the three main groups of blood vessels?

Blood Circuits

The vessels together may be subdivided into two groups or circuits: pulmonary and systemic. The vessels in these two circuits are shown in Figure 15-1; the anatomic relation of the circuits to the heart is shown in Figure 14-2 in Chapter 14.

The Pulmonary Circuit
The *pulmonary circuit* eliminates carbon dioxide from the blood and replenishes its supply of oxygen. The pulmonary vessels that carry blood to and from the lungs include the following:

- The pulmonary artery and its branches, which carry blood from the right ventricle to the lungs
- The capillaries in the lungs, through which gases are exchanged
- The pulmonary veins, which carry blood back to the left atrium

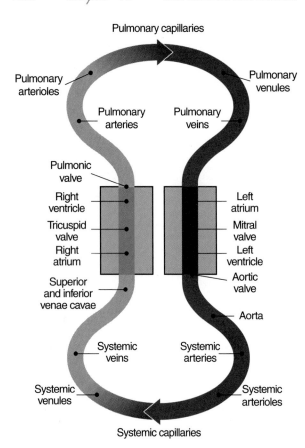

FIGURE **15•1** Blood vessels form a closed system for the flow of blood. Blood high in oxygen (oxygenated) is shown in red; blood low in oxygen (deoxygenated) is shown in blue. Changes in oxygen content occur as blood flows through capillaries.

The pulmonary vessels differ from those in the systemic circuit in that the pulmonary arteries carry blood that is *low* in oxygen, and the pulmonary veins carry blood that is *high* in oxygen. All the remaining arteries carry highly oxygenated blood, and all remaining veins carry blood that is low in oxygen.

The Systemic Circuit

The *systemic* (sis-TEM-ik) *circuit* serves the rest of the body. These vessels supply nutrients and oxygen to all the tissues and carry waste materials away from the tissues for disposal. The systemic vessels include the following:

- The aorta, which receives blood from the left ventricle and then branches into the

systemic arteries carrying blood to the tissues
- The systemic capillaries, through which materials are exchanged
- The systemic veins, which carry blood back toward the heart. The venous blood flows into the right atrium of the heart through the superior vena cava and inferior vena cava.

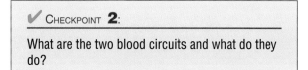

✔ CHECKPOINT **2**:

What are the two blood circuits and what do they do?

Vessel Structure

Artery Walls

The arteries have thick walls because they must be strong enough to receive blood pumped under pressure from the ventricles of the heart (Fig. 15-2). The three coats (tunics) of the arteries resemble the three tissue layers of the heart:

- The innermost membrane of simple, flat epithelial cells makes up the ***endothelium*** (en-do-THE-le-um), forming a smooth surface over which the blood flows easily.
- The middle and thickest layer is made of smooth (involuntary) muscle, which is under the control of the autonomic nervous system. Elastic tissue between the layers of the arterial wall allows these vessels to stretch when receiving blood and then return to their original size. The amount of elastic tissue diminishes as the arteries branch and become smaller.
- An outer tunic is made of a supporting connective tissue.

The largest artery, the ***aorta*** (a-OR-tah), is about 2.5 cm (1 inch) in diameter and has the thickest wall because it receives blood under the highest pressure from the left ventricle. The smallest subdivisions of arteries, the arterioles, have thinner walls in which there is little elastic connective tissue but relatively more smooth muscle.

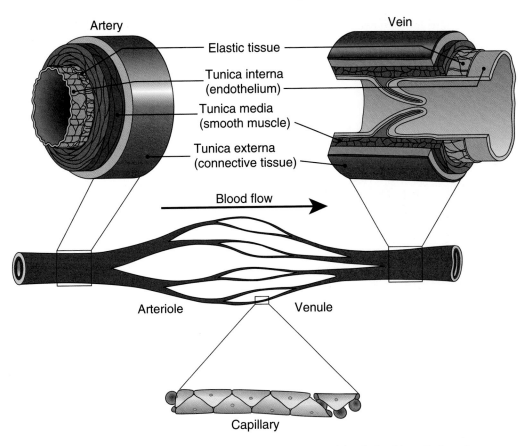

Artery

Vein

Elastic tissue

Tunica interna
(endothelium)

Tunica media
(smooth muscle)

Tunica externa
(connective tissue)

Blood flow

Arteriole

Venule

Capillary

FIGURE **15•2** Sections of small blood vessels showing the thick arterial wall, the thin wall of a vein, and the single-layered wall of a capillary. A venous valve also is shown. The arrow indicate the direction of blood flow.

Capillary Walls

The microscopic branches of these tiny connecting vessels have the thinnest walls of any vessels: one cell layer. The capillary walls are transparent and are made of smooth, platelike cells that continue from the lining of the arteries. Because of the thinness of these walls, exchanges between the blood and the body cells are possible. The capillary boundaries are the most important center of activity for the entire circulatory system. Their function is explained later in this chapter.

Vein Walls

The smallest veins, the **venules,** are formed by the union of capillaries, and their walls are only slightly thicker than those of the capillaries. As veins become larger, their walls become thicker.

The wall of a vein, however, is much thinner than the wall of an artery of comparable size and has less elastic tissue. As a result, the blood within the veins is carried under much lower pressure.

Although there are the same three layers of tissue in the walls of the larger veins, as in the artery walls, the middle tunic is relatively thin in the veins. Therefore, veins are easily collapsed, and only slight pressure on a vein by a tumor or other mass may interfere with return blood flow. Most veins are equipped with one-way valves that permit blood to flow in only one direction: toward the heart (see Fig. 15-2). Such valves are most numerous in the veins of the extremities.

Figure 15-3 is a cross-section of an artery and a vein as seen through a microscope.

smooth muscle

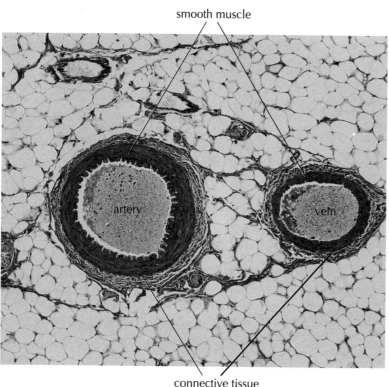

artery

vein

connective tissue

FIGURE **15•3** Cross section of an artery and a vein as seen through a microscope. (Cormack DH: Essential Histology, Plate 11–1. Philadelphia, JB Lippincott, 1993)

15

✔ CHECKPOINT **3**:

What type of tissue makes up the middle layer of arteries and veins, and how is this tissue controlled?

SYSTEMIC ARTERIES

The Aorta and Its Parts

The aorta extends upward and to the right from the left ventricle. Then it curves backward and to the left. It continues down behind the heart just in front of the vertebral column, through the diaphragm, and into the abdomen (Figs. 15-4 and 15-5). The aorta is one continuous artery, but it may be divided into sections:

- The **ascending aorta** is near the heart and inside the pericardial sac.
- The **aortic arch** curves from the right to the left and also extends backward.
- The **thoracic aorta** lies just in front of the

vertebral column behind the heart and in the space behind the pleura.
- The **abdominal aorta** is the longest section of the aorta, spanning the abdominal cavity.

The thoracic and abdominal aorta together make up the descending aorta.

Branches of the Ascending Aorta and Aortic Arch

The first, or ascending, part of the aorta has two branches near the heart, called the **left** and **right coronary arteries,** which supply the heart muscle. These form a crown around the base of the heart and give off branches to all parts of the myocardium.

The arch of the aorta, located immediately beyond the ascending aorta, gives off three large branches.

- The **brachiocephalic** (brak-e-o-seh-FAL-ik) **trunk** is a short artery formerly called the *innominate.* Its newer name means that it supplies the head and the arm.

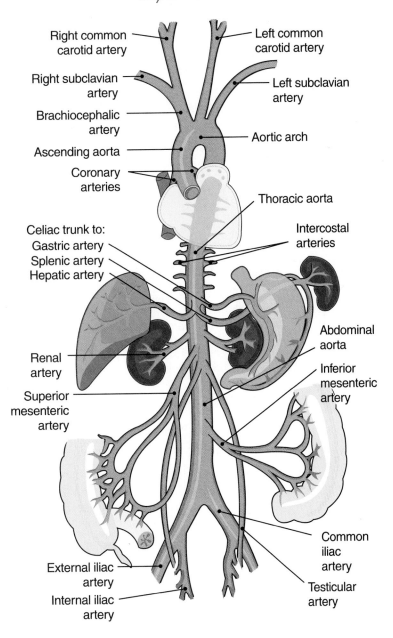

Right common carotid artery

Left common carotid artery

Right subclavian artery

Left subclavian artery

Brachiocephalic artery

Aortic arch

Ascending aorta

Coronary arteries

Thoracic aorta

Celiac trunk to:
Gastric artery
Splenic artery
Hepatic artery

Intercostal arteries

Renal artery

Abdominal aorta

Inferior mesenteric artery

Superior mesenteric artery

Common iliac artery

External iliac artery

Testicular artery

Internal iliac artery

Figure **15•4** Aorta and its branches.

After extending upward somewhat less than 5 cm (2 inches), it divides into the **right subclavian** (sub-KLA-ve-an) **artery,** which supplies the right upper extremity (arm), and the **right common carotid** (kah-ROT-id) **artery,** which supplies the right side of the head and the neck. Note that the brachiocephalic artery is unpaired.

• The **left common carotid artery** extends upward from the highest part of the aortic arch. It supplies the left side of the neck and the head.

• The **left subclavian artery** extends under the left (collar bone) clavicle and supplies the left upper extremity. This is the last branch of the aortic arch.

Branches of the Thoracic Aorta

The thoracic aorta supplies branches to the chest wall, to the **esophagus** (e-SOF-ah-gus), and to the bronchi (the subdivisions of the

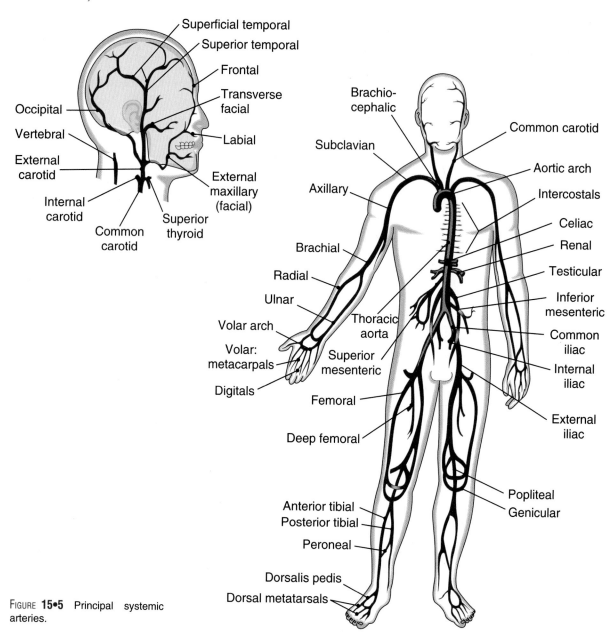

FIGURE **15•5** Principal systemic arteries.

15

trachea) and their treelike subdivisions in the lungs. There are usually 9 to 10 pairs of **intercostal** (in-ter-KOS-tal) **arteries** that extend between the ribs, sending branches to the muscles and other structures of the chest wall.

Branches of the Abdominal Aorta

As in the case of the thoracic aorta, there are unpaired branches extending forward and paired arteries extending toward the side. The unpaired vessels are large arteries that supply the abdominal viscera. The most important of these visceral branches are as follows:

- The **celiac** (SE-le-ak) **trunk** is a short artery about 1.25 cm (½ inch) long that subdivides into three branches: the **left gastric artery** goes to the stomach, the **splenic** (SPLEN-ik) **artery** goes to the spleen, and the **hepatic** (heh-PAT-ik) **artery** carries oxygenated blood to the liver.

- The *superior mesenteric* (mes-en-TER-ik) *artery,* the largest of these branches, carries blood to most of the small intestine and to the first half of the large intestine.
- The much smaller *inferior mesenteric artery,* located below the superior mesenteric and near the end of the abdominal aorta, supplies the second half of the large intestine.

The paired lateral branches of the abdominal aorta include the following right and left vessels:

- The *phrenic* (FREN-ik) *arteries* supply the diaphragm.
- The *suprarenal* (su-prah-RE-nal) *arteries* supply the adrenal (suprarenal) glands.
- The *renal* (RE-nal) *arteries,* the largest in this group, carry blood to the kidneys.
- The *ovarian arteries* in the female and *testicular* (tes-TIK-u-lar) *arteries* in the male (formerly called the *spermatic arteries*), supply the sex glands.
- Four pairs of *lumbar* (LUM-bar) *arteries* extend into the musculature of the abdominal wall.

> ✔ CHECKPOINT **4**:
>
> What are the subdivisions of the aorta, the largest artery?

The Iliac Arteries and Their Subdivisions

The abdominal aorta finally divides into two *common iliac* (IL-e-ak) *arteries.* Both of these vessels, about 5 cm (2 inches) long, extend into the pelvis, where each one subdivides into an *internal* and an *external iliac artery.*

The internal iliac vessels then send branches to the pelvic organs, including the urinary bladder, the rectum, and some of the reproductive organs.

Each external iliac artery continues into the thigh as the *femoral* (FEM-or-al) *artery.* This vessel gives off branches in the thigh and then becomes the *popliteal* (pop-LIT-e-al) *artery,* which subdivides below the knee. The subdivi-

sions include the *tibial artery* and the *dorsalis pedis* (dor-SA-lis PE-dis), which supply the leg and the foot.

Arteries That Branch to the Head and Arm

Each common carotid artery gives off branches to the thyroid gland and other structures in the neck before dividing into the *external* and *internal carotid arteries,* which supply parts of the head.

The arm and hand receive blood from the *subclavian* (sub-KLA-ve-an) *artery*, which becomes the *axillary* (AK-sil-ar-e) *artery* in the axilla (armpit). The longest part of this vessel, the *brachial* (BRA-ke-al) *artery,* is in the arm proper. It subdivides into two branches near the elbow: the *radial artery,* which continues down the thumb side of the forearm and wrist, and the *ulnar artery,* which extends along the medial or little finger side into the hand.

Just as the larger branches of a tree give off limbs of varying sizes, so the arterial tree has a multitude of subdivisions. Hundreds of names might be included. We have mentioned only some of them.

Anastomoses

A communication between two vessels is called an *anastomosis* (ah-nas-to-MO-sis). By means of arterial anastomoses, blood reaches vital organs by more than one route. Some examples of such unions of end arteries are as follows:

- The *circle of Willis* (Fig. 15-6) receives blood from the two internal carotid arteries and from the *basilar* (BAS-il-ar) *artery,* which is formed by the union of two vertebral arteries. This arterial circle lies just under the center of the brain and sends branches to the cerebrum and other parts of the brain.
- The *volar* (VO-lar) *arch* is formed by the union of the radial and ulnar arteries in the hand. It sends branches to the hand and the fingers.

15

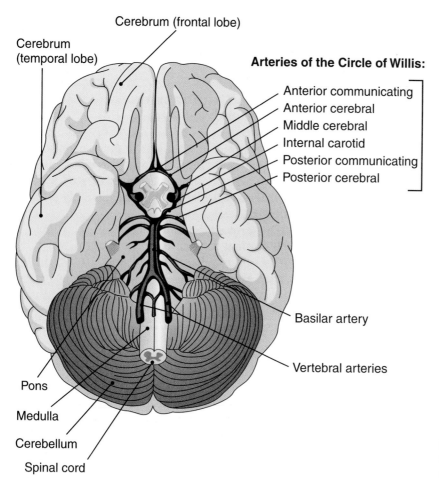

Cerebrum (frontal lobe)

Cerebrum (temporal lobe)

Arteries of the Circle of Willis:

Anterior communicating
Anterior cerebral
Middle cerebral
Internal carotid
Posterior communicating
Posterior cerebral

Basilar artery

Vertebral arteries

Pons

Medulla

Cerebellum

Spinal cord

FIGURE **15•6** Arteries that supply the brain, showing the arteries that make up the circle of Willis.

- The **mesenteric arches** are made of communications between branches of the vessels that supply blood to the intestinal tract.
- **Arterial arches** are formed by the union of branches of the tibial arteries in the foot. Similar anastomoses are found in other parts of the body.

Arteriovenous anastomoses are blood shunts found in a few areas, including the external ears, the hands, and the feet. Vessels with muscular walls connect arteries directly with veins and thus bypass the capillaries (Fig. 15-7). This provides a more rapid flow and a greater volume of blood to these areas than elsewhere, thus protecting these exposed parts from freezing in cold weather.

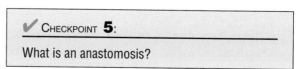

✔ CHECKPOINT **5**:

What is an anastomosis?

SYSTEMIC VEINS

Whereas most arteries are located in protected and rather deep areas of the body, many veins are found near the surface (Fig. 15-8). The most important of these **superficial veins** are in the extremities. These include the following:

- The veins on the back of the hand and at the front of the elbow. Those at the elbow are often used for removing blood samples for test purposes as well as for intravenous

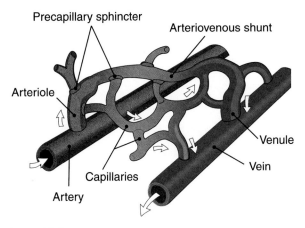

FIGURE **15•7** Capillary network showing an arteriovenous shunt (anastomosis).

injections. The largest of this group of veins are the **cephalic** (seh-FAL-ik), the **basilic** (bah-SIL-ik), and the **median cubital** (KU-bih-tal) **veins.**

- The **saphenous** (sah-FE-nus) **veins** of the lower extremities, which are the longest veins of the body. The great saphenous vein begins in the foot and extends up the medial side of the leg, the knee, and the thigh. It finally empties into the femoral vein near the groin.

The **deep veins** tend to parallel arteries and usually have the same names as the corresponding arteries. Examples of these include the **femoral** and the **iliac** vessels of the lower part of the body and the **brachial, axillary,** and **subclavian** vessels of the upper extremities. Exceptions are found in the veins of the head and the neck. The **jugular** (JUG-u-lar) **veins** drain the areas supplied by the carotid arteries. Two **brachiocephalic** (innominate) **veins** are formed, one on each side, by the union of the subclavian and the jugular veins. (Remember, there is only *one* brachiocephalic artery.)

The Venae Cavae and Their Tributaries

The veins of the head, neck, upper extremities, and chest all drain into the **superior vena cava** (VE-nah KA-vah), which goes to the

heart. It is formed by the union of the right and left brachiocephalic veins, which drain the head, neck, and upper extremities. The **azygos** (AZ-ih-gos) **vein** drains the veins of the chest wall and empties into the superior vena cava just before the latter empties into the heart (see Fig. 15-8).

The **inferior vena cava,** which is much longer than the superior vena cava, returns the blood from the parts of the body below the diaphragm. It begins in the lower abdomen with the union of the two common iliac veins. It then ascends along the back wall of the abdomen, through a groove in the posterior part of the liver, through the diaphragm, and finally through the lower thorax to empty into the right atrium of the heart.

Drainage into the inferior vena cava is more complicated than drainage into the superior vena cava. The large veins below the diaphragm may be divided into two groups:

- The right and left veins that drain paired parts and organs. They include the **iliac veins** from near the groin, four pairs of **lumbar veins** from the dorsal part of the trunk and from the spinal cord, the **testicular veins** from the testes of the male and the **ovarian veins** from the ovaries of the female, the **renal** and **suprarenal veins** from the kidneys and adrenal glands near the kidneys, and finally the large **hepatic veins** from the liver. For the most part, these vessels empty directly into the inferior vena cava. The left testicular in the male and the left ovarian in the female empty into the left renal vein, which then takes this blood to the inferior vena cava; these veins thus constitute exceptions to the rule that the paired veins empty directly into the vena cava.
- Unpaired veins that come from the spleen and from parts of the digestive tract (stomach and intestine) empty into a vein called the **hepatic portal vein.** Unlike other lower veins, which empty into the inferior vena cava, the hepatic portal vein is part of a special system that enables blood to circulate through the liver before returning to the heart.

15

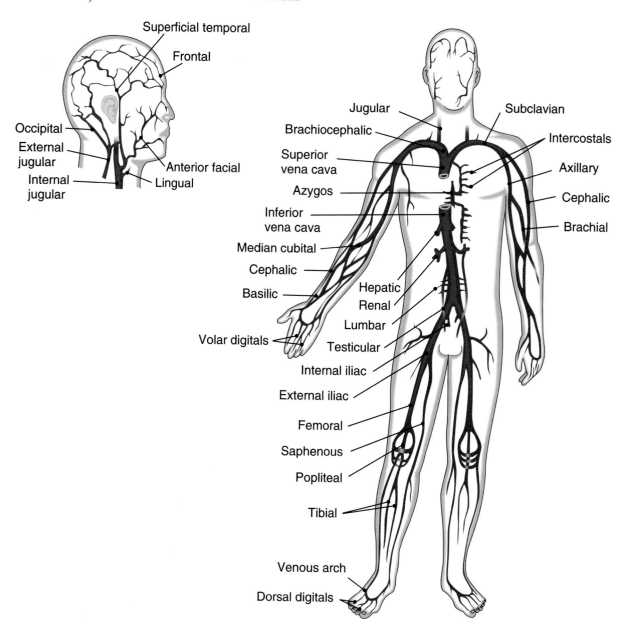

FIGURE **15•8** Principal systemic veins.

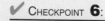

✔ CHECKPOINT **6**:

Veins are described as superficial or deep. What does superficial mean?

Venous Sinuses

The word *sinus* means "space" or "hollow." A *venous sinus* is a large channel that drains de-oxygenated blood but does not have the usual tubular structure of the veins.

One example of a venous sinus is the ***coronary sinus,*** which receives most of the blood from the veins of the heart wall (see Fig. 14-4 in Chap. 14). It lies between the left atrium and left ventricle on the posterior surface of the heart, and it empties directly into the right atrium along with the two venae cavae.

Other important venous sinuses are the ***cra-***

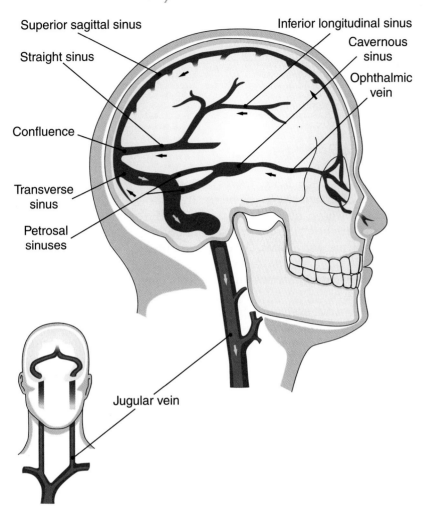

Superior sagittal sinus

Straight sinus

Confluence

Transverse sinus

Petrosal sinuses

Inferior longitudinal sinus

Cavernous sinus

Ophthalmic vein

Jugular vein

FIGURE **15•9** Cranial venous sinuses. The paired transverse sinuses, which carry blood from the brain to the jugular veins, are shown in the inset.

15

nial venous sinuses, which are located inside the skull and drain the veins that come from all over the brain (Fig. 15-9). The largest of the cranial venous sinuses are the following:

- The two ***cavernous sinuses,*** situated behind the eyeballs, serve to drain the ***ophthalmic*** (of-THAL-mik) ***veins*** of the eyes.
- The ***superior sagittal*** (SAJ-ih-tal) ***sinus*** is a single long space located in the midline above the brain and in the fissure between the two hemispheres of the cerebrum. It ends in an enlargement called the ***confluence*** (KON-flu-ens) ***of sinuses.***
- The two ***transverse sinuses,*** also called the ***lateral sinuses,*** are large spaces be-

tween the layers of the dura mater (the outermost membrane around the brain). They begin posteriorly, in the region of the confluence of sinuses, and then extend toward either side. As each sinus extends around the inside of the skull, it receives blood draining those parts not already drained by the superior sagittal and other sinuses that join the back portions of the transverse sinuses. This means that nearly all the blood that comes from the veins of the brain eventually empties into one or the other of the transverse sinuses. On either side, the sinus extends far enough forward to empty into an internal jugular vein, which then passes through a hole in the skull to continue downward in the neck.

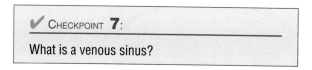

✔ CHECKPOINT **7**:

What is a venous sinus?

The Hepatic Portal System

Almost always, when blood leaves a capillary bed, it flows directly back to the heart. In a portal system, however, blood circulates through a second capillary bed, usually in a second organ, before it returns to the heart. A portal system is a kind of detour in the pathway of venous return that transports materials directly from one organ to another.

The largest portal system in the body is the *hepatic portal system,* which carries blood from the abdominal organs to the liver (Fig. 15-10). In a similar fashion, a small, local portal system is located in the brain to carry substances from the hypothalamus to the pituitary (see Chap. 12). The hepatic portal system includes the veins that drain blood from capillaries in the spleen, stomach, pancreas, and intestine. Instead of emptying their blood directly into the inferior vena cava, they deliver it by way of the hepatic portal vein to the liver. The largest tributary of the portal vein is the *superior mesenteric vein,* which drains blood from the proximal portion of the intestine. It is joined by the *splenic vein* just under the liver. Other tributaries of the portal circulation are the *gastric, pancreatic,* and *inferior mesenteric veins.*

On entering the liver, the portal vein divides and subdivides into ever smaller branches. Eventually, the portal blood flows into a vast network of sinuslike vessels called *sinusoids* (SI-nus-oyds). These enlarged capillary channels allow liver cells close contact with the

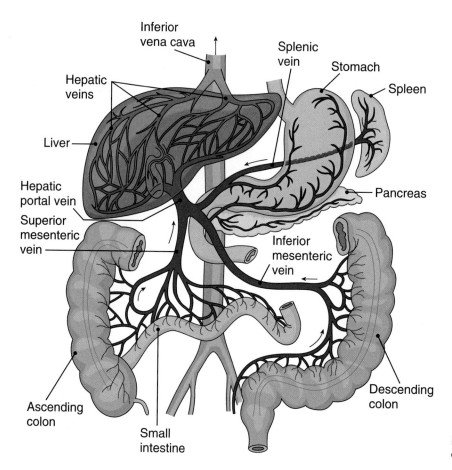

FIGURE **15•10** Hepatic portal circulation.

blood coming from the abdominal organs. (Similar blood channels are found in the spleen and endocrine glands, including the thyroid and adrenals.) After leaving the sinusoids, blood is finally collected by the hepatic veins, which empty into the inferior vena cava.

The purpose of the hepatic portal system of veins is to transport blood from the digestive organs and the spleen to the liver sinusoids, so that the liver cells can carry out their functions. For example, when food is digested, most of the end products are absorbed from the small intestine into the bloodstream and transported to the liver by the portal system. In the liver, these nutrients are processed, stored, and released as needed into the general circulation.

> ✔ CHECKPOINT **8**:
>
> The hepatic portal system takes blood from the abdominal organs to what organ?

THE PHYSIOLOGY OF CIRCULATION

In a general way, the circulating blood might be compared to a train that travels around the country, loading and unloading freight in each of the cities it serves. For example, as blood flows through capillaries surrounding the air sacs in the lungs, it picks up oxygen and unloads carbon dioxide. Later, when this oxygenated blood is pumped to capillaries in other parts of the body, it unloads the oxygen and picks up carbon dioxide and other substances resulting from cellular activities (Fig. 15-11). The microscopic capillaries are of fundamental importance in these activities. It is only through and between the cells of these thin-walled vessels that the necessary exchanges can occur. See The Blood–Brain Barrier.

All living cells are immersed in a slightly salty liquid called *tissue fluid* or *interstitial fluid*. Looking again at Figure 15-11, one can see how this fluid serves as "middleman" between the capillary membrane and the neighboring cells. As water, oxygen, and other materials necessary for cellular activity pass

The Blood—Brain Barrier

The blood–brain barrier (BBB) is an adaptation of the circulation that protects the central nervous system from harmful substances traveling in the blood. It acts as a barrier to hormones, drugs, neurotransmitters, and other substances that might harm the brain or adversely affect its function. The barrier is formed by special cells in the brain capillaries. These cells are joined by tight junctions that limit the passage of materials between them. Also contributing to this barrier are astrocytes, specialized glial (connective tissue) cells that wrap around the capillaries to limit their permeability.

Pathogens are excluded by the blood–brain barrier, although some viruses, including poliovirus and herpesvirus, can get around it by traveling along peripheral nerves into the central nervous system. Also, some streptococci have the ability to get through the tight capillary junctions.

The blood–brain barrier can be an obstacle to getting drugs into the brain. Some antibiotics can cross the barrier, whereas others cannot. In Parkinson's disease, there is a deficiency of the neurotransmitter dopamine in the brain. The neurotransmitter itself will not pass through the barrier, but a related compound, L-dopa, is administered instead. L-dopa can cross the blood–brain barrier and is then converted to dopamine in the brain.

through the capillary walls, they enter the tissue fluid. Then, these substances make their way by diffusion to the cells. At the same time, carbon dioxide and other end products of cell metabolism come from the cells and move in the opposite direction. These substances enter the capillary and are carried away in the bloodstream, to reach other organs or to be eliminated from the body.

Capillary Exchange

Diffusion is the main process by which substances move between the cells and the capillary blood. A secondary force is the pressure of the blood as it flows through the capillaries. Blood pressure acts to filter, or "push," water

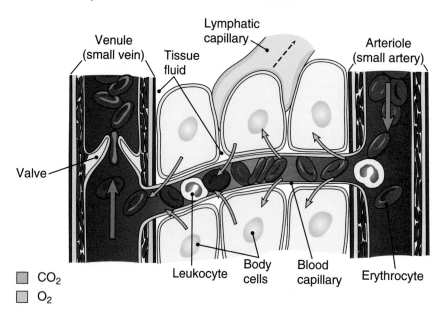

FIGURE **15•11** Diagram showing the connection between the small blood vessels through capillaries. Note the lymphatic capillary, which aids in tissue drainage.

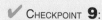 CO$_2$
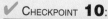 O$_2$

and dissolved materials out of the capillary into the tissue fluid. Fluid is drawn back into the capillary by osmotic pressure, the "pulling force" of substances dissolved and suspended in the blood. Osmotic pressure is maintained by plasma proteins (mainly albumin), which are too large to go through the capillary wall. These processes result in the constant exchange of fluids across the capillary wall.

The movement of blood through the capillaries is relatively slow, owing to the much larger size of the cross-sectional area of the capillaries compared with that of the larger vessels from which capillaries branch. This slow progress through the capillaries allows time for exchanges to occur.

✔ CHECKPOINT **9**:

As materials diffuse back and forth between the blood and tissue fluid across the capillary wall, what force helps to push materials out of the capillary? What force helps to draw materials into the capillary?

The Dynamics of Blood Flow

The flow of blood is carefully regulated to supply the needs of the tissues without unnecessary burden on the heart. Some organs, such as

the brain, liver, and kidneys, require large quantities of blood even at rest. The requirements of some tissues, such as those of skeletal muscles and digestive organs, increase greatly during periods of activity. (The blood flow in muscle can increase 25 times during exercise.) The volume of blood flowing to a particular organ can be regulated by changing the size of the blood vessels supplying that organ.

An increase in the diameter of a blood vessel is called *vasodilation.* This change allows for the delivery of more blood to an area. *Vasoconstriction* is a decrease in the diameter of a blood vessel, causing a decrease in blood flow. These *vasomotor activities* result from the contraction or relaxation of smooth muscle in the walls of the blood vessels, mainly the arterioles. A *vasomotor center* in the medulla of the brain stem regulates these activities, sending its messages through the autonomic nervous system.

The flow of blood into an individual capillary is regulated by a *precapillary sphincter* of smooth muscle that encircles the entrance to the capillary (see Fig. 15-7). This widens to allow more blood to enter when tissues need oxygen.

✔ CHECKPOINT **10**:

Where are vasomotor activities regulated?

Return of Blood to the Heart

By the time blood arrives in the veins, little force remains from the pumping action of the heart. Also, because the veins tend to expand under pressure, considerable amounts of blood are stored in the venous system. Blood is moved back toward the heart by several mechanisms:

- **Contraction of skeletal muscles**. As skeletal muscles contract, they compress the veins and squeeze blood forward.
- **Valves** in the veins prevent backflow and keep blood flowing toward the heart.
- **Breathing**. Changes in pressures in the abdominal and thoracic cavities during breathing also promote return of blood in the venous system. During inhalation, the diaphragm flattens and puts pressure on the large abdominal veins. At the same time, expansion of the chest causes pressure to drop in the thorax. Together, these actions serve to both push and pull blood through these cavities and return it to the heart.

As evidence of these effects, if a person stands completely motionless, especially on a hot day when the superficial vessels dilate, enough blood can accumulate in the lower extremities to cause fainting from insufficient oxygen to the brain.

The Pulse

The ventricles pump blood into the arteries regularly about 70 to 80 times a minute. The force of ventricular contraction starts a wave of increased pressure that begins at the heart and travels along the arteries. This wave, called the ***pulse***, can be felt in any artery that is relatively close to the surface, particularly if the vessel can be pressed down against a bone. At the wrist, the radial artery passes over the bone on the thumb side of the forearm, and the pulse is most commonly obtained here. Other vessels sometimes used for obtaining the pulse are the carotid artery in the neck and the dorsalis pedis on the top of the foot.

Normally, the pulse rate is the same as the heart rate. Only if a heartbeat is abnormally weak, or if the artery is obstructed, may the beat not be detected as a pulse. In checking the pulse of another person, it is important to use your second or third finger. If you use your thumb, you may find that you are getting your own pulse. When taking a pulse, it is important to gauge the strength as well as the regularity and the rate.

Pulse Rate

Various factors may influence the pulse rate. We describe just a few here:

- The pulse is somewhat faster in small people than in large people and usually is slightly faster in women than in men.
- In a newborn infant, the rate may be from 120 to 140 beats/minute. As the child grows, the rate tends to become slower.
- Muscular activity influences the pulse rate. During sleep, the pulse may slow down to 60 beats/minute, whereas during strenuous exercise, the rate may go up to well over 100 beats/minute. For a person in good condition, the pulse does not go up as rapidly as it does in an inactive person, and it returns to a resting rate more quickly after exercise.
- Emotional disturbances may increase the pulse rate.
- In many infections, the pulse rate increases with the increase in temperature.
- An excessive amount of secretion from the thyroid gland may cause a rapid pulse.

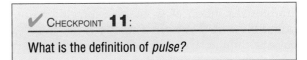

✔ CHECKPOINT **11**:

What is the definition of *pulse?*

Blood Pressure

Blood pressure is the force exerted by the blood against the walls of the vessels. Blood pressure is the product of the output of the heart and the resistance in the vessels. The output of the heart is influenced by the following factors:

- Strength of the contraction of the heart
- Total blood volume, which controls the volume each beat pushes out

The resistance in the vessels is affected by the following factors:

- Vasomotor changes. Vasoconstriction increases resistance to flow; vasodilation lowers resistance.
- Elasticity of blood vessels. Blood vessels lose elasticity and often become hard as a part of aging, thus increasing resistance.
- Thickness of the blood, called *viscosity*. Increased numbers of red blood cells increase viscosity.

Measurement of Blood Pressure

The measurement and careful interpretation of blood pressure may prove a valuable guide in the care and evaluation of a person's health. Because blood pressure decreases as the blood flows from arteries into capillaries and finally into veins, measurements ordinarily are made of arterial pressure only. The instrument used is called a **sphygmomanometer** (sfig-mo-mah-NOM-eh-ter), and two variables are measured:

- **Systolic pressure,** which occurs during heart muscle contraction, averages about 120 and is expressed in millimeters of mercury (mmHg).
- **Diastolic pressure,** which occurs during relaxation of the heart muscle, averages about 80 mmHg.

The sphygmomanometer is essentially a graduated column of mercury connected to an inflatable cuff. The cuff is wrapped around the patient's upper arm and inflated with air until the brachial artery is compressed and the blood flow is cut off. Then, listening with a stethoscope, the doctor or nurse slowly lets air out of the cuff until the first pulsations are heard. At this point, the pressure in the cuff is equal to the systolic pressure, and this pressure is read off the mercury column. Then, more air is let out until a characteristic muffled sound indicates the point at which the diastolic pressure is to be read. Considerable experience is required to ensure an accurate reading. The blood pressure is reported as a fraction, with the systolic pressure above and the diastolic pressure below, such as 120/80 mmHg. Note that blood pressure varies throughout the day, so a single reading does not give a complete picture.

See Special Methods for Measuring Blood Pressure.

✔ CHECKPOINT **12**:

What is the definition of blood pressure?

Abnormal Blood Pressure

Lower-than-normal blood pressure is called **hypotension** (hi-po-TEN-shun). Because of individual variations in normal pressure levels, however, what would be a low pressure for one person might be normal for someone else. For this reason, hypotension is best evaluated in terms of how well the body tissues are being supplied with blood. A person whose systolic blood pressure drops to below his or her normal range may experience episodes of fainting because of inadequate blood flow to the brain. The sudden lowering of blood pressure below a per-

Special Methods for Measuring Blood Pressure

Measurement of blood pressure with a simple inflatable cuff cannot reflect the pressure in all parts of the cardiovascular system. In specialized hospital units, more specific readings can be obtained by using a catheter (thin tube) inserted directly into the heart and large vessels. One type commonly used is the Swan-Ganz catheter, which has an inflatable balloon at the tip. This device is threaded through a nearby vein into the right side of the heart, where atrial and ventricular pressures can be recorded. As the catheter continues into the pulmonary artery, pressure in this vessel can be read. When the balloon is inflated, the catheter becomes wedged in a branch of the pulmonary artery, blocking blood flow. The reading obtained is called the **pulmonary capillary wedge (PCW) pressure.** It gives information on pressure in the left side of the heart and on resistance in the lungs. Combined with other tests, it can be used to diagnose cardiac and pulmonary disorders.

son's normal level is one symptom of shock; it may also occur in certain chronic diseases and in heart block.

Hypertension, or high blood pressure, has received a great deal of attention. Often, it occurs temporarily as a result of excitement or exertion. It may be persistent in a number of conditions, including the following:

- Kidney disease and uremia (nitrogen waste in the blood) or other toxic conditions
- Endocrine disorders, such as hyperthyroidism and acromegaly
- Arterial disease, including hardening of the arteries (atherosclerosis), which reduces elasticity of the vessels
- Tumors of the central portion (medulla) of the adrenal gland

Hypertension that has no apparent medical cause is called ***essential hypertension.*** This condition, which is fairly common, may cause stroke, heart failure, or kidney damage. Excess of an enzyme produced in the kidney, called ***renin*** (RE-nin), appears to play a role in the severity of this kind of hypertension. Renin raises blood pressure by causing blood vessels to constrict and by promoting the retention of salt and water by the kidneys.

Although emphasis is often placed on the systolic blood pressure, in many cases, the diastolic pressure is even more important because the total volume of fluid in the vascular system and the condition of small arteries may have more of an effect on diastolic pressure.

Treatment of Hypertension

Even though there is much individual variation in blood pressure, guidelines have been established for the diagnosis and treatment of hypertension. The first stage of hypertension begins at 140/90 mmHg. Treatment at this point should be based on diet, exercise, and weight loss, if necessary. People with pressure reading above 159/99 mmHg should add drug therapy to this regimen. Drugs used to treat hypertension include the following:

- Diuretics, which promote water loss
- Drugs that limit production of renin
- Drugs that relax blood vessels

✔ CHECKPOINT **13**:

What is meant by hypertension and hypotension?

DISORDERS INVOLVING THE BLOOD VESSELS

Arterial Degeneration

As a result of age or other degenerative changes, materials may be deposited within the walls of the arteries. These deposits cause an irregular thickening of the artery wall at the expense of the lumen (space inside the vessel) as well as a loss of elasticity. In some cases, calcium salts and scar tissue may cause this hardening of the arteries, technically called ***arteriosclerosis*** (ar-te-re-o-skle-RO-sis). The most common form of this disorder is ***atherosclerosis*** (ath-er-o-skle-RO-sis) (Fig. 15-12), in which areas of yellow, fatlike material, called ***plaque*** (PLAK), accumulate in the vessels and separate the muscle and elastic connective tissue. Sometimes, the lining of the artery is also damaged, leading to possible formation of a blood clot (thrombus). The thrombus may partially or

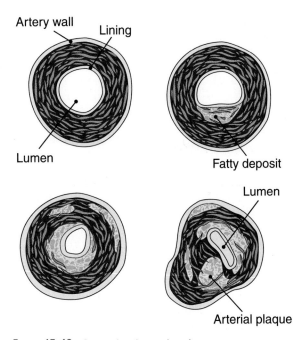

FIGURE **15•12** Stages in atherosclerosis.

completely obstruct the vessel, as it sometimes does in coronary thrombosis. A diet high in fats, particularly saturated fats, is known to contribute to atherosclerosis. Cigarette smoking also increases the extent and severity of this disorder (see Keeping Your Arteries Clean).

Arterial damage may be present for years without causing any noticeable symptoms. As the thickening of the wall continues and the diameter of the passage for blood flow is decreased, a variety of symptoms can appear. The nature of these disturbances varies with the parts of the body affected and with the extent of the changes in the arterial walls. Some examples are listed below:

- Leg cramps, pain, and sudden lameness while walking may be due to insufficient blood supply to the lower extremities as a result of artery wall damage.
- Headaches, dizziness, and mental disorders may be the result of cerebral artery sclerosis.
- Hypertension may result from a decrease in size of the lumina (central openings) within many arteries throughout the body. Although hypertension may be present in young people with no apparent artery damage, and atherosclerosis may be present without causing hypertension, the two are often found together in elderly people.
- Palpitations, dyspnea (difficulty in breathing), paleness, weakness, and other symptoms may be the result of arteriosclerosis of the coronary arteries. The severe pain of angina pectoris may follow the lack of oxygen and myocardial damage associated with sclerosis of the vessels that supply the heart.
- An increase in the amount of urine with the appearance of albumin. Albumin is a normal plasma protein usually found in the urine only if there is kidney damage. Other symptoms referable to the kidneys may be due to damage to the renal arteries.

Keeping Your Arteries Clean

The first step in the buildup of plaque deposits is thought to be microscopic damage to the inner wall of the arteries, the endothellium. This damage is thought to be caused by direct contact with LDL (the "bad" cholesterol), oxidizing chemicals, such as free-radicals, and some proteins. LDL invades the endothelium, causing an accumulation of lipids in the wall of the artery. This is followed by aggregation of platelets and macrophages. The endothelium starts to divide in an attempt to seal itself off. This leads to the incorporation of all of the above substances within the arterial wall. The wall soon bulges into the lumen and obstructs blood flow. This obstruction then leads to the formation of clots that may further close off the flow of blood through the vessel. Arteries in the heart, brain, kidneys, and the extremities seem to be especially vulnerable to this process. To help slow this degenerative process, one should:

- Reduce fat intake; cut intake of foods high in LDL—the saturated fats
- Increase intake of soluble fibers, such as oat, bran, and fruit fibers, which have been shown to decrease cholesterol levels in the blood
- Take in adequate amounts of vitamin E, vitamin C, folic acid, and calcium; each has been shown to have beneficial effects on the heart
- Add vitamins B_6 and B_{12} to your diet; both are thought to help the heart by lowering levels of an enzyme considered to be harmful to the heart
- Take one low-dose aspirin a day (check with your doctor first!); aspirin helps to block platelet aggregation in the arterial wall, preventing clot formation.

Gradual narrowing of the interior of the arteries, with a consequent reduction in the volume of blood that passes through them, gives rise to *ischemia* (is-KE-me-ah), a lack of blood. Those parts that are supplied by the damaged artery suffer from an inadequate blood supply, the result being that vital cells in these organs gradually die. The death of cells, for whatever cause, is called *necrosis* (neh-KRO-sis).

Once vital cells die, the organ loses its effectiveness. One example of necrosis due to ischemia is the death of certain cells of the brain, with mental disorders as a possible result. Another example is the chain of complications resulting from gradual closure of the arteries of the leg or (rarely) of the arm. The circulation of blood in the toes or the fingers, never too brisk even at the best of times, may cease altogether. Necrosis occurs; the dead tissue is invaded by bacteria, and putrefaction sets in. This condition, called **gangrene** (GANG-grene), can result from a number of disorders that may injure the arteries, such as diabetes. Diabetic gangrene is a fairly common occurrence in elderly diabetic patients.

Aneurysm

An **aneurysm** (AN-u-rizm) is a bulging sac in the wall of a blood vessel due to a localized weakness in that part of the vessel. The aorta and vessels in the brain are common sites of aneurysm. The damage to the wall may be congenital or due to hardening of the arteries. Whatever the cause, the aneurysm may continue to grow in size. As it swells, it may cause some derangement of other structures, in which case, definite symptoms are present. If undiagnosed, the walls of the weakened area eventually yield to the pressure, and the aneurysm bursts like a balloon, usually causing immediate death. Surgical replacement of the damaged segment with a synthetic graft may be lifesaving.

Hemorrhage

A profuse escape of blood from the vessels is known as **hemorrhage,** a word that means "a bursting forth of blood." Such bleeding may be external or internal, may be from vessels of any size, and may involve any part of the body. Capillary oozing usually is stopped by the normal process of clot formation.

First Aid for Hemorrhage

The loss of a small amount of blood will cause no problem for a healthy adult, but loss of one liter of blood or more is life-threatening. The first step to control bleeding is the application of direct pressure to the wound using a clean cloth. An assisting person should wear gloves to protect from blood-borne diseases. A bleeding extremity should be elevated above the level of the heart. In cases of severe, persistent bleeding, application of pressure where a local artery can be pressed against a bone slows the bleed-

ing. The most important of these "pressure points" are the following:

- The **facial artery,** which may be pressed against the lower jaw for hemorrhage around the nose, mouth, and cheek. The pulse of the facial artery can be felt in the depression about 1 inch anterior to the angle of the lower jaw.
- The **temporal artery,** which may be pressed against the side of the skull just in front of the ear to stop hemorrhage on the side of the face and around the ear
- The **common carotid artery** in the neck, which may be pressed back against the spinal column for bleeding in the neck and the head. Avoid prolonged compression, which can result in lack of oxygen to the brain.
- The **subclavian artery,** which may be pressed against the first rib by a downward push with the thumb to stop bleeding from the shoulder or arm
- The **brachial artery,** which may be pressed against the humerus (arm bone) by a push inward along the natural groove between the two large muscles of the arm. This stops hand, wrist, and forearm hemorrhage.
- The **femoral artery** (in the groin), which may be pressed to avoid serious hemorrhage of the lower extremity.

It is important not to leave the pressure on too long, as this may cause damage to tissues supplied by arteries past the pressure point.

Shock

The word **shock** has a number of meanings. In terms of the circulating blood, it refers to a life-threatening condition in which there is inadequate blood flow to the tissues of the body. The factor common to all cases of shock is inadequate output by the heart. Shock can be instigated by a wide range of conditions that reduce the effective circulation. The exact cause of shock is often not known; however, a widely used classification is based on causative factors, the most important of which include the following:

- **Cardiogenic** (kar-de-o-JEN-ik) **shock,** sometimes called *pump failure,* is often a complication of heart muscle damage, as occurs in myocardial infarction. It is the leading cause of shock death.
- **Septic shock** is second only to cardiogenic shock as a cause of shock death. It is usually due to an overwhelming bacterial infection.
- **Hypovolemic** (hi-po-vo-LE-mik) **shock** is due to a decrease in the volume of circulating blood and may follow severe hemorrhage or burns.
- **Anaphylactic** (an-ah-fih-LAK-tik) **shock** is a severe allergic reaction to foreign substances to which the person has been sensitized.

When the cause is not known, shock is classified according to its severity.

In **mild shock**, regulatory mechanisms act to relieve the circulatory deficit. Symptoms are often subtle changes in heart rate and blood pressure. Constriction of small blood vessels and the detouring of blood away from certain organs increase the effective circulation. Mild shock may develop into a severe, life-threatening circulatory failure.

Severe shock is characterized by poor circulation, which causes further damage and deepening of the shock. Symptoms of late shock include clammy skin, anxiety, low blood pressure, rapid pulse, and rapid, shallow breathing. Contractions of the heart are weakened, owing to the decrease in blood supply to the heart muscle. The muscles in the blood vessel walls also are weakened, so that they dilate. The capillaries become more permeable and lose fluid, owing to the accumulation of metabolic wastes.

The victim of shock should first be placed in a horizontal position and covered with a blanket. If there is bleeding, it should be stopped. The patient's head should be kept turned to the side to prevent aspiration (breathing in) of vomited material, an important cause of death in shock cases. Further treatment of shock depends largely on treatment of the causative factors. For example, shock due to fluid loss, such as hemorrhage or burns, is best treated with blood products or plasma expanders (intravenous fluids). Shock due to heart failure should be treated with drugs that improve the contractions of the heart muscle. In any case, all measures are aimed at supporting the circulation and improving the output of the heart. Oxygen is frequently administered to improve the delivery of oxygen to the tissues.

✔ CHECKPOINT **14**:
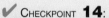

With regard to the circulation, what is meant by shock?

Thrombosis

Formation of a blood clot in a vessel is **thrombosis** (throm-BO-sis). A blood clot in a vein, termed *deep venous thrombosis* (DVT), most commonly develops in the deep veins of the calf muscle, although it may appear elsewhere. Thromboses typically occur in people who are recovering from surgery, injury, or childbirth or those who are bedridden. Clot formation may also be associated with some diseases, with obesity, and with certain drugs, such as hormonal medications. Symptoms are pain and swelling, often with warmth and redness below or around the clot. Thrombosis can be diagnosed with ultrasound or with magnetic resonance imaging (MRI).

A dangerous complication of thrombosis is formation of an **embolus** (EM-bo-lus), a piece of the clot that becomes loose and floats in the blood. An embolus is carried through the circulatory system until it lodges in a vessel. If it reaches the lungs, sudden death from **pulmonary embolism** (EM-bo-lizm) may result. Prevention of infection, early activity to ensure circulation after an injury or an operation, and the use of anticoagulant drugs when appropriate have greatly reduced the incidence of this condition.

Phlebitis (fleh-BI-tis), inflammation of a vein, may contribute to formation of a clot, in which case the condition is called **thrombophlebitis** (throm-bo-fleh-BI-tis).

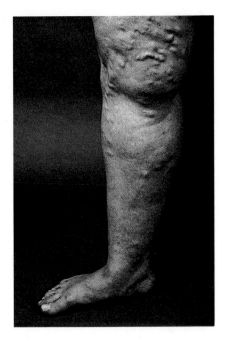

FIGURE **15•13** Varicose veins. (Bates B: Guide to Physical Examination and History Taking, 6th ed, p. 439. Philadelphia, JB Lippincott, 1995)

Varicose Veins

Varicose veins are superficial veins that have become swollen, tortuous, and ineffective. They may be a problem in the esophagus or in the rectum, but the veins most commonly involved are the saphenous veins of the lower extremities (Fig. 15-13). This condition is found frequently in people who spend a great deal of time standing, such as salespeople. Pregnancy, with its accompanying pressure on the veins in the pelvis, may also be a predisposing cause. Varicose veins in the rectum are called *hemorrhoids* (HEM-o-royds), or *piles*. The general term for varicose veins is *varices* (VAR-ihseze); the singular form is *varix* (VAR-iks).

Stasis Dermatitis and Ulcers

Stasis means a standing still or stoppage in normal blood flow. Often, the valves in the veins of the lower extremity become incompetent, and blood is not returned from the legs. The skin becomes inflamed and undergoes scaling; fissures (cracks) form, followed by ulcers. Treatment of the causes and attention to the local lesions should be in the hands of a physician, and patient cooperation is most important.

Arterial Obstruction

When the lumen of an artery is completely blocked by arteriosclerosis, the condition is known as *arteriosclerosis obliterans* (o-BLITer-ans). The complete obstruction to blood flow causes intense pain; if the disease is allowed to progress and is not treated, the affected part or parts may become ulcerated or gangrenous.

Small areas of blockage can be relieved by direct surgical removal of the obstruction. In other cases, the affected vessel can be dilated by angioplasty with a balloon catheter. When the obstruction cannot be relieved by these methods, a bypass graft is placed surgically. The most successful of these grafts uses the saphenous vein from the patient's own body.

Summary

I. **Blood vessels**
 A. Types of blood vessels
  1. Arteries—carry blood away from heart
   a. Arterioles—small arteries
  2. Veins—carry blood toward heart
   a. Venules—small veins
  3. Capillaries—allow for exchanges between blood and tissues, or blood and air in lungs; connect arterioles and venules
 B. Blood circuits
  1. Pulmonary circuit—carries blood to and from lungs
  2. Systemic circuit—carries blood to and from rest of body
 C. Vessel structure
  1. Artery walls—layers
   a. Innermost—single layer of flat epithelial cells (endothelium)
   b. Middle—thicker layer of smooth muscle and elastic connective tissue
   c. Outer—connective tissue
  2. Arterioles—thinner walls, less elastic tissue, more smooth muscle
  3. Capillaries—only endothelium; single layer of cells
  4. Venules—wall slightly thicker than capillary wall
  5. Veins—all three layers; thinner walls than arteries, less elastic tissue

II. **Systemic arteries**
 A. The aorta and its parts
  1. Largest artery
  2. Divisions
   a. Ascending aorta
    1. Left and right coronary arteries
   b. Aortic arch
    1. Brachiocephalic trunk—branches to head and arm
    2. Left common carotid artery—supplies left side of neck and the head
    3. Left subclavian artery—supplies left arm
   c. Descending aorta
    1. Thoracic aorta—branches to chest wall, esophagus, bronchi
    2. Abdominal aorta—supplies abdominal viscera
 B. Iliac arteries and their subdivisions
  1. Final divisions of aorta
  2. Branch to pelvis and legs
 C. Arteries that branch to the head and arm—carotid, subclavian, brachial
 D. Anastomoses—communications between vessels

III. **Systemic veins**
  1. Superficial—near surface
  2. Deep—usually parallel to arteries with same names as corresponding arteries
 A. The venae cavae and their tributaries
  1. Superior vena cava—drains upper part of body
  2. Inferior vena cava—drains lower part of body
 B. Venous sinuses—enlarged venous channels
 C. Hepatic portal system—carries blood from abdominal organs to liver, where it is processed before returning to heart

IV. **The physiology of circulation**
 A. Capillary exchange
  1. Primary method—diffusion
  2. Medium—tissue fluid
  3. Blood pressure—drives fluid into tissues
  4. Osmotic pressure—pulls fluid into capillary
 B. Dynamics of blood flow
  1. Vasomotor activities
   a. Vasodilation—increase in diameter of blood vessel
   b. Vasoconstriction—decrease in diameter of blood vessel
   c. Vasomotor center—in medulla; controls contraction and relax-

ation of smooth muscle in vessel wall

2. Precapillary sphincter—regulates blood flow into capillary

3. Return of blood to heart
   a. Pumping action of heart
   b. Pressure of skeletal muscles on veins
   c. Valves in veins
   d. Breathing—changes in pressure move blood toward heart

C. The pulse
1. Wave of pressure that travels along arteries as ventricles contract
2. Rate affected by size, age, sex, activity, and other factors

D. Blood pressure
1. Force exerted by blood against vessel walls
2. Product of cardiac output, vascular resistance
3. Measured in arm with sphygmomanometer
   a. Systolic pressure
      (1) Occurs during heart contraction
      (2) Averages 120 mmHg
   b. Diastolic pressure
      (1) Occurs during heart relaxation
      (2) Averages 80 mmHg

E. Abnormal blood pressure
1. Hypotension—low blood pressure
2. Hypertension—high blood pressure
   a. Essential hypertension—has no apparent medical cause

b. May involve renin, enzyme released from kidneys

V. Disorders involving the blood vessels
   A. Arterial degeneration
   1. Arteriosclerosis—hardening of arteries with scar tissue, calcium salts, or fatty deposits; may result in ischemia and cell necrosis
      a. Atherosclerosis—deposits of fatty material (plaque) in vessels
      b. May result in thrombosis (blood clot), ischemia (lack of blood supply), and necrosis (cell death)
   2. Aneurysm—weakness and bulging of a vessel; may burst

   C. Hemorrhage
      a. Profuse loss of blood
      b. First aid measures: direct pressure, elevation of limb, pressure on artery

   D. Shock—inadequate output of blood from heart

   E. Thrombosis—formation of blood clot in a vessel
   1. Embolus—piece of a clot traveling in circulation
      a. Pulmonary embolism—clot lodged in lung
   2. Phlebitis—inflammation of a vein; may lead to thrombophlebitis

   F. Varicose veins—swelling and loss of function in superficial veins, usually in legs and rectum (hemorrhoids)

   G. Stasis dermatitis and ulcers

   H. Arterial obstruction

Questions for Study and Review

1. Name the three main groups of blood vessels and describe their functions.
2. Compare the oxygen content of blood in the pulmonary and systemic vessels.
3. How does the structure of the vessels correlate with their function?
4. Name the main branches of the aorta.
5. Describe an arterial anastomosis and give several examples.
6. Trace a drop of blood through the shortest possible route from the capillaries of the foot to the capillaries of the head.

15

7. What are the names and functions of some cranial venous sinuses? Where is the coronary venous sinus and what does it do?
8. What large vessels drain the blood low in oxygen from most of the body into the right atrium? What vessels carry blood high in oxygen into the left atrium?
9. Trace a drop of blood from capillaries in the wall of the small intestine to the right atrium. What is the purpose of going through the liver on this trip?
10. Define *portal system*. Name the largest portal system in the body.
11. What is the purpose of interstitial fluid?
12. What substances diffuse into the tissues from the capillaries? into the capillaries from the tissues?
13. What force pushes fluid out of the capillaries? What force pulls fluid back into the capillaries?
14. What actions help force blood back to the heart?
15. What is meant by *pulse?* Where is the pulse usually determined? If a large part of the body were burned, leaving only the lower extremities accessible for obtaining the pulse, what vessel would you try to use?
16. What are some factors that cause an increase in the pulse rate?
17. List five factors that can change blood pressure.
18. What instrument is used for measuring blood pressure? What are the two values usually obtained called and what does each represent?
19. What are some examples of disorders that cause hypertension of a persistent kind? Of what importance is the diastolic blood pressure reading?
20. What are some symptoms of arteriosclerosis and how are these produced?
21. What is the meaning of *hemorrhage?* What vessels cause the most serious bleeding if they are cut? What are some of the most effective ways of stopping hemorrhage?
22. What is shock and why is it so dangerous? Name some symptoms of shock and identify four types of shock.
23. What are some conditions that can lead to thrombosis?
24. In what organs are varicose veins most commonly found?
25. Explain the difference between the terms in the following pairs:
    a. *pulmonary circuit* and *systemic circuit*
    b. *arteriole* and *venule*
    c. *vasodilation* and *vasoconstriction*
    d. *hypotension* and *hypertension*
    e. *thrombus* and *embolus*

✔ ANSWERS TO CHECKPOINTS

1. The three main groups of blood vessels are arteries, veins, and capillaries.
2. The pulmonary circuit carries blood from the heart to the lungs and back to the heart; the systemic circuit carries blood to and from all remaining tissues in the body.
3. Smooth muscle makes up the middle layer of arteries and veins. Smooth muscle is involuntary muscle controlled by the autonomic nervous system.
4. The aorta is divided into the ascending aorta, aortic arch, thoracic aorta, and abdominal aorta.
5. An anastomosis is a communication between two vessels.
6. Superficial means near the surface.
7. A venous sinus is a large channel that drains deoxygenated blood.
8. The hepatic portal system takes blood from the abdominal organs to the liver.
9. As materials diffuse across the capillary wall, blood pressure helps to push materials out of the capillaries, and osmotic pressure of the blood helps to draw materials into the capillaries.
10. Vasomotor activities are regulated in the medulla of the brain stem.
11. The pulse is the wave of pressure that begins at the heart and travels along the arteries.
12. Blood pressure is the force exerted by blood against the walls of the vessels.
13. Hypertension is high blood pressure, and hypotension is low blood pressure.
14. Circulatory shock is inadequate blood flow to the tissues due to inadequate output by the heart.

The Lymphatic System and Lymphoid Tissue

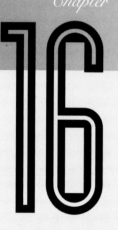

Chapter

16

SELECTED KEY TERMS

The following terms are defined in the Glossary:

chyle

lacteal

lymph

lymphadenitis

lymphadenopathy

lymphangitis

lymphatic duct

lymph node

spleen

thymus

tonsil

BEHAVIORAL OBJECTIVES

After careful study of this chapter, you should be able to:

1. List the functions of the lymphatic system

2. Explain how lymphatic capillaries differ from blood capillaries

3. Name the two main lymphatic ducts and describe the area drained by each

4. List the major structures of the lymphatic system and give the locations and functions of each

5. Describe the composition and function of the reticuloendothelial system

6. Describe the major disorders of the lymphatic system

THE LYMPHATIC SYSTEM

As noted in the preceding chapter, body cells live in tissue fluid, a liquid derived from the bloodstream. Water and dissolved substances, such as oxygen and nutrients, are constantly filtering through capillary walls into the spaces between cells and constantly adding to the volume of tissue fluid. Under normal conditions, fluid is also constantly removed, so that it does not accumulate in the tissues. Part of this fluid simply diffuses back into the capillary bloodstream, taking with it some of the end products of cellular metabolism, including carbon dioxide and other substances. A second pathway for the drainage of tissue fluid involves the *lymphatic system* (Fig. 16-1).

In the tissues, in addition to the blood-carrying capillaries, there are microscopic vessels called *lymphatic capillaries*, which drain excess fluid that does not return to the blood. The lymphatic capillaries also absorb any proteins suspended in this interstitial (tissue) fluid and return them to the bloodstream. Figure 16-2 shows the lymphatic capillaries and the pathway of lymphatic drainage within the tissues.

Lymph

As soon as tissue fluid enters the lymphatic capillary, it is called *lymph.* The lymphatic capillar-

ies join to form the larger lymphatic vessels, or ducts, and these vessels (which we shall have a closer look at in a moment) eventually empty into veins near the heart. Before the lymph reaches these veins, it flows through a series of filters called *lymph nodes,* where bacteria and other foreign particles are trapped and destroyed. The lymph nodes may be compared in a simple way to the oil filter in an automobile.

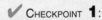

> ✔ CHECKPOINT **1**:
>
> What are some functions of the lymphatic system?

Lymphatic Capillaries

The lymphatic capillaries resemble the blood capillaries in that they are made of one layer of flattened (squamous) epithelial cells, also called *endothelium,* which allows for easy passage of soluble materials and water (Fig. 16-3). The gaps between these endothelial cells in the lymphatic capillaries are larger than those of the blood capillaries to allow easier entrance of proteins and other relatively large suspended particles (see How Lymphatic Capillaries Work). They are more permeable than the blood capillaries; that is, materials can pass through them more easily.

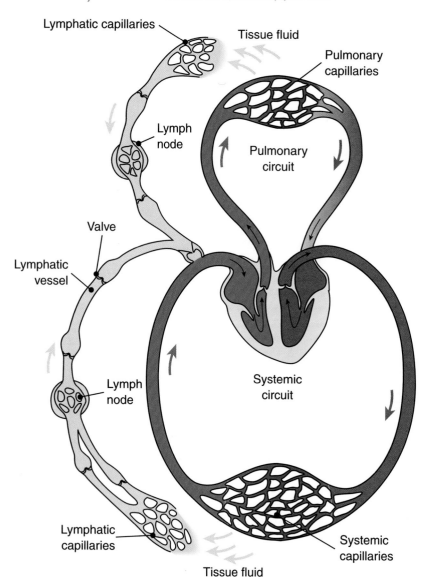

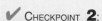

FIGURE **16•1** The lymphatic system in relation to the cardiovascular system.

Unlike the capillaries of the bloodstream, the lymphatic capillaries begin blindly; that is, they are closed at one end and do not serve to bridge two larger vessels. Instead, one end simply lies within a lake of tissue fluid, and the other communicates with a larger lymphatic vessel that transports the lymph toward the heart (see Fig. 16-1).

In the small intestine are some specialized lymphatic capillaries, called *lacteals* (LAK-te-als), which act as a pathway for the transfer of digested fats into the bloodstream. This process is covered in the chapter on the digestive system (see Chap. 19).

✔ CHECKPOINT **2**:

What are two differences between blood capillaries and lymphatic capillaries?

Lymphatic Vessels

The lymphatic vessels are thin walled and delicate and have a beaded appearance because of indentations where valves are located (see Fig. 16-1). These valves prevent backflow in the same way as do those found in some veins.

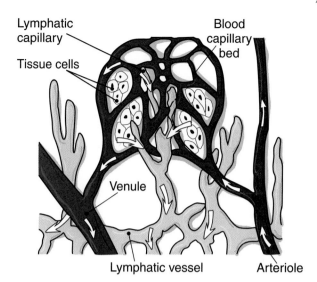

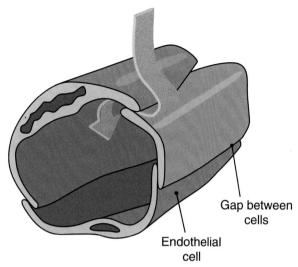

FIGURE **16•2**   Pathway of lymphatic drainage in the tissues.

FIGURE **16•3**   Structure of a lymphatic capillary.

Lymphatic vessels (Fig. 16-4) include **superficial** and **deep** sets. The surface lymphatics are immediately below the skin, often lying near the superficial veins. The deep vessels are usually larger and accompany the deep veins.

Lymphatic vessels are named according to location. For example, those in the breast are called **mammary** lymphatic vessels, those in the thigh **femoral** lymphatic vessels, and those in the leg **tibial** lymphatic vessels. All the lymphatic vessels form networks, and at certain points, they carry lymph into the regional nodes (the nodes that "service" a particular area). For example, nearly all the lymph from the upper extremity and the breast passes through the **axillary lymph nodes,** whereas that from the lower extremity passes through the **inguinal nodes.** Lymphatic vessels carrying lymph away from the regional nodes eventually drain into one of the two terminal vessels, the right lymphatic duct or the thoracic duct, both of which empty into the bloodstream.

The **right lymphatic duct** is a short vessel about 1.25 cm (½ inch) long that receives only the lymph that comes from the upper right quadrant of the body: the right side of the head, neck, and thorax, as well as the right upper extremity. It empties into the right subclavian vein. Its opening into this vein is guarded by two pocketlike semilunar valves to prevent blood from entering the duct. The rest of the body is drained by the thoracic duct.

The Thoracic Duct

The **thoracic duct** is the larger of the two terminal vessels; it is about 40 cm (16 inches) in length. As shown in Figure 16-4, the thoracic duct receives lymph from all parts of the body except those above the diaphragm on the right side. This duct begins in the posterior part of the abdominal cavity, below the attachment of the diaphragm. The first part of this duct is enlarged to form a cistern, or temporary storage

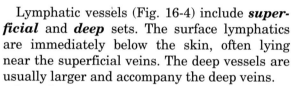

How Lymphatic Capillaries Work

Lymphatic capillaries are more permeable than blood capillaries because the junctions between the cells are wider and because there is less basement membrane underlying the cells. Proteins and other large molecules that escape from the bloodstream can enter the lymphatic capillaries more easily than they can return to the blood capillaries.

Why don't substances that get into the lymphatic capillaries flow right out again? The cells that form the capillary wall overlap slightly to function as one-way valves. Pressure outside the vessel forces materials in. Once fluid enters the capillary, pressure against the cells in the capillary wall blocks its return.

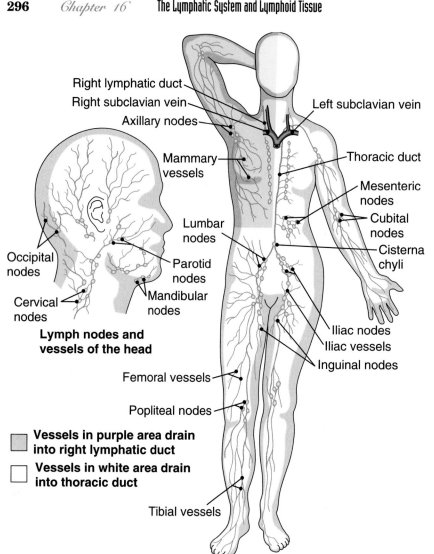

Right lymphatic duct
Right subclavian vein
Axillary nodes
Left subclavian vein
Mammary vessels
Thoracic duct
Mesenteric nodes
Cubital nodes
Lumbar nodes
Cisterna chyli
Occipital nodes
Parotid nodes
Cervical nodes
Mandibular nodes
Lymph nodes and vessels of the head
Iliac nodes
Iliac vessels
Inguinal nodes
Femoral vessels
Popliteal nodes

☐ **Vessels in purple area drain into right lymphatic duct**
☐ **Vessels in white area drain into thoracic duct**

Tibial vessels

FIGURE **16•4** Lymphatic system.

pouch, called the *cisterna chyli* (sis-TER-nah KI-li). *Chyle* (kile) is the milky fluid, formed by the combination of fat globules and lymph, that comes from the intestinal lacteals. Chyle passes through the intestinal lymphatic vessels and the lymph nodes of the mesentery, finally entering the cisterna chyli. In addition to chyle, all the lymph from below the diaphragm empties into the cisterna chyli by way of the various clusters of lymph nodes and then is carried by the thoracic duct into the bloodstream.

The thoracic duct extends upward through the diaphragm and along the back wall of the thorax up into the root of the neck on the left side. Here, it receives the left jugular lymphatic vessels from the head and neck, the left subclavian vessels from the left upper extremity, and other lymphatic vessels from the thorax and its parts. In addition to the valves along the duct, there are two valves at its opening into the left subclavian vein to prevent the passage of blood into the duct.

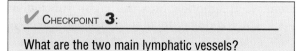

✔ CHECKPOINT **3**:

What are the two main lymphatic vessels?

Movement of Lymph

The segments of lymphatic vessels located between the valves contract rhythmically, propelling the lymph along. The rate of these contractions is related to the volume of fluid in the vessel—the more fluid, the more rapid the contractions of the vessel.

Lymph is also moved by the same mechanisms that promote venous return of blood to the heart. As skeletal muscles contract during movement, they compress the lymphatic vessels and drive lymph forward. Changes in pressures within the abdominal and thoracic cavities due to breathing aid the movement of lymph during passage through these body cavities.

See When Lymph Does Not Flow: Lymphedema.

LYMPHOID TISSUE

The previous section was a brief survey of the system of lymph vessels and lymph transport. Although the lymph nodes were mentioned, they are described in greater detail in this section, along with discussion of other organs made of similar tissue.

Lymphoid (LIM-foyd) *tissue* is distributed throughout the body and makes up the specialized organs of the lymphatic system. We will look at some of these organs, but first let us consider some properties of lymphoid tissue to see what characteristics these organs have in common.

Some of the general functions of lymphoid tissue include the following:

* Removal of impurities, such as carbon particles, cancer cells, pathogenic organisms, and dead blood cells. These materials are filtered out of body fluids and then destroyed by phagocytes that ingest and destroy foreign matter.
* Processing of lymphocytes, cells of the immune system. Some of these lymphocytes produce antibodies, substances in the blood that aid in combating infection; others attack foreign invaders directly. Lympho-

When Lymph Does Not Flow: Lymphedema

We often take for granted that fluid balance in the body remains within an acceptable range, with fluid appropriately distributed between the cardiovascular system, lymphatic system, and the tissues. When the balance is tipped toward excess fluid in the tissues, a condition known as *edema*, the first suspicion is usually heart failure. However, disturbances in lymphatic fluid flow can easily create a form of edema known as *lymphedema.*

Lymphedema occurs as a buildup of fluid in the subcutaneous tissues, usually in the lower extremities, and is usually present only in one leg (heart failure causes swelling of both extremities). Lymphedema (more common in women) is usually worse during warm weather, before menstruation, and after long periods of standing or sitting. It may occur as primary lymphedema, which is often present at birth and is caused by a lack of development of lymphatic vessels. Secondary lymphedema is caused by trauma to a limb, surgery, or disease processes that either destroy or obstruct lymphatic flow. One of the most common causes of lymphedema is the removal of axillary lymph nodes during mastectomy. Another cause is infection in the lymphatic system itself, known as lymphangitis.

The primary treatment for lymphedema is to elevate the affected limb, firmly wrapping the limb to apply compression. Diuretics may help excess tissue fluid reabsorb into the capillaries rather than lymphatic vessels. Lymphangitis requires the use of appropriate antibiotics.

cytes and the immune system are discussed further in Chapter 17.

Lymph Nodes

The lymph nodes, as we have seen, are designed to filter the lymph once it is drained from the tissues (Fig. 16-5). The lymph nodes are small, rounded masses varying from pinhead size to as long as 2.5 cm (1 inch). Each has a fibrous con-

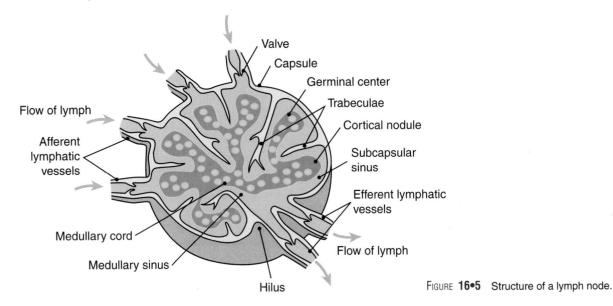

FIGURE **16•5** Structure of a lymph node.

nective tissue capsule from which partitions (trabeculae) extend into the substance of the node. Inside the node are masses of lymphatic tissue, which include lymphocytes and macrophages, white blood cells active in immunity.

At various points in the surface of the node, afferent lymphatic vessels pierce the capsule to carry lymph into the spaces inside the pulplike nodal tissue. An indented area called the *hilus* (HI-lus) serves as the exit for efferent lymphatic vessels carrying lymph out of the node. At this region, other structures, including blood vessels and nerves, connect with the node.

Lymph nodes are seldom isolated. As a rule, they are massed together in groups, the number in each group varying from 2 or 3 to well over 100. Some of these groups are placed deeply, whereas some are superficial. The main groups include the following:

- *Cervical nodes,* located in the neck in deep and superficial groups, drain various parts of the head and neck. They often become enlarged during upper respiratory infections.
- *Axillary nodes,* located in the axillae (armpits), may become enlarged after infections of the upper extremities and the breasts. Cancer cells from the breasts often metastasize (spread) to the axillary nodes.
- *Tracheobronchial* (tra-ke-o-BRONG-ke-al) *nodes* are found near the trachea and

around the larger bronchial tubes. In people living in highly polluted areas, these nodes become so filled with carbon particles that they are solid black masses resembling pieces of coal.
- *Mesenteric* (mes-en-TER-ik) *nodes* are found between the two layers of peritoneum that form the mesentery (membrane around the intestines). There are some 100 to 150 of these nodes.
- *Inguinal nodes,* located in the groin region, receive lymph drainage from the lower extremities and from the external genital organs. When they become enlarged, they are often referred to as *buboes* (BU-bose), from which bubonic plague got its name.

See Cancer and the Lymphatic System.

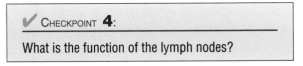

✔ CHECKPOINT **4**:

What is the function of the lymph nodes?

The Tonsils

There are masses of lymphoid tissue that are designed to filter not lymph, but tissue fluid. Found beneath certain areas of moist epithelium that are exposed to the outside, and hence

Cancer and the Lymphatic System

Ordinarily, the lymphatic system is one of our primary defenses against disease. In cancer, however, it can be a vehicle for the spread (metastasis) of disease. Tumor cells that enter the lymphatic vessels can be carried to other parts of the body. In breast cancer, for example, the degree of invasion of nearby lymph nodes is an important factor in diagnosis and treatment. In mastectomies, in addition to removing breast tissue, it is sometimes necessary to remove lymphatic vessels and nodes. This may interfere with normal lymph flow from the arm, resulting in lymphedema and an increased risk of infection. To minimize node removal, surgeons now use radioactive tracers to identify the node that receives lymph from the area of a tumor. Biopsy of this "sentinel node" reveals whether tumor cells are present and helps to determine how many nodes need to be removed and what type of treatment should follow surgery.

to contamination, these masses include parts of the digestive, urinary, and respiratory tracts. Associated with the latter system are those well-known masses of lymphoid tissue called the *tonsils,* which include the following:

- The *palatine* (PAL-ah-tine) *tonsils,* oval bodies located at each side of the soft palate. These are generally meant when one refers to "the tonsils."
- The *pharyngeal* (fah-RIN-je-al) *tonsil,* commonly referred to as the *adenoids* (from a general term that means "gland-like"). It is located behind the nose on the back wall of the upper pharynx.
- The *lingual* (LING-gwal) *tonsils,* little mounds of lymphoid tissue at the back of the tongue.

Any or all of these tonsils may become so loaded with bacteria that the pathogens gain the upper hand; removal then is advisable. A slight enlargement of any of them is not an indication for surgery. All lymphoid tissue masses tend to be larger in childhood, so that the physician must consider the patient's age in determining

whether these masses are enlarged abnormally. Because the tonsils function in immunity during early childhood, efforts are made *not* to remove them unless absolutely necessary.

> ✔ CHECKPOINT **5**:
>
> Tonsils filter tissue fluid. What is the general location of the tonsils?

The Thymus

Because of its appearance under the microscope, the *thymus* (THI-mus), located in the upper thorax beneath the sternum, has been considered part of the lymphoid system. Recent studies, however, suggest that this structure has a much wider function than other lymphoid tissue. It appears that the thymus plays a key role in the development of the immune system before birth and during the first few months of infancy. Certain lymphocytes must mature in the thymus gland before they can perform their functions in the immune system (see Chap. 17). These T cells (T lymphocytes) develop under the effects of the hormone from the thymus gland called *thymosin* (THI-mo-sin), which also promotes the growth and activity of lymphocytes in lymphoid tissue throughout the body. Removal of the thymus causes a decrease in the production of T cells as well as a decrease in the size of the spleen and of lymph nodes throughout the body.

The thymus is most active during early life. After puberty, the tissue undergoes changes; it shrinks in size and is replaced by connective tissue and fat.

> ✔ CHECKPOINT **6**:
>
> What kind of immune system cells develop in the thymus?

The Spleen

The spleen is an organ that contains lymphoid tissue designed to filter blood. It is located in the upper left hypochondriac region of the abdomen, high up under the dome of the diaphragm, and normally is protected by the lower part of the rib cage. The spleen is a soft, purplish, and somewhat flattened organ about 12.5 to 16 cm (5 to 6 inches) long and 5 to 7.5 cm (2 to 3 inches) wide. The capsule of the spleen, as well as its framework, is more elastic than that of the lymph nodes. It contains involuntary muscle, which enables the splenic capsule to contract and also to withstand some swelling.

The spleen has an unusually large blood supply, considering its size. The organ is filled with a soft pulp, one of the functions of which is to filter out worn-out red blood cells. The spleen also harbors phagocytes, which engulf bacteria and other foreign particles. The spleen is classified as part of the lymphatic system because it contains prominent masses of lymphoid tissue. However, it has wider functions than other lymphatic structures, including the following:

- Cleansing the blood by filtration and phagocytosis
- Destroying old, worn-out red blood cells. The iron and other breakdown products of hemoglobin are carried to the liver by the hepatic portal system to be reused or eliminated from the body.
- Producing red blood cells before birth
- Serving as a reservoir for blood, which can be returned to the bloodstream in case of hemorrhage or other emergency

Splenectomy (sple-NEK-to-me), or surgical removal of the spleen, is usually well tolerated. Although the spleen is the largest unit of lymphoid tissue in the body, other lymphoid tissues can take over its functions. The human body has thousands of lymphoid units, and the loss of any one unit or group ordinarily is not a threat to life.

✔ CHECKPOINT **7**:

What is filtered by the spleen?

THE RETICULOENDOTHELIAL SYSTEM

The *reticuloendothelial* (reh-tik-u-lo-en-do-THE-le-al) *system* consists of related cells concerned with the destruction of worn-out blood cells, bacteria, cancer cells, and other foreign substances that are potentially harmful to the body. Included among these cells are monocytes, relatively large white blood cells (see Fig. 13-1 in Chap. 13) that are formed in the bone marrow and then circulate in the bloodstream to various parts of the body. On entering the tissues, monocytes develop into *macrophages* (MAK-ro-faj-ez), a term that means "big eaters."

Some monocytes are given special names; *Kupffer's* (KOOP-ferz) *cells,* for example, are located in the lining of the liver sinusoids (blood channels). Other parts of the reticuloendothelial system are found in the spleen, bone marrow, lymph nodes, and brain. Some macrophages are located in the lungs, where they are called *dust cells* because they ingest solid particles that enter the lungs; others are found in soft connective tissues all over the body.

This widely distributed protective system has been called by several other names, including *tissue macrophage system, mononuclear phagocyte system,* and *monocyte-macrophage system.* These names describe the type of cells found in this system.

DISORDERS OF THE LYMPHATIC SYSTEM AND LYMPHOID TISSUE

Lymphangitis

Lymphangitis (lim-fan-JI-tis), which is inflammation of lymphatic vessels, usually begins in the region of an infected and neglected injury and can be seen as red streaks extending along an extremity. Such inflamed vessels are a sign that bacteria have spread into the lymphatic system. If the lymph nodes are not able to stop the infection, pathogens may enter the bloodstream, causing *septicemia* (sep-tih-SE-me-ah), or blood poisoning. Streptococci often are the invading organisms in such cases.

Lymphadenitis

In *lymphadenitis* (lim-fad-en-I-tis), or inflammation of the lymph nodes, the nodes become enlarged and tender. This condition reflects the body's attempt to combat an infection. Cervical lymphadenitis occurs during measles, scarlet fever, septic sore throat, diphtheria, and, frequently, the common cold. Chronic lymphadenitis may be due to the bacillus that causes tuberculosis. Infections of the upper extremities cause enlarged axillary nodes, as does cancer of the mammary glands. Infections of the external genitals or the lower extremities may cause enlargement of the inguinal lymph nodes.

Lymphadenopathy

Lymphadenopathy (lim-fad-en-OP-ah-the) is a term meaning "disease of the lymph nodes." Enlarged lymph nodes are a common symptom in a number of infectious and cancerous diseases. For example, generalized lymphadenopathy is an early sign of infection with human immunodeficiency virus (HIV), the virus that causes acquired immunodeficiency syndrome (AIDS). *Infectious mononucleosis* (mon-o-nu-kle-O-sis) is an acute viral infection, the hallmark of which is a marked enlargement of the cervical lymph nodes. Mononucleosis is fairly common among college students. Enlarged lymph nodes are commonly referred to as *glands,* as in "swollen glands." However, they do not produce secretions and are not glands.

Splenomegaly

Enlargement of the spleen, known as *splenomegaly* (sple-no-MEG-ah-le), accompanies certain acute infectious diseases, including scarlet fever, typhus fever, typhoid fever, and syphilis. Many tropical parasitic diseases cause splenomegaly. A certain blood fluke (flatworm) that is fairly common among workers in Japan and other parts of Asia causes marked splenic enlargement.

Splenic anemia is characterized by enlargement of the spleen, hemorrhages from the stomach, and accumulation of fluid in the abdomen. In this disease and others of the same nature, splenectomy appears to constitute a cure.

Lymphoma

Lymphoma (lim-FO-mah) is any tumor, benign or malignant, that occurs in lymphoid tissue.

Two examples of malignant lymphoma are described next.

Hodgkin's Disease

Hodgkin's disease is a chronic malignant disorder, most common in young men, that is characterized by enlargement of the lymph nodes. The nodes in the neck particularly, and often those in the armpit, thorax, and groin, enlarge. The spleen may become enlarged as well. Chemotherapy and radiotherapy, either separately or in combination, have been used with good results, affording patients many years of life.

Non-Hodgkin's Lymphoma

Non-Hodgkin's lymphoma is more common than Hodgkin's disease and generally appears in an older age range of adults. This category includes widely varied malignant diseases involving lymphoid tissues. Enlargement of the lymph nodes (lymphadenopathy), especially in the cervical (neck) region, is an early sign in many cases. These disorders are often initially widespread and respond poorly to therapy.

Elephantiasis

As mentioned in Chapter 5, *elephantiasis* is a great enlargement of the lower extremities resulting from blockage of lymphatic vessels by small worms called *filariae* (fi-LA-re-e). These tiny parasites, carried by insects such as flies and mosquitoes, invade the tissues as embryos or immature forms. They then grow in the lymph channels and thus obstruct the flow of lymph. The swelling of the legs or, as sometimes happens in men, the scrotum, may be so great that the victim becomes incapacitated. This disease is especially common in certain parts of Asia and in some of the Pacific islands. No cure is known.

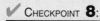

✔ CHECKPOINT **8**:

What is lymphoma and what are two examples of malignant lymphoma?

Summary

I. Lymphatic system
  1. Functions
    a. Drainage of excess fluid and protein from tissues
    b. Filtration of body fluids
    c. Absorption of fats from small intestine
  A. Lymph—fluid in lymphatic system
  B. Lymphatic capillaries—made of endothelium (simple squamous epithelium)
  C. Lymphatic vessels
    a. Superficial
    b. Deep
    c. Right lymphatic duct—drains upper right part of body and empties into right subclavian vein
    d. Thoracic duct—drains remainder of body and empties into left subclavian vein
  D. Movement of lymph
    1. Valves in vessels
    2. Contraction of vessels
    3. Muscle contraction
    4. Breathing

II. Lymphoid tissue—distributed throughout body
  1. General functions
    a. Removal of impurities by filtration and phagocytosis

    b. Processing of lymphocytes of immune system
  A. Lymph nodes—filtration of lymph
  B. Tonsils—filtration of tissue fluid
  C. Thymus
    1. Processing of T lymphocytes (T cells)
    2. Secretion of thymosin—stimulates T lymphocytes in lymphoid tissue
  D. Spleen
    1. Filtration of blood
    2. Destruction of old red cells
    3. Production of red cells before birth
    4. Storage of blood

III. The reticuloendothelial system—cells throughout body that remove impurities

IV. Disorders of the lymphatic system and lymphoid tissue
  A. Lymphangitis—inflammation of lymphatic vessels
  B. Lymphadenitis—inflammation of lymph nodes that occurs during infection
  C. Lymphadenopathy—disease of lymph nodes
  D. Splenomegaly—enlargement of the spleen
  E. Lymphoma—tumor of lymphoid tissue
    1. Hodgkin's disease—chronic malignancy with enlarged lymph nodes
    2. Non-Hodgkin's lymphoma—more common in older adults
  F. Elephantiasis—blockage of lymphatic vessels by parasitic worms

Questions for Study and Review

1. What is lymph? How is it formed?
2. Briefly describe the system of lymph circulation.
3. Describe the lymphatic vessels with respect to structure and location.
4. Name the two main lymphatic ducts. What part of the body does each drain, and into what blood vessel does each empty?
5. Describe two functions of lymphoid tissue
6. What is the cisterna chyli and what are its purposes?
7. Describe the structure of a typical lymph node.

8. Describe the location of the main groups of lymph nodes.
9. Name some conditions that cause enlargement of lymph nodes in specific regions.
10. What are the different tonsils called and where are they located? What is the purpose of these structures?
11. What is the function of the thymus?
12. Give the location of the spleen and name several of its functions.
13. Describe the reticuloendothelial system.
14. What is lymphangitis? lymphadenitis? lymphadenopathy?
15. What is splenomegaly and what can cause it?
16. Describe two forms of lymphoma.
17. Describe elephantiasis and its cause.

✔ ANSWERS TO CHECKPOINTS

1. The lymphatic system drains excess fluid and proteins from the tissues and filters impurities from body fluids.
2. The lymphatic capillaries are more permeable than blood capillaries and begin blindly. They are closed at one end and do not bridge two vessels.
3. The two main lymphatic vessels are the right lymphatic duct and the thoracic duct.
4. The lymph nodes filter lymph.
5. Tonsils are located in the vicinity of the throat (pharynx).
6. T cells of the immune system develop in the thymus.
7. Blood is filtered by the spleen.
8. Lymphoma is any tumor of lymphoid tissue. Two examples of malignant lymphoma are Hodgkin's disease and non-Hodgkin's lymphoma.

16

Body Defenses, Immunity, and Vaccines

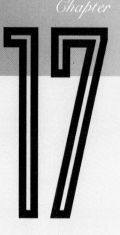

Chapter

17

BEHAVIORAL OBJECTIVES

After careful study of this chapter, you should be able to:

1. List the factors that determine the occurrence of infection

2. Differentiate between nonspecific and specific body defenses and give examples of each

3. Briefly describe the inflammatory reaction

4. List several types of inborn immunity

5. Define *antigen* and *antibody*

6. Compare T cells and B cells with respect to development and type of activity

7. Explain the role of macrophages in immunity

8. Describe the reaction between an antigen and an antibody

9. Differentiate between naturally acquired and artificially acquired immunity

10. Differentiate between active and passive immunity

11. Define the term *vaccine* and give several examples of vaccines

12. Define the term *immune serum* and give several examples of immune sera

13. List several disorders of the immune system

14. Explain the possible role of the immune system in preventing cancer

Chapter 5 presents a rather frightening list of harmful organisms that surround us in our environment. Fortunately, most of us survive contact with these invaders and even become more resistant to disease in the process. The job of protecting us from these harmful agents belongs in part to certain blood cells and to the lymphatic system, which together make up our *immune system.*

The immune system is part of our general body defenses against disease. Some of these defenses are *nonspecific;* that is, they are effective against any harmful agent that enters the body. Other defenses are referred to as *specific;* that is, they act only against a certain agent and no other.

FACTORS IN THE OCCURRENCE OF INFECTION

Although the body is constantly exposed to pathogenic invasion, many conditions determine whether an infection will actually occur. Pathogens have a decided preference for certain body tissues and must have access to these tissues. Some viruses attack only nervous tissue. The poliovirus, for example, may be inhaled or swallowed in large numbers and therefore may be in direct contact with the mucous membranes lining the respiratory and digestive tracts, yet it causes no apparent disorder of these tissues. In contrast, the viruses that cause influenza and the common cold do attack these mucous membranes. HIV, the virus that causes AIDS, attacks a certain type of white blood cell, known as a T cell, which has surface receptors for the virus.

The *portal of entry* is an important condition influencing the occurrence of infection. The respiratory tract is a common entrance route for pathogens. Other important avenues of entry include the digestive system and the tubes that open into the urinary and reproductive systems. Any break in the skin or in a mucous membrane allows organisms such as staphylococci easy access to deeper tissues and may lead to infection, whereas unbroken skin or mucous membrane is usually not affected.

The *virulence* (VIR-u-lens) of an organism, or the power of the organism to overcome the defenses of its host, must also be considered. Virulence has two aspects: one may be thought of as "aggressiveness," or invasive power; the other is the ability of the organism to produce *toxins* (poisons) that damage the body. Different organisms vary in virulence. The virulence of a specific organism also can change; the influenza virus, for example, can be more dangerous in some years than in others. Organisms may gain virulence as they pass from one infected host to another.

The ***dose*** (number) of pathogens that invade the body also has much to do with whether an infection develops. Even if the virulence of a particular organism happens to be low, infection may occur if a large number of them enters the body.

Finally, the condition, or ***predisposition,*** of the individual to infection is also important. Disease organisms are around us all the time. Why does a person only occasionally get a cold, flu, or other infection? Part of the answer lies in the person's condition, as influenced by general physical and emotional health, nutrition, living habits, and age.

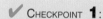

CHECKPOINT **1**:

What are some factors that influence the occurrence of infection?

NONSPECIFIC DEFENSES

The features that protect the body against disease are usually considered as successive "lines of defense," beginning with the relatively simple or outer barriers and proceeding through progressively more complicated responses until the ultimate defense mechanism—immunity—is reached.

Chemical and Mechanical Barriers

Part of the first line of defense against invaders is the skin, which serves as a mechanical barrier as long as it remains intact. A serious danger to burn victims, for example, is the risk of infection as a result of destruction of the skin.

The mucous membranes that line the passageways leading into the body also act as barriers, trapping foreign material in their sticky secretions. The cilia in membranes in the upper respiratory tract help to sweep impurities out of the body.

Body secretions, such as tears, perspiration, and saliva, wash away microorganisms and may contain acids, enzymes, or other chemicals that destroy invaders. Digestive juices destroy many ingested bacteria and their toxins.

Certain reflexes aid in the removal of pathogens. Sneezing and coughing, for instance, tend to remove foreign matter, including microorganisms, from the upper respiratory tract. Vomiting and diarrhea are ways in which toxins and bacteria may be expelled.

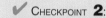

CHECKPOINT **2**:

What tissues constitute the first line of defense against the invasion of pathogens?

Phagocytosis

Phagocytosis is part of the second line of defense against invaders. In the process of phagocytosis, white blood cells take in and destroy waste and foreign material (see Fig. 13-2 in Chap. 13). Neutrophils and macrophages are the main phagocytic white blood cells. Neutrophils are a type of granular leukocyte. Macrophages are derived from monocytes, a type of agranular leukocyte. Both types of cells travel in the blood to sites of infection. Some of the macrophages remain fixed in the tissues, for example, in the skin, liver, lungs, lymphoid tissue, and bone marrow, to fight infection and remove debris.

Natural Killer Cells

The ***natural killer (NK) cell*** is a type of lymphocyte different from those active in immunity, which are described below. NK cells can recognize body cells with abnormal membranes, such as tumor cells and cells infected with virus, and, as their name indicates, can destroy them on contact. NK cells are found in the lymph nodes, spleen, bone marrow, and blood. They destroy abnormal cells by secreting a protein that breaks down the cell membrane, but the way in which they find their targets is not yet completely understood.

Inflammation

Inflammation is the body's effort to get rid of anything that irritates it (or, if this proves impossible, to limit the harmful effects of the irritant). Inflammation can occur as a result of any irritant, not only microorganisms. Friction, fire, chemicals, x-rays, and cuts or blows can all be classed as irritants. If the irritant is due to pathogenic invasion, the resulting inflammation is termed an *infection.* With the entrance of pathogens and their subsequent multiplication, a whole series of defensive processes begins. This *inflammatory reaction* is accompanied by four classic symptoms: heat, redness, swelling, and pain, as described below.

When tissues are injured, *histamine* (HIS-tah-mene) and other substances are released from the damaged cells, causing the small blood vessels to dilate (widen). More blood then flows into the area, resulting in heat, redness, and swelling.

With the increased blood flow come a vast number of leukocytes. Now a new phenomenon occurs: the walls of the tiny blood vessels become "coarsened" in texture (as does a piece of cloth when it is stretched). Blood flow slows down, and the leukocytes move through these altered walls and into the tissue, where they can get at the irritant directly. Fluid from the blood plasma also leaks out of the vessels into the tissues and begins to clot.

When this response occurs in a local area, it helps prevent the spread of the foreign agent. The mixture of leukocytes and fluid, the *inflammatory exudate,* causes pressure on the nerve endings; this, combined with the increased amount of blood in the vessels, causes the pain of inflammation.

As the phagocytes do their work, large numbers of them are destroyed, so that eventually the area becomes filled with dead leukocytes. The mixture of exudate, living and dead white blood cells, pathogens, and destroyed tissue cells is *pus.*

Meanwhile, the lymphatic vessels begin to drain fluid from the inflamed area and carry it toward the lymph nodes for filtration. The regional lymph nodes become enlarged and tender, a sign that they are performing their protective function by working overtime to produce phagocytic cells that "clean" the lymph flowing through them.

Fever

An increase in body temperature above the normal range can be a sign that body defenses are at work. When phagocytes are exposed to infecting organisms, they release substances that act to raise body temperature. Fever boosts the immune system in several ways. It stimulates phagocytes, increases metabolism, and decreases the ability of certain organisms to multiply.

Advertisers would have the public believe that fever is a dangerous symptom that should always be eliminated. Control of fever in itself does little to alter the course of an illness. The health care worker should, however, always be alert to the development of fever as a possible sign of a serious disorder and should recognize that an increased metabolic rate may have adverse effects on the heart of a weak person or an elderly ill person.

Interferon

Cells infected with viruses and certain other agents produce a substance that prevents the infection of other cells. This substance was first found in cells infected with influenza virus, and it was called *interferon* because it "interferes" with multiplication of the virus. Interferon, now known to be a group of substances, is also of interest because it nonspecifically stimulates the immune system. It has been used with varying success to boost the immune system in the treatment of malignancies and infections.

The remainder of this chapter is devoted to the immune system, our specific defense against disease.

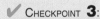 CHECKPOINT **3**:

What are some nonspecific factors that help to control infection?

IMMUNITY

Immunity is the final line of defense against disease. Immunity can be defined as "the power of an individual to resist or overcome the effects of a particular disease or other harmful agent." Immunity is a selective process; that is, immunity to one disease does not necessarily cause immunity to another. This selective characteristic is called **specificity** (spes-ih-FIS-ih-te).

There are two main categories of immunity:

- **Inborn immunity** is inherited along with other characteristics in a person's genes.
- **Acquired immunity** develops after birth. Acquired immunity may be obtained by **natural** or **artificial** means; in addition, acquired immunity may be either **active** or **passive.**

Figure 17-1 is a summary of the different types of immunity. Refer to this diagram as we investigate each category in turn.

Inborn Immunity

Both humans and animals have what is called a **species immunity** to many of each other's diseases. Although certain diseases found in animals may be transmitted to humans, many infections, such as chicken cholera, hog cholera, distemper, and other animal diseases, do not affect human beings. However, the constitutional differences that make human beings immune to these disorders also make them susceptible to others that do not affect the lower animals. Such infections as measles, scarlet fever, diphtheria, and influenza do not appear to affect animals in contact with humans who have these illnesses.

Another form of inborn immunity is **population immunity.** Some groups appear to have a greater inborn immunity to certain diseases than others. Although measles, for example, is generally a mild disease in Europeans, it became a serious and often fatal disease among people of the Pacific Islands when foreigners

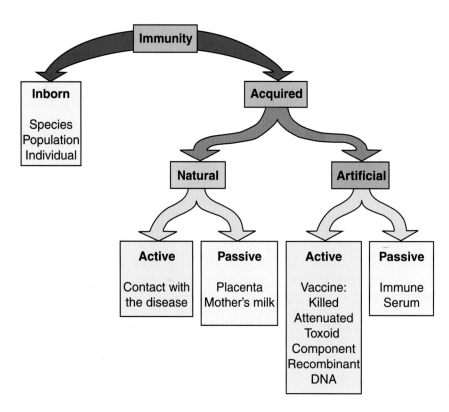

FIGURE **17•1** Types of immunity.

brought it there. These populations had never been exposed to the measles virus and had not developed genetic resistance to the disease over time. When poliomyelitis was a public health threat in the United States, American blacks were apparently more resistant to the disease than whites. Some populations are more resistant to malaria and yellow fever than others.

Of course, it is often difficult to tell how much of this variation in resistance to infection is due to environment and how much is due to inborn traits of the various groups.

Some members of a given group have a more highly developed *individual immunity* to specific diseases. For example, some people are prone to cold sores (fever blisters) caused by herpes virus, whereas others have never experienced this type of infection. Newspapers and magazines sometimes feature the advice of an elderly person who is asked to give her secret for living to a ripe old age. One elderly person may say that he practiced temperance and lived a carefully regulated life with the right amount of rest, exercise, and work, whereas the next may boast of her use of alcoholic beverages, constant smoking, lack of exercise, and other kinds of reputedly unhealthy behavior. However, it is possible that the latter person had lived through the onslaughts of toxins and disease organisms, resisted infection, and maintained health despite her habits, rather than because of them, thanks to the resistance factors and immunity to disease she inherited.

✔ CHECKPOINT **4**:

What are some types of inborn immunity?

Acquired Immunity

Unlike inborn immunity, which is due to inherited factors, acquired immunity develops during a person's lifetime as that person encounters various specific harmful agents.

If the following description of the immune system seems complex, bear in mind that from infancy on, your immune system is able to protect you from millions of foreign substances, even synthetic compounds and substances not found in nature. All the while, the system is kept in check, so that it does not usually overreact to produce allergies or mistakenly attack and damage your own body tissues.

Antigens
An *antigen* (AN-te-jen) *(Ag)* is any foreign substance that enters the body and induces an immune response. Most antigens are large protein molecules, but carbohydrates and some lipids may act as antigens. Antigens may be found on the surface of pathogenic organisms, on the surface of red blood cells and tissue cells, on pollens, in toxins, and in foods. The critical feature of any substance described as an antigen is that it stimulates the activity of certain lymphocytes classified as T or B cells.

T Cells
Both T and B cells come from stem cells in bone marrow, as do all blood cells. They differ, however, in their development and their method of action. Some of the immature stem cells migrate to the thymus gland and become T cells, which constitute about 80% of the lymphocytes in the circulating blood. While in the thymus, these T lymphocytes multiply and become capable of combining with specific foreign antigens, at which time they are described as *sensitized.* These thymus-derived cells produce an immunity that is said to be *cell-mediated immunity.*

There are several types of T cells, each with different functions. Some of these functions and the T cell type involved in each are as follows:

- To destroy foreign cells directly. These are the *cytotoxic T cells.*
- To release substances known as *interleukins* (in-ter-LU-kinz) that stimulate other lymphocytes and macrophages and thereby assist in the destruction of foreign cells. There are several subtypes of these *helper T cells,* one of which is infected and destroyed by the AIDS virus (HIV). These targeted cells have a special surface receptor (CD_4) to which the virus attaches.
- To suppress the immune response in order to regulate it. These *suppressor T cells* may inhibit or destroy active lymphocytes.
- To remember an antigen and start a rapid

response if that antigen is met again. These are *memory T cells.*

The T cell portion of the immune system is generally responsible for defense against cancer cells, certain viruses, and other pathogens that grow within cells (intracellular parasites), as well as for the rejection of tissue transplanted from another person.

The Role of Macrophages

Macrophages are phagocytic white blood cells derived from monocytes (their name means "big eater"). They ingest foreign proteins, such as disease organisms, and break them down. For a T cell to react with an antigen, that antigen must be presented to the T cell on the surface of a macrophage in combination with proteins that the T cell can recognize as belonging to the "self" (Fig. 17-2). Self antigens are known as MHC (major histocompatibility complex) antigens because of their importance in cross-matching for tissue transplantation. They are also known as HLAs (human leukocyte antigens) because white blood cells are used in testing tissues for compatibility. Macrophages and other cells that present antigens to T cells are known as APCs (antigen-presenting cells).

After combining with T cells, the macrophages also release interleukins (the name means "between white blood cells"). These substances stimulate the growth of T cells and have been used medically in efforts to boost the immune system.

✔ CHECKPOINT **5**:
_____

What is the difference between inborn and acquired immunity?

✔ CHECKPOINT **6**:
_____

What is an antigen?

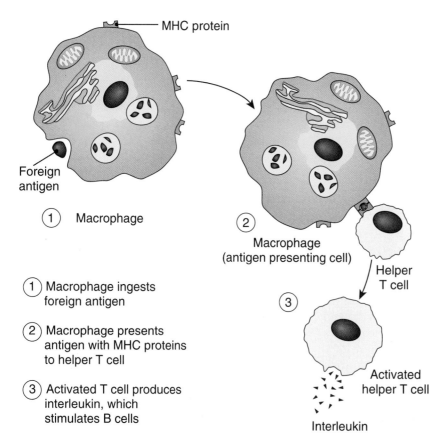

— MHC protein

Foreign antigen

① Macrophage

② Macrophage (antigen presenting cell)

Helper T cell

③

Activated helper T cell

Interleukin

① Macrophage ingests foreign antigen

② Macrophage presents antigen with MHC proteins to helper T cell

③ Activated T cell produces interleukin, which stimulates B cells

FIGURE **17•2** Activation of a helper T cell by a macrophage.

B Cells and Antibodies

An ***antibody (Ab),*** also known as an ***immunoglobulin (Ig),*** is a substance produced in response to an antigen. Antibodies are manufactured by ***B cells*** (B lymphocytes), another type of lymphocyte active in the immune system. These cells must mature in the fetal liver or in lymphoid tissue before becoming active in the blood.

B cells have surface receptors that bind with a specific type of antigen (Fig. 17-3). Exposure to the antigen stimulates the cells to multiply rapidly and produce large numbers (clones) of ***plasma cells***. Plasma cells produce antibodies against the original antigen and release these antibodies into the blood, providing the form of immunity described as ***humoral immunity*** (the term humoral refers to body fluids) (see Antibodies).

Humoral immunity generally protects against circulating antigens and bacteria that grow outside the cells (extracellular parasites). All antibodies are contained in a portion of the blood plasma called the ***gamma globulin*** fraction.

Some antibodies produced by B cells remain in the blood to give long-term immunity. In addition, some of the activated B cells do not become plasma cells but, like certain T cells, become memory cells. On repeated contact with

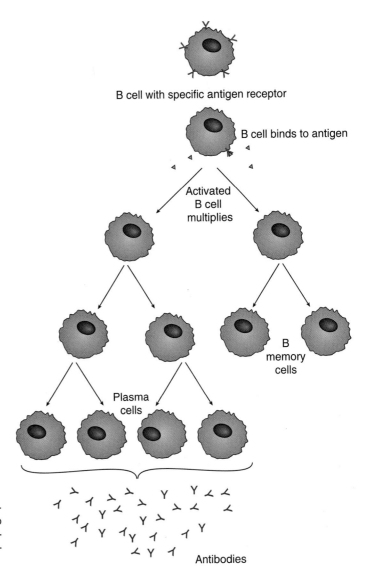

B cell with specific antigen receptor

B cell binds to antigen

Activated
B cell
multiplies

B
memory
cells

Plasma
cells

Antibodies

FIGURE **17•3**   Activation of B cells. The B cell combines with a specific antigen. The cell divides to form plasma cells, which produce antibodies. Memory cells are also formed; these protect against reinfection.

Antibodies

Antibodies are substances produced in response to specific antigens. They are all contained in a fraction of the blood plasma known as *gamma globulin.* Because the plasma contains other globulins as well, antibodies have become known as *immunoglobulins (Ig).* Immunologic studies have shown that there are several classes of immunoglobulins that vary in molecular size and in function. Studies of these antibody fractions can be of help in diagnosis. For example, high levels of IgM antibodies, because they are the first to be produced in an immune response, indicate a recent infection. Briefly described, these classes are as follows:

IMMUNO-GLOBULIN	PERCENTAGE OF ANTIBODIES	FUNCTION
IgG	75	Protect against bacteria and viruses; the only antibodies that can pass through the placenta
IgA	15	Local protection in mucous membranes
IgM	5–10	The first antibodies to be secreted after infection
IgD	<1	Help to activate B cells
IgE	<0.1	Active in allergic reactions and parasitic infections

an antigen, these cells are ready to produce antibodies immediately. Because of this "immunologic memory," one is usually immune to a childhood disease after having it.

✔ CHECKPOINT **7**:

Immunity is based on the actions of two types of lymphocytes. What are these two types of cells called?

The Antigen–Antibody Reaction

The antibody that is produced in response to a specific antigen, such as a bacterial cell or a toxin, has a shape that matches some part of that antigen, much in the same way that the shape of a key matches the shape of its lock. The antibody can bind specifically to the antigen that caused its production and thereby destroy or inactivate it. In the laboratory, this can be seen as a settling (precipitation) or a clumping (agglutination) of the antigen–antibody combination, as is seen in the typing of red blood cells.

Complement

The destruction of foreign cells sometimes requires the enzymatic activity of a group of nonspecific proteins in the blood, together called *complement.* Complement proteins boost immunity by lysing (destroying) organisms that have been coated with antibody. They can also attract and activate phagocytes.

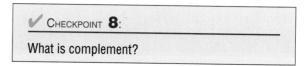

✔ CHECKPOINT **8**:

What is complement?

Naturally Acquired Immunity

Active

Immunity may be acquired naturally through contact with a specific disease organism. In this case, antibodies manufactured by the infected person's cells act against the infecting agent or its toxins. The infection that calls forth the immunity may be a subclinical or inapparent infection that is so mild as to cause no symptoms. Nevertheless, it stimulates the host's cells to produce an active immunity.

Each time a person is invaded by disease organisms, his or her cells manufacture antibodies that provide immunity against the infection. Such immunity may last for years and in some cases lasts for life. Because the host is actively involved in the production of antibodies, this type of immunity is called *active immunity.*

See Stress and the Immune System.

Stress and the Immune System

The effects of stress on the immune system may be the most wide ranging and significant of its many effects on the body. Stressors such as trauma, infection, debilitating disease, surgery, pain, extreme environmental conditions, and emotional distress all have significant effects on the immune system's ability to function fully and correctly.

The predominant effects of stress on the immune system are caused by an increase in the hormone cortisol, which is secreted in response to ACTH from the anterior pituitary. This increase parallels the release of norepinephrine and epinephrine from the sympathetic nervous system. The combined effect of these secretions is to increase the total number of white blood cells in circulation. The increase, however, occurs primarily in neutrophils, while eosinophils and basophils are reduced. In addition, lymphocyte maturation in the lymph nodes is halted since epinephrine decreases blood flow to the nodes in favor of flow to the heart, lungs, brain and muscles. Cortisol also reduces production of interleukins and antibodies, affecting both cellular and humoral immunity. These changes leave the body less capable of fighting off the effects of injury and disease, and, indeed, stress itself.

The increase in cortisol levels, initiated by stress, is an integral part of one's immediate ability to fight off a life-or-death stressor. Continued stress, however, even at low levels, leads to accumulated decreases in immune function.

Passive

Immunity also may be acquired naturally by the passage of antibodies from a mother to her fetus through the placenta. Because these antibodies come from an outside source, this type of immunity is called *passive immunity.* The antibodies obtained in this way do not last as long as actively produced antibodies, but they do help protect the infant for about 6 months, at which time the child's own immune system begins to function. Nursing an infant can lengthen this period of protection owing to the presence of specific antibodies in breast milk and colostrum (the first breast secretion). These are the only known examples of naturally acquired passive immunity.

✓ CHECKPOINT **9**:

What is the difference between the active and passive forms of naturally acquired immunity?

Artificially Acquired Immunity

Active Immunization

A person who has not been exposed to repeated small doses of a particular organism has no antibodies against that organism and is defenseless against a heavy infection. Therefore, artificial measures may be taken to cause a person's tissues to manufacture antibodies. The administration of virulent pathogens obviously would be dangerous. Instead, the harmful agent is treated to reduce its virulence and then administered. In this way, the immune system is made to produce antibodies without causing a serious illness. This protective process is known as *vaccination* (vak-sin-A-shun), or *immunization,* and the solution used is called a *vaccine* (vak-SENE). Ordinarily, the administration of a vaccine is a preventive measure designed to provide protection in anticipation of invasion by a certain disease organism.

Types of Vaccines

Vaccines can be made with live organisms or with organisms killed by heat or chemicals. If live organisms are used, they must be nonvirulent for humans, such as the cowpox virus used for smallpox immunization, or they must be treated in the laboratory to weaken them as human pathogens. An organism weakened for use in vaccines is described as *attenuated.* In some cases, just an antigenic component of the pathogen is used as a vaccine. Another type of vaccine is made from a form of the toxin produced by a disease organism. The toxin is altered with heat or chemicals to reduce its harmfulness, but it can still function as an antigen to induce immunity. Such an altered toxin is called a *toxoid.*

The newest types of vaccines are produced from antigenic components of pathogens or by genetic engineering. By techniques of **recombinant DNA,** the genes for specific disease antigens are inserted into the genetic material of harmless organisms. The antigens produced by these organisms are extracted and purified and used for immunization. The hepatitis B vaccine is produced in this manner.

Examples of Vaccines

Originally, the word *vaccination* meant inoculation against smallpox. (The term even comes from the Latin word for *cow,* referring to cowpox, which is used to vaccinate against smallpox.) According to the World Health Organization, however, smallpox has now been eliminated as a result of widespread immunization programs. Mandatory vaccination has been discontinued because the chance of adverse side effects from the vaccine is thought to be greater than the probability of contraction of the disease.

Because of the seriousness of whooping cough in young infants, early inoculation with whooping cough, or **pertussis** (per-TUS-is), vaccine, is recommended. A new form of the vaccine containing pertussis toxoid causes fewer adverse reactions than older types that contained heat-killed organisms. This acellular (aP) vaccine usually is given in a mixture with diphtheria toxoid and tetanus toxoid. The combination, referred to as *DTaP,* may be given as early as the second month of life and should be followed by additional injections at 4, 6, and 15 months and again when the child enters day care, a school, or any other environment in which he or she might be exposed to one of these contagious diseases.

Routine inoculation against *Haemophilus influenzae* type B (Hib) has nearly eliminated the life-threatening meningitis caused by this organism among preschool children. Hib also causes pneumonia and recurrent ear infections in young children.

Viral Vaccines

Intensive research on viruses has resulted in the development of vaccines for an increasing number of viral diseases. Spectacular results in eliminating poliomyelitis have been obtained by the use of vaccines. The first of these vaccines was made with killed poliovirus (Salk vaccine). A more convenient oral vaccine (Sabin vaccine) made with live attenuated virus was then developed. Both types of vaccines are presently used in immunization programs.

MMR, made with live attenuated viruses, protects against measles (rubeola), mumps, and rubella (German measles). Rubella is a very mild disease, but it causes birth defects in a developing fetus (see Table 3 in Appendix 4).

Infants are now routinely immunized against hepatitis B, receiving the first of three shots just after birth and two more before the age of 18 months. A vaccine against hepatitis A virus has been approved and is recommended for travelers and others at high risk for infection.

A vaccine against chicken pox (varicella) has been available since 1995. Children who have not had the disease by 1 year of age should be vaccinated. Although chicken pox is usually a mild disease, infection in pregnant women can cause congenital malformation of the fetus. Because varicella is the same virus that causes shingles, vaccination may prevent this late life sequel.

A number of vaccines have been developed against influenza, which is caused by a variety of different strains of the virus. A new vaccine is produced each year against what is hoped to be the most common strains in the population.

Rotavirus causes an intestinal infection that may result in severe diarrhea among preschool children. An oral vaccine against rotavirus is available for early immunization.

The rabies vaccine is an exception to the rule that a vaccine should be given before the invasion of the disease organism. Rabies is a viral disease transmitted by the bite of wild animals such as raccoons, bats, foxes, and skunks. Mandatory vaccination of domestic animals has practically eliminated this source of rabies in some countries, including the United States, but worldwide, a variety of wild and domestic animals are host to the virus. There is no cure for rabies; it is fatal in nearly all cases. The disease develops so slowly, however, that affected people vaccinated after transmission of the organism still have time to develop an active immunity. The vaccine may be given preventively to people who work with animals.

Boosters

A final word about the long-term efficacy of vaccines: in many cases, an active immunity acquired by artificial (or even natural) means does not last a lifetime. Circulating antibodies can decline with time. To help maintain a high titer (level) of antibodies in the blood, repeated inoculations, called *booster shots,* are administered at intervals. The number of booster injections recommended varies with the disease and with the environment or range of exposure of the individual.

The successful completion of childhood immunizations can be a public health concern. States have different requirements for preschool immunizations and for vaccinations and boosters for older children. On occasion, epidemics in high schools or colleges may prompt recommendations for specific boosters.

> ✔ CHECKPOINT **10**:
> What are some bacterial diseases for which there are vaccines?

> ✔ CHECKPOINT **11**:
> What are some viral diseases for which there are vaccines?

Passive Immunization

It takes several weeks to produce a naturally acquired active immunity and even longer to produce an artificial active immunity through the administration of a vaccine. Therefore, a person who receives a large dose of virulent organisms and has no established immunity to them is in great danger. To prevent illness, the person must quickly receive a counteracting dose of borrowed antibodies. This is accomplished through the administration of an *immune serum,* or *antiserum.* The "ready-made" serum gives short-lived but effective protection against the invaders in the form of an artificially acquired passive immunity. Immune sera

are used in emergencies, that is, in situations in which there is no time to wait until an active immunity has developed.

Preparation of Antisera

Sera prepared for immune purposes are often derived from animals, mainly horses. It has been found that the tissues of the horse produce large quantities of antibodies in response to the injection of organisms or their toxins. After repeated injections, the horse is bled according to careful sterile technique; because of the size of the animal, it is possible to remove large quantities of blood without causing injury. The blood is allowed to clot, and the serum is removed and packaged in sterile containers.

Injecting humans with serum derived from animals is not without its problems. The foreign proteins in animal sera may cause an often serious sensitivity reaction, called *serum sickness.* To avoid this problem, human antibody in the form of gamma globulin may be used.

> ✔ CHECKPOINT **12**:
> What is an immune serum and when are immune sera used?

Examples of Antisera

Some immune sera contain antibodies, known as *antitoxins,* that neutralize toxins but have no effect on the toxic organisms themselves. Certain antibodies act directly on pathogens, engulfing and destroying them or preventing their continued reproduction. Some antisera are obtained from animal sources, others from human sources. Examples of immune sera are:

- Diphtheria antitoxin, obtained from immunized horses
- Tetanus immune globulin, effective in preventing lockjaw (tetanus), which is often a complication of neglected wounds. Because tetanus immune globulin is of human origin, there is decreased chance of adverse reactions with it than with sera obtained from horses.
- Immune globulin (human) is given to peo-

ple exposed to hepatitis A, measles, polio, or chicken pox. It is also given on a regular basis to people with congenital (present at birth) immune deficiencies.

- Hepatitis B immune globulin, used after hepatitis B exposure, is given principally to infants born to mothers who have hepatitis.
- The immune globulin Rh$_o$(D) (trade name RhoGAM), a concentrated human antibody given to prevent the formation of Rh antibodies by an Rh-negative mother. It is given during pregnancy with, and after the birth of, an Rh-positive infant (or even after a miscarriage of a presumably Rh-positive fetus) (see Chap. 13). It is also given when Rh transfusion incompatibilities occur.
- Anti–snake bite sera, or *antivenins* (an-te-VEN-ins), used to combat the effects of bites of certain poisonous snakes
- Botulism antitoxin, from horses, an antiserum that offers the best hope for botulism victims, although only if given early
- Rabies antiserum, from humans or horses, used with vaccine to treat victims of bites of rabid animals

DISORDERS OF THE IMMUNE SYSTEM

Allergy

Allergy involves antigens and antibodies, and its chemical processes are much like those of immunity. Allergy—a broader term for which is *hypersensitivity*—can be defined informally as a tendency to react unfavorably to the presence of certain substances that are normally harmless to most people.

These reaction-producing substances are called *allergens* (AL-er-jens), and like most antigens, they are usually proteins. Examples of typical allergens are pollens, house dust, horse dander (*dander* is the term for the minute scales that are found on hairs and feathers), and certain food proteins.

When the tissues of a susceptible person are repeatedly exposed to an allergen—for example, exposure of the nasal mucosa to pollens—those tissues become *sensitized;* that is, antibodies are produced in them. When the next invasion

of the allergen occurs, there is an antigen–antibody reaction. Normally, this type of reaction takes place in the blood without harm, as in immunity. In allergy, however, the antigen–antibody reaction takes place within the cells of the sensitized tissues, with results that are disagreeable and sometimes dangerous. In the case of the nasal mucosa that has become sensitized to pollen, the allergic manifestation is *hay fever,* with symptoms much like those of the common cold. Many drugs can bring about the allergic state, particularly aspirin, barbiturates, and antibiotics (especially penicillin).

Serum sickness is an example of an allergic manifestation that may occur in response to various sera. People who are allergic to the proteins in serum derived from the horse or some other animal show such symptoms as fever, vomiting, joint pain, enlargement of the regional lymph nodes, and hives, or *urticaria* (ur-tih-KA-re-ah). This type of allergic reaction can be severe but is rarely fatal.

The antigen–antibody reaction in sensitive individuals may cause the release of excessive amounts of histamine. The histamine causes dilation and leaking from capillaries as well as contraction of involuntary muscles (*e.g.*, in the bronchi). A group of drugs called *antihistamines* is effective in treating the symptoms of certain allergies. Sometimes, it is possible to desensitize an allergic person by means of repeated injections of the offending allergen at short intervals. Unfortunately, this form of protection does not last long.

Autoimmunity

The term *autoimmunity* refers to an abnormal reactivity to one's own tissues. In autoimmunity, the immune system reacts to the body's own cells, described as "self," as if they were foreign substances, or "nonself." Normally, the immune system learns before birth to ignore (tolerate) the body's own tissues by eliminating or inactivating those lymphocytes that will attack them. The loss of this immune tolerance may be a cause of rheumatoid arthritis, multiple sclerosis, lupus erythematosus, Graves' disease, glomerulonephritis, and juvenile diabetes, among others.

Immune Deficiency Diseases

An immune deficiency is some failure of the immune system. This failure may involve any part of the system, such as T cells, B cells, or the thymus gland, and it may vary in severity. Such disorders may be congenital (present at birth) or may be acquired as a result of malnutrition, infection, or treatment with x-rays or certain drugs.

The disease **AIDS (acquired immunodeficiency syndrome)** is a devastating example of an infection that attacks the immune system. It is caused by **HIV (human immunodeficiency virus),** which destroys the specific helper T cells that have a receptor (CD_4) for the virus. The disease appeared in the United States in the early 1980s among homosexual men and intravenous drug abusers, but it has now spread to heterosexual populations of all ages. It is spread through unprotected sexual activity and the use of contaminated needles and can also be transmitted from a mother to her fetus. The testing of donated blood has eliminated the spread of AIDS through blood transfusions.

Patients with AIDS succumb easily to disease, including rare diseases such as parasitic (*Pneumocystis carinii*) pneumonia and an especially malignant skin cancer, **Kaposi's** (KAP-o-seze) **sarcoma**.

Drugs active against HIV stop growth of the virus at different stages of replication (see Retroviruses). These drugs, often used in combination, can slow the progress of AIDS, but so far, do not cure it. An obstacle to the development of a vaccine against HIV is the tremendous variability of the virus.

✔ CHECKPOINT **13**:

What are some disorders of the immune system?

THE IMMUNE SYSTEM AND CANCER

Cancer cells differ slightly from normal body cells and therefore should be recognized as "nonself" by the immune system. The fact that

Retroviruses

HIV, the virus that causes AIDS, belongs to a group of viruses that is unique in its method of reproduction. Their name, *retroviruses,* means "backward viruses" because they reverse the common order of genetic action. Retroviruses have RNA instead of DNA as their genetic material. Unlike other RNA viruses, however, they transcribe (copy) the RNA into DNA to reproduce inside the host cell. To accomplish this unusual feat, the virus has an enzyme called *reverse transcriptase.*

The DNA formed using reverse transcriptase enters the nucleus of the host cell and becomes part of the cell's genetic material. Here, it may direct the formation of more viruses or lie dormant and undetected for long periods, even years, before being triggered to multiply and cause disease. Some retroviruses can transform the DNA of the host cell and produce cancer. These viruses have been identified with leukemia in both humans and animals and with other types of tumors in animals.

One type of drug used against retroviruses, AZT for example, acts by inhibiting reverse transcriptase and interrupting the replication cycle of the virus.

people with AIDS and other immune deficiencies develop cancer at a higher than normal rate suggests that this is so. Cancer cells probably form continuously in the body but normally are destroyed by NK cells and the immune system, a process called **immune surveillance** (sur-VAY-lans). As a person ages, cell-mediated immunity declines and cancer is more likely to develop.

Some efforts are being made to treat cancer by stimulating the patient's immune system, a practice called **immunotherapy.** In one approach, T cells have been removed from the patient, activated with interleukin, and then reinjected. This method has given some positive results, especially in treatment of melanoma, a highly malignant form of skin cancer. In the future, a vaccine against cancer may become a reality. Vaccines that target specific proteins produced by cancer cells have already been tested in a few forms of cancer.

17

TRANSPLANTATION AND THE REJECTION SYNDROME

Transplantation is the grafting to a recipient of an organ or tissue from an animal or other human to replace an injured or incompetent part of the body. Much experimental work preceded transplantation surgery in humans. Transplantation by grafting of bone marrow, lymphoid tissue, skin, corneas, parathyroid glands, ovaries, kidneys, lungs, heart, liver, and uterus are among those that have been attempted.

The natural tendency of every organism to destroy foreign substances, including tissues from another person or any other animal, has been the most formidable obstacle to complete success. This normal antigen–antibody reaction has, in this case, been called the ***rejection syndrome.***

In all cases of transplantation or grafting, the tissues of the donor, the person donating the part, should be typed in much the same way that blood is typed when a transfusion is given. Blood type antigens are much fewer in number than tissue antigens; thus, the process of obtaining matching blood is much less involved than is the process of obtaining matching tissues. Tissue typing is being done in a number of laboratories, and an effort is being made to obtain donors whose tissues contain relatively few antigens that might cause transplant rejection in a recipient (the person receiving the part).

Because it is impossible to match all the antigens of a donor with those of the recipient, drugs that suppress the immune reaction to the transplanted tissue are given to the recipient. As you must now realize, these drugs also leave the patient unprotected from infection. Because T cells cause much of the reaction against the foreign material in transplants, efforts are being made, using drugs and antibodies, to suppress the action of these lymphocytes without damaging the B cells. B cells produce circulating antibodies and are most important in preventing infections. Success with transplantation will increase when methods are found to suppress selectively the immune attack on transplants without destroying the recipient's ability to combat disease.

> ✓ CHECKPOINT **14**:
>
> What is the greatest obstacle to transplantation of tissues from one individual to another?

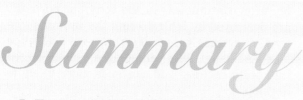

Summary

I. Factors in the occurrence of infection
1. Tissue preference of pathogen
2. Portal of entry of pathogen
3. Virulence of pathogen
   a. Invasive power
   b. Production of toxins (poisons)
4. Dose (number) of pathogens
5. Predisposition of host

II. Nonspecific defenses
  A. Chemical and mechanical barriers
    1. Skin
    2. Mucous membranes
    3. Body secretions
    4. Reflexes—coughing, sneezing
  B. Phagocytosis—mainly by neutrophils and macrophages
  C. Natural killer (NK) cells—attack tumor cells and virus-infected cells
  D. Inflammation
  E. Fever
  F. Interferon—substances released from virus-infected cells that prevent infection of other cells and stimulate the immune response

III. Immunity—specific defense against disease
  A. Inborn immunity—inherited

1. Types: species, population, individual
B. Acquired immunity—develops after birth
  1. Antigens—stimulate lymphocyte activity
  2. Antibodies—inactivate pathogens or neutralize toxins
  3. T cells (T lymphocytes)
    a. Processed in thymus
    b. Types: cytotoxic, helper, suppressor, memory
    c. Helper T cells produce interleukins (immune stimulants)
    d. Involved in cell-mediated immunity
  4. Macrophages
    a. Derived from monocytes
    b. Present antigen to T cells in combination with MHC ("self") proteins
  5. B cells (B lymphocytes)
    a. Mature in lymphoid tissue
    b. Develop into plasma cells that produce circulating antibodies
    c. Also develop into memory cells
    d. Involved in humoral immunity
C. The antigen–antibody reaction
  1. Shape of antibody matches shape of antigen
  2. Complement—group of proteins
    a. Aids in destroying foreign cells
    b. Boosts immune response
D. Naturally acquired immunity
  1. Active—acquired through contact with the disease

2. Passive—acquired from antibodies obtained through placenta and mother's milk
E. Artificially acquired immunity
  1. Active—immunization with vaccines
    a. Types: live (attenuated), killed, toxoid, recombinant DNA
    b. Boosters—keep antibody titers high
  2. Passive—administration of immune serum (antiserum)

IV. Disorders of the immune system
  A. Allergy—hypersensitivity to normally harmless substances (allergens)
  B. Autoimmunity—abnormal response to body's own tissues
  C. Immune deficiency disease—failure in the immune system
    1. Congenital (present at birth)
    2. Acquired (*e.g.*, AIDS)

V. The immune system and cancer
  1. Immune surveillance—ability of immune system to find and destroy abnormal cells (*e.g.*, cancer cells)
  2. Immunotherapy—stimulating the immune system to treat cancer

VII. Transplantation
  1. Grafting of an organ or tissue to replace injured or incompetent part
  2. Requirements
    a. Tissue typing
    b. Suppression of immune system

17

Questions for Study and Review

1. Name five conditions that determine whether an infection will occur in the body.
2. What is meant by a *nonspecific defense*? Give several examples.
3. Define *phagocytosis*. Name cells active in phagocytosis.
4. Describe the process of inflammation.
5. Define *immunity.*
6. Give three examples of inborn immunity.
7. What is the difference between inborn and acquired immunity?

8. Define *antigen* and *antibody*. Why is the reaction between and antigen and antibody described as specific?
9. How do T and B cells differ? In what ways are they the same?
10. Name four types of T cells and briefly describe the function of each type.
11. What is the role of macrophages in immunity?
12. Define: *interferon, complement, interleukin.*
13. Compare active and passive immunity.
14. What is a vaccine? a toxoid? Give examples of each. What is a booster shot?
15. What is an immune serum? Give examples. Define *antitoxin.*
16. Name two sources of antisera. Why is one sometimes used in preference to another?
17. Define *allergy.* How is the process of allergy like that of immunity, and how do they differ?
18. What is an allergen? Give some examples.
19. Name and describe some typical allergic disorders.
20. What does *autoimmunity* mean? Name four disorders caused by autoimmunity.
21. What does *AIDS* stand for? Name the virus that causes AIDS.
22. What role does the immune system play in preventing cancer?
23. What is meant by *rejection syndrome,* and what is being done to offset this syndrome?

✔ ANSWERS TO CHECKPOINTS

1. Factors that influence the occurrence of infection include access to preferred body tissues, the portal of entry, virulence, dose, and the predisposition of the individual to infection.
2. The unbroken skin and mucous membranes constitute the first line of defense against the invasion of pathogens.
3. Some nonspecific factors that help to control infection are chemical and mechanical barriers, phagocytosis, natural killer cells, inflammation, fever, and interferon.
4. Some types of inborn immunity are species, population, and individual immunity.
5. Inborn immunity is inherited in a person's genetic material; acquired immunity develops during an individual's lifetime.
6. An antigen is any foreign substance, usually a protein, that induces an immune response.
7. The cells active in immunity are T cells and B cells.
8. Complement is a group of proteins in the blood that sometimes is required for the destruction of foreign cells.
9. The active form of naturally acquired immunity comes from contact with a disease organism; the passive form comes from the passage of antibodies from a mother to her fetus through the placenta or breast milk.
10. Bacterial diseases for which there are vaccines include smallpox, whooping cough (pertussis), diphtheria, tetanus, and *Haemophilus influenzae* type b (Hib).
11. Viral diseases for which there are vaccines include polio, measles (rubeola), mumps, rubella (German measles), hepatitis A and B, chicken pox (varicella), and rabies.
12. An immune serum is an antiserum prepared in an animal; immune sera can be used in emergencies to provide passive immunization.
13. Disorders of the immune system include allergy, autoimmunity, and immune deficiency diseases.
14. The tendency of every organism to destroy foreign substances is the greatest obstacle to transplantation of tissues from one individual to another.

17

It is the purpose of the five chapters of this unit to show how oxygen and nutrients are processed, taken up by the body fluids, and used by the cells to yield energy. This unit also describes how the stability of body functions (homeostasis) is maintained and how waste products are eliminated.

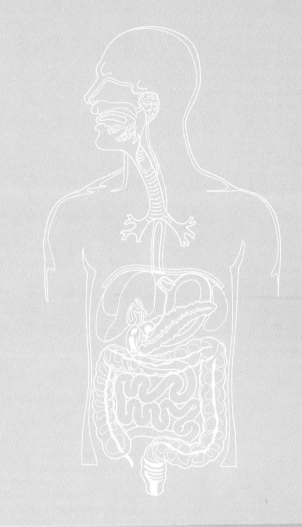

Unit

ENERGY: SUPPLY AND USE

Respiration

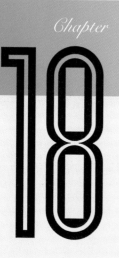

Chapter

18

BEHAVIORAL OBJECTIVES

After careful study of this chapter, you should be able to:

1. Define *respiration* and describe the three phases of respiration

2. Name and describe all the structures of the respiratory system

3. Explain the mechanism for pulmonary ventilation

4. List the ways in which oxygen and carbon dioxide are transported in the blood

5. Describe the ways in which respiration is regulated

6. Give several examples of abnormal respiration

7. List and define four conditions that result from inadequate breathing

8. Describe four types of respiratory infection

9. Name the diseases involved in chronic obstructive pulmonary disease (COPD)

10. Describe the equipment used to treat respiratory disorders

Most people think of respiration simply as the process by which air moves into and out of the lungs, that is, *breathing*. By scientific definition, respiration is the process by which oxygen is obtained from the environment and delivered to the cells. Carbon dioxide is transported to the outside in a reverse pathway.

Respiration includes three phases:

- ***Pulmonary ventilation,*** which is the exchange of air between the atmosphere and the air sacs of the lungs. This is normally accomplished by the inspiration and expiration of breathing.
- The ***diffusion*** of gases, which includes the passage of oxygen from the air sacs into the blood and the passage of carbon dioxide out of the blood
- The ***transport*** of gases in the circulating blood. Oxygen is carried to the cells and carbon dioxide is transported from the cells to the lungs.

In the process of ***cellular respiration,*** oxygen is taken into the cell and used in the breakdown of nutrients with the release of energy. Carbon dioxide is the waste product of cellular respiration.

✔ CHECKPOINT **1**:

What are the three phases of respiration?

THE RESPIRATORY SYSTEM

The respiratory system is an intricate arrangement of spaces and passageways that conduct air into the lungs (Fig. 18-1). These spaces include the ***nasal cavities;*** the ***pharynx*** (FAR-inks), which is common to the digestive and respiratory systems; the voice box, or ***larynx*** (LAR-inks); the windpipe, or ***trachea*** (TRA-ke-ah); and the ***lungs*** themselves, with their conducting tubes and air sacs. The entire system might be thought of as a pathway for air between the atmosphere and the blood.

The Nasal Cavities

Air makes its initial entrance into the body through the openings in the nose called the ***nostrils.*** Immediately inside the nostrils, located between the roof of the mouth and the cranium, are the two spaces known as the ***nasal cavities.*** These two spaces are separated from each other by a partition, the ***nasal septum.*** The superior portion of the septum is formed by a thin plate of the ethmoid bone that extends down-

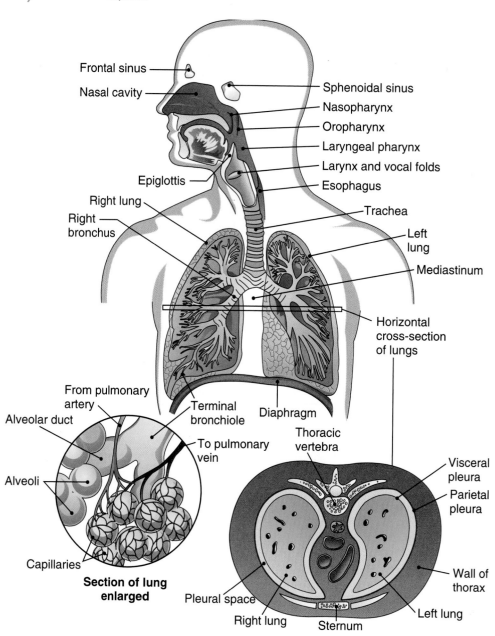

Frontal sinus
Nasal cavity
Sphenoidal sinus
Nasopharynx
Oropharynx
Laryngeal pharynx
Larynx and vocal folds
Epiglottis
Esophagus
Right lung
Trachea
Right bronchus
Left lung
Mediastinum
Horizontal cross-section of lungs
From pulmonary artery
Alveolar duct
Terminal bronchiole
Diaphragm
Thoracic vertebra
To pulmonary vein
Visceral pleura
Parietal pleura
Alveoli
Capillaries
Section of lung enlarged
Pleural space
Right lung
Sternum
Left lung
Wall of thorax

FIGURE **18•1**   Respiratory system.

ward, and the inferior portion is formed by the vomer (see Fig. 7-3A in Chap. 7). An anterior extension of the septum is made of hyaline cartilage. The septum and the walls of the nasal cavity are covered with mucous membrane. On the lateral (side) walls of each nasal cavity are three projections called the ***conchae*** (KONG-ke) (see Figs. 7-3A and 7-6 in Chap. 7). The shell-like conchae greatly increase the surface over which air must travel on its way through the nasal cavities.

The mucous membrane lining the nasal cavities contains many blood vessels that deliver heat and moisture. The cells of this membrane secrete a large amount of fluid—up to 1 quart each day. The following changes are produced in the air as it comes in contact with the lining of the nose:

- Foreign bodies, such as dust particles and pathogens, are filtered out by the hairs of the nostrils or caught in the surface mucus.
- Air is warmed by the blood in the vascular membrane.
- Air is moistened by the liquid secretion.

To allow for these protective changes to occur, it is preferable to breathe through the nose rather than through the mouth.

The ***sinuses*** are small cavities lined with mucous membrane in the bones of the skull. The sinuses communicate with the nasal cavities, and they are highly susceptible to infection.

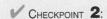

✔ CHECKPOINT **2**:

What happens to air as it passes over the nasal mucosa?

The Pharynx

The muscular ***pharynx,*** or throat, carries air into the respiratory tract and carries foods and liquids into the digestive system (see Fig. 18-1). The upper portion, located immediately behind the nasal cavity, is called the ***nasopharynx*** (na-zo-FAR-inks); the middle section, located behind the mouth, is called the ***oropharynx*** (o-ro-FAR-inks); and the lowest portion is called the ***laryngeal*** (lah-RIN-je-al) ***pharynx.*** This last section opens into the larynx toward the front and into the esophagus toward the back.

The Larynx

The ***larynx,*** commonly called the *voice box* (Fig. 18-2), is located between the pharynx and the trachea. It has a framework of cartilage, part of which is the thyroid cartilage that protrudes in the front of the neck. The projection formed by the thyroid cartilage is popularly called the *Adam's apple* because it is considerably larger in the male than in the female.

On both sides at the upper end of the larynx are folds of mucous membrane used in producing speech. These are the vocal folds, or ***vocal cords*** (Fig. 18-3). They are set into vibration by the flow of air from the lungs. A difference in the size of the larynx is what accounts for the difference between male and female voices; because a man's larynx is larger than a woman's, his voice is lower in pitch. The nasal cavities,

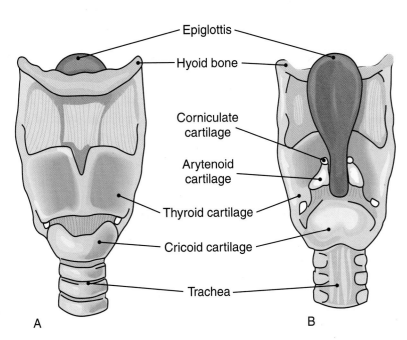

FIGURE **18•2** The larynx. **(A)** Anterior view. **(B)** Posterior view.

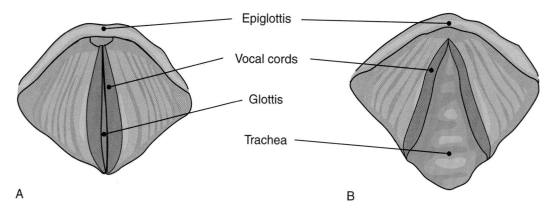

FIGURE **18•3**   The vocal cords viewed from above. **(A)** The glottis in closed position. **(B)** The glottis in open position.

the sinuses, and the pharynx all serve as resonating chambers for speech, just as the cabinet does for an audio speaker.

The space between the vocal cords is called the **glottis** (GLOT-is), and the little leaf-shaped cartilage that covers the larynx during swallowing is called the **epiglottis** (ep-ih-GLOT-is). The glottis and epiglottis help keep food and liquids out of the remainder of the respiratory tract. As the larynx moves upward and forward during swallowing, the epiglottis moves downward, covering the opening into the larynx. The glottis assists by closing during swallowing. You can feel the larynx move upward toward the epiglottis during this process by placing the flat ends of your fingers on your larynx as you swallow.

The Trachea

The **trachea,** commonly called the *windpipe,* is a tube that extends from the lower edge of the larynx to the upper part of the chest above the heart. The purpose of the trachea is to conduct air between the larynx and the lungs.

The trachea has a framework of cartilages to keep it open. These cartilages, shaped somewhat like a tiny horseshoe or the letter C, are found along the entire length of the trachea. The open sections in the cartilages are lined up in the back so that the esophagus can bulge into this region during swallowing.

✔ CHECKPOINT **3**:

What are the scientific names for the throat, the voice box, and the windpipe?

The Bronchi

At its inferior end, the trachea divides into two primary, or main-stem, **bronchi** (BRONG-ki), which enter the lungs. The right bronchus is considerably larger in diameter than the left and extends downward in a more vertical direction. Therefore, if a foreign body is inhaled, it is likely to enter the right lung. Each bronchus enters the lung at a notch or depression called the **hilus** (HI-lus) or **hilum** (HI-lum). Blood vessels and nerves also connect with the lung in this region.

The Lining of the Air Passageways

The bronchi and other conducting passageways of the respiratory tract are lined with a special type of epithelium (Fig. 18-4). Basically, it is simple columnar epithelium, but the cells are arranged in such a way that they appear stratified. The tissue is thus described as *pseudostratified,* meaning "falsely stratified." These epithelial cells have cilia to filter out impurities and to create movement of fluids within the conducting tubes. The cilia beat to drive impuri-

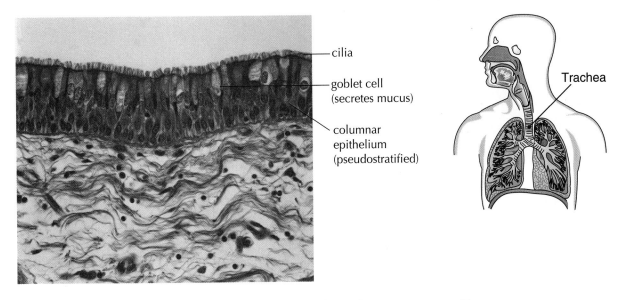

cilia

goblet cell
(secretes mucus)

columnar
epithelium
(pseudostratified)

Trachea

FIGURE **18•4** Microscopic view of the ciliated epithelium that lines the respiratory passageways. (Cormack DH: Essential Histology, Plate 4-1D, Philadelphia, JB Lippincott, 1993)

ties toward the throat, where they can be eliminated by coughing, sneezing, or blowing the nose.

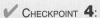 CHECKPOINT **4**:

The cells that line the respiratory passageways help to keep impurities out of the lungs. What feature of these cells enables them to filter impurities and move fluids?

The Lungs

The *lungs* are the organs in which the diffusion of gases takes place through the extremely thin and delicate lung tissues. The two lungs are set side by side in the thoracic (chest) cavity. On its medial side, the left lung has an indentation that accommodates the heart.

Each primary bronchus enters the lung at the hilus and immediately subdivides. The right bronchus divides into three secondary bronchi, each of which enters one of the three lobes of the right lung. The left bronchus gives rise to two secondary bronchi, which enter the two lobes of the left lung. Because the subdivisions

of the bronchi resemble the branches of a tree, they have been given the common name *bronchial tree*. The bronchi subdivide again and again, becoming progressively smaller as they branch through lung tissue.

The smallest of these conducting tubes are called **bronchioles** (BRONG-ke-oles). The bronchi contain small bits of cartilage, which give firmness to the walls and serve to hold the passageways open so that air can pass in and out easily. As the bronchi become smaller, however, the cartilage decreases in amount. In the bronchioles, there is no cartilage at all; what remains is mostly smooth muscle, which is under the control of the autonomic (involuntary) nervous system.

The Alveoli

At the end of the **terminal bronchioles,** the smallest subdivisions of the bronchial tree, are the clusters of tiny air sacs in which most gas exchange takes place. These sacs are known as **alveoli** (al-VE-o-li). The wall of each alveolus is made of a single-cell layer of squamous (flat) epithelium. This thin wall provides easy passage for the gases entering and leaving the blood as the blood circulates through the millions of tiny capillaries covering the alveoli.

18

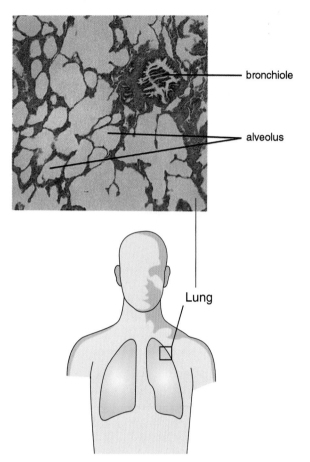

FIGURE **18•5** Lung tissue as seen through a microscope, (Courtesy of Dana Morse Bittus and B.J. Cohen)

Certain cells in the alveolar wall produce *surfactant* (sur-FAK-tant), a substance that reduces the surface tension ("pull") of the fluids that line the alveoli. This surface action prevents collapse of the alveoli and eases expansion of the lungs.

There are millions of alveoli in the human lung. The resulting surface area in contact with gases approximates 60 square meters, about three times as much lung tissue as is necessary for life. Because of the many air spaces, the lung is light in weight; normally, a piece of lung tissue dropped into a glass of water will float. Figure 18-5 shows a microscopic view of lung tissue.

The pulmonary circuit brings blood to and from the lungs. In the lungs, the blood passes through the capillaries around the alveoli, where the gas exchange takes place (see Fig. 18-7, shown later).

The Lung Cavities and Pleura

The lungs occupy a considerable portion of the thoracic cavity, which is separated from the abdominal cavity by the muscular partition known as the *diaphragm.* A continuous doubled sac, known as the *pleura,* covers each lung. Each layer of the pleura is named according to its location. The portion of the pleura that is attached to the chest wall is the *parietal pleura,* and the portion that is attached to the surface of the lung is called the *visceral pleura.* Each closed sac completely surrounds the lung, except in the place where the bronchus and blood vessels enter the lung, a region known as the *root* of the lung.

Between the two layers of the pleura is the *pleural space,* in which there is a thin film of fluid that lubricates the membranes. The effect is the same as between two flat pieces of glass joined by a film of water; that is, the surfaces slide easily on each other but strongly resist separation. Thus, the lungs are able to move and enlarge effortlessly in response to changes in the thoracic volume that occur during breathing.

The region between the lungs, the *mediastinum* (me-de-as-TI-num), contains the heart, great blood vessels, esophagus, trachea, and lymph nodes.

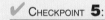

✔ CHECKPOINT **5**:

What is the name of the membrane that encloses the lung?

THE PROCESS OF RESPIRATION

Pulmonary Ventilation

Ventilation is the movement of air into and out of the lungs, as in breathing. There are two phases of ventilation (Fig. 18-6):

- *Inhalation* is the drawing of air into the lungs.

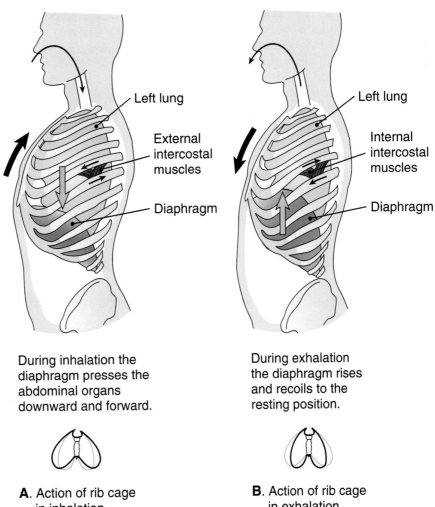

Left lung

External intercostal muscles

Diaphragm

During inhalation the diaphragm presses the abdominal organs downward and forward.

A. Action of rib cage in inhalation

Left lung

Internal intercostal muscles

Diaphragm

During exhalation the diaphragm rises and recoils to the resting position.

B. Action of rib cage in exhalation

FIGURE **18•6** Pulmonary ventilation. **(A)** Inhalation. **(B)** Exhalation.

- ***Exhalation*** is the expulsion of air from the lungs.

In ***inhalation,*** the active phase of breathing, the respiratory muscles contract to enlarge the thoracic cavity. During quiet breathing, the movement of the diaphragm accounts for most of the increase in thoracic volume. The diaphragm is a strong, dome-shaped muscle attached to the body wall around the base of the rib cage. The contraction and flattening of the diaphragm cause a pistonlike downward motion that results in an increase in the vertical dimension of the chest. Other muscles that participate in enlarging the chest cavity during inhalation are the intercostal muscles. These muscles run at angles in two layers between the ribs. As they contract, they lift the rib cage upward and outward. Put the palms of your hands on either side of the rib cage to feel this action as you inhale. During exertion, the rib cage is moved further up and out by contraction of muscles in the neck and chest wall.

As the thoracic cavity increases in size, gas pressure within the cavity decreases. When the pressure drops to slightly below atmospheric pressure, air is drawn into the lungs, as by suction.

The ease with which the lungs and thorax can

be expanded is termed **compliance**. Normal elasticity of the lung tissue, aided by surfactant, allows the lungs to expand under pressure and fill adequately with air during inhalation. Compliance is decreased when the lungs resist expansion. Conditions that can decrease compliance include diseases that damage or scar lung tissue, accumulation of fluid in the lungs, deficiency of surfactant, and interference with the action of breathing muscles.

In **exhalation,** the passive phase of breathing, the muscles of respiration relax, allowing the ribs and diaphragm to return to their original positions. The tissues of the lung are elastic and recoil during exhalation. During forced exhalation, the internal intercostal muscles in the posterior of the rib cage and the muscles of the abdominal wall contract, pulling the bottom of the rib cage in and down, pushing the abdominal viscera upward against the relaxed diaphragm.

Air enters the respiratory passages and flows through the ever-dividing tubes of the bronchial tree. As the air traverses this passage, it moves more and more slowly through the great number of bronchial tubes until there is virtually no forward flow as it reaches the alveoli. Here, the incoming air mixes with the existing air so that the gases soon are evenly distributed. Each breath causes relatively little change in the gas composition of the alveoli, but normal continuous breathing ensures the presence of adequate oxygen and the removal of carbon dioxide. See The Air We Breathe.

Table 18-1 gives the definitions and average values for some of the breathing volumes and capacities that are important in any evaluation of respiratory function. A lung *capacity* is a sum of volumes.

The Air We Breathe

The air we breathe comes under close inspection because of our increasing awareness of air pollution, both indoors and out. Automobile exhaust and industrial smoke pollute the air in many populated areas. The pronounced increase in asthma among children observed since 1980 is explained in part by increased exposure to allergens both within the home and in the general environment. Air in agricultural areas may include smoke from burning fields and drift of airborne pesticide applications far from the intended target. Lumber operations may burn scrap. Wind carries dust and pollen everywhere. Much work is being carried out to decrease these sources of airborne pollution.

Air inside homes or offices often carries a less visible burden of pollution. Many products give off invisible gases that tend to accumulate in modern buildings, which usually are tightly sealed. Unless adequate amounts of clean air are supplied, the occupants often complain of vague illnesses. Attention needs to be given to processing the air not only for temperature but also for humidity. Most important, the air must be filtered, so that undesirable pollutants are removed.

✔ CHECKPOINT **6**:

What are the two phases of breathing? Which is active and which is passive?

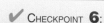

Table 18•1	**Lung Volumes and Capacities**	

VOLUME	DEFINITION	AVERAGE VALUE (mL)
Tidal volume	The amount of air moved into or out of the lungs in quiet, relaxed breathing	500
Residual volume	The volume of air that remains in the lungs after maximum exhalation	1200
Vital capacity	The volume of air that can be expelled from the lungs by maximum exhalation after maximum inhalation	4800
Total lung capacity	The total volume of air that can be contained in the lungs after maximum inhalation	6000
Functional residual capacity	The amount of air remaining in the lungs after normal exhalation	2400

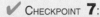

Liquid Ventilation

Researchers have been attempting for years to develop a fluid that could carry high concentrations of oxygen in the body. Such a fluid could substitute for blood in transfusions or be used to carry oxygen into the lungs. Early work on liquid ventilation climaxed dramatically in the mid-1960s when a pioneer in this field submerged a laboratory mouse in a beaker of fluid and the animal survived total immersion for more than 10 minutes. The fluid was a synthetic substance that could hold as much oxygen as does air. A newer version of this fluid, a fluorine-containing chemical known as *PFC*, has been tested to ventilate the collapsed lungs of premature babies. The fluid is less damaging to delicate lung tissue than is air, which has to be pumped in under higher pressure. Other possible uses include treatment of people whose lungs have been damaged by infection or inhalation of toxins.

Gas Exchange in the Lungs

The barrier that separates alveolar air from the blood is composed of the wall of the alveolus and the wall of the capillary, both of which are extremely thin. This respiratory membrane is not only very thin, it is also moist. The moisture is important because the oxygen and carbon dioxide must go into solution before they can diffuse across the membrane. Recall that *diffusion* refers to the movement of molecules from an area in which they are in higher concentration to an area in which they are in lower concentration. Normally, inspired air contains about 21% oxygen and 0.04% carbon dioxide; expired air has only 16% oxygen and 3.5% carbon dioxide. These figures illustrate that a two-way diffusion takes place through the walls of the alveoli and capillaries.

In the tissues, also by the process of diffusion, oxygen leaves the blood, and carbon dioxide enters. Therefore, blood returning from the tissues and entering the lung capillaries is relatively low in oxygen. Oxygen then diffuses from the alveolus, where its concentration is higher, into the blood. Again, based on relative concentration, carbon dioxide diffuses out of the blood into the air of the alveolus (Fig. 18-7). See Liquid Ventilation.

✔ CHECKPOINT **7**:

Gases move between the alveoli and the blood by the process of diffusion. What is the definition of diffusion?

Gas Transport

Transport of Oxygen

Almost all the oxygen that diffuses into the capillary blood in the lungs is bound to the *hemoglobin* of the red blood cells. A small percentage is carried in solution in the plasma. The hemoglobin molecule is a large protein with four small iron-containing "heme" regions. The oxygen is bound to these heme portions.

Arterial blood (in systemic arteries and pulmonary veins) is 97% saturated with oxygen, whereas venous blood (in systemic veins and pulmonary arteries) is about 70% saturated with oxygen. This 27% difference represents the oxygen that has been taken up by the cells.

Note that in clinical practice, gas concentrations are expressed as pressure in millimeters of mercury (mmHg), just as blood pressure is reported. Because air is a mixture of gases, each gas exerts only a portion of the total pressure, or a *partial pressure* (P). The partial pressures of oxygen and carbon dioxide are symbolized as P_{O_2} and P_{CO_2} respectively.

To enter the cells, oxygen must separate from hemoglobin. Normally, the bond between oxygen and hemoglobin is easily broken, and oxygen is released as blood travels into areas where the oxygen concentration is relatively low. Cells are constantly using oxygen in metabolism and obtaining fresh supplies by diffusion from the blood.

The Effect of Carbon Monoxide

Carbon monoxide (CO) at low partial pressure binds with hemoglobin at the same sites as does oxygen. However, it binds more tightly and displaces oxygen. Even a small amount of carbon monoxide causes a serious reduction in the ability of the blood to carry oxygen.

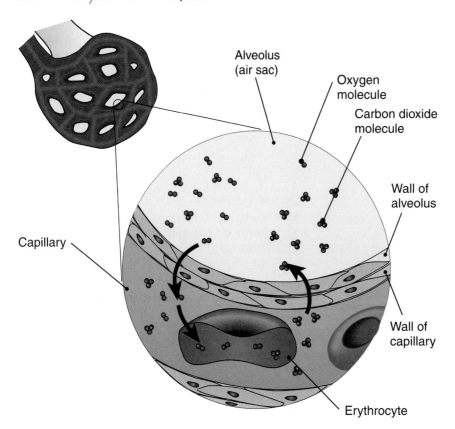

Alveolus
(air sac)

Oxygen
molecule

Carbon dioxide
molecule

Wall of
alveolus

Capillary

Wall of
capillary

Erythrocyte

FIGURE **18•7** Diagram illustrating the diffusion of gas molecules in the lungs.

✔ CHECKPOINT **8**:

What substance in red blood cells carries almost all of the oxygen in the blood?

Transport of Carbon Dioxide

Carbon dioxide is produced continuously in the tissues as a byproduct of metabolism. It diffuses from the cells into the blood to be transported to the lungs in three ways:

- About 10% is dissolved in the plasma and the fluid in red blood cells.
- About 20% is combined with the protein portion of hemoglobin and plasma proteins.
- About 70% is transported as an ion, known as a ***bicarbonate ion,*** which is formed when carbon dioxide dissolves in blood fluids.

The bicarbonate ion is formed slowly in the plasma but much more rapidly inside the red blood cells, where an enzyme called ***carbonic***

anhydrase increases the speed of the reaction. The bicarbonate formed in the red blood cells moves to the plasma and then is carried to the lungs. Here, the process is reversed as bicarbonate reenters the red blood cells and releases carbon dioxide for diffusion into the alveoli and exhalation.

Carbon dioxide is important in regulating the pH (acid–base balance) of the blood. As a bicarbonate ion is formed from carbon dioxide in the plasma, a hydrogen ion (H^+) is also produced. Therefore, the blood becomes more acidic as the amount of carbon dioxide in the blood increases. The exhalation of carbon dioxide shifts the pH of the blood more toward the alkaline (basic) range. The bicarbonate ion is also an important buffer in the blood, acting chemically to help keep the pH of body fluids at a steady pH of 7.4.

✔ CHECKPOINT **9**:

What is the main form in which carbon dioxide is carried in the blood?

18

Regulation of Respiration

The respiratory pattern is controlled by centers in the central nervous system as modified in response to chemical stimuli detected by special receptors.

Nervous Control

Regulation of respiration is a complex process that must keep pace with moment-to-moment changes in cellular oxygen requirements and carbon dioxide production. Regulation depends primarily on a respiratory control center located partly in the medulla and partly in the pons of the brain stem. The main part of the control center, located in the medulla, sets the basic pattern of respiration. This pattern can be modified by centers in the pons. Breathing is regulated continuously, so that levels of oxygen, carbon dioxide, and acid are kept within normal limits.

✔ CHECKPOINT **10**:

What part of the brain stem sets the basic pattern of respiration?

From the respiratory center in the medulla, motor nerve fibers extend into the spinal cord. From the cervical (neck) part of the cord, these nerve fibers continue through the ***phrenic*** (FREN-ik) ***nerve*** to the diaphragm. The diaphragm and the other muscles of respiration are voluntary in the sense that they can be regulated consciously by messages from the higher brain centers, notably the cortex. It is possible for a person to deliberately breathe more rapidly or more slowly or to hold his or her breath and not breathe at all for a while. Most of the time, however, we breathe without thinking about it, and the respiratory center in the brain stem is in control.

✔ CHECKPOINT **11**:

What is the name of the motor nerve that controls the diaphragm?

Chemical Control

Of vital importance in the control of respiration are ***chemoreceptors*** (ke-mo-re-SEP-tors), which, like the receptors for taste and smell, are sensitive to chemicals dissolved in body fluids. The receptors that regulate respiration are found in structures called the *carotid* and *aortic bodies* as well as outside the medulla of the brain stem. The carotid bodies are located near the bifurcation (forking) of the common carotid arteries in the neck, whereas the aortic bodies are located in the aortic arch. These bodies contain many small blood vessels and sensory neurons that respond to increases in carbon dioxide and acidity (H^+) and to decreases in oxygen supply.

Changes in the composition of the blood generate nerve impulses that are then sent to the brain. Because there is usually an ample reserve of oxygen in the blood, carbon dioxide has the most immediate effect in regulating respiration. When carbon dioxide levels increase, breathing must be increased to blow off the excess. It is only when oxygen levels fall considerably that this gas becomes a controlling factor. The receptor cells outside the medulla actually respond to the concentration of hydrogen ions in cerebrospinal fluid (CSF). The level of hydrogen ion increases as carbon dioxide dissolves in the blood.

✔ CHECKPOINT **12**:

What gas is the main chemical controller of respiration?

Abnormal Ventilation

In ***hyperventilation***, an increased amount of air enters the alveoli. This condition results from deep and rapid respiration that occurs commonly during anxiety attacks. It causes an increase in the oxygen level and a decrease in the carbon dioxide level of the blood. The loss of carbon dioxide increases the pH of the blood (alkalosis), resulting in dizziness and tingling sensations. Breathing may stop because the respiratory control center is not stimulated. Gradually, the carbon dioxide level returns to normal, and a regular breathing pattern is resumed. Breathing into a paper bag to increase the carbon dioxide level in the blood may relieve symptoms of hyperventilation.

In **hypoventilation,** an insufficient amount of air enters the alveoli. The many possible causes of this condition include respiratory obstruction, lung disease, injury to the respiratory center, depression of the respiratory center, as by drugs, and chest deformity. Hypoventilation results in an increase in the concentration of carbon dioxide in the blood, leading to a decrease in blood pH (acidosis).

Breathing Patterns

Normal rates of breathing vary from 12 to 20 times per minute for adults. In children, rates may vary from 20 to 40 times per minute, depending on age and size. In infants, the respiratory rate may be more than 40 times per minute. Changes in respiratory rates are important in various disorders and should be recorded carefully. To determine the respiratory rate, the health care worker counts the client's breathing for at least 30 seconds, usually by watching the rise and fall of the chest with each inhalation and exhalation. The count is then multiplied to obtain the rate in breaths per minute. It is best if the person does not realize that he or she is being observed because awareness of the measurement may cause a change in the breathing rate.

Some Terms for Altered Breathing
The following is a list of terms designating various abnormalities of respiration. These are symptoms, not diseases. Note that the word ending -*pnea* refers to breathing.

* **Hyperpnea** (hi-PERP-ne-ah) refers to an abnormal increase in the depth and rate of respiration.
* **Tachypnea** (tak-IP-ne-ah) is an excessive rate of breathing that may be normal, as in exercise.
* **Apnea** (AP-ne-ah) is a temporary cessation of breathing, as may occur during sleep.

* **Dyspnea** (disp-NE-ah) is a subjective feeling of difficult or labored breathing.
* **Orthopnea** (or-THOP-ne-ah) refers to a difficulty in breathing that is relieved by sitting in an upright position, either against two pillows in bed or in a chair.
* **Cheyne-Stokes** (CHANE-stokes) **respiration** is a rhythmic variation in the depth of respiratory movements alternating with periods of apnea. It is due to depression of the breathing centers and is seen in certain critically ill patients.

Results of Inadequate Breathing
Conditions that may result from decreased respiration include the following:

* **Cyanosis** (si-ah-NO-sis) is a bluish color of the skin and mucous membranes caused by an insufficient amount of oxygen in the blood.
* **Hypoxia** (hi-POK-se-ah) means a lower than normal level of oxygen in the tissues. The term *anoxia* (ah-NOK-se-ah) is sometimes used instead but is not as accurate because it means a total lack of oxygen.
* **Hypoxemia** (hi-pok-SE-me-ah) refers to a lower than normal concentration of oxygen in arterial blood.
* **Suffocation** is the cessation of respiration, often the result of a mechanical blockage of the respiratory passages.

DISORDERS OF THE RESPIRATORY SYSTEM

Disorders of the Nasal Cavities and Related Structures

The sinuses are located close to the nasal cavities and in one case near the ear. Infection may easily travel into these sinuses from the mouth, the nose, and the throat along the mucous membranes lining these cavities. The resulting inflammation is called **sinusitis.** Long-standing (chronic) sinus infection may cause changes in the epithelial cells, resulting in tumor formation. Some of these growths have a grapelike appearance and cause obstruction of the air pathway; these tumors are called **polyps** (POL-ips).

The partition separating the two nasal cavities is called the *nasal septum.* Because many of us have minor structural defects, it is not surprising that the nasal septum is rarely exactly in the midline. If it is markedly to one side, it is described as a **deviated septum.** In this condition, one nasal space may be considerably smaller than the other. If an affected person has an attack of hay fever or develops a cold with accompanying swelling of the mucosa, the smaller nasal cavity may be completely closed. Sometimes, the septum is curved in such a way that both nasal cavities are occluded, forcing the person to breathe through the mouth. Such an occlusion may also prevent proper drainage from the sinuses and aggravate a case of sinusitis.

The most common cause of nosebleed, also called **epistaxis** (ep-e-STAK-sis), is an injury or blow to the nose. Other causes include inflammation and ulceration such as may occur after a persistent discharge from a sinusitis. Growths, including polyps, can also cause epistaxis. Rarely, abnormally high blood pressure causes the vessels in the nasal lining to break, resulting in varying degrees of hemorrhage.

To stop a nosebleed, the affected person should remain quiet with the head slightly elevated. Pressure applied to the nostril of the bleeding side and cold compresses over the nose are usually helpful. In some cases, it may be necessary to insert a plug into the bleeding side to encourage adequate clotting. If these methods fail, a physician should be consulted.

Infection

The mucosa of the respiratory tract is one of the most important portals of entry for disease-producing organisms. The transfer of disease organisms from the respiratory system of one human being to that of another occurs most rapidly in crowded places, such as schools, theaters, and institutions. Droplets from one sneeze may be loaded with many billions of disease-producing organisms.

To a certain extent, the mucous membranes can protect themselves by producing larger quantities of mucus. The runny nose, an unpleasant symptom of the common cold, is an attempt on the part of nature to wash away the pathogens and so protect the deeper tissues from further infection. If the resistance of the mucous membrane is reduced, however, the membrane may act as a pathway for the spread of disease. The infection may travel along the membrane into the nasal sinuses, into the middle ear, or into the lung.

Among the infections transmitted through the respiratory passageways are the common cold, diphtheria, chicken pox, measles, influenza, pneumonia, and tuberculosis. Any infection that is confined to the nose and throat is called an **upper respiratory infection** (often called *URI*). Very often, an upper respiratory infection is the first evidence of infectious disease in children. Such an infection may precede the onset of a serious disease, such as rheumatic fever.

The respiratory passageways may become infected one by one as organisms travel along the lining membrane. Each infection is named according to the part involved, such as pharyngitis (commonly called a *sore throat*), laryngitis, or bronchitis.

The Common Cold

The common cold is the most widespread of all respiratory diseases—of all communicable diseases, for that matter. More time is lost from school and from work because of the common cold than because of any other disorder. The causative agents are viruses that probably number more than 200 different types. Because there are so many organisms involved, the production of an effective vaccine against colds seems unlikely. Medical science has yet to establish the effectiveness of any method of preventing the common cold.

The symptoms of the common cold are familiar: first the swollen and inflamed mucosa of the nose and the throat, then the copious discharge of watery fluid from the nose, and finally the thick and ropy discharge that occurs when the cold is subsiding. The scientific name for the common cold is **acute coryza** (ko-RI-zah); the word *coryza* can also mean simply "a nasal discharge."

Influenza

Influenza, or "flu," is an acute contagious disease characterized by an inflammatory condition of the upper respiratory tract accompanied by generalized aches and pains. It is caused by a virus and may spread to the sinuses and downward to the lungs. Inflammation of the trachea and the bronchi causes the characteristic cough of influenza, and the general infection causes an extremely weakened condition. The great danger of influenza is its tendency to develop into a particularly severe form of pneumonia. At intervals in history, there have been tremendous epidemics of influenza in which millions of people have died. Vaccines have been effective, although the protection is of short duration.

Pneumonia

Pneumonia is an inflammation of the lungs in which the air spaces become filled with fluid. A variety of organisms, including staphylococci, pneumococci, streptococci, *Legionella pneumophila* (as in Legionnaires' disease), chlamydiae, and viruses may be responsible. Many of these pathogens may be carried by a healthy person in the mucosa of the upper respiratory tract. If the person remains in good health, these pathogens may be carried for an indefinite period with no ill effect. If the patient's resistance to infection is lowered, however, the pathogens may invade the tissues and cause disease.

Susceptibility to pneumonia is increased in patients with chronic, debilitating illness or chronic respiratory disease, in smokers, and in people with alcoholism. It is also increased in cases of exposure to toxic gases, suppression of the immune system, or viral respiratory infections.

There are two main kinds of pneumonia as determined by the extent of lung involvement and other factors:

- **Bronchopneumonia,** in which the disease process is scattered here and there throughout the lung. The cause may be infection with a staphylococcus, gram-negative *Proteus* species, colon bacillus (not normally pathogenic), or a virus. Bronchopneumonia most often is secondary to an infection or to some agent that has lowered the patient's resistance to disease. This is the most common form of pneumonia.
- **Lobar pneumonia,** in which an entire lobe of the lung is infected at one time. The organism is usually a pneumococcus, although other pathogens may also cause this disease. *Legionella* is the causative agent of a severe lobar pneumonia that occurs mostly in localized epidemics.

A characteristic of most types of pneumonia is the formation of a fluid, or **exudate,** in the infected alveoli; this fluid consists chiefly of serum and pus, products of infection. Some red blood cells may be present, as indicated by red streaks in the sputum. Sometimes, so many air sacs become filled with fluid that the victim finds it hard to absorb enough oxygen to maintain life.

Tuberculosis

Tuberculosis (TB) is an infectious disease caused by the bacillus *Mycobacterium tuberculosis*. Although the tubercle bacillus may invade any tissue in the body, the lung is the usual site of growth. Tuberculosis remains a leading cause of death from communicable disease, primarily because of the relatively large numbers of cases among recent immigrants, elderly people, and poor people in metropolitan areas. The spread of AIDS has been linked with a rising incidence of TB because this viral disease weakens host defenses.

The name of the disease comes from the small lesions, or tubercles, that form where the organisms grow. If unchecked, these lesions degenerate and may even liquefy to cause cavities within an organ. In early stages, the disease may lie dormant, only to flare up at a later time. The tuberculosis organism can readily spread into the lymph nodes or into the blood to be carried to other organs. The lymph nodes in the thorax, especially those surrounding the trachea and the bronchi, are frequently involved. Infection of the pleura results in tuberculous pleurisy (inflammation of the pleura). In this case, a collection of fluid, known as an **effusion** (e-FU-zhun), accumulates in the pleural space.

Drugs can be used successfully in many cases of tuberculosis, although strains of the TB organism that are resistant to multiple antibiotics have appeared recently. The best results have been obtained by use of a combination of several drugs, with prompt, intensive, and uninterrupted treatment once such a program is begun. Such therapy is usually continued for a minimum of 6 to 18 months; therefore, close supervision by the health care practitioner is important. Adverse drug reactions are rather common, necessitating changes in the drug combinations. Drug treatment of patients whose infection has not progressed to active disease is particularly effective.

Hay Fever and Asthma

Hypersensitivity to plant pollens, dust, certain foods, and other allergens may lead to **hay fever** or **asthma** or both. Hay fever, known medically as *allergic rhinitis*, is characterized by a watery discharge from the eyes and nose. Hay fever often appears in a seasonal pattern due to pollen allergy. The response may be chronic if the allergen is present year round. The symptoms of asthma are due to reversible changes, which include inflammation of airway tissues and spasm of the involuntary muscle of the bronchial tube walls. Spasm constricts the tubes so that the patient cannot exhale easily. He or she experiences a sense of suffocation and has labored breathing (dyspnea). Treatment may include inhaled steroids to prevent inflammation and inhaled bronchodilators to open airways during acute episodes.

Patients vary considerably in their responses, and most cases of asthma involve multiple causes. Respiratory infection, noxious fumes, or drug allergy can initiate episodes, but one of the more common triggers for asthma attacks is exercise. The rapid movement of air in sensitive airways causes smooth muscle spasm in the breathing passages.

A great difficulty in the treatment of hay fever or asthma is identification of the particular substance to which the patient is allergic. Usually, a number of skin tests are given, but in most cases, the results of these tests are far from conclusive. People with allergies may benefit from treatment with a series of injections to reduce their sensitivity to specific substances.

COPD

Chronic obstructive pulmonary disease (COPD) is the term used to describe several lung disorders, including **chronic bronchitis** and **emphysema**. Most affected patients have symptoms and lung damage characteristic of both diseases. In chronic bronchitis, the linings of the airways are chronically inflamed and produce excessive secretions. Emphysema is characterized by dilation and finally destruction of the alveoli.

In COPD, respiratory function is impaired by obstruction to normal air flow, by air trapping and overinflation of parts of the lungs, and by reduced exchange of oxygen and carbon dioxide. In the early stages of these diseases, the small airways are involved, and several years may pass before symptoms become evident. Later, the affected person develops dyspnea as a result of the difficulty of exhaling air through the obstructed air passages.

In certain smokers, COPD may result in serious disability and death within 10 years of the onset of symptoms. Giving up smoking may reverse progression of the disorder, especially when it is diagnosed early and other respiratory irritants also are eliminated. Sometimes, the word *emphysema* is used to mean COPD.

✓ CHECKPOINT **13**:

What does COPD mean and what two diseases are commonly involved in COPD?

Atelectasis

Atelectasis (at-e-LEK-tah-sis) is the incomplete expansion of a lung or portion of a lung. This disorder may affect scattered groups of alveoli or an entire lobe, causing its collapse. Symptoms are hypoxia and dyspnea. Obstruction by mucous plugs in COPD, by foreign bodies, or by lung cancer is a cause of atelectasis. Another cause is the insufficient production of surfactant, as in *respiratory distress syndrome* (RDS), also called *hyaline membrane disease,* seen in premature newborns. Atelectasis is also seen in cases of external compression of the lung or interference with deep breathing, for example, with pain from fractured ribs.

Lung Cancer

Cancer of the lungs is the most common cause of cancer deaths in both men and women. The incidence rate in women continues to increase, whereas the rate in men has been decreasing recently. By far, the most important cause of lung cancer is cigarette smoking. Smokers suffer from lung cancer 10 times as often as do nonsmokers. The risk of getting cancer of the lungs is increased in people who started smoking early in life, who smoke large numbers of cigarettes daily, and who inhale deeply. Smokers who are exposed to toxic chemicals or particles in the air have an even higher rate of lung cancer. Smoking has also been linked with an increase in COPD and cancers of respiratory passages. See Recovering From Smoking: Yes You Can!

A common form of lung cancer is ***bronchogenic*** (brong-ko-JEN-ik) ***carcinoma,*** so called because the malignancy originates in a bronchus. The tumor may grow until the bronchus is blocked, cutting off the supply of air to that lung. The lung then collapses, and the secretions trapped in the lung spaces become infected, with a resulting pneumonia or formation of a lung abscess. Such a lung cancer can spread, causing secondary growths in the lymph nodes of the chest and neck and in the brain and other parts of the body. A treatment that offers a possibility of cure, before secondary growths have had time to form, is complete removal of the lung. This operation is called a ***pneumonectomy*** (nu-mo-NEK-to-me).

Malignant tumors of the stomach, breast, and other organs may spread to the lungs as secondary growths (metastases).

Recovering From Smoking: Yes You Can!

The damage to your respiratory system caused by smoking tobacco products is not necessarily permanent. Many studies have documented the following benefits of stopping smoking:

- Risk of having a heart attack returns to that of a nonsmoker within about 1 to 2 years.
- Risk of having a stroke returns to that of a nonsmoker within 1 to 3 years
- Rate of deterioration of lung function returns to that caused simply by age within about 3 years
- Risk of developing lung cancer returns to baseline in as little as 10 years
- Risk of developing rapidly advancing chronic obstructive pulmonary disease (COPD) returns to baseline after 5 years.

Of all patients who stop smoking each year, 90% do so with no medical assistance. However, in any given year, only 3.6% of all smokers succeed in their efforts to stop. To increase the chance of successful cessation, doctors advise the following:

- Select a specific quit date
- Use behavior modification to substitute for your normal cues to smoking
- Quit "cold turkey;" it works better than tapering off
- Manage tobacco withdrawal; nicotine gum or patches should be started on the quit date; the antidepressant medication buproprion may be started 1–2 weeks before the quit date

Disorders Involving the Pleural Space

Pleurisy (PLUR-ih-se), or inflammation of the pleura, usually accompanies a lung infection—particularly pneumonia or tuberculosis. This condition can be quite painful because the inflammation produces a sticky exudate that roughens the pleura of both the lung and the chest wall; when the two surfaces rub together during ventilation, the roughness causes acute irritation. The sticking together of two surfaces is called an ***adhesion*** (ad-HE-zhun).

Infection of the pleura also causes an increase in the amount of pleural fluid. This fluid may accumulate in the pleural space in quantities large enough to compress the lung, resulting in an inability to obtain enough air.

Pneumothorax is an accumulation of air in the pleural space. The lung on the affected side collapses, causing the patient to have great difficulty breathing. Pneumothorax may be caused by a wound in the chest wall or by rupture of lung air spaces. In a pneumothorax caused by a penetrating wound in the chest wall, an airtight cover over the opening prevents further air from entering. The remaining lung can then function to provide adequate amounts of oxygen.

Blood in the pleural space, a condition called **hemothorax,** is also caused by penetrating wounds of the chest. In such cases, the first priority is to stop the bleeding.

The abnormal accumulation of fluid or air in the pleural space from any of the above conditions may call for procedures to promote lung expansion. In *thoracentesis* (thor-ah-sen-TE-sis) a large-bore needle is inserted between ribs into the pleural space below the lung to remove fluid. The presence of both air and fluid in the pleural space may require insertion of a chest tube, a large tube with several openings along the internal end. The tube is securely connected to a water-seal chest drainage system. These procedures restore negative pressure in the pleural space and allow re-expansion of the lung.

AGE AND THE RESPIRATORY TRACT

With age, the tissues of the respiratory tract lose elasticity and become more rigid. Similar rigidity in the chest wall, combined with arthritis and loss of strength in the breathing muscles, results in an overall decrease in compliance and in lung capacity. Reduction in protective mechanisms, such as phagocytosis in the lungs, leads to increased susceptibility to infection. The incidence of emphysema increases with age, hastened by cigarette smoking and by exposure to other environmental irritants. Although there is much individual variation, especially related to how much activity one is accustomed to, these changes gradually lead to reduced capacity for exercise.

SPECIAL EQUIPMENT FOR RESPIRATORY TREATMENT

The *bronchoscope* (BRONG-ko-skope) is a rigid or flexible fiberoptic tubular instrument used for inspection of the primary bronchi and the larger bronchial tubes. Most bronchoscopes are now attached to video recording equipment. The bronchoscope is passed into the respiratory tract by way of the mouth and the pharynx. It may be used to remove foreign bodies, to inspect and take tissue samples (biopsies) from tumors, or to collect other specimens. Children inhale a variety of objects, such as pins, beans, pieces of nuts, and small coins, all of which may be removed with the aid of a bronchoscope. If such items are left in the lung, an abscess or other serious complication may result and can cause death.

Oxygen therapy is used to sustain life when some condition interferes with adequate oxygen supply to the tissues. The oxygen must first have moisture added by being bubbled through water that is at room temperature or heated. Oxygen may be delivered to the patient by mask, catheter, or nasal prongs. Because there is danger of fire when oxygen is being administered, no one in the room should smoke.

A *suction apparatus* is used for removing mucus or other substances from the respiratory tract by means of negative pressure. A container to trap secretions is located between the patient and the machine. The tube leading to the patient has an opening to control application of the suction. When suction is applied, the drainage flows from the patient's respiratory tract into the collection container.

A *tracheostomy* (tra-ke-OS-to-me) *tube* is used if the pharynx or the larynx is obstructed. It is a small metal or plastic tube that is inserted through a cut made in the trachea, and it acts as an artificial airway for ventilation. The procedure for the insertion of such a tube is a *tracheostomy*. The word *tracheotomy* (tra-ke-OT-o-me) refers to the incision in the trachea.

18

Artificial respiration is used when a patient has temporarily lost the capacity to perform the normal motions of respiration. Such emergencies include cases of smoke asphyxiation, electric shock, and drowning.

Classes are offered by many public agencies in the techniques of mouth-to-mouth respiration and cardiac massage to revive people experiencing respiratory or cardiac arrest. This technique is known as *cardiopulmonary resuscitation,* or *CPR.* Part of these classes is instruction in emergency airway clearance using abdominal thrusts (Heimlich maneuver), chest thrusts, or back blows to open obstructed airways.

Summary

I. The respiratory system
A. Nasal cavities—filter, warm, and moisten air
B. Pharynx (throat)—carries air into respiratory tract and food into digestive tract
C. Larynx (voice box)—contains vocal cords
   1. Epiglottis—covers larynx on swallowing to help prevent food from entering
D. Trachea (windpipe)
E. Bronchi—branches of trachea that enter lungs and then subdivide
   1. Bronchioles—smallest subdivisions
F. Lungs
   1. Organs of gas exchange
   2. Lobes: three on right; two on left
   3. Alveoli
      a. Tiny air sacs where gases are exchanged
      b. Surfactant—reduces surface tension in alveoli; eases expansion of lungs
   4. Pleura—membrane that encloses the lung
      a. Visceral pleura—attached to surface of lung
      b. Parietal pleura—attached to chest wall
      c. Pleural space—between layers
   5. Mediastinum—space and organs between lungs

II. The process of respiration
A. Pulmonary ventilation
   1. Inhalation—drawing of air into lungs
      a. Compliance—ease with which lungs and thorax can be expanded
   2. Exhalation—expulsion of air from lungs
   3. Lung volumes—used to evaluate respiratory function (*e.g.,* vital capacity, total lung capacity)
B. Gas exchange in the lungs
   1. Gases diffuse from area of higher concentration to area of lower concentration
   2. In lungs—oxygen enters blood and carbon dioxide leaves
   3. In tissues—oxygen leaves blood and carbon dioxide enters
C. Gas transport
   1. Oxygen—almost totally bound to heme portion of hemoglobin in red blood cells; separates from hemoglobin when oxygen concentration is low (in tissues)
      a. Carbon monoxide replaces oxygen on hemoglobin
   2. Carbon dioxide—most carried as bicarbonate ion; regulates pH of blood
D. Regulation of respiration
   1. Normal ventilation
      a. Controlled by center in medulla and pons
      b. Chemoreceptors detect changes in gas composition of blood
E. Abnormal ventilation

1. Hyperventilation—rapid, deep respiration
2. Hypoventilation—inadequate air in alveoli

F. Breathing patterns
1. Normal—12 to 20 times per minute in adult
2. Types of altered breathing
   a. Hyperpnea—increase in depth and rate of breathing
   b. Tachypnea—excessive rate of breathing
   c. Apnea—temporary cessation of breathing
   d. Dyspnea—difficulty in breathing
   e. Orthopnea—difficulty relieved by upright position
   f. Cheyne-Stokes—irregularity found in critically ill
3. Possible results—cyanosis, hypoxia (anoxia), hypoxemia, suffocation

III. Disorders of the respiratory system
A. Disorders of the nasal cavities and related structures—sinusitis, polyps, deviated septum, nosebleed (epistaxis)
B. Infection—colds, influenza, pneumonia, tuberculosis
C. Hay fever and asthma—hypersensitivity (allergy)

D. COPD—involves emphysema and bronchitis
E. Atelectasis—collapse of lung or portion of lung; seen in respiratory distress syndrome due to lack of surfactant
F. Lung cancer—smoking a major causative factor
G. Disorders involving the pleural space
1. Pleurisy—inflammation of pleura
2. Pneumothorax—air in pleural space
3. Hemothorax—blood in pleural space

IV. Age and the respiratory tract

V. Special equipment for respiratory treatment
1. Bronchoscope—tube used to examine air passageways and remove foreign bodies
2. Oxygen therapy
3. Suction apparatus—removes mucus and other substances
4. Tracheostomy—artificial airway
   a. Tracheotomy—incision into trachea
5. Artificial respiration—cardiopulmonary resuscitation (CPR)

Questions for Study and Review

1. What is the definition of *respiration* and what are its three phases?
2. Trace the pathway of air from outside the body into the blood.
3. What is the purpose of the cilia on the cells that line the respiratory passageways?
4. What are the advantages of breathing through the nose?
5. What muscles are used for inhalation? forceful exhalation?
6. How is oxygen transported in the blood? What causes its release to the tissues?
7. How is carbon dioxide transported in the blood?
8. How does the pH of the blood change as the level of carbon dioxide increases? decreases?
9. Why does hyperventilation cause a cessation of breathing?
10. What are chemoreceptors and how do they function to regulate breathing?
11. Name and describe six types of abnormal breathing.
12. Define five volumes or capacities used to measure breathing.
13. Name several conditions that may result from inadequate breathing.
14. What are *sinusitis, polyps,* and *deviated septum?* What is the effect of each?
15. What are some causes of nosebleed?

16. Give some examples and describe the effects of upper respiratory infections.
17. What triggers hay fever and asthma?
18. What changes occur in the lungs in chronic obstructive lung disease?
19. What are the symptoms of atelectasis?
20. What are some possible causes of lung cancer?
21. What is pleurisy? What are its complications?
22. Describe pneumothorax.
23. Name and describe several devices used in treatment of the respiratory tract.
24. Define:
    a. *epiglottis*
    b. *alveolus*
    c. *surfactant*
    d. *pleura*
    e. *mediastinum*
    f. *compliance*

✔ ANSWERS TO CHECKPOINTS

1. The three phases of respiration are pulmonary ventilation, diffusion of gases, and transport of gases in the blood.
2. As air passes over the nasal mucosa, it is filtered, warmed, and moistened.
3. The scientific name for the throat is pharynx, for the voice box is larynx, and for the windpipe is trachea.
4. The cells that line the respiratory passageways have cilia to filter impurities and to move fluids.
5. The pleura is the membrane that encloses the lung.
6. The two phases of breathing are inhalation, which is active, and exhalation, which is passive.
7. Diffusion is the movement of molecules from an area in which they are in higher concentration to an area where they are in lower concentration.
8. The substance in red blood cells that carries almost all of the oxygen in the blood is hemoglobin.
9. The main form in which carbon dioxide is carried in the blood is as bicarbonate ion.
10. The medulla of the brain stem sets the basic pattern of respiration.
11. The phrenic nerve is the motor nerve that controls the diaphragm.
12. Carbon dioxide is the main chemical controller of respiration.
13. Influenza, pneumonia, colds, and tuberculosis are some infectious diseases of the respiratory tract.

Digestion

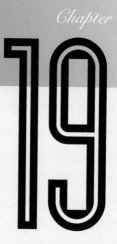

Chapter

19

SELECTED KEY TERMS

The following terms are defined in the Glossary:

absorption

bile

chyle

chyme

colon

defecation

deglutition

digestion

duodenum

emulsify

enzyme

esophagus

hydrolysis

lacteal

mastication

peristalsis

peritoneum

saliva

sphincter

ulcer

villi

BEHAVIORAL OBJECTIVES

After careful study of this chapter, you should be able to:

1. Name the two main functions of the digestive system
2. Describe the four layers of the digestive tract wall
3. Differentiate between the two layers of the peritoneum
4. Name and describe the functions of the organs of the digestive tract
5. Name and describe the functions of the accessory organs of digestion
6. Describe how bile functions in digestion
7. Name the ducts that carry bile from the liver into the digestive tract
8. Explain the role of enzymes in digestion and give examples of enzymes
9. Name the digestion products of fats, proteins, and carbohydrates
10. Define *absorption*
11. Define *villi* and state how villi function in absorption
12. Explain the use of feedback in regulating digestion and give several examples
13. List several hormones involved in regulating digestion
14. Describe common disorders of the digestive tract and the accessory organs

FUNCTION AND DESIGN OF THE DIGESTIVE SYSTEM

Every body cell needs a constant supply of nutrients to provide energy and to provide the building blocks for the manufacture of body substances. Food as we take it in, however, is too large to enter the cells. It must first be broken down into particles small enough to pass through the plasma membrane of the cell. This breakdown process is known as *digestion.*

After digestion, food must be carried to the cells in every part of the body by the circulation. The transfer of food into the circulation is called *absorption*. Digestion and absorption are the two chief functions of the digestive system.

For our purposes, the digestive system may be divided into two groups of organs:

* The *digestive tract,* a continuous passageway beginning at the mouth, where food is taken in, and terminating at the anus, where the solid waste products of digestion are expelled from the body
* The *accessory organs,* which are necessary for the digestive process but are not a direct part of the digestive tract. They release substances into the digestive tract through ducts. These organs are the salivary glands, liver, gallbladder, and pancreas.

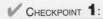

✔ CHECKPOINT **1**:

Why does food have to be digested before it can be used by cells?

Before describing the individual organs of the digestive tract, we will pause to discuss the general pattern of the organs and also the large membrane (peritoneum) that lines the abdominopelvic cavity in which most of the digestive organs are contained.

The Wall of the Digestive Tract

Although modified for specific tasks in different organs, the wall of the digestive tract, from the esophagus to the anus, is similar in structure throughout. The general pattern consists of four layers:

* Mucous membrane
* Submucosa
* Smooth muscle
* Serous membrane

Refer to the diagram of the small intestine in Figure 19-1 as we describe the layers of this wall from the innermost to the outermost surface.

First is the *mucous membrane,* or *mucosa*, so called because its epithelial layer contains many mucus-secreting cells. From the mouth through the esophagus, and also in the anus,

19

345

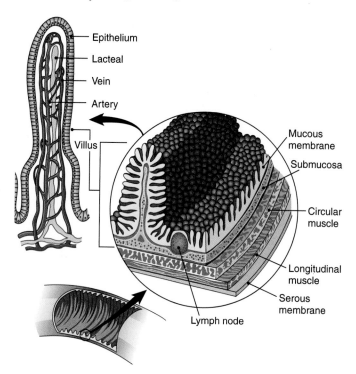

- Epithelium
- Lacteal
- Vein
- Artery

Villus

Mucous membrane

Submucosa

Circular muscle

Longitudinal muscle

Serous membrane

Lymph node

FIGURE **19•1** Diagram of the wall of the small intestine showing numerous villi. At the left is an enlarged drawing of a single villus.

the epithelium consists of multiple layers of squamous (flat) cells, which aid in protection of deeper tissues. Throughout the remainder of the digestive tract, the type of epithelium in the mucosa is simple columnar. Figure 19-2 is a microscopic view of the small intestine; the

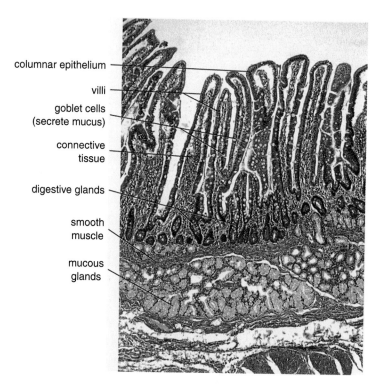

columnar epithelium

villi

goblet cells (secrete mucus)

connective tissue

digestive glands

smooth muscle

mucous glands

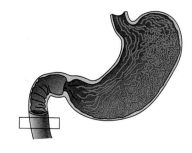

FIGURE **19•2** Microscopic view of the small intestine (duodenum). (Cormack DH: Essential Histology, Plate 13-48. Philadelphia, JB Lippincott, 1993)

mucus-secreting cells appear as clear areas between epithelial cells.

The layer of connective tissue beneath the mucosa is the **submucosa,** which contains blood vessels and some of the nerves that help regulate digestive activity.

The next layer is composed of **smooth muscle**. Most of the digestive organs have two layers of smooth muscle: an inner layer of circular fibers, and an outer layer of longitudinal fibers. The alternate contractions of these muscles create the wavelike movement that propels food through the digestive tract and mixes it with digestive juices. This movement is called **peristalsis** (per-ih-STAL-sis).

The esophagus differs slightly from this pattern in having striated muscle in its upper portion, and the stomach has an additional third layer of smooth muscle in its wall to add strength for churning food.

The digestive organs in the abdominopelvic cavity have an outermost layer of **serous membrane,** a thin, moist tissue composed of simple squamous epithelium and loose connective tissue. This membrane forms part of the peritoneum (per-i-to-NE-um). The esophagus above the diaphragm has instead an outer layer composed of fibrous connective tissue.

✔ CHECKPOINT **2:**

Most of the digestive tract has a wall that is similar throughout its length and is composed of four layers. What are the typical four layers of this wall?

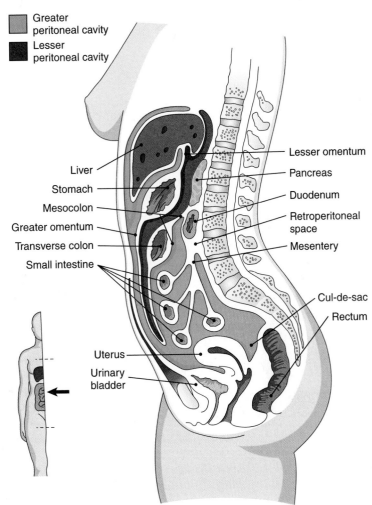

Greater peritoneal cavity

Lesser peritoneal cavity

Liver

Stomach

Mesocolon

Greater omentum

Transverse colon

Small intestine

Uterus

Urinary bladder

Lesser omentum

Pancreas

Duodenum

Retroperitoneal space

Mesentery

Cul-de-sac

Rectum

FIGURE **19•3** Diagram of the abdominal cavity showing the peritoneum.

19

The Peritoneum

The abdominopelvic cavity is lined with a thin, shiny serous membrane that also folds back to cover most of the organs contained within the cavity (Fig. 19-3). The outer portion of this membrane, the layer that lines the cavity, is called the ***parietal peritoneum;*** that covering the organs is called the ***visceral peritoneum***. The peritoneum carries blood vessels, lymphatic vessels, and nerves. In some places, it serves to support the organs and to bind them to each other. Subdivisions of the peritoneum around the various organs have special names.

Subdivisions of the Peritoneum

The ***mesentery*** (MES-en-ter-e) is a double-layered portion of the peritoneum shaped somewhat like a fan. The handle portion is attached to the back wall, and the expanded long edge is attached to the small intestine. Between the two layers of membrane that form the mesentery are the vessels and nerves that supply the intestine. The section of the peritoneum that extends from the colon to the back wall is the ***mesocolon*** (mes-o-KO-lon).

A large double layer of the peritoneum containing much fat hangs like an apron over the front of the intestine. This ***greater omentum*** (o-MEN-tum) extends from the lower border of the stomach into the pelvic part of the abdomen and then loops back up to the transverse colon. There is also a smaller membrane, called the ***lesser omentum,*** that extends between the stomach and the liver.

> ✔ CHECKPOINT **3**:
>
> What is the name of the large serous membrane that lines the abdominopelvic cavity and covers the organs it contains?

Peritonitis

Inflammation of the peritoneum, termed ***peritonitis*** (per-ih-to-NI-tis), is a serious complication that may follow infection of one of the organs covered by the peritoneum—often, the appendix. The frequency and severity of peritonitis have been greatly reduced by the use of antibiotics. The disorder still occurs, however, and can be dangerous. If the infection is kept in one area, it is said to be *localized peritonitis*. A *generalized peritonitis,* as may be caused by a ruptured appendix, a perforated ulcer, or a penetrating wound, may lead to the growth of so many disease organisms and the release of so much bacterial toxin as to be fatal. Immediate surgery to repair the rupture and medical care are needed.

ORGANS OF THE DIGESTIVE TRACT

As we study the organs of the digestive system, locate each in Figure 19-4.

The digestive tract is a muscular tube extending through the body. It is composed of several parts: the ***mouth, pharynx, esophagus, stomach, small intestine,*** and ***large intestine.*** The digestive tract is sometimes called the ***alimentary tract,*** derived from a Latin word that means "food." It is more commonly referred to as the ***gastrointestinal (GI) tract*** because of the major importance of the stomach and intestine in the process of digestion.

The Mouth

The mouth, also called the ***oral cavity,*** is where a substance begins its travels through the digestive tract (Fig. 19-5). The mouth has three digestive functions:

* To receive food, a process called ***ingestion***
* To prepare food for digestion
* To begin the digestion of starch

Digestive activities in the mouth require saliva, a secretion that is produced by the salivary glands and secreted into the mouth. The salivary glands are described with the other accessory organs.

The tongue, a muscular organ that projects into the mouth, is used as an aid in chewing and in swallowing and is one of the principal organs of speech. The tongue has on its surface a number of special organs, called *taste buds,* by

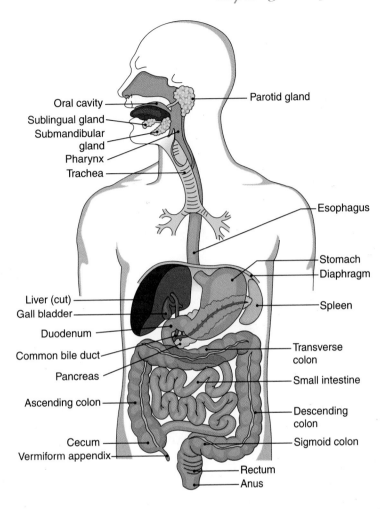

Figure **19•4** Digestive system.

means of which taste sensations (bitter, sweet, sour, or salty) can be differentiated.

The Teeth

The oral cavity also contains the teeth (see Fig. 19-5). A child between 2 and 6 years of age has 20 teeth, known as the baby teeth or ***deciduous*** (de-SID-u-us) teeth. (The word *deciduous* means "falling off at a certain time," such as the leaves that fall off the trees in autumn.) A complete set of adult permanent teeth numbers 32. Among these, the cutting teeth, or ***incisors,*** occupy the front part of the oral cavity, whereas the larger grinding teeth, the ***molars,*** are in the back.

The first eight deciduous (baby) teeth to appear through the gums are the incisors. Later, the ***cuspids*** (commonly called *canines* or *eyeteeth*) and molars appear. Usually, the 20 baby teeth have all appeared by the time a child has

reached the age of 2 to 3 years. During the first 2 years, the permanent teeth develop within the upper jaw (maxilla) and lower jaw (mandible) from buds that are present at birth. The first permanent tooth to appear is the important 6-year molar. This permanent tooth comes in before the baby incisors are lost. Because decay and infection of adjacent deciduous molars may spread to and involve new, permanent teeth, deciduous teeth need proper care.

As a child grows, the jawbones grow, making space for additional teeth. After the 6-year molars have appeared, the baby incisors loosen and are replaced by permanent incisors. Next, the baby canines (cuspids) are replaced by permanent canines, and finally, the baby molars are replaced by the bicuspids (premolars) of the permanent teeth.

Now the larger jawbones are ready for the appearance of the 12-year, or second, permanent

19

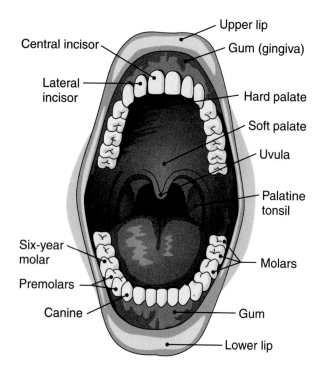

FIGURE **19•5** The mouth, showing the teeth and tonsils.

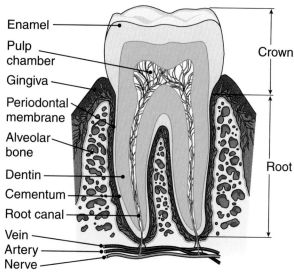

FIGURE **19•6** A molar tooth. (Cohen B: Medical Terminology: An Illustrated Guide, 3rd ed, p. 226. Philadelphia, Lippincott-Raven, 1998)

molar teeth. During or after the late teens, the third molars, or so-called *wisdom teeth,* may appear. In some cases, the jaw is not large enough for these teeth, or there are other abnormalities, so that the third molars may not erupt or may have to be removed. Figure 19-6 shows the parts of a molar.

✓ CHECKPOINT **4**:

How many baby teeth are there and what is the scientific name for the baby teeth?

Diseases of the Mouth and Teeth

Tooth decay is also termed dental *caries* (KA-reze), which means "rottenness." It has a number of causes, including diet, heredity, mechanical problems, and endocrine disorders. People who ingest a lot of sugar are particularly prone to this disease. Because a baby's teeth begin to develop before birth, the diet of the mother during pregnancy is important in ensuring the formation of healthy teeth in her baby.

Any infection of the gum is called *gingivitis* (jin-jih-VI-tis). If such an infection continues and is untreated, it may lead to a more serious condition, *periodontitis* (per-e-o-don-TI-tis), which involves not only the gum tissue but also the supporting bone of the teeth. Loosening of the teeth and destruction of the supporting bone follow unless the process is halted by proper treatment and improved dental hygiene. Periodontitis is responsible for nearly 80% of loss of teeth in people older than 45 years of age.

Vincent's disease, a kind of gingivitis caused by a spirochete or a bacillus, is most prevalent in teenagers and young adults. Characterized by inflammation, ulceration, and infection of the mucous membranes of the mouth and gums, this disorder is highly contagious, particularly by oral contact.

Patients on antibiotic therapy are more likely than normal to develop fungal infections of the mouth and tongue because these drugs may destroy the normal bacteria of the mouth and allow other organisms to grow.

Leukoplakia (lu-ko-PLA-ke-ah) is characterized by thickened white patches on the mucous membranes of the mouth. It is common in smokers and is considered precancerous.

The Pharynx

The **pharynx** (FAR-inks) is commonly referred to as the *throat* (see Fig. 18-1 in Chap. 18). The oral part of the pharynx, the oropharynx, is visible when you look into an open mouth and depress the tongue. The palatine tonsils may be seen at either side of the oropharynx. The pharynx also extends upward to the nasal cavity as the nasopharynx and downward to the level of the larynx as the laryngeal pharynx. The **soft palate** is tissue that forms the back of the roof of the oral cavity. From it hangs a soft, fleshy, V-shaped mass called the **uvula** (U-vu-lah), which is used in speech production.

In swallowing, a **bolus,** a small portion of chewed food mixed with saliva, is pushed by the tongue into the pharynx. When the food reaches the pharynx, swallowing occurs rapidly by an involuntary reflex action. At the same time, the soft palate and uvula are raised to prevent food and liquid from entering the nasal cavity, and the tongue is raised to seal the back of the oral cavity. The entrance of the trachea is guarded during swallowing by a leaf-shaped cartilage, the **epiglottis,** which covers the opening of the larynx. The swallowed food is then moved into the esophagus.

The Esophagus

The **esophagus** (eh-SOF-ah-gus) is a muscular tube about 25 cm (10 inches) long. In the esophagus, food is lubricated with mucus and moved by peristalsis into the stomach. No additional digestion occurs in the esophagus.

Before joining the stomach, the esophagus must pass through the diaphragm. It travels through a space in the diaphragm called the **esophageal hiatus** (eh-sof-ah-JE-al hi-A-tus). If there is a weakness in the diaphragm at this point, a portion of the stomach or other abdominal organ may protrude through the space, a condition called **hiatal hernia.**

The esophagus is prone to develop to varicose veins in cases of liver disease. These varices are subject to severe bleeding.

The Stomach

The stomach is an expanded J-shaped organ in the upper left region of the abdominal cavity (Fig. 19-7). In addition to the two muscle layers already described, it has a third, inner oblique (angled) layer that aids in grinding food and mixing it with digestive juices. The left-facing arch of the stomach is the **greater curvature,** whereas the right surface forms the **lesser curvature.**

Sphincters

A muscular ring, or **sphincter** (SFINK-ter), that permits the passage of substances in only one direction guards each end of the stomach.

Between the esophagus and the stomach is the **lower esophageal sphincter (LES).** This valve has also been called the **cardiac sphincter** because it separates the esophagus from the region of the stomach that is close to the heart. We are sometimes aware of the existence of this sphincter; sometimes, it does not relax as it should, producing a feeling of being unable to swallow past that point.

Between the distal, or far, end of the stomach and the small intestine is the **pyloric** (pi-LOR-ik) **sphincter**. The region of the stomach leading into this sphincter, the **pylorus** (pi-LOR-us), is important in regulating how rapidly food moves into the small intestine.

Functions of the Stomach

The stomach serves as a storage pouch, digestive organ, and churn. When the stomach is empty, the lining forms many folds called **rugae** (RU-je). These folds disappear as the stomach expands. (It may be stretched to hold one half of a gallon of food and liquid.) Special cells in the lining of the stomach secrete substances that mix together to form **gastric juice,** the two main components of which are the following:

* Hydrochloric acid (HCl), a strong acid that softens the connective tissue in meat and destroys foreign organisms
* Pepsin, a protein-digesting enzyme produced in an inactive form and activated only when food enters the stomach and HCl is produced

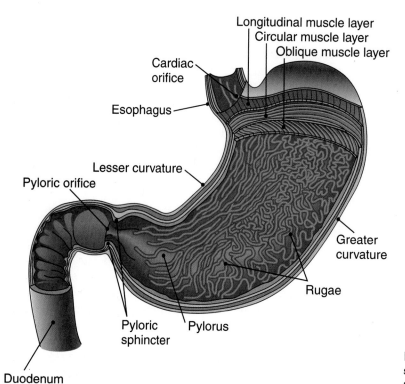

FIGURE **19•7** Longitudinal section of the stomach and a portion of the duodenum showing the interior.

Longitudinal muscle layer
Circular muscle layer
Oblique muscle layer
Cardiac orifice
Esophagus
Lesser curvature
Pyloric orifice
Pyloric sphincter
Pylorus
Duodenum
Greater curvature
Rugae

The semiliquid mixture of gastric juice and food that leaves the stomach to enter the small intestine is called *chyme* (kime).

✔ CHECKPOINT **5**:

What type of food is digested in the stomach?

Disorders Involving the Stomach

A burning sensation in the region of the esophagus and stomach, popularly known as *heartburn,* is often caused by the sudden intake of a large amount of fluid or food, resulting in excessive stretching of the lower esophagus. This interferes with the functioning of the lower esophageal sphincter, allowing gastric acid to enter the esophagus. Contrary to popular belief, heartburn is not due to hyperacidity of the stomach contents.

Nausea is an unpleasant sensation that may follow distention or irritation of the lower esophagus or of the stomach as a result of various nervous and mechanical factors. It may be a symptom of interference with the normal forward peristaltic motion of the stomach and intestine and thus may be followed by vomiting.

Vomiting is the expulsion of gastric (and sometimes intestinal) contents through the mouth by reverse peristalsis. The contraction of the abdominal wall muscles forcibly empties the stomach. Vomiting is frequently caused by overeating or by inflammation of the stomach lining, a condition called *gastritis* (gas-TRI-tis). Gastritis results from irritation of the mucosa by certain drugs, food, or drinks. For example, the long-term use of aspirin, highly spiced foods, or alcohol can lead to gastritis. The nicotine in cigarettes can also cause gastritis.

Flatus (FLA-tus) usually refers to excessive amounts of air (gas) in the stomach or intestine. The resulting condition is referred to as *flatulence* (FLAT-u-lens). In some cases, it may be necessary to insert a tube into the stomach or rectum to aid the patient in expelling flatus.

Stomach Cancer

Although stomach cancer has become rare in the United States, it is common in many parts of the world, and it is an important disorder because of the high death rate associated with it.

Males are more susceptible than females to stomach cancer. The tumor nearly always develops from the epithelial or mucosal lining of the stomach and is often of the type called ***adenocarcinoma*** (ad-en-o-kar-sih-NO-mah). Sometimes, the victim has suffered from long-standing indigestion but has failed to consult a physician until the cancer has spread to other organs, such as the liver or lymph nodes, in which there may be several metastases. Persistent indigestion is one of the important warning signs of cancer of the stomach.

Peptic Ulcer

An ulcer is an area of the skin or mucous membrane in which the tissues are gradually destroyed. ***Peptic ulcers*** (named for the enzyme pepsin) occur in the mucous membrane of the esophagus, stomach, or duodenum (the first part of the small intestine) and are most common in people between the ages of 30 and 45 years. Peptic ulcers in the stomach are *gastric ulcers;* those in the duodenum are *duodenal* (du-o-DE-nal) *ulcers.*

Smoking cigarettes and taking aspirin or other anti-inflammatory drugs are major causative factors. Recently, it has been found that infection with a bacterium, *Helicobacter pylori,* is a factor in causing peptic ulcers. The organism is associated with inflammation of the stomach and duodenum, and most people with ulcers who have this infection are cured when the organism is eliminated with antibiotics. Drugs that inhibit the secretion of stomach acids are often an effective aid in treatment.

Pyloric Stenosis

Normally, the stomach contents are moved through the pyloric sphincter within about 2 to 6 hours after eating. Some infants, however, most often boys, are born with an obstruction of the pyloric sphincter, a condition called ***pyloric stenosis*** (steh-NO-sis). Usually, surgery is required in these cases to modify the muscle, so that food can pass from the stomach into the duodenum.

The Small Intestine

The small intestine is the longest part of the digestive tract. It is known as the small intestine because, although it is longer than the large in-

testine, it is smaller in diameter, with an average width of about 2.5 cm (1 inch). After death, when relaxed to its full length, the small intestine is about 6 m (20 feet) long. In life, the small intestine averages 3 m (10 feet) in length. The first 25 cm (10 inches) or so of the small intestine make up the ***duodenum*** (du-o-DE-num). Beyond the duodenum are two more divisions: the ***jejunum*** (je-JU-num), which forms the next two fifths of the small intestine, and the ***ileum*** (IL-e-um), which constitutes the remaining portion.

Functions of the Small Intestine

The wall of the duodenum contains glands that secrete large amounts of mucus to protect the small intestine from the strongly acidic chyme entering from the stomach. Cells of the small intestine also secrete enzymes that digest proteins and carbohydrates. In addition, digestive juices from the liver and pancreas enter the small intestine through a small opening in the duodenum. Most of the digestive process takes place in the small intestine under the effects of these juices.

Most absorption of digested food also occurs through the walls of the small intestine. To increase the surface area of the organ for this purpose, the mucosa is formed into millions of tiny, fingerlike projections, called ***villi*** (VIL-li) (see Fig. 19-1), which give the inner surface a velvety appearance. In addition, each epithelial cell has small projecting folds of the cell membrane known as ***microvilli***. These create a remarkable increase in the total surface area available in the small intestine for the absorption of nutrients (see Surface Area and Transport).

> ✔ CHECKPOINT **6**:
>
> How does the small intestine function in the digestive process?

The Large Intestine

Any material that cannot be digested as it passes through the digestive tract must be eliminated from the body. In addition, most of the water secreted into the digestive tract for

Surface Area and Transport

Whenever materials pass from one system to another, they must travel through a cellular membrane. A major factor in how much transport can occur per unit of time is the total surface area of the membrane.

The problem of packing a large amount of surface into a small space is solved in the body by folding the membranes. We do the same thing in everyday life. Imagine trying to store a bed sheet in the closet without folding it!

In the small intestine, where digested food must move into the bloodstream, there is folding of membranes down to the level of the single cells.

- The organ as a whole is coiled to fit its length into the abdominal cavity.
- The inner wall of the organ forms circular folds called *plicae circulares.*
- The projecting villi provide more surface area than a flat membrane would.
- The individual cells that line the small intestine have microvilli, tiny fingerlike folds of the cell membrane, that increase surface area tremendously.

Can you name other portions of the digestive tract or other systems that show this folding pattern and explain why it is there?

proper digestion must be reabsorbed into the bloodstream to prevent dehydration. The storage and elimination of undigested waste and the reabsorption of water are the functions of the large intestine.

The large intestine is about 6.5 cm (2.5 inches) in diameter and about 1.5 m (5 feet) long. The outer longitudinal muscle fibers in its wall form three separate bands on the surface. These bands draw up the wall of the organ to give it its distinctive puckered appearance.

Subdivisions of the Large Intestine

The large intestine begins in the lower right region of the abdomen. The first part is a small pouch called the *cecum* (SE-kum). Between the ileum of the small intestine and the cecum is a sphincter, the *ileocecal* (il-e-o-SE-kal) *valve,* that prevents food from traveling backward into the small intestine. Attached to the cecum is a small, blind tube containing lymphoid tissue; its full name is *vermiform* (VER-mih-form) *appendix* (*vermiform* means "wormlike"). Inflammation of this tissue as a result of infection or obstruction is *appendicitis*.

The second portion, the *ascending colon,* extends upward along the right side of the abdomen toward the liver. The large intestine then bends and extends across the abdomen, forming the *transverse colon*. At this point, it bends sharply and extends downward on the left side of the abdomen into the pelvis, forming the *descending colon.* The lower part of the colon bends posteriorly in an S shape and continues downward as the *sigmoid colon*. The sigmoid colon empties into the *rectum,* which serves as a temporary storage area for indigestible or nonabsorbable food residue (see Fig. 19-4). Enlargement of the veins in this area constitutes *hemorrhoids*. A narrow portion of the distal large intestine is called the *anal canal*. This leads to the outside of the body through an opening called the *anus* (A-nus).

Functions of the Large Intestine

The large intestine secretes large quantities of mucus but no enzymes. Food is not digested in this organ, but water is reabsorbed, and undigested food is stored, formed into solid waste material called *feces* (FE-seze) or stool, and then eliminated.

At intervals, usually after meals, the involuntary muscles within the walls of the large intestine propel solid waste toward the rectum. Stretching of the rectum stimulates contraction of smooth muscle in the rectal wall. Aided by voluntary contractions of the diaphragm and the abdominal muscles, the feces are eliminated from the body in a process called *defecation* (def-e-KA-shun). An anal sphincter provides voluntary control over defecation.

While the food residue is stored in the large intestine, bacteria that normally live in the colon act on it to produce vitamin K and some of the B-complex vitamins. As mentioned, systemic antibiotic therapy may destroy these symbiotic (helpful) bacteria and others living in the large intestine, causing undesirable side effects.

✓ CHECKPOINT **7**:

What are the functions of the large intestine?

Intestinal Disorders

Inflammatory Diseases

Two similar diseases are included under the heading of *inflammatory bowel disease (IBD)*: *Crohn's* (kronz) *disease* and *ulcerative colitis*. Both occur mainly in adolescents and young adults and cause similar symptoms of pain, diarrhea, weight loss, and rectal bleeding. Crohn's disease usually involves inflammation of the lower part of the small intestine. It may be an autoimmune disease and may be in part hereditary. Ulcerative colitis involves inflammation and ulceration of the lining of the colon and usually the rectum.

Irritable bowel syndrome (IBS) is a common gastrointestinal disorder seen typically in young to middle-aged women. Symptoms include pain and constipation or diarrhea, sometimes both conditions in alternation. In IBS, the intestine is overly sensitive to stimulation, often brought on by stress. Although the condition is chronic and causes much pain, frustration, and anxiety, it is not life-threatening and does not develop into more serious diseases of the bowel.

Difficulties with digestion or absorption may be due to *enteritis* (en-ter-I-tis), an intestinal inflammation. When both the stomach and the small intestine are involved, the disorder is called *gastroenteritis* (gas-tro-en-ter-I-tis). The symptoms of gastroenteritis include nausea, vomiting, and diarrhea as well as acute abdominal pain (colic). The disorder may be caused by a variety of pathogenic organisms, including viruses, bacteria, and protozoa. Chemical irritants, such as alcohol, certain drugs (*e.g.,* aspirin), and other toxins, have been known to cause this disorder as well.

Diarrhea

Diarrhea is a symptom characterized by abnormally frequent watery bowel movements. The danger of diarrhea is dehydration and loss of salts, especially in infants. Diarrhea may result from excess activity of the colon, faulty absorption, or infection. Infections resulting in diarrhea include cholera, dysentery, and food poisoning. Tables 1 and 4 in Appendix 4 list some of the organisms causing these diseases. Such infections are often spread by poor sanitation and by contaminated food, milk, or water. An examination of the stool may be required to establish the cause of diarrhea; examination may reveal the presence of pathogenic organisms, worm eggs, or blood.

Constipation

Millions of dollars are spent each year in an effort to remedy a condition called *constipation.* What is constipation? Many people erroneously think they are constipated if they go a day or more without having a bowel movement. Actually, what is normal varies greatly; one person may normally have a bowel movement only once every 2 or 3 days, whereas another may normally have more than one movement daily. The term *constipation* is also used to refer to hard stools or difficulty with defecation.

On the basis of its onset, constipation may be classified as acute or chronic. Acute constipation occurs suddenly and may be due to an intestinal obstruction, such as a tumor associated with cancer or an inflammation of the saclike bulges (diverticula) of the intestinal wall, as seen in *diverticulitis* (di-ver-tik-u-LI-tis). Laxatives and enemas should be avoided, and a physician should be consulted at once. Chronic constipation, in contrast, has a more gradual onset and may be divided into two groups:

- *Spastic constipation,* in which the intestinal musculature is overstimulated so that the canal becomes narrowed and the space (lumen) inside the intestine is not large enough to permit the passage of fecal material
- *Flaccid* (FLAK-sid) *constipation,* which is characterized by a lazy, or *atonic* (ah-TON-ik), intestinal muscle. Elderly people and those on bed rest are particularly susceptible to this condition. Often, it results from repeated denial of the urge to defecate.

How to Increase Fiber in Your Diet

Fiber in the diet has been deemed to be of benefit in decreasing colon cancer, improving bowel habits, and easing weight loss. Inadequate fiber is a predisposing cause in diverticulosis, bulging pouches in the large intestine.

Fiber is of plant origin and is a type of carbohydrate not digested by the gastrointestinal tract. The amount of fiber recommended for a 2000-calorie diet is 25 grams per day, but most people in the United States tend to get only half of this amount. Fiber-rich foods should be eaten throughout the day to meet the requirement. Note that it is best to increase fiber in the diet gradually to avoid unpleasant symptoms, such as intestinal bloating and flatulence. If your diet lacks fiber, try adding the following foods over a period of several weeks:

- Whole grain bread, cereals, pasta, and brown rice. These add 1 to 3 more grams of fiber per serving than the "white" product.
- Legumes, which include beans, peas, and lentils. These add 4 to 12 grams of fiber per serving.
- Fruits and vegetables. Whole, raw, unpeeled versions contain the most fiber, juices the least. Apple juice has no fiber, whereas a whole apple has 3 grams.
- Unprocessed bran. This can be sprinkled over almost any food: cereal, soups, casseroles. One tablespoon adds 2 grams of fiber. Be sure to take adequate fluids with bran.

Regular bowel habits, moderate exercise, an increase in the ingestion of vegetables and other bulky foods, and an increase in fluid may help people who have sluggish intestinal muscles (see How to Increase Fiber in Your Diet).

The chronic use of laxatives and enemas should be avoided. The streams of fluid used in enemas may injure the lining of the intestine by removing the normal protective mucus. In addition, enemas aggravate hemorrhoids. Enemas should be done only on the order of a physician, and sparingly.

Cancer of the Colon and Rectum

Tumors of the colon and rectum are among the six most common types of cancer in the United States. These tumors are usually adenocarcinomas that arise from the mucosal lining. The occurrence of colon cancer is evenly divided between the sexes, but malignant tumors of the rectum are more common in men than in women.

Tumors may be detected by direct examination of the rectum and lower colon with an instrument called a *sigmoidoscope* (sig-MOY-do-skope) (named for the sigmoid colon). A *colonoscope* (ko-LON-o-skope) is used to examine deeper regions of the colon (see Endoscopy). The presence of blood in the stool may indicate cancer of the bowel or some other gastrointestinal disturbance. A simple chemical test can detect extremely small quantities of blood in the stool, referred to as *occult* ("hidden") *blood*. Early detection and treatment are the keys to increasing survival rates.

Endoscopy

A goal of modern medicine is to find out what is going on inside the body without resorting to invasive surgery. An instrument that has made this possible in many cases is the *endoscope* (EN-do-skope), which is used for examining the interior of a tube or hollow organ. Most endoscopes in use today are *fiberoptic* (fi-ber-OP-tik) *endoscopes,* which contain flexible bundles of glass or plastic that propagate light and can show the lining of internal organs or cavities. Endoscopy is used to detect structural abnormalities, bleeding, ulcers, inflammation, and tumors in organs of the digestive system. In addition to their use for viewing the interior of organs, endoscopes can be used to remove samples of fluid or tissue biopsy specimens. Some surgery can even be done with an endoscope, such as the removal of polyps from the colon or the opening of a sphincter. Other examples of endoscopes are the cystoscope, used for the urinary bladder, and the bronchoscope, which is used to examine the airways, obtain specimens for testing, or remove foreign objects from the respiratory tree.

THE ACCESSORY ORGANS

The Salivary Glands

While food is in the mouth, it is mixed with *saliva*, one purpose of which is to moisten the food and facilitate the processes of chewing, or *mastication* (mas-tih-KA-shun), and swallowing, or *deglutition* (deg-lu-TISH-un). Saliva also helps keep the teeth and mouth clean and helps reduce bacterial growth.

This watery mixture contains mucus and an enzyme called *salivary amylase* (AM-ih-laze), which begins the digestive process by converting starch to sugar. It is manufactured mainly by three pairs of glands that function as accessory organs (see Fig. 19-4):

- The *parotid* (pah-ROT-id) *glands,* the largest of the group, are located below and in front of the ear.
- The *submandibular* (sub-man-DIB-u-lar), or *submaxillary* (sub-MAK-sih-ler-e), *glands* are located near the body of the lower jaw.
- The *sublingual* (sub-LING-gwal) *glands* are under the tongue.

All these glands empty by means of ducts into the oral cavity.

The contagious disease commonly called *mumps* is a viral infection of the parotid salivary glands. This type of *parotitis* (par-o-TI-tis), or inflammation of the parotid glands, may lead to inflammation of the testicles by the same virus. Males affected after puberty are at risk for permanent damage to these sex organs, resulting in sterility. Another complication of mumps that occurs in about 10% of cases is meningitis. Like many contagious diseases, mumps is now preventable by use of a vaccine given to children early in life.

The Liver

The liver, often referred to by the word root *hepat,* is the largest glandular organ of the body (Fig. 19-8). It is located in the upper right portion of the abdominal cavity under the dome of the diaphragm. The lower edge of a normal-sized liver is level with the lower margin of the ribs. The human liver is the same reddish brown color as the animal liver seen in the supermarket. It has a large right lobe and a smaller left lobe; the right lobe includes two in-

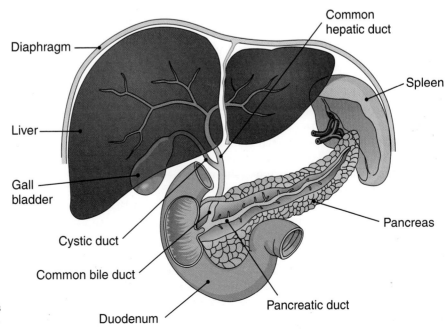

FIGURE **19•8** Accessory organs of digestion.

ferior smaller lobes. The liver is supplied with blood through two vessels: the portal vein and the hepatic artery. These vessels deliver about 1½ quarts of blood to the liver every minute. The hepatic artery carries oxygenated blood, whereas the portal system of veins carries blood that is rich in the end products of digestion. This most remarkable organ has so many functions that only some of its major activities can be listed here:

- The storage of glucose (simple sugar) in the form of *glycogen,* the animal equivalent of the starch found in plants. When the blood sugar level falls below normal, liver cells convert glycogen to glucose, which is released into the bloodstream; this serves to restore the normal concentration of blood sugar.
- The formation of blood plasma proteins, such as albumin, globulins, and clotting factors
- The synthesis of *urea* (u-RE-ah), a waste product of protein metabolism. Urea is released into the blood and transported to the kidneys for elimination.
- The modification of fats, so that they can be used more efficiently by cells all over the body
- The manufacture of bile, a substance needed for the digestion of fats
- The destruction of old red blood cells and the recycling or elimination of their breakdown products. One byproduct, a pigment called *bilirubin* (BIL-ih-ru-bin), is eliminated in bile and gives the stool its characteristic dark color.
- The *detoxification* (de-tok-sih-fih-KA-shun) (removal of the poisonous properties) of harmful substances, such as alcohol and certain drugs
- The storage of some vitamins and iron

The main digestive function of the liver is the production of *bile*. The salts contained in bile act like a detergent to *emulsify* fat, that is, to break up fat into small droplets that can be acted on more effectively by digestive enzymes. Bile also aids in the absorption of fat from the small intestine.

Bile leaves the lobes of the liver by two ducts that merge to form the *common hepatic duct.* After collecting bile from the gallbladder, this duct, now called the *common bile duct,* delivers bile into the duodenum. These and the other accessory ducts are shown in Figure 19-8.

Diseases of the Liver
Hepatitis

Inflammation of the liver, called *hepatitis* (hep-ah-TI-tis), may be caused by drugs, alcohol, or infection (see Table 3 in Appendix 4). The known viruses that cause hepatitis are named A through G. These vary in route (pathway) of infection, severity, and complications. All types of hepatitis are marked by hepatic cell destruction and such symptoms as loss of appetite, jaundice, and liver enlargement. In most patients, the liver cells regenerate with little residual damage. The types of hepatitis and their primary routes of transmission are as follows:

Hepatitis A: commonly transmitted in fecal matter and contaminated food and water. There is a vaccine for hepatitis A, which is recommended for people traveling to areas where this disease is a threat.

Hepatitis B: transmitted by direct exchange of blood or body fluids, although it also can be spread by fecal contamination. This is the most prevalent form of hepatitis, and it is usually transmitted by use of improperly sterilized needles. A vaccine is available that is now recommended for childhood immunization and for people working in health care and child care.

Hepatitis C: transmitted primarily by direct exchange of blood with evidence of limited sexual exchange

Hepatitis D: transmitted by direct exchange of blood. It occurs only in those with hepatitis B infection.

Hepatitis E: transmitted by fecal contamination of water. Most cases have been linked to epidemics in the Middle East and Asia.

Hepatitis G: transmitted by direct exchange of blood

There is no specific treatment for hepatitis.

Cirrhosis

Cirrhosis (sih-RO-sis) of the liver is a chronic disease in which active liver cells are replaced by inactive connective (scar) tissue. The most common type of cirrhosis is alcoholic (portal) cirrhosis. Alcohol has a direct damaging effect on liver cells that is compounded by malnutrition. Destruction of the liver cells hampers the portal circulation, causing blood to accumulate in the spleen and gastrointestinal tract and causing fluid (ascites) to accumulate in the peritoneal cavity.

Jaundice

Damage to the liver or blockage in any of the bile ducts may cause bile pigment to accumulate in the blood. As a result, the stool may become pale in color and the skin and sclera of the eyes may become yellowish; this symptom is called **jaundice** (JAWN-dis). Jaundice may also be caused by excess destruction of red blood cells. In addition, it is often seen in newborns, in whom the liver is immature and not yet functioning efficiently.

Cancer

The spread (metastasis) of cancer to the liver is common in cases that begin as cancer in one of the abdominal organs; the tumor cells are carried in the blood through the portal system to the liver.

The Gallbladder

The gallbladder is a muscular sac on the inferior surface of the liver that serves as a storage pouch for bile. Although the liver may manufacture bile continuously, the body is likely to need it only a few times a day. Consequently, bile from the liver flows into the hepatic ducts and then up through the **cystic** (SIS-tik) **duct** connected with the gallbladder. When chyme enters the duodenum, the gallbladder contracts, squeezing bile through the cystic duct and into the common bile duct leading to the duodenum.

The most common disease of the gallbladder is the formation of stones, or **cholelithiasis** (ko-le-lih-THI-ah-sis). Stones are formed from the substances contained in bile, mainly choles-

terol. They may remain in the gallbladder or may lodge in the bile ducts, causing extreme pain. Cholelithiasis is usually associated with inflammation of the gallbladder, or **cholecystitis** (ko-le-sis-TI-tis).

The Pancreas

The pancreas is a long gland that extends from the duodenum to the spleen (see Fig. 19-8). The pancreas produces enzymes that digest fats, proteins, carbohydrates, and nucleic acids. The protein-digesting enzymes are produced in inactive forms, which must be converted to active forms in the small intestine by other enzymes.

The pancreas also produces large amounts of alkaline fluid, which neutralizes the chyme in the small intestine, thus protecting the lining of the digestive tract. These juices collect in a main duct that joins the common bile duct or empties into the duodenum near the common bile duct. Most people have an additional smaller duct that opens into the duodenum.

The pancreas also functions as an endocrine gland, producing the hormones insulin and glucagon that regulate sugar metabolism. These secretions of the islet cells are released directly into the blood.

Pancreatitis

Because they are usually confined to proper channels, pancreatic enzymes do not damage body tissues. If the bile ducts become blocked, however, pancreatic enzymes back up into the pancreas. Also, in some cases of stomach inflammation from excess alcohol consumption or in gallbladder disease, irritation may extend to the pancreas and cause abnormal activation of the pancreatic enzymes. In either circumstance, the pancreas suffers destruction by its own juice, and the outcome can be fatal; this condition is known as **acute pancreatitis**.

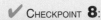

✔ CHECKPOINT **8**:

What are the names of the accessory organs of digestion?

THE PROCESS OF DIGESTION

Enzymes

Although the different organs of the digestive tract are specialized for digesting different types of food, the basic chemical process of digestion is the same for fats, proteins, and carbohydrates. In every case, this process requires enzymes. Enzymes are catalysts, substances that speed the rate of chemical reactions but that are not themselves changed or used up in the reaction.

All enzymes are proteins, and they are highly specific in their actions. In digestion, an enzyme acts only in a certain type of reaction involving a certain type of food molecule. For example, the carbohydrate-digesting enzyme amylase only splits starch into the disaccharide (double sugar) maltose. Another enzyme is required to split maltose into two molecules of the monosaccharide (simple sugar) glucose. Other enzymes split fats into their building blocks, glycerol and fatty acids, and still others split proteins into their building blocks, amino acids.

The Role of Water

Because water is added to nutrient molecules as they are split by enzymes, the process of digestion is referred to chemically as *hydrolysis* (hi-DROL-ih-sis), which means "splitting by means of water." You can now understand why a large amount of water is needed in digestion. Water not only is used to produce digestive juices and to dilute food, so that it can move more easily through the digestive tract, but also is used in the chemical process of digestion itself.

Digestion, Step-by-Step

Let us see what happens to a mass of food from the time it is taken into the mouth to the moment that it is ready to be absorbed.

In the mouth, the food is chewed and mixed with saliva, softening it so that it can be swallowed easily. Salivary amylase initiates the process of digestion by changing some of the starches into sugar (see Table 19-1).

Digestion in the Stomach

When the food reaches the stomach, it is acted on by gastric juice, which contains hydrochloric acid (HCl) and enzymes. The hydrochloric acid has the important function of breaking down proteins and preparing them for digestion. In addition, HCl activates the enzyme pepsin, which is secreted by the cells of the gastric lining in an inactive form. Once activated by hydrochloric acid, pepsin works to digest protein; this enzyme is the first to digest nearly every type of protein in the diet. The stomach also secretes a fat-digesting enzyme (lipase), but it is of little importance in adults.

The food, gastric juice, and mucus (which is also secreted by cells of the gastric lining) are mixed to form the semiliquid substance chyme. Chyme is moved from the stomach to the small intestine for further digestion.

Table 19•1	**Summary of Digestion**		
ORGAN	ACTIVITY	NUTRIENTS DIGESTED	ACTIVE SECRETIONS
Mouth	Food chewed and mixed with saliva; formed into bolus for swallowing	Starch	Salivary amylase
Esophagus	Moves food by peristalsis into stomach	—	—
Stomach	Stores food; churns food and mixes it with digestive juices	Proteins	Hydrochloric acid; pepsin
Small intestine	Secretes enzymes; neutralizes acidity; receives secretions from pancreas and liver; absorbs food into bloodstream or lymph	Fats, proteins, carbohydrates, nucleic acids	Intestinal enzymes; pancreatic enzymes; bile from liver
Large intestine	Reabsorbs water; forms, stores, and eliminates stool	—	—

Digestion in the Small Intestine

In the duodenum, the first part of the small intestine, chyme is mixed with the greenish yellow bile delivered from the liver and the gallbladder through the common bile duct. Bile does not contain enzymes; instead, it contains salts that emulsify (split) fats into smaller particles to allow the powerful pancreatic secretions to act on them most efficiently. The pancreatic juice contains a number of enzymes, including the following:

Lipase. After the physical division of fats into tiny particles by the action of bile, the highly active pancreatic enzyme lipase digests almost all of the fats. In this process, fats are usually broken down into two simpler compounds, glycerol (glycerin) and fatty acids, which are more readily absorbable. If pancreatic lipase is absent, fats are expelled with the feces in undigested form.

Amylase. This enzyme changes starch to sugar.

Trypsin (TRIP-sin). This enzyme splits proteins into amino acids, which are small enough to enter the bloodstream.

Nucleases (NU-kle-ases). These enzymes digest the nucleic acids DNA and RNA.

The intestinal juice contains a number of enzymes, including three that act on complex sugars to transform them into the simpler form in which they are absorbed. These are **maltase, sucrase,** and **lactase.** It must be emphasized that most of the chemical changes in foods occur in the intestinal tract because of the pancreatic juice, which has the ability to digest all types of foods. When pancreatic juice is absent, serious digestive disturbances always occur.

Table 19-2 summarizes the main substances used in digestion. Note that, except for HCl, sodium bicarbonate, and bile salts, all the substances listed are enzymes.

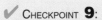

✔ CHECKPOINT **9**:

What organ produces the most complete digestive secretions?

ABSORPTION

The means by which the digested nutrients reach the blood is known as **absorption**. Most absorption takes place through the mucosa of the small intestine by means of the villi (see Fig. 19-1). Within each villus are a small artery and a small vein bridged with capillaries. Simple sugars, amino acids, some simple fatty acids, and water are absorbed into the blood through the capillary walls in the villi. From here, they pass by way of the portal system to the liver, to be stored or released and used as needed.

19

ORGAN	MAIN DIGESTIVE JUICES SECRETED	ACTION
Salivary glands	Salivary amylase*	Begins starch digestion
Stomach	Hydrochloric acid (HCl)	Breaks down proteins
	Pepsin*	Begins protein digestion
Small intestine	Peptidases*	Digest proteins to amino acids
	Lactase, maltase, sucrase*	Digest disaccharides to monosaccharides
Pancreas	Sodium bicarbonate	Neutralizes HCl
	Amylase*	Digests starch
	Trypsin*	Digests protein to amino acids
	Lipases*	Digest fats to fatty acids and glycerol
	Nucleases*	Digest nucleic acids
Liver	Bile salts	Emulsify fats

Table 19•2 **Digestive Juices Produced by the Organs of the Digestive Tract and the Accessory Organs**

*Enzymes.

Absorption of Fats

Most fats have an alternative method of reaching the blood. Instead of entering the blood capillaries, they are absorbed by lymphatic capillaries in the villi that are called **lacteals**. The fat droplets give the lymph a milky appearance (the word *lacteal* means "like milk"). The mixture of lymph and fat globules that is drained from the small intestine after a quantity of fat has been digested is called **chyle** (kile). It circulates in the lymph and eventually enters the bloodstream near the heart.

Absorption of Vitamins and Minerals

Minerals and vitamins taken in with food are also absorbed from the small intestine. The minerals and some of the vitamins dissolve in water and are absorbed directly into the blood. Other vitamins are incorporated in fats and are absorbed along with the fats. Some B vitamins and vitamin K are produced by the action of bacteria in the colon and are absorbed from the large intestine.

CONTROL OF DIGESTION

As food moves through the digestive tract, its rate of movement and the activity of each organ it passes through must be carefully regulated. If food moves too slowly or digestive secretions are inadequate, the body will not get enough nourishment. If food moves too rapidly or excess secretions are produced, digestion may be incomplete or the lining of the digestive tract may be damaged.

There are two types of control over digestion: nervous and hormonal. Both illustrate the principles of feedback control.

The nerves that control digestive activity are located in the submucosa and between the muscle layers of the organ walls. Instructions for action come from the autonomic (visceral) nervous system. In general, parasympathetic stimulation increases activity, and sympathetic stimulation decreases activity. Excess sympathetic stimulation, as in stress, can block the movement of food through the digestive tract and inhibit secretion of the mucus that is so important in protecting the lining of the digestive tract.

The digestive organs themselves produce the hormones involved in regulation of digestion. Let us look at some examples of these controls (Table 19-3).

The sight, smell, thought, taste, or feel of food in the mouth stimulates, through the nervous system, the secretion of saliva and the release of gastric juice. Once in the stomach, food stimulates the release into the blood of the hormone **gastrin,** which promotes stomach secretions and movement.

When chyme enters the duodenum, nerve impulses inhibit movement of the stomach, so that food will not move too rapidly into the small intestine. This action is a good example of negative feedback. At the same time, hormones released from the duodenum feed back to the stomach to reduce its activity. One of these hormones, **secretin** (se-KRE-tin), also stimulates the pancreas to release water and bicarbonate to dilute and neutralize the chyme. Another hormone, **cholecystokinin** (ko-le-sis-to-KI-nin) **(CCK),** stimulates the release of enzymes from the pancreas and causes the gallbladder to release bile.

Table 19•3	**Hormones Active in Digestion**	
HORMONE	SOURCE	ACTION
Gastrin	Stomach	Stimulates release of gastric juice
Gastric-inhibitory peptide (GIP)	Small intestine	Inhibits release of gastric juice
Secretin	Duodenum	Stimulates release of water and bicarbonate from pancreas; stimulates release of bile from liver; inhibits the stomach
Cholecystokinin (CCK)	Duodenum	Stimulates release of digestive enzymes from pancreas; stimulates release of bile from gallbladder; inhibits the stomach

✔ CHECKPOINT **10**:

What are the two types of control over the digestive process?

Hunger and Appetite

Hunger is the desire for food and can be satisfied by the ingestion of a filling meal. Hunger is regulated by centers in the hypothalamus that respond to the levels of nutrients in the blood. When these levels are low, the hypothalamus stimulates a sensation of hunger. Strong, mildly painful contractions of the empty stomach may stimulate a feeling of hunger. Messages received by the hypothalamus reduce hunger as food is chewed and swallowed and begins to fill the stomach. The short-term regulation of food intake works to keep the amount of food taken in within the limits of what can be processed by the intestine. The long-term regulation of food intake maintains appropriate blood levels of certain nutrients.

Appetite differs from hunger in that, although it is basically a desire for food, it often has no relationship to the need for food. Even after an adequate meal that has relieved hunger, a person may still have an appetite for additional food.

A variety of factors, such as emotional state, cultural influences, habit, and memories of past food intake, can affect appetite. The regulation of appetite is not well understood.

Eating Disorders

A chronic loss of appetite, called ***anorexia*** (an-o-REK-se-ah), may be due to a great variety of physical and mental disorders. Because the hypothalamus and the higher brain centers are involved in the regulation of hunger, it is possible that emotional and social factors contribute to the development of anorexia.

Anorexia nervosa is a psychological disorder that mainly afflicts young women. In a desire to be excessively thin, affected people literally starve themselves, sometimes to the point of death. A related disorder, ***bulimia*** (bu-LIM-e-ah), is also called the *binge-purge syndrome*. Affected individuals take in huge quantities of food at one time and then induce vomiting or take large doses of laxatives to prevent absorption of the food.

✔ CHECKPOINT **11**:

What is the difference between hunger and appetite?

AGING AND THE DIGESTIVE SYSTEM

With age, receptors for taste and smell deteriorate, leading to a loss of appetite and decreased enjoyment of food. A decrease in saliva and poor gag reflex make swallowing more difficult. Loss of teeth or poorly fitting dentures may make chewing food more difficult.

Activity of the digestive organs decreases. These changes can be seen in poor absorption of certain vitamins and poor digestion of protein foods. Slowing of peristalsis in the large intestine and increased consumption of easily chewed, refined foods contribute to the common occurrence of constipation.

The tissues of the digestive system require constant replacement. Slowing of this process contributes to a variety of digestive disorders, including gastritis, ulcers, and diverticulosis. As with many body systems, tumors and cancer occur more frequently with age.

19

Summary

I. **Function and design of the digestive system**
   1. Functions—digestion and absorption
   2. Two groups of organs—digestive tract and accessory organs
   A. The wall of the digestive tract—mucous membrane (mucosa), submucosa, smooth muscle, serosa
   B. The peritoneum—serous membrane that lines the abdominal cavity and folds over organs
      1. Peritonitis—peritoneal inflammation

II. **Organs of the digestive tract**
   A. Mouth
      1. Functions
         a. Ingest food
         b. Prepare food for digestion
         c. Begin digestion of starch with salivary amylase
      2. Structures
         a. Tongue—aids chewing (mastication) and swallowing; has taste buds
         b. Teeth
            (1) Deciduous (baby) teeth—20 (incisors, canines, molars)
            (2) Permanent teeth—32 (incisors, canines, premolars, molars)
      3. Diseases of mouth and teeth—caries, gingivitis, periodontitis, Vincent's disease, leukoplakia
   B. Pharynx (throat)—moves portion of food (bolus) into esophagus by reflex swallowing (deglutition)
   C. Esophagus—long muscular tube that carries food to stomach by peristalsis
   D. Stomach
      1. Functions
         a. Storage of food
         b. Breakdown of food by churning
         c. Liquefaction of food with hydrochloric acid (HCl) to form chyme
         d. Digestion of protein with enzyme pepsin
      2. Disorders—nausea, vomiting, gastritis, flatus
      3. Diseases—cancer, ulcer, pyloric stenosis
   E. Small intestine
      1. Functions
         a. Digestion of food
         b. Absorption of food through villi (small projections of intestinal lining)
      2. Divisions—duodenum, jejunum, ileum
   F. Large intestine
      1. Functions
         a. Storage and elimination of waste (defecation)
         b. Reabsorption of water
      2. Divisions—cecum; ascending, transverse, descending, and sigmoid colons; rectum; anus
   G. Intestinal disorders—inflammatory diseases (Crohn's, ulcerative colitis, irritable bowel, enteritis), diarrhea, constipation, cancer

III. **Accessory organs**
   A. Salivary glands—secrete saliva
      1. Functions of saliva
         a. Moistening food—aids chewing and swallowing
         b. Cleaning of mouth and teeth
         c. Digestion of starch with amylase
      2. Three pairs—parotid, submandibular, sublingual
   B. Liver
      1. Functions
         a. Storage of glucose
         b. Formation of blood plasma proteins
         c. Synthesis of urea
         d. Modification of fats
         e. Manufacture of bile
         f. Destruction of old red blood cells
         g. Detoxification of harmful substances
         h. Storage of vitamins and iron

2. Diseases of the liver—hepatitis, cirrhosis, jaundice, cancer
C. Gallbladder
  1. Function—storage of bile until needed for digestion
  2. Diseases—gallstones (cholelithiasis), inflammation (cholecystitis)
D. Pancreas
  1. Secretes powerful digestive juice
  2. Secretes neutralizing fluid

IV. **The process of digestion**
A. Enzymes—catalysts that speed reactions
  1. Products
     a. Simple sugars (monosaccharides) from carbohydrates
     b. Amino acids from proteins
     c. Glycerol and fatty acids from fats
B. The role of water
  1. Used to split foods (hydrolysis)
  2. Lubricates and dilutes food
C. Digestion, step by step
  1. Mouth—starch

2. Stomach—protein
3. Small intestine—remainder of food

V. **Absorption**—movement of nutrients into the circulation

VI. **Control of digestion**
  1. Nervous control
     a. Parasympathetic system—generally increases activity
     b. Sympathetic system—generally decreases activity
  2. Hormonal control
     a. Stimulation of digestive activity
     b. Feedback to inhibit stomach activity
     c. Examples—gastrin, secretin, CCK
A. Hunger and appetite

VII. **Aging and the digestive system**

Questions for Study and Review

1. Describe the layers of the digestive tract wall.
2. Trace the path of a mouthful of food through the digestive tract.
3. What is the peritoneum? Name the two layers and describe the location of each. Name and locate four subdivisions of the peritoneum.
4. Differentiate between deciduous and permanent teeth with respect to kinds and numbers.
5. What is the pharynx and what are its three subdivisions?
6. What is peristalsis? Name some structures in which it occurs.
7. Name the purposes of the acid in gastric juice.
8. Define an enzyme and give several examples of enzymes.
9. Where does absorption occur, and what structures are needed for absorption?
10. What types of digested materials are absorbed into the blood?
11. What types of digested materials are absorbed into the lymph?
12. Name the accessory organs of digestion and the functions of each.
13. Name five functions of the liver.
14. Give examples of negative feedback in the control of digestion.
15. Name several hormones that regulate digestion.
16. Name several diseases that involve the organs of digestion.
17. List several forms of inflammatory diseases of the intestine.
18. Describe what happens in the formation of a peptic ulcer and list some causes of peptic ulcers.

19

19. What is an important symptom of stomach cancer?
20. How is hunger regulated?

✔ ANSWERS TO CHECKPOINTS

1. Food must be broken down by digestion into particles small enough to pass through the plasma membrane.
2. Most of the organs of the digestive tract have a wall composed of a mucous membrane, a submucosa, smooth muscle, and a serous membrane.
3. The peritoneum is the large serous membrane that lines the abdominopelvic cavity and covers the organs it contains.
4. There are 20 baby teeth, which are also called deciduous teeth.
5. Proteins are digested in the stomach.
6. Most digestion takes place in the small intestine under the effects of digestive juices from the small intestine and the accessory organs. Most absorption of digested food also occurs in the small intestine.
7. The large intestine serves to reabsorb water and to store, form, and eliminate the stool. It also houses bacteria that provide some vitamins.
8. The accessory organs of digestion are the salivary glands, liver, gallbladder, and pancreas.
9. The pancreas produces the most complete digestive secretions.
10. The two types of control over the digestive process are nervous control and hormonal control.
11. Hunger is the desire for food that can be satisfied by the ingestion of a filling meal. Appetite is a desire for food that is unrelated to a need for food.

19

Metabolism, Nutrition, and Body Temperature

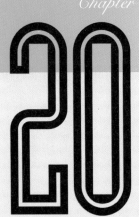

Chapter

20

BEHAVIORAL OBJECTIVES

After careful study of this chapter, you should be able to:

1. Differentiate between catabolism and anabolism
2. Differentiate between the anaerobic and aerobic phases of cellular respiration and give the end products and the relative amount of energy released from each
3. Define *metabolic rate*
4. Name several factors that affect the metabolic rate
5. Explain the role of glucose in metabolism
6. Compare the energy contents of fats, proteins, and carbohydrates
7. Define *essential amino acid*
8. Explain the roles of minerals and vitamins in nutrition and give examples of each
9. List the recommended percentages of fats, carbohydrates, and protein in the diet
10. List some adverse effects of alcohol consumption
11. Explain how heat is produced in the body
12. List the ways in which heat is lost from the body
13. Describe the role of the hypothalamus in regulating body temperature
14. Define *fever*
15. Describe some adverse effects of exces-

METABOLISM

The end products of digestion are used for all the cellular activities of the body, which together make up *metabolism*. These activities fall into two categories:

- *Catabolism,* which is the breakdown of complex compounds into simpler compounds. Catabolism includes the digestion of food into small molecules and the release of energy from these molecules within the cell.
- *Anabolism,* which is the building of simple compounds into substances needed for cellular activities and the growth and repair of tissues.

Through the steps of catabolism and anabolism, there is a constant turnover of body materials as energy is consumed, cells function and grow, and waste products are generated.

> ✔ CHECKPOINT **1**:
>
> What are the two phases of metabolism?

How Cells Obtain Energy From Food

Cellular Respiration
Energy is released from nutrients in a series of reactions called *cellular respiration* (Table 20-1). Early studies on cellular respiration were done with *glucose* as the starting compound. Glucose is a simple sugar that is the main energy source for the body.

The Anaerobic Phase
The first steps in the breakdown of glucose do not require oxygen; that is, they are *anaerobic*. This phase of catabolism, known as *glycolysis* (gli-KOL-ih-sis), occurs in the cytoplasm of the cell. It yields a small amount of energy, which is used to make ATP (adenosine triphosphate), the energy compound of the cells.

The anaerobic breakdown of glucose is incomplete and ends with formation of an organic product called *pyruvic* (pi-RU-vik) *acid*. This end product is further metabolized in the next phase of cellular respiration. In muscle cells operating briefly under anaerobic conditions, pyruvic acid is converted to lactic acid, which accumulates while the cells build up an oxygen debt, as described in Chapter 8. The body must soon rest, so that cells can restore their oxygen supplies and continue with cellular respiration.

The Aerobic Phase
To generate enough energy for survival, the body's cells must break glucose down completely. Further oxygen-requiring, or *aerobic,* reactions occur within the mitochondria of the cell, and these reactions transfer much of the energy remaining in the nutrients to ATP.

20

Table 20•1 Capsule Summary of Cellular Respiration of Glucose			
PHASE	LOCATION IN CELL	END PRODUCT(S)	ENERGY YIELD/GLUCOSE
Anaerobic (glycolysis)	Cytoplasm	Pyruvic acid	2 ATP
Aerobic	Mitochondria	Carbon dioxide and water	34–36 ATP

In the course of the aerobic steps of cellular respiration, carbon dioxide is released and must be transported to the lungs for elimination. In addition, water is formed by the combination of oxygen with hydrogen obtained from nutrient molecules. Because of the type of chemical reactions involved, and because oxygen is used in the final steps, cellular respiration is described as an **oxidation** of nutrients. Note that enzymes are required as catalysts in all the reactions of cellular respiration. Many of the vitamins and minerals described later in this chapter are parts of these enzymes.

Although the oxidation of food is often compared to the burning of fuel, this comparison is inaccurate. Burning results in a sudden and often wasteful release of energy in the form of heat and light. In contrast, metabolic oxidation occurs in steps, and much of the energy released is stored as ATP for later use by the cells; some of the energy is released as heat, which is used to maintain body temperature, as discussed later in this chapter.

For those who know how to read chemical equations, the net balanced equation for cellular respiration, starting with glucose, is as follows:

$$C_6 H_{12} O_6 \ + \ 6O_2 \ \rightarrow \ 6CO_2 \ + \ 6H_2O$$

(glucose)   (oxygen)   (carbon dioxide)   (water)

✔ CHECKPOINT **2**:

What name is given to the series of reactions that releases energy from nutrients?

Metabolic Rate

Metabolic rate refers to the rate at which energy is released from nutrients in the cells. It is affected by a person's size, body fat, sex, age, activity, and hormones, especially thyroid hormone (thyroxine).

Basal metabolism is the amount of energy needed to maintain life functions while the body is at rest. Metabolic rate is high in children and adolescents and decreases with age. See Estimation of Daily Energy Needs for an explanation of how to calculate basal energy needs and

Estimation of Daily Energy Needs

Basal energy requirements for a day can be estimated with a simple formula.

An average female requires 0.9 kcal/kg/hour (1.0 kcal/kg/hour for a male). By multiplying 0.9 by your weight in kilograms,* by 24 (or 1.0 x kg x 24 for a male), you get your daily basal energy requirement. For example, for a female weighing 132 pounds; the equation would be as follows:

132 pounds ÷ 2.2 = 60 kg

0.9 × 60 kg = 54 kcal/hour

54 × 24 = 1296 kcal/day

To estimate your total energy needs for a day, basal requirements must be multiplied by a factor based on your activity level—couch potato to serious athlete. For a female with moderate activity levels, basal energy requirements are multiplied by 1.6; for a male by 1.7. Following the example given above, the following equation applies:

1296 × 1.6 = 2073.6
(about 2075 kcal/day)

*To convert pounds to kilograms, divide weight in pounds by 2.2

total energy needs for an individual who exercises moderately.

The unit used to measure the energy in food is the **kilocalorie** (kcal), which is the amount of heat needed to raise 1 kilogram of water 1°C.

The Use of Nutrients for Energy

As noted, the main source of energy in the body is glucose. Most of the carbohydrates in the diet are converted to glucose in the course of metabolism. Glucose circulates in the blood to provide energy for all the cells. Reserves of glucose are stored in liver and muscle cells as **glycogen** (GLI-ko-jen), a compound built from glucose molecules. When glucose is needed for energy, glycogen is broken down to yield glucose.

Glycerol and fatty acids (from fat digestion) and amino acids (from protein digestion) can also be used for energy, but they enter the breakdown process at different points.

Fat in the diet yields more than twice as much energy as protein or carbohydrate (it is more "fattening"); fat yields 9 kcal of energy per gram, whereas protein and carbohydrate each yield 4 kcal per gram. Food that is ingested in excess of need is converted to fat and stored in adipose tissue.

Before they are oxidized for energy, amino acids must have their nitrogen (amine) groups removed. This removal, called *deamination,* occurs in the liver, where the nitrogen groups are then formed into urea by combination with carbon dioxide. The bloodstream transports the urea to the kidneys to be eliminated.

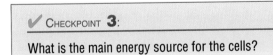

✔ CHECKPOINT **3**:

What is the main energy source for the cells?

Anabolism

Nutrient molecules are built into body materials by anabolic steps, all of which are catalyzed by enzymes.

Essential Amino Acids
Eleven of the 20 amino acids needed to build proteins can be manufactured internally by

metabolic reactions. These 11 amino acids are described as *nonessential* because they need not be taken in with food. The remaining 9 amino acids cannot be made by the body and therefore must be taken in with the diet; these are the **essential amino acids**. Most animal proteins supply all of the essential amino acids and are described as **complete proteins**. Vegetables may be lacking in one or more of the essential amino acids. People on strict vegetarian diets must learn to combine foods, such as beans with rice or wheat, to obtain all the essential amino acids each day.

Essential Fatty Acids
There are also two essential fatty acids that must be taken in with food. These are easily obtained through a healthful, balanced diet.

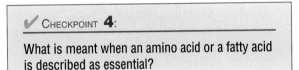

✔ CHECKPOINT **4**:

What is meant when an amino acid or a fatty acid is described as essential?

Minerals and Vitamins

In addition to needing fats, proteins, and carbohydrates, the human body requires minerals and vitamins.

Minerals are chemical elements needed for body structure, fluid balance, and such activities as muscle contraction, nerve impulse conduction, and blood clotting. Some minerals are components of vitamins. A list of the main minerals needed in a proper diet is given in Table 20-2. Some additional minerals not listed are also required for good health. Minerals needed in extremely small amounts are referred to as **trace elements**.

Vitamins are complex organic substances needed in very small quantities. Vitamins are parts of enzymes or other substances essential for metabolism, and vitamin deficiencies lead to a variety of nutritional diseases.

The water-soluble vitamins are the B vitamins and vitamin C. These are not stored in the body and must be taken in regularly with food. The fat-soluble vitamins are A, D, E, and K. These vitamins are kept in reserve in fatty tissue. Excess intake of the fat-soluble vitamins

Table 20•2 **Minerals**			
MINERAL	FUNCTIONS	SOURCES	RESULTS OF DEFICIENCIES
Calcium (Ca)	Formation of bones and teeth, blood clotting, nerve conduction, muscle contraction	Dairy products, eggs, green vegetables, legumes (peas and beans)	Rickets, tetany, osteoporosis
Phosphorus (P)	Formation of bones and teeth; found in ATP, nucleic acids	Meat, fish, poultry, egg yolk, dairy products	Osteoporosis, abnormal metabolism
Sodium (Na)	Fluid balance; nerve impulse conduction, muscle contraction	Most foods, especially processed foods, table salt	Weakness, cramps, diarrhea, dehydration
Potassium (K)	Fluid balance, nerve and muscle activity	Fruits, meats, seafood, milk, vegetables, grains	Muscular and neurologic disorders
Chloride (Cl)	Fluid balance, hydrochloric acid in stomach	Meat, milk, eggs, processed foods, table salt	Rarely occur
Iron (Fe)	Oxygen carrier (hemoglobin, myoglobin)	Meat, eggs, fortified cereals, legumes, dried fruit	Anemia, dry skin, indigestion
Iodine (I)	Thyroid hormones	Seafood, iodized salt	Hypothyroidism, goiter
Magnesium (Mg)	Catalyst for enzyme reactions, carbohydrate metabolism	Green vegetables, grains, nuts, legumes	Spasticity, arrhythmia, vasodilation
Manganese (Mn)	Catalyst in actions of calcium and phosphorus; facilitator of many cell processes	Many foods	Possible reproductive disorders
Copper (Cu)	Necessary for absorption and use of iron in formation of hemoglobin; part of some enzymes	Meat, water	Anemia
Chromium (Cr)	Works with insulin to regulate blood glucose levels	Meat, unrefined food, fats and oils	Inability to use glucose
Cobalt (Co)	Part of vitamin B_{12}	Animal products	Pernicious anemia
Zinc (Zn)	Promotes carbon dioxide transport and energy metabolism; found in enzymes	Meat, fish, poultry, grains, vegetables	Alopecia (baldness); possibly related to diabetes
Fluoride (F)	Prevents tooth decay	Fluoridated water, tea, seafood	Dental caries

can lead to toxicity. A list of vitamins is given in Table 20-3.

✔ CHECKPOINT **5**:

Both vitamins and minerals are needed in metabolism. What is the difference between vitamins and minerals?

NUTRITION GUIDELINES

Good nutrition is absolutely essential for the maintenance of health (see Food as Good Medicine). If any vital food material is missing from the diet, the body will suffer from *malnutrition*. One commonly thinks of a malnourished person as one who does not have enough to eat, but malnutrition can also occur from eating too much of the wrong foods.

The simplest and perhaps best advice for maintaining a healthful diet is to eat a wide variety of fresh, wholesome foods daily. The U.S. Department of Agriculture (USDA) presently recommends a distribution of food in the diet as shown in Figure 20-1. The "Food Guide Pyramid" emphasizes grains, fruits, and vegetables, with limited intake of fats, oils, and sugars.

Carbohydrates, Fats, and Proteins

Because proteins, unlike carbohydrates and fats, are not stored, protein foods should be taken in on a regular basis. The average U.S. diet, however, contains more than enough protein and too much fat, especially animal fat. It

Table 20•3 Vitamins

VITAMINS	FUNCTIONS	SOURCES	RESULTS OF DEFICIENCIES
A (retinol)	Required for healthy epithelial tissue and for eye pigments; involved in reproduction and immunity	Orange fruits and vegetables, liver, eggs, dairy products, dark green vegetables	Night blindness; dry, scaly skin; decreased immunity
B_1 (thiamin)	Required for enzymes involved in oxidation of nutrients; nerve function	Pork, cereal, grains, meats, legumes, nuts	Beriberi, a disease of nerves
B_2 (riboflavin)	In enzymes required for oxidation of nutrients	Milk, eggs, liver, green leafy vegetables, grains	Skin and tongue disorders
B_3 (niacin, nicotinic acid)	Involved in oxidation of nutrients	Yeast, meat, liver, grains, legumes, nuts	Pellagra with dermatitis, diarrhea, mental disorders
B_6 (pyridoxine)	Amino acid and fatty acid metabolism; formation of niacin; manufacture of red blood cells	Meat, fish, poultry, fruit, grains, legumes, vegetables	Anemia, irritability, convulsions, muscle twitching, skin disorders
Pantothenic acid	Essential for normal growth; energy metabolism	Yeast, liver, eggs, and many other foods	Sleep disturbances, digestive upset
B_{12} (cyanocobalamin)	Production of cells; maintenance of nerve cells; fatty acid and amino acid metabolism	Animal products	Pernicious anemia
Biotin	Involved in fat and glycogen formation, amino acid metabolism	Peanuts, liver, tomatoes, eggs, and many other foods	Lack of coordination, dermatitis, fatigue
Folate (folic acid)	Required for amino acid metabolism, DNA synthesis, maturation of red blood cells	Vegetables, liver, legumes, seeds	Anemia, digestive disorders, neural tube defects in the embryo
C (ascorbic acid)	Maintains healthy skin and mucous membranes; involved in synthesis of collagen; antioxidant	Citrus fruits, green vegetables, potatoes, orange fruits	Scurvy, poor wound healing, anemia, weak bones
D (calciferol)	Aids in absorption of calcium and phosphorus from intestinal tract	Fatty fish, liver, eggs, fortified milk	Rickets, bone deformities
E (tocopherol)	Protects cell membranes; antioxidant	Seeds, green vegetables, nuts, grains, oils, eggs	Anemia, muscle and liver degeneration, pain
K	Synthesis of blood clotting factors, bone formation	Bacteria in digestive tract, liver, cabbage, and leafy green vegetables	Hemorrhage

is currently recommended that calories from the three types of food be distributed as follows:

- Carbohydrate: 58%
- Fat: 30%
- Protein: 12%

The carbohydrates should be mainly complex, naturally occurring carbohydrates, and refined sugars should be kept to a minimum.

Fats are subdivided into saturated and unsaturated forms. Most *saturated fats* are from animal sources and are solid at room temperature, such as butter and lard. Also included in

this group are the so-called "tropical oils": coconut oil and palm oil. *Unsaturated fats* are derived from plants. They are liquid at room temperature and are generally referred to as *oils*.

No more than one third of the fats in the diet should be saturated fats. Diets high in saturated fats are associated with a higher than normal incidence of cancer, heart disease, and cardiovascular problems, although the relation between these factors is not fully understood.

Many commercial products contain fats that are artificially saturated to prevent rancidity and provide a more solid consistency. These are

Food as Good Medicine

Does an apple a day keep the doctor away? This adage reflects what people have long known—that the foods we eat have a profound effect on our health. The apple has fiber, which is known to reduce the risk of colon cancer by diluting carcinogens in the bowel and reducing their contact with the bowel wall. It is also lacking in fats, which should be controlled in the diet, especially saturated fats. People with diets rich in fruits and vegetables have lower incidences of diabetes, cardiovascular disease, and several types of cancer. Vegetables in the mustard family, such as broccoli, cabbage, and kale, appear to contain compounds that inhibit the growth of cancer cells. Studies are now underway to identify which components of the various vegetables may provide this protection.

listed on food labels as partially hydrogenated vegetable oils and are found in baked goods, processed peanut butter, vegetable shortening, and solid margarine. Evidence shows that components of hydrogenated fats, known as *transfatty acids*, may be just as harmful, if not more so, than natural saturated fats and should be avoided.

A weight loss diet should follow the same guidelines as given above with a reduction in portion sizes. Exercise is also recommended. (See Obesity.)

Vitamin and Mineral Supplements

The need for mineral and vitamin supplements to the diet is a subject of controversy. Some researchers maintain that adequate amounts of these substances can be obtained from a varied, healthful diet; others hold that pollution, depletion of the soils, and the storage, refining, and processing of foods make supplementation beneficial. Most agree, however, that children, elderly people, pregnant and lactating women, and teenagers, who often do not get enough of the proper foods, would profit from additional minerals and vitamins.

When required, supplements should be selected by a physician or nutritionist to fit the particular needs of the individual. Megavitamin dosages may cause unpleasant reactions and in some cases are hazardous. Vitamins A and D have both been found to cause serious toxic effects when taken in excess.

Food Allergies

The subject of allergies has received much attention. Some people develop clear allergic (hypersensitive) symptoms if they eat certain foods. The most common food allergens are wheat, yeast, milk, and eggs, but almost any food might cause an allergic reaction in a given individual. Although food allergies may be responsible for symptoms with no other known cause, most people can probably eat all types of foods.

Alcohol

Alcohol yields energy, in the amount of 7 kcal per gram, but it is not considered a nutrient because it does not yield useful end products. In

Obesity

Obesity is usually defined as being 20% or more above normal weight. Its causes are complex and include social, psychological, and hereditary components. Obesity has been linked with high blood pressure, diabetes, cardiovascular problems, and breast cancer.

People in the United States spend millions of dollars each year in the effort to lose weight. Unfortunately, for most people, reducing diets do not work, especially if they are viewed as temporary measures. Usually, the lost weight is regained—and more. When faced with very-low-calorie diets, the body's metabolic rate actually declines in an effort to save energy, making weight loss even more difficult. For most people, a varied diet eaten in moderation and regular exercise are the surest ways to avoid obesity.

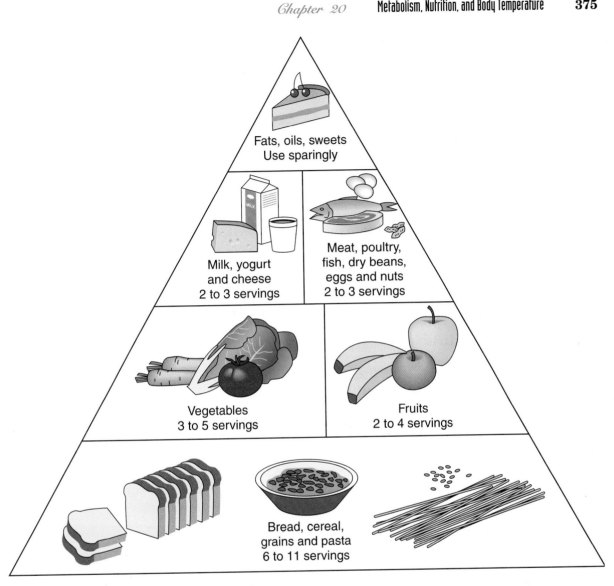

Fats, oils, sweets
Use sparingly

Milk, yogurt
and cheese
2 to 3 servings

Meat, poultry,
fish, dry beans,
eggs and nuts
2 to 3 servings

Vegetables
3 to 5 servings

Fruits
2 to 4 servings

Bread, cereal,
grains and pasta
6 to 11 servings

FIGURE **20•1**   Guide to daily food choices. (Taylor C, Lillis C, LeMone P: Fundamentals of Nursing: The Art and Science of Nursing Care, 2nd ed, p. 805. Philadelphia, JB Lippincott, 1993)

fact, alcohol interferes with metabolism and contributes to a variety of disorders.

The body can metabolize about one half ounce of pure alcohol (ethanol) per hour. This amount translates into one glass of wine, one can of beer, or one shot of hard liquor. Consumed at a more rapid rate, alcohol enters the bloodstream and affects many cells, notably in the brain.

Alcohol is rapidly absorbed through the stomach and small intestine and is detoxified by the liver. When delivered in excess to the liver, alcohol can lead to the accumulation of fat and to cirrhosis. Metabolism of alcohol ties up enzymes needed for oxidation of nutrients and also results in byproducts that acidify body fluids. Other effects of alcoholism include obesity, malnutrition, cancer, ulcers, and fetal alcohol syndrome. Pregnant women are advised not to drink any alcohol. In addition, alcohol impairs judgment and leads to increased involvement in accidents.

Although consumption of alcohol is compatible with good health and may even have a beneficial effect on the cardiovascular system, alcohol should be consumed only in moderation.

Nutrition and Aging

With age, a person may find it difficult to maintain a balanced diet. Often, the elderly lose interest in buying and preparing food or are unable to do so. Because metabolism generally slows, and less food is required to meet energy needs, nutritional deficiencies may develop. Medications may interfere with appetite and with the absorption and use of specific nutrients.

It is important for older people to seek out foods that are "nutrient dense," that is, foods that have a high proportion of nutrients in comparison to the number of calories they provide. Exercise helps to boost appetite and maintains muscle tissue, which is more active metabolically.

BODY TEMPERATURE

Heat is an important byproduct of the many chemical activities constantly going on in tissues all over the body. Heat is always being lost through a variety of outlets. Because of a number of regulatory devices, however, under normal conditions, body temperature remains constant within quite narrow limits. Maintenance of a constant temperature despite both internal and external influences is one phase of homeostasis, the tendency of all body processes to maintain a normal state despite forces that tend to alter them.

Heat Production

Heat is produced when nutrients are oxidized in the cells. Thus, heat is a byproduct of the cellular reactions that generate energy. The amount of heat produced by a given organ varies with the kind of tissue and its activity.

Sources of Heat
Tissues vary in the amount of heat they generate at rest and during activity. While at rest, muscles may produce as little as 25% of total body heat, but when muscles contract, heat production is greatly multiplied, owing to the increase in metabolic rate. Under basal conditions (at rest), the liver and other abdominal organs produce about 50% of total body heat. The brain produces only 15% of body heat at rest, and an increase in nervous tissue activity produces little increase in heat production.

Although it would seem from this description that some parts of the body would tend to become much warmer than others, the circulating blood distributes the heat fairly evenly.

Factors Affecting Heat Production
The rate at which heat is produced is affected by a number of factors, including exercise, hormone production, food intake, and age.

Hormones, such as thyroxine from the thyroid gland and epinephrine (adrenaline) from the medulla of the adrenal gland, increase the rate of heat production.

The intake of food is also accompanied by increased heat production. The nutrients that enter the blood after digestion are available for increased cellular metabolism. In addition, the glands and muscles of the digestive system generate heat as they set to work. These responses do not account for all the increase, however, nor do they account for the much greater increase in metabolism after a meal containing a large amount of protein. Although the reasons are not entirely clear, the intake of food definitely increases metabolism and thus adds to heat production.

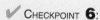

✔ CHECKPOINT **6**:

What are some factors that affect heat production in the body?

Heat Loss

More than 80% of heat loss occurs through the skin. The remaining 15% to 20% is dissipated by the respiratory system and with the urine and feces.

Heat Loss Through the Skin
Networks of blood vessels in the dermis (deeper part) of the skin can bring considerable quantities of blood near the surface, so that heat can be dissipated to the outside. This can occur in several ways.

- Heat can be transferred to the surrounding air by means of the process of **conduction**.
- Heat also travels from its source in the form of heat waves or rays, a process termed **radiation.**
- If the air is moving, so that the layer of heated air next to the body is constantly being carried away and replaced with cooler air (as by an electric fan), the process is known as **convection**.
- Finally, heat loss may be produced by **evaporation,** the process by which liquid changes to the vapor state.

To illustrate evaporation, rub some alcohol on your skin; it evaporates rapidly, using so much heat from the skin that your arm feels cold. Perspiration does the same thing, although not as quickly. The rate of heat loss through evaporation depends on the humidity of the surrounding air. When this exceeds 60% or so, perspiration does not evaporate so readily, making one feel generally miserable unless one can resort to some other means of heat loss, such as convection caused by a fan.

Prevention of Heat Loss
Factors that play a part in heat loss through the skin include the volume of tissue compared with the amount of skin surface. A child loses heat more rapidly than does an adult. Such parts as fingers and toes are affected most by exposure to cold because they have a great amount of skin compared with total tissue volume.

If the temperature of the surrounding air is lower than that of the body, excessive heat loss is prevented by both natural and artificial means.

Clothing checks heat loss by trapping "dead air" in both its material and its layers. This noncirculating air is a good insulator.

An effective natural insulation against cold is the layer of fat under the skin. Even when skin temperature is low, this fatty tissue prevents the deeper tissues from losing much heat. On the average, this layer is slightly thicker in females than in males. Naturally, there are individual variations, but as a rule, the degree of insulation depends on the thickness of this layer of subcutaneous fat.

Temperature Regulation

Given that body temperature remains almost constant despite wide variations in the rate of heat production or loss, there must be internal mechanisms for regulating temperature.

The Role of the Hypothalamus
Many areas of the body take part in this heat-regulating process, but the most important center is the area inside the brain, located just above the pituitary gland, the **hypothalamus**.

Some of the cells in the hypothalamus control the production of heat in the body tissues, whereas another group of cells controls heat loss. This control comes about in response to the temperature of the blood circulating through the brain as well as in response to nerve impulses from temperature receptors in the skin.

Conservation of Heat
If these two factors indicate that too much heat is being lost, impulses are sent quickly from the hypothalamus to the autonomic (involuntary) nervous system, which in turn causes constriction of the skin blood vessels to reduce heat loss. Other impulses are sent to the muscles to cause shivering, a rhythmic contraction of many body muscles, which results in increased heat production. Furthermore, the output of epinephrine may be increased if necessary. Epinephrine increases cell metabolism for a short period, and this in turn increases heat production.

Release of Heat
If there is danger of overheating, the hypothalamus transmits impulses that stimulate the sweat glands to increase their activity and dilate the blood vessels in the skin, so that increased blood flow results in greater loss of heat. The hypothalamus may also encourage the relaxation of muscles and thus minimize the production of heat in these organs.

The Role of Muscles
Muscles are especially important in temperature regulation because variations in the amount of activity in these large masses of tissue can readily increase or decrease the total

amount of heat produced. Because muscles form roughly one third of the bulk of the body, either an involuntary or a purposeful increase in the activity of this big group of organs can form enough heat to offset a considerable decrease in the temperature of the environment.

✔ CHECKPOINT **7**:

What part of the brain is responsible for regulating body temperature?

Age Factors

Very young and very old people are limited in their ability to regulate body temperature when exposed to extremes in environment. The body temperature of a newborn infant decreases if the infant is exposed to a cool environment for a long period. Elderly people also are not able to produce enough heat to maintain body temperature in a cool environment.

With regard to overheating in these age groups, heat loss mechanisms are not fully developed in the newborn. The elderly do not lose as much heat from their skin. Both groups should be protected from extreme temperatures.

Normal Body Temperature

The normal temperature range obtained by either a mercury or an electronic thermometer may extend from 36.2°C to 37.6°C (97°F to 100°F). Body temperature varies with the time of day. Usually, it is lowest in the early morning because the muscles have been relaxed and no food has been taken in for several hours. Temperature tends to be higher in the late afternoon and evening because of physical activity and consumption of food.

Normal temperature also varies in different parts of the body. Skin temperature obtained in the axilla (armpit) is lower than mouth temperature, and mouth temperature is a degree or so lower than rectal temperature. It is believed that, if it were possible to place a thermometer inside the liver, it would register a degree or more higher than rectal temperature. The tem-

perature within a muscle might be even higher during its activity.

Although the Fahrenheit scale is used in the United States, in most parts of the world, temperature is measured with the **Celsius** (SEL-se-us) thermometer. On this scale, the ice point is at 0° and the normal boiling point of water is at 100°, the interval between these two points being divided into 100 equal units. The Celsius scale is also called the **centigrade scale** (think of 100 cents in a dollar). See Appendix 2 for a comparison of the Celsius and Fahrenheit scales and formulas for converting from one to the other.

✔ CHECKPOINT **8**:

What is normal body temperature?

Abnormal Body Temperature

Fever

Fever is a condition in which the body temperature is higher than normal. An individual with a fever is described as **febrile** (FEB-ril). Usually, the presence of fever is due to an infection, but there can be many other causes, such as malignancies, brain injuries, toxic reactions, reactions to vaccines, and diseases involving the central nervous system (CNS). Sometimes, emotional upsets can bring on a fever. Whatever the cause, the effect is to reset the body's thermostat in the hypothalamus.

Curiously enough, fever usually is preceded by a chill—that is, a violent attack of shivering and a sensation of cold that such measures as blankets and heating pads seem unable to relieve. As a result of these reactions, heat is being generated and stored in the body, and when the chill subsides, the body temperature is elevated.

The old adage that a fever should be starved is completely wrong. During a fever, there is an increase in metabolism that is usually proportional to the amount of fever. In addition to the use of available sugar and fat, there is an increase in the use of protein, and during the first week or so of a fever, there is definite evidence of destruction of body protein. A high-calorie diet with plenty of protein is therefore desirable.

When a fever ends, sometimes the drop in temperature to normal occurs very rapidly. This sudden fall in temperature is called the ***crisis,*** and it is usually accompanied by symptoms indicating rapid heat loss: profuse perspiration, muscular relaxation, and dilation of blood vessels in the skin. A gradual drop in temperature, in contrast, is known as ***lysis***. A drug that reduces fever is described as ***antipyretic*** (an-ti-pi-RET-ik).

The mechanism of fever production is not completely understood, but we might think of the hypothalamus as a thermostat that is set higher during fever than normally. This change in the heat-regulating mechanism often follows the injection of a foreign protein or the entrance into the bloodstream of bacteria or their toxins. Substances that produce fever are called ***pyrogens*** (PI-ro-jens).

Up to a point, fever may be beneficial because it steps up phagocytosis (the process by which white blood cells surround, engulf, and digest bacteria and other foreign bodies), inhibits the growth of certain organisms, and increases cellular metabolism, which may help recovery from disease.

Extreme Outside Temperatures

The body's heat-regulating devices are efficient, but there is a limit to what they can accomplish.

Excess Heat

High outside temperature may overcome the body's heat loss mechanisms, in which case body temperature rises and cellular metabolism and accompanying heat production increase. When body temperature rises, the affected person is apt to suffer from a series of disorders: heat cramps are followed by heat exhaustion, which, if untreated, is followed by heat stroke.

In ***heat cramps,*** there is localized muscle cramping of the extremities and occasionally of the abdomen. The condition abates with rest in a cool environment and adequate fluids.

With further heat retention and more fluid loss, ***heat exhaustion*** occurs. Symptoms of this disorder include headache, tiredness, vomiting, and a rapid pulse. There may be a decrease in circulating blood volume and lowered blood pressure. Heat exhaustion may also be treated by rest and fluid replacement.

Heat stroke (also called *sunstroke*) is a medical emergency. Heat stroke can be recognized by a body temperature of up to 41°C (105°F); hot, dry skin; and CNS symptoms, including confusion, dizziness, and loss of consciousness. The body has responded to the loss of fluid from the circulation by reducing blood flow to the skin and sweat glands.

It is important to lower the sunstroke victim's body temperature immediately by removing the individual's clothing, placing him or her in a cool environment, and cooling the body with cold water or ice. The patient should be treated with appropriate fluids containing the vital electrolytes, including sodium, potassium, calcium, and chloride. Supportive medical care is also necessary because heat stroke can cause fatal complications.

✔ CHECKPOINT **9**:

What are some conditions brought on by excessive heat?

Excess Cold

The body is no more capable of coping with prolonged exposure to cold than with prolonged exposure to heat. If, for example, the body is immersed in cold water for a time, the water (a better heat conductor than air) removes more heat from the body than can be replaced, and body temperature falls. This can happen too, of course, in cold air, particularly when clothing is inadequate. The main effects of an excessively low body temperature, termed ***hypothermia*** (hi-po-THER-me-ah), are uncontrolled shivering, lack of coordination, and decreased heart and respiratory rates. Speech becomes slurred, and there is overpowering sleepiness, which may lead to coma and death.

Outdoor activities in cool, not necessarily cold, weather cause many unrecognized cases of hypothermia. Wind, fatigue, and depletion of water and energy stores all play a part.

When the body is cooled below a certain point, cellular metabolism is slowed, and heat production is inadequate for maintaining a normal body temperature. The person must then be warmed by heat from an outside source. The best first aid measure is to remove the person's clothing and put him or her in a warmed sleeping bag with an unclothed companion until shivering stops. Administration of hot, sweetened fluids also helps.

Exposure to cold, particularly to moist cold, may result in *frostbite,* which can cause permanent local tissue damage. The areas most likely to be affected by frostbite are the face, ears, and extremities. The causes of damage include the formation of ice crystals and the reduction of blood supply to the area. Necrosis (death) of the tissues with gangrene can result. The very young, the very old, and those who suffer from disease of the circulatory system are particularly susceptible to cold injuries.

A frostbitten area should *never* be rubbed; rather, it should be rapidly thawed by immersion in warm water or by contact with warm bare skin. The affected area should be treated gently; a person with frostbitten feet should not be permitted to walk. People with cold-damaged extremities frequently have some lowering of body temperature. Warming of the whole person should not be neglected during warming of the affected part.

Hypothermia is employed in certain types of surgery. In such cases, the hypothalamus is depressed by drugs and the body temperature reduced to as low as 25°C (77°F) before the operation is begun. In the case of heart surgery, further cooling to 20°C (68°F) is accomplished as the blood goes through the heart-lung machine. This method has been successful even in infants suffering from congenital heart abnormalities.

✔ CHECKPOINT **10**:

What is the term for excessively low body temperature?

Summary

I. **Metabolism**—life-sustaining reactions that occur in the living cell
  1. Catabolism—breakdown of complex compounds into simpler compounds
  2. Anabolism—building of simple compounds into substances needed for cellular activities, growth, and repair
  A. How cells obtain energy from food
    1. Cellular respiration—a series of reactions in which food is oxidized for energy
      a. Anaerobic phase—does not require oxygen
        (1) Location—cytoplasm
        (2) Yield—small amount of energy
        (3) End product—organic (*i.e.,* pyruvic acid)
      b. Aerobic phase-requires oxygen
        (1) Location—mitochondria
        (2) Yield—almost all remaining energy in food
        (3) End products—carbon dioxide and water
    2. Metabolic rate—rate at which energy is released from food in the cells
      a. Basal metabolism—amount of energy needed to maintain life functions while at rest
  B. Use of nutrients for energy
    1. Glucose—main energy source
    2. Fats—highest energy yield
    3. Proteins—can be used for energy after removal of nitrogen
  C. Anabolism
    1. Essential amino acids and fatty acids must be taken in with food
      a. Complete proteins contain all the essential amino acids
  D. Minerals and vitamins
    1. Minerals—elements needed for body structure and cell activities

a. Trace elements—elements needed in extremely small amounts

2. Vitamins—organic substances needed in small amounts

II. Nutrition guidelines
1. Malnutrition—too little food or inadequate amounts of specific foods
2. Components of healthy diet
   a. USDA Food Guide Pyramid
   b. Less than 10% of total daily calories in form of saturated fats
A. Vitamin and mineral supplements
B. Food allergies
C. Alcohol
D. Nutrition and aging

III. Body temperature
A. Heat production
1. Most heat produced in muscles and glands
2. Distributed by the circulation
3. Affected by exercise, hormones, food, age
B. Heat loss
1. Avenues—skin, urine, feces, respiratory system
2. Mechanisms—conduction, radiation, convection, evaporation
C. Temperature regulation
1. Hypothalamus—main temperature-regulating center; responds to temperature of blood and temperature receptors in skin
2. Responses to decrease in body temperature

a. Constriction of blood vessels in skin
b. Shivering
c. Increased release of epinephrine
3. Responses to increase in body temperature
   a. Dilation of skin vessels
   b. Sweating
   c. Relaxation of muscles
D. Normal body temperature—ranges from 36.2°C to 37.6°C; varies with time of day and location measured
E. Abnormal body temperature
1. Fever—higher than normal body temperature resulting from infection, injury, toxin, damage to CNS, etc.
   a. Pyrogen—substance that produces fever
   b. Antipyretic—drug that reduces fever
2. Extreme outside temperatures
   a. Excessive heat—heat cramps, heat exhaustion, heat stroke
   b. Excessive cold
      (1) Hypothermia—low body temperature
         (a) Results—coma and death
         (b) Uses—surgery
      (2) Frostbite—reduction of blood supply to areas such as face, ears, toes, fingers
         (a) Results—necrosis and gangrene

Questions for Study and Review

1. Define *cellular respiration.*
2. In what part of the cell does anaerobic respiration occur? What are its end products?
3. In what part of the cell does aerobic respiration occur? What are its end products?
4. Define *metabolic rate.* What factors affect the metabolic rate?
5. What is the definition of *basal metabolism?*
6. About how many kilocalories are released from a gram of butter? a gram of egg white? a gram of sugar?

7. Gelatin is not a complete protein. What are the dangers of eating flavored gelatin as a sole source of protein?

8. Name the foods that are emphasized in the USDA Food Guide Pyramid; which are to be eaten sparingly?

9. If you eat 2000 kcal a day, how many kilocalories should come from carbohydrates? from fats? from proteins?

10. What organ metabolizes alcohol?

11. How is heat produced in the body? What structures produce the most heat during increased activity?

12. Name four factors that affect heat production.

13. How is heat lost from the body?

14. Name four ways in which heat escapes to the environment.

15. In what ways is heat kept in the body?

16. Name the main temperature regulator and describe what it does when the body is too hot and when it is too cold. What parts do muscles play?

17. What is the normal body temperature range? How does it vary with respect to the time of day and the part of the body?

18. Define *fever.* Name some aspects of fever's course, and list some of fever's beneficial and harmful effects.

19. Name and describe two consequences of excessive outside heat. Why do these conditions occur? What is the prime emergency measure for sunstroke?

20. What is hypothermia? Under what circumstances does it usually occur? List some of its effects.

21. Name and describe two common injuries resulting from cold. What happens in the body to bring these conditions about?

22. Differentiate between the terms in each of the following pairs:
    a. *catabolism* and *anabolism*
    b. *aerobic* and *anaerobic*
    c. *mineral* and *vitamin*
    d. *saturated fats* and *unsaturated fats*
    e. *crisis* and *lysis*

20

✔ ANSWERS TO CHECKPOINTS

1. The two phases of metabolism are catabolism, the breakdown phase of metabolism, and anabolism, the building phase of metabolism.

2. Cellular respiration is the series of reactions that releases energy from nutrients in the cell.

3. Glucose is the main energy source for the cells.

4. An essential amino acid or fatty acid cannot be made metabolically and must be taken in with the diet.

5. Minerals are chemical elements, and vitamins are complex organic substances.

6. Some factors that affect heat production are exercise, hormone production, food intake, and age.

7. The hypothalamus of the brain is responsible for regulating body temperature.

8. Normal body temperature is 36.2°C to 37.6°C (97°F to 100°F).

9. Heat cramps, heat exhaustion, and heat stroke are brought on by excessive heat.

10. Excessively low body temperature is hypothermia.

Body Fluids

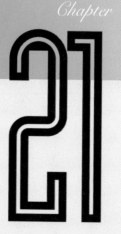

Chapter

21

SELECTED KEY TERMS

The following terms are defined in the Glossary:

acidosis
alkalosis
ascites
buffer
dehydration
edema
effusion
electrolyte
extracellular
interstitial
intracellular
pH

BEHAVIORAL OBJECTIVES

After careful study of this chapter, you should be able to:

1. Compare intracellular and extracellular fluids

2. List four types of extracellular fluids

3. Name the systems that are involved in water balance

4. Define *electrolytes* and describe some of their functions

5. Describe the role of hormones in electrolyte balance

6. Describe three methods for regulating the pH of body fluids

7. Describe five disorders involving body fluids

8. Specify fluids used in therapy

THE IMPORTANCE OF WATER

Water is important to living cells as a solvent, as a transport medium, and as a participant in metabolic reactions. The normal proportion of body water varies from 50% to 70% of a person's weight. It is highest in the young and in thin, muscular individuals. As the amount of fat increases, and as a person ages, the percentage of water in the body decreases.

Various electrolytes (salts), nutrients, gases, waste, and special substances, such as enzymes and hormones, are dissolved or suspended in body water. The composition of body fluids is an important factor in homeostasis. Whenever the volume or chemical makeup of these fluids deviates even slightly from normal, disease results. (See Appendix 3 for normal values.) The constancy of body fluids is maintained in the following ways:

- The thirst mechanism, which maintains the volume of water at a constant level
- Kidney activity, which regulates the volume and composition of body fluids (see Chap. 22)
- Hormones, which serve to regulate fluid volume and electrolytes
- Regulators of pH (acidity), including buffers, respiration, and kidney function

FLUID COMPARTMENTS

Although body fluids have much in common no matter where they are located, there are some important differences between fluid inside and fluid outside cells. Accordingly, fluids are grouped into two main compartments:

- *Intracellular fluid* is contained within the cells. About two thirds to three fourths of all body fluids are in this category.
- *Extracellular fluid* includes all body fluids outside of cells. In this group are included the following:
  - *Blood plasma,* which constitutes about 4% of a person's body weight
  - *Interstitial* (in-ter-STISH-al) *fluid,* or more simply, tissue fluid. This fluid is located in the spaces between the cells in tissues all over the body. It is estimated that tissue fluid constitutes about 15% of body weight.
  - *Lymph,* the fluid that drains from the tissues into the lymphatic system
- *Fluid in special compartments,* such as cerebrospinal fluid, the aqueous and vitreous humors of the eye, serous fluid, and synovial fluid. Together, these make up about 1% to 3% of total body fluids.

Fluids are not locked into one compartment. There is a constant interchange between com-

21

385

partments as fluids are transferred across semi-permeable cell membranes by diffusion and osmosis (Fig. 21-1).

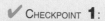

✔ CHECKPOINT **1**:

What are the two main compartments into which body fluids are grouped?

WATER BALANCE

In a person whose health is normal, the quantity of water taken in (intake) is about equal to the quantity lost (output). The quantity of water consumed in a day varies considerably. The average adult in a comfortable environment takes in about 2500 mL of water (about 2½ quarts) daily (see How Much to Drink).

About half of this quantity comes from drinking water and other beverages, and about half comes from foods—fruits, vegetables, and soups.

Water is constantly being lost from the body by the following routes:

- The **skin.** Although sebum and keratin help prevent dehydration, water is constantly evaporating from the surface of the skin. Larger amounts of water are lost from the skin in the form of sweat when it is necessary to cool the body.
- The **lungs** expel water along with carbon dioxide.
- The **intestinal tract** eliminates water along with the feces.
- The **kidneys** excrete the largest quantity of water lost each day. About 1 to 1.5 liters of water are eliminated daily in the urine.

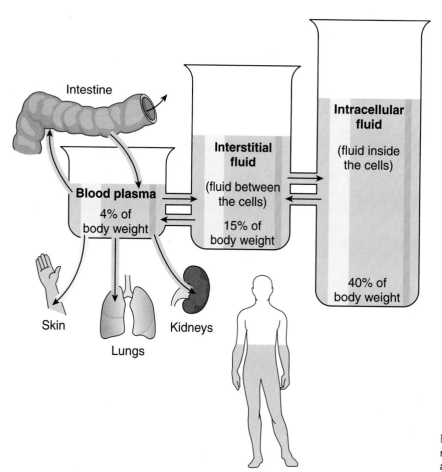

FIGURE **21•1** Main fluid compartments showing the relative percentage of body fluid in each.

How Much to Drink

Most people engaging in routine activities drink 6 to 8 cups of fluid daily to meet their needs. This may be in the form of water, juices, or milk. Beverages containing alcohol or caffeine should not be included in this total because they act as diuretics and increase water loss. The thirst center of the brain should stimulate enough drinking to balance fluids, but this is not always the case. When exercising vigorously, especially in hot weather, the body can dehydrate rapidly. People may not drink enough to replace needed fluids. In addition, if plain water is consumed, the dilution of body fluids may depress the thirst center. Athletes exercising very strenuously may need to drink beverages with some carbohydrates for energy and also some electrolytes to keep fluids in balance.

Osmoreceptors

Osmoreceptors are specialized neurons that help to maintain water balance by detecting changes in the concentration of extracellular fluid (ECF). They are located in the hypothalamus of the brain in an area adjacent to the third ventricle. Here they monitor the osmotic pressure (concentration) of the circulating blood plasma.

The osmoreceptors respond primarily to small increases in sodium, the most common ion in ECF. As the blood becomes more concentrated, sodium draws water out of the cells, initiating nerve impulses. Traveling to different regions of the hypothalamus, these impulses may have two different but related effects:

- The hypothalamus is stimulated to produce antidiuretic hormone (ADH), which is then released from the posterior pituitary. ADH travels to the kidneys and causes these organs to conserve water.
- The thirst center of the hypothalamus is stimulated, causing increased consumption of water.

Both these mechanisms serve to dilute the blood and other body fluids. Either mechanism alone can maintain water balance. If both fail, a person soon becomes dehydrated.

In many disorders, it is important for the health care team to know whether a patient's intake and output are about equal; in such a case, a 24-hour intake–output record is kept. The intake record includes *all* the liquid the patient has taken in. This means fluids administered intravenously as well as those consumed by mouth. The health care worker must account for water, other beverages, and liquid foods, such as soup and ice cream. The output record includes the quantity of urine excreted in the same 24-hour period as well as an estimation of fluid losses due to fever, vomiting, diarrhea, bleeding, wound discharge, or other causes.

✔ CHECKPOINT **2**:

What are three routes for water loss from the body?

Sense of Thirst

The control center for the sense of thirst is located in the hypothalamus of the brain (see Osmoreceptors). This center plays a major role in the regulation of total fluid volume. A decrease in fluid volume or an increase in the concentration of body fluids stimulates the thirst center

and thus causes an individual to drink water or other fluids containing large amounts of water. Dryness of the mouth also causes a sensation of thirst. Excessive thirst, such as that caused by excessive urine loss in cases of diabetes, is called ***polydipsia*** (pol-e-DIP-se-ah).

✔ CHECKPOINT **3**:

Where is the control center for the sense of thirst located?

ELECTROLYTES AND THEIR FUNCTIONS

Electrolytes are important constituents of body fluids. These are compounds that separate in solution into positively and negatively charged ions. Positively charged ions are called *cations;* negatively charged ions are called *anions.* Electrolytes are so-named because they conduct an electrical current in solution. A few of the most important ions are reviewed next:

- Positive ions (cations)
  - *Sodium* is chiefly responsible for maintaining osmotic balance and body fluid volume. It is the main positive ion in extracellular fluids. Sodium is required for nerve impulse conduction and is important in maintaining acid–base balance.
  - *Potassium* is also important in the transmission of nerve impulses and is a major positive ion in intracellular fluids. Potassium is involved in cellular enzyme activities, and it helps regulate the chemical reactions by which carbohydrate is converted to energy and amino acids are converted to protein.
  - *Calcium* is required for bone formation, muscle contraction, nerve impulse transmission, and blood clotting.
- Negative ions (anions)
  - *Phosphate* is essential in the metabolism of carbohydrates, bone formation, and acid–base balance. Phosphates are found in the cell membrane and in the nucleic acids (DNA and RNA).
  - *Chloride* is essential for the formation of the hydrochloric acid in the gastric juice.

✔ CHECKPOINT **4:**

What is the main cation in extracellular fluid? In intracellular fluid?

Electrolyte Balance

Electrolytes must be kept in the proper concentration in both intracellular and extracellular fluids. The maintenance of water and electrolyte balance is one of the most difficult problems for health workers in caring for patients. Although some electrolytes are lost in the feces and through the skin as sweat, the job of bal-

ancing electrolytes is left mainly to the kidneys, as described in Chapter 22. (See Sodium and Potassium Imbalances.)

The Role of Hormones

Several hormones are involved in balancing electrolytes. Aldosterone, produced by the adrenal cortex, promotes the reabsorption of sodium (and water) and the elimination of potassium. In **Addison's disease,** a disease in which the adrenal cortex does not produce enough aldosterone, there is a loss of sodium and water and an excess of potassium.

When the blood concentration of sodium rises above the normal range, the pituitary secretes more antidiuretic hormone (ADH). This hormone increases the reabsorption of water in the kidney to dilute the excess sodium.

Hormones from the parathyroid and thyroid glands regulate calcium and phosphate levels. Parathyroid hormone increases blood calcium levels by causing the bones to release calcium and by causing the kidneys to reabsorb calcium. The thyroid hormone calcitonin lowers blood

---

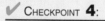

Sodium and Potassium Imbalances

The concentrations of sodium and potassium in body fluids are important measures of water and electrolyte balance. An excess of sodium in body fluids is termed **hypernatremia** (hi-per-nah-TRE-me-ah), taken from the Latin name for sodium, *natrium.* This condition accompanies dehydration and severe vomiting. **Hyponatremia,** a deficiency of sodium in body fluids, can come from water intoxication, heart failure, kidney failure, cirrhosis of the liver, pH imbalance, or endocrine disorders.

The term **hyperkalemia** (hi-per-kah-LE-me-ah) is taken from the Latin name for potassium, *kalium.* It refers to excess potassium in body fluids, which may result from kidney failure, dehydration, and other causes. **Hypokalemia,** or low potassium in body fluids, may result from taking diuretics, which cause potassium to be lost along with water. It may also result from pH imbalance or secretion of too much aldosterone from the adrenal cortex.

calcium by causing calcium to be deposited in the bones.

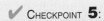

> ✓ CHECKPOINT **5**:
>
> What are some mechanisms for regulating electrolytes in body fluids?

ACID–BASE BALANCE

The pH scale is a measure of how acidic or basic (alkaline) a solution is. Body fluids are slightly alkaline at about pH 7.4. These fluids must be kept within a narrow range of pH, or damage, even death, will result.

Regulation of pH

Several systems act together to maintain acid–base balance. These are as follows:

- *Buffer systems.* Buffers are substances that prevent sharp changes in hydrogen ion (H^+) concentration and thus maintain a relatively constant pH. Buffers work by accepting or releasing these ions as needed to keep the pH steady. The main buffer systems in the body are bicarbonate buffers, phosphate buffers, and proteins, such as hemoglobin in red blood cells and plasma proteins.
- *Respiration.* The role of respiration in controlling pH was described in Chapter 18. Recall that the release of carbon dioxide from the lungs acts to make the blood more alkaline by reducing the amount of carbonic acid formed. In contrast, retention of carbon dioxide makes the blood more acidic. Respiratory rate can adjust pH for short-term regulation.
- *Kidney function.* The kidneys serve to regulate pH by reabsorbing or eliminating hydrogen ions as needed. The kidneys are responsible for the long-term regulation of pH. The activity of the kidneys is described in Chapter 22.

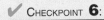

> ✓ CHECKPOINT **6**:
>
> What are three mechanisms for maintaining the acid—base balance of body fluids?

Abnormal pH

If shifts in pH cannot be controlled, either acidosis or alkalosis results.

Acidosis (as-ih-DO-sis) is a condition produced by a drop in the pH of body fluids. Acidosis may result from respiratory obstruction, lung disease, kidney failure, or prolonged diarrhea, which drains the alkaline contents of the intestine.

Acidosis may also result from inadequate carbohydrate metabolism, as occurs in diabetes mellitus, ingestion of a low-carbohydrate diet, or starvation. In these cases, the body metabolizes too much fat and protein from food or body materials, leading to the production of excess acid. When acidosis results from the accumulation of ketone bodies, as in the case of diabetes, the condition is more accurately described as *ketoacidosis.*

Alkalosis (al-kah-LO-sis) results from an increase in pH. Its possible causes include hyperventilation (the release of too much carbon dioxide), ingestion of antacids, and prolonged vomiting with loss of stomach acids.

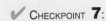

> ✓ CHECKPOINT **7**:
>
> What are conditions that arise from abnormally low or high pH of body fluids?

DISORDERS OF BODY FLUIDS

Edema is the accumulation of excessive fluid in the intercellular spaces. Some causes of edema are as follows:

- Interference with normal fluid return to the heart, as caused by congestive heart failure or blockage in the venous or lymphatic sys-

21

tems. A backup of fluid in the lungs, ***pulmonary edema,*** is a serious potential consequence of congestive heart failure.

- Lack of protein in the blood. This deficiency may result from protein loss or ingestion of too little dietary protein for an extended period. It may also result from failure of the liver to manufacture adequate amounts of the protein albumin, as frequently occurs in liver disease. The decrease in protein lowers the osmotic pressure of the blood and reduces the return of fluid to the circulation. Diminished fluid return results in accumulation of fluid in the tissues.
- Kidney failure, a common clinical cause of edema, resulting from the inability of the kidneys to eliminate adequate amounts of urine
- Increased loss of fluid through the capillaries, as caused by injury, allergic reaction, or certain infections.

Water intoxication involves dilution of body fluids in both the intracellular and extracellular compartments. Transport of water into the cells results in swelling. In the brain, the swelling of cells may lead to convulsions, coma, and finally death. Causes of water intoxication include an excess of ADH and intake of excess fluids by mouth or by intravenous injection.

Effusion (e-FU-zhun) is the escape of fluid into a cavity or a space. An example is pleural effusion, fluid within the pleural space; in this condition fluid compresses the lung, so that normal breathing is not possible. Tuberculosis, cancer, and some infections may give rise to effusion.

Effusion into the pericardial sac, which encloses the heart, may occur in autoimmune disorders, such as lupus erythematosus and rheumatoid arthritis. Infection is another cause of pericardial effusion. The fluid may interfere with normal heart contractions and can cause death.

Ascites (ah-SI-teze) is effusion with accumulation of fluid within the abdominal cavity. It may occur in disorders of the liver, kidneys, and heart, as well as in cancers and infection.

Dehydration (de-hi-DRA-shun), a severe deficit of body fluids, will result in death if it is prolonged. The causes include vomiting, diarrhea, drainage from burns or wounds, excessive perspiration, and too little fluid intake, as in cases of damage to the thirst mechanism. In such cases, it may be necessary to administer intravenous fluids to correct fluid and electrolyte imbalances.

✔ CHECKPOINT **8**:

What is edema?

FLUID THERAPY

Fluids are administered into a vein under a wide variety of conditions to help maintain normal body functions when natural intake is not possible. Fluids are also administered to correct specific fluid and electrolyte imbalances in cases of losses due to disease or injury.

The first fluid started in emergencies is normal saline, which contains 0.9% sodium chloride, a concentration equal to that of plasma. Because it is isotonic, this type of solution does not change the distribution of ions in the body fluid compartments.

Frequently, the patient receives 5% dextrose (glucose) in ½ normal saline. This solution is hypertonic when infused but becomes hypotonic after the sugar is used. Another common fluid is 5% dextrose in water. This solution is slightly hypotonic when infused. The amount of sugar contained in a liter of this fluid is equal to 170 calories. The sugar is soon used up, resulting in a fluid that is effectively pure water. Use of these hypotonic fluids is not advisable for long-term therapy because of the common occurrence of water intoxication. Both these dextrose solutions increase the plasma fluid volume. Small amounts of potassium chloride are often added to replace electrolytes lost by vomiting or diarrhea.

Ringer's lactate solution contains sodium, potassium, calcium, chloride, and lactate. In this formulation, the electrolyte concentrations are equal to normal plasma values. The lactate is metabolized to bicarbonate, which acts as a buffer. This fluid is given when the need is for additional plasma volume with the electrolyte concentration equal to that of the blood.

Serum albumin 25% contains the plasma protein albumin in a concentration five times normal. This hypertonic solution draws fluid from the interstitial spaces into the circulation.

Fluids containing varied concentrations of dextrose, sodium chloride, potassium, and other electrolytes and substances are manufactured. These fluids are used to correct specific imbalances. Nutritional solutions containing concentrated sugar, protein, and fat are available for administration when oral intake is not possible for an extended period.

Summary

I. The importance of water
  1. Functions
     a. Solvent
     b. Transport medium
     c. Participant in metabolic reactions
  2. 50% to 70% of body
  3. Contains electrolytes, nutrients, gases, wastes, hormones, and other substances
  4. Important in homeostasis

II. Fluid compartments
  1. Intracellular fluid—contained within the cells
  2. Extracellular fluid—outside the cells
     a. Blood plasma
     b. Interstitial (tissue) fluid
     c. Lymph
     d. Fluid in special compartments

III. Water balance
  1. Output—through skin, lungs, intestinal tract, kidneys
  2. Intake—through beverages, food, intravenous fluid
  A. Sense of thirst—control center in hypothalamus

IV. Electrolytes and their functions
  1. Electrolytes release ions in solution
     a. Positive ions (cations)—e.g., sodium, potassium, calcium
     b. Negative ions (anions)—phosphate, chloride
  A. Electrolyte balance
     1. Kidneys—main regulators
     2. Role of hormones
        a. Aldosterone (from adrenal cortex)
           (1) Promotes reabsorption of sodium
           (2) Promotes excretion of potassium
        b. ADH (from pituitary)
           (1) Causes kidney to retain water
        c. Parathyroid hormone (from parathyroid glands)
           (1) Increases blood calcium level
        d. Calcitonin (from thyroid)
           (1) Decreases blood calcium level

V. Acid–base balance
  1. Normal pH is 7.4
  A. Regulation of pH
     1. Buffers—maintain constant pH
     2. Respiration—release of carbon dioxide increases alkalinity; retention of carbon dioxide increases acidity
     3. Kidney—regulates amount of hydrogen ion excreted
  B. Abnormal pH
     1. Acidosis—decrease in pH; causes respiratory obstruction, lung disease, kidney failure, diarrhea, diabetes mellitus
     2. Alkalosis—increase in pH; causes hyperventilation, ingestion of antacids, prolonged vomiting

VI. Disorders of body fluids

1. Edema—accumulation of fluid in tissues
    a. Causes
        (1) Interference with fluid return to heart
        (2) Lack of proteins in blood
        (3) Kidney failure
        (4) Fluid loss from capillaries
2. Water intoxication—dilution of body fluids
3. Effusion—escape of fluid into a cavity or space
4. Ascites—accumulation of fluid in abdominal cavity
5. Dehydration—deficiency of fluid

VII. Fluid therapy

1. Purpose
    a. Correct fluid balance
    b. Correct electrolyte balance
    c. Provide nourishment
2. Commonly used solutions
    a. Normal saline
    b. 5% dextrose (glucose) in 1/2 normal saline
    c. 5% dextrose in water
    d. Ringer's lactate
    e. 25% serum albumin

Questions for Study and Review

1. List four types of extracellular fluid.
2. In a healthy person, what is the ratio of fluid intake to output?
3. Explain the role of the hypothalamus in water balance.
4. Name five common ions in the body. How is each used?
5. Name three hormones involved in electrolyte balance and explain what each does.
6. Define *buffer* and name the three main buffer systems in the body.
7. How does the respiratory system help regulate pH?
8. Describe five disorders involving body fluids.
9. List some causes of edema.
10. List several reasons for administering intravenous fluids.
11. When is normal saline used for treatment?
12. List the contents of some other fluids commonly used for treatment.
13. Compare the terms in each of the following pairs:
    a. *intracellular fluid* and *extracellular fluid*
    b. *acidosis* and *alkalosis*

✔ ANSWERS TO CHECKPOINTS

1. Body fluids are grouped into intracelluar fluid and extracellular fluid.
2. Water is lost from the body through the skin, the lungs, the intestinal tract, and the kidneys.
3. The control center for the sense of thirst is located in the hypothalamus of the brain.
4. Sodium is the main cation in extracellular fluid. Potassium is the main cation in intracellular fluid.
5. Some electrolytes are lost through the feces and through sweat. The kidneys have the main job of balancing electrolytes. Several hormones, such as aldosterone, parathyroid hormone, and calcitonin, are also involved.
6. The acid–base balance of body fluids is maintained by buffer systems, respiration, and kidney function.
7. Abnormally low pH of body fluids results in acidosis; abnormally high pH of body fluids results in alkalosis.
8. Edema is the accumulation of excessive fluid in the intercellular spaces.

The Urinary System

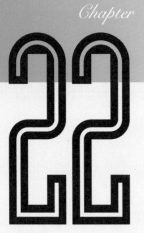

Chapter

22

SELECTED KEY TERMS

The following terms are defined in the Glossary:

angiotensin

antidiuretic hormone (ADH)

cystitis

dialysis

erythropoietin

excretion

glomerular filtrate

glomerulonephritis

glomerulus

hemodialysis

kidney

micturition

nephron

renin

urea

ureter

urethra

urinalysis

urinary bladder

urine

BEHAVIORAL OBJECTIVES

After careful study of this chapter, you should be able to:

1. List the systems that eliminate waste and name the substances eliminated by each

2. Describe the parts of the urinary system and give the functions of each

3. Trace the path of a drop of blood as it flows through the kidney

4. Describe a nephron

5. Describe the components and the functions of the juxtaglomerular apparatus

6. Name the four processes involved in urine formation and describe how each functions

7. Identify the role of ADH in urine formation

8. Describe the process of micturition

9. List the common disorders of the urinary system

10. List six signs of chronic renal failure

11. Explain the principle and the purpose of kidney dialysis

12. Name three normal and six abnormal constituents of urine

The urinary system is also called the *excretory system* because one of its main functions is to remove waste products from the blood and eliminate them from the body. It has many other functions as well, including regulation of the volume, acid–base balance (pH), and electrolyte composition of body fluids.

Although the focus of this chapter is the urinary system, certain aspects of other systems are also discussed because body systems work interdependently to maintain homeostasis (balance). The systems active in excretion and some of the substances that they eliminate are the following:

- The *urinary system* excretes water, waste products containing nitrogen, and salts. These are all constituents of the urine.
- The *digestive system* eliminates water, some salts, bile, and the residue of digestion, all of which are contained in the feces. The liver is important in eliminating the products of red blood cell destruction and in breaking down certain drugs and toxins.
- The *respiratory system* eliminates carbon dioxide and water. The latter appears as vapor, as can be demonstrated by breathing on a windowpane.
- The skin, or *integumentary system*, excretes water, salts, and very small quanti-

ties of nitrogenous wastes. These all appear in perspiration, although evaporation of water from the skin may go on most of the time without our being conscious of it.

✔ CHECKPOINT **1**:

The main function of the urinary system is to eliminate waste. What are some other systems that eliminate waste?

ORGANS OF THE URINARY SYSTEM

The main parts of the urinary system, shown in Figure 22-1, are as follows:

- Two *kidneys.* These organs extract wastes from the blood, balance body fluids, and form urine.
- Two *ureters* (U-re-ters). These tubes conduct urine from the kidneys to the urinary bladder.
- A single *urinary bladder*. This reservoir receives and stores the urine brought to it by the two ureters.
- A single *urethra* (u-RE-thrah). This tube conducts urine from the bladder to the outside of the body for elimination.

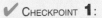

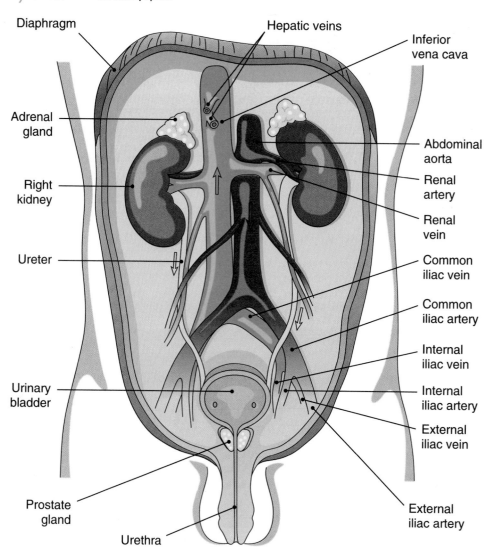

FIGURE **22•1** Urinary system, with blood vessels.

Labels (clockwise from top): Diaphragm, Hepatic veins, Inferior vena cava, Abdominal aorta, Renal artery, Renal vein, Common iliac vein, Common iliac artery, Internal iliac vein, Internal iliac artery, External iliac vein, External iliac artery, Urethra, Prostate gland, Urinary bladder, Ureter, Right kidney, Adrenal gland

---

✓ CHECKPOINT **2**:

What are the organs of the urinary system?

THE KIDNEYS

Location of the Kidneys

The two kidneys lie against the muscles of the back in the upper abdomen. They are up under the dome of the diaphragm and are protected by the lower ribs and the rib (costal) cartilages. Each kidney is enclosed in a membranous capsule that is made of fibrous connective tissue; this capsule adheres loosely to the kidney itself. In addition, there is a crescent of fat called the *adipose capsule* around the organ. An outer layer of fascia (connective tissue) anchors the kidney to the peritoneum and abdominal wall. The kidneys, as well as the ureters, lie behind the peritoneum. Thus, they are not in the peritoneal cavity but rather in an area known as the ***retroperitoneal*** (ret-ro-per-ih-to-NE-al) ***space***.

Blood Supply to the Kidney

The blood supply to the kidney is illustrated in Figure 22-2. Blood is brought to the kidney by a short branch of the abdominal aorta called the ***renal artery***. After entering the kidney, the renal artery subdivides into smaller and smaller branches, which eventually make contact with the functional units of the kidney, the ***nephrons*** (NEF-ronz) (Figs. 22-3 and 22-4). Blood leaves the kidney by vessels that finally merge to form the ***renal vein***, which carries blood into the inferior vena cava for return to the heart.

✔ CHECKPOINT **3**:

The kidneys are located in the retroperitoneal space. Where is this space?

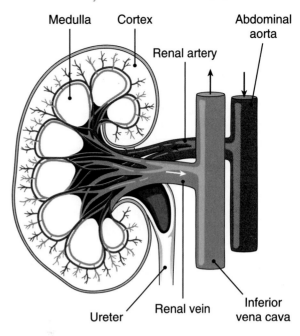

FIGURE **22•2**   Blood supply and circulation of the kidney.

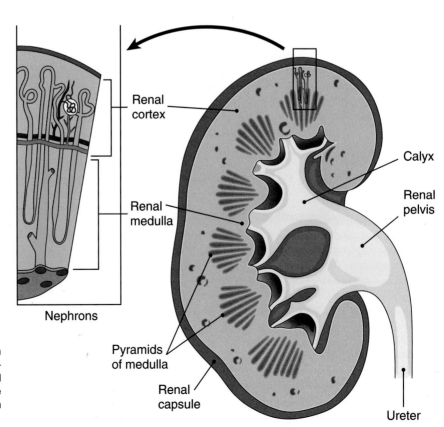

FIGURE **22•3** Longitudinal section through the kidney showing its internal structure and an enlarged diagram of a nephron. There are more than 1 million nephrons in each kidney.

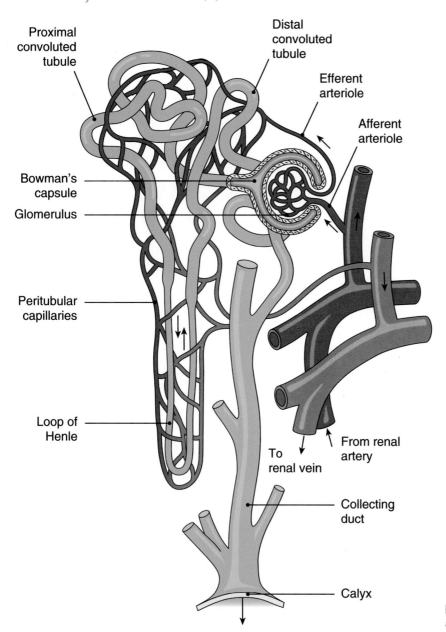

Proximal
convoluted
tubule

Distal
convoluted
tubule

Efferent
arteriole

Afferent
arteriole

Bowman's
capsule

Glomerulus

Peritubular
capillaries

Loop of
Henle

To
renal vein

From renal
artery

Collecting
duct

Calyx

FIGURE **22•4**   Simplified diagram of
a nephron.

Structure of the Kidney

The kidney is a somewhat flattened organ about
10 cm (4 inches) long, 5 cm (2 inches) wide, and
2.5 cm (1 inch) thick. On the inner, or medial,

border there is a notch called the **hilus,** at
which region the renal artery, the renal vein,
and the ureter connect with the kidney. The
outer, or lateral, border is convex (curved outward), giving the entire organ a bean-shaped
appearance.

The kidney is divided into two regions: the
renal cortex and the renal medulla (see Fig. 22-
3). The **renal cortex** is the outer portion of the
kidney. The **renal medulla** contains the tubes
in which urine is formed and collected. These

tubes form a number of cone-shaped structures called **renal pyramids**. The tips of the pyramids point toward the **renal pelvis**, a funnel-shaped basin that forms the upper end of the ureter. Cuplike extensions of the renal pelvis surround the tips of the pyramids and collect urine; these extensions are called **calyces** (KA-lih-seze) (sing., **calyx** [KA-liks]). The urine that collects in the pelvis then passes down the ureters to the bladder.

The Nephron

As is the case with most organs, the most fascinating aspect of the kidney is too small to be seen with the naked eye. This basic unit of the kidney, where the kidney's work is actually done, is the **nephron** (see Fig. 22-4). The nephron is essentially a tiny coiled tube with a bulb at one end. This bulb, known as **Bowman's capsule**, surrounds a cluster of capillaries called the **glomerulus** (glo-MER-u-lus) (pl., *glomeruli* [glo-MER-u-li]). Each kidney contains about 1 million nephrons; if all these coiled tubes were separated, straightened out, and laid end to end, they would span some 120 kilometers (75 miles)! Figure 22-5 is a microscopic view of kidney tissue showing several glomeruli, each surrounded by a Bowman's capsule. It also shows sections through the tubular portions of the nephrons.

A small blood vessel, called the **afferent arteriole**, supplies the glomerulus with blood; another small vessel, called the **efferent arteriole**, carries blood from the glomerulus. When blood leaves the glomerulus, it does not head immediately back toward the heart. Instead, it flows into a capillary network that surrounds the tubular portion of the nephron. These small vessels, **peritubular capillaries**, are named for their location around the nephron.

The tubular part of the nephron consists of several portions. The coiled portion leading from Bowman's capsule is called the **proximal convoluted** (KON-vo-lu-ted) **tubule (PCT)**. The tubule then uncoils to form a hairpin-shaped segment called the **loop of Henle**. Continuing from the loop, the tubule coils once again into the **distal convoluted tubule (DCT)**, so called because it is farther along the tubule from Bowman's capsule than is the PCT. The distal end of each tubule empties into a collecting duct, which then continues through the medulla toward the renal pelvis.

The glomerulus, Bowman's capsule, and the proximal and distal convoluted tubules of the nephrons are within the renal cortex. The loops of Henle and collecting ducts extend into the medulla (see Fig. 22-3).

The Juxtaglomerular Apparatus

The first portion of the DCT curves back toward the glomerulus to pass between the afferent and efferent arterioles (Fig. 22-6). At the point where the DCT makes contact with the afferent arteriole, there are specialized cells in each that together make up the **juxtaglomerular** (juks-tah-glo-MER-u-lar) **(JG) apparatus.** The name means "near the glomerulus," which describes the location of this structure. The JG apparatus helps to regulate kidney function. When blood pressure falls, cells in the wall of the afferent arteriole secrete the enzyme **renin** (RE-nin), which raises blood pressure by a mechanism described later.

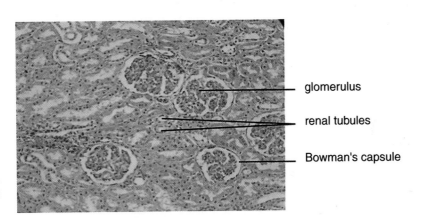

glomerulus

renal tubules

Bowman's capsule

FIGURE 22•5 Microscopic view of the kidney. (Courtesy of Dana Morse Bittus and B. J. Cohen)

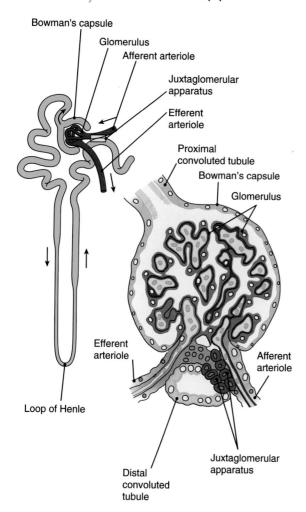

Bowman's capsule
Glomerulus
Afferent arteriole
Juxtaglomerular apparatus
Efferent arteriole
Proximal convoluted tubule
Bowman's capsule
Glomerulus
Efferent arteriole
Afferent arteriole
Loop of Henle
Juxtaglomerular apparatus
Distal convoluted tubule

FIGURE 22•6   Structure of the juxtaglomerular apparatus. Note how the distal convoluted tubule contacts the afferent arteriole.

✔ CHECKPOINT **5**:

What is the functional unit of the kidney called?

Functions of the Kidney

The kidneys are involved in the following processes:

- Excretion of unwanted substances, such as waste products from cell metabolism, excess salts, and toxins. One product of amino acid metabolism is nitrogen-containing waste material, a chief form of which is **urea** (u-RE-ah). Urea is produced in the liver and transported in the bloodstream to the kidneys for elimination. The kidneys provide a specialized mechanism for the elimination of urea and other nitrogenous (ni-TROJ-en-us) wastes.

- Maintenance of water balance. Although the amount of water consumed in a day can vary tremendously, the kidneys can adapt to these variations, so that the volume of body water remains remarkably stable from day to day. Water is constantly lost in many ways: from the skin, from the respiratory system during exhalation, and from the intestinal tract. Normally, the amount of water taken in or produced (intake) is about equal to the amount lost (output).

- Regulation of the acid–base balance of body fluids. Acids are constantly being produced by cell metabolism, and certain foods can cause acids or bases to be formed in the body. Bases in the form of antacids, such as baking soda, may also be ingested. However, if the body is to function normally, a certain critical proportion of acids and bases must be maintained at all times.

- Regulation of blood pressure. If blood pressure falls too low for effective filtration through the glomerulus, the cells of the JG apparatus release the enzyme renin. In the blood, renin activates a protein called **angiotensin** (an-je-o-TEN-sin) that causes blood vessels to constrict, thus raising blood pressure.

- Regulation of red blood cell production. When the kidneys do not get enough oxygen, they produce the hormone **erythropoietin** (eh-rith-ro-POY-eh-tin) **(EPO),** which stimulates the production of red blood cells in the red bone marrow. EPO made by genetic engineering is now available to reduce severe anemia, such as occurs in the end stage of kidney failure.

✔ CHECKPOINT **6**:

What substance is produced by the JG apparatus and under what conditions is it produced?

Formation of Urine

Glomerular Filtration

The process of urine formation begins with the glomerulus in Bowman's capsule. The membranes that form the walls of the glomerular capillaries are sievelike and permit the free flow of water and soluble materials through them. Like other capillary walls, however, they are impermeable (im-PER-me-abl) to blood cells and large protein molecules, and these components remain in the blood (Fig. 22-7).

Because the diameter of the afferent arteriole is slightly larger than the diameter of the efferent arteriole (see Fig. 22-7), blood can enter the glomerulus more easily than it can leave. Thus, the pressure of the blood in the glomerulus is about three to four times as high as it is in other body capillaries. To understand this effect, think of placing your thumb over the end of a garden hose as water comes through. Because the diameter of the opening is made smaller, water is forced out under higher pressure. As a result of this increased pressure in the glomerulus, materials are constantly being pushed out of the blood and into Bowman's capsule of the nephron. This movement of materials under pressure from the blood into Bowman's capsule is known as ***glomerular filtration***.

The fluid that enters Bowman's capsule, called the ***glomerular filtrate,*** begins its journey along the tubular system of the nephron. In addition to water and the normal soluble substances in the blood, other substances, such as drugs, may also be filtered and become part of the glomerular filtrate.

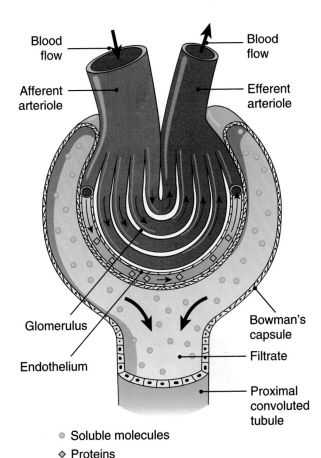

Blood flow

Blood flow

Afferent arteriole

Efferent arteriole

Glomerulus

Endothelium

Bowman's capsule

Filtrate

Proximal convoluted tubule

● Soluble molecules
◇ Proteins

FIGURE 22•7 Diagram showing the process of filtration in the formation of urine. Blood pressure inside the glomerulus forces water and dissolved substances into Bowman's capsule. Blood cells and proteins remain behind in the blood. The smaller caliber of the efferent arteriole as compared with that of the afferent arteriole maintains pressure.

✔ CHECKPOINT **7**:

The first step in urine formation is glomerular filtration. What is glomerular filtration?

Tubular Reabsorption

About 160 to 180 liters of filtrate are formed each day in the kidneys. However, only 1 to 1.5 liters of urine are eliminated daily. Clearly, most of the water that enters the nephron is not excreted with the urine but rather is returned to the circulation. In addition to water, many substances that are needed by the body, such as nutrients and ions, also pass into the nephron as part of the filtrate. These must be returned to the body as well. Therefore, the process of filtration that occurs in Bowman's capsule is followed by a process of ***tubular reabsorption***. As the filtrate travels through the tubular system of the nephron, water and other needed substances leave the tubule by diffusion and active transport and enter the surrounding tissue fluids. They then enter the blood in the peritubular capillaries and return to the circulation. In contrast, most of the urea and other nitrogenous waste materials are kept within the tubule to be eliminated with the urine (see The Transport Maximum).

22

The Transport Maximum

The kidney works very efficiently to return valuable substances to the blood after glomerular filtration. However, the carriers that are needed for active transport of these substances can become overloaded. There is a limit to the amount of each substance that can be reabsorbed in a given time period. The limit of this rate of reabsorption is called the **transport maximum (Tm)** for that substance, and it is measured in milligrams (mg) per minute.

If a substance is present in excess in the blood, it may exceed its transport maximum and then, because it cannot be totally reabsorbed, some will be excreted in the urine. For example, if the concentration of glucose in the blood exceeds 180 mg/dL, glucose will begin to appear in the urine, a condition called **glucosuria** (glu-ko-SU-re-ah). The most common cause of glucosuria is uncontrolled diabetes mellitus.

Tubular Secretion

Before the filtrate leaves the body as urine, final adjustments in composition are made by the process of *tubular secretion*. In this process, some substances are actively moved from the blood into the nephron. Notably, potassium ions are moved into the urine by this process. Also, by the active secretion of hydrogen ions, the kidneys regulate the acid–base (pH) balance of body fluids.

Concentration of the Urine

The amount of water that is eliminated with the urine is regulated by a complex mechanism within the nephron that is influenced by *antidiuretic hormone (ADH),* a hormone released from the posterior portion of the pituitary gland. The process is called the *countercurrent mechanism* because it involves fluid traveling in opposite directions within the loop of Henle. The countercurrent mechanism is illustrated in Figure 22-8. Its essentials are described as follows.

As the filtrate passes through the loop of Henle, salts, especially sodium, are actively pumped out by the cells of the nephron, with the result that the interstitial fluid of the medulla becomes increasingly concentrated. Because the nephron is not very permeable to water at this point, the fluid within the nephron becomes increasingly dilute. As the fluid passes through the more permeable DCT and through the collecting duct, water is drawn out by the concentrated fluids around the nephron and returned to the blood. (Remember, according to the laws of diffusion, water follows salt.) In this manner, the urine becomes more concentrated, and its volume is reduced.

ADH

The role of ADH is to make the walls of the DCT and collecting tubule more permeable to water, so that more water will be reabsorbed and less will be excreted with the urine. The release of ADH from the pituitary is regulated by a feedback system. As the blood becomes more concentrated, the hypothalamus causes more ADH to be released from the posterior pituitary; as the blood becomes more dilute, less ADH is released. In the disease diabetes insipidus, there is inadequate secretion of ADH from the hypothalamus. This results in the elimination of large amounts of dilute urine accompanied by excessive thirst.

Summary of Urine Formation

The processes involved in urine formation are summarized below and illustrated in Figure 22-9.

* Glomerular filtration allows all diffusible materials to pass from the blood into the nephron.
* Tubular reabsorption moves useful substances back into the blood while keeping waste products in the nephron to be eliminated in the urine.
* Tubular secretion moves additional substances from the blood into the nephron for elimination. Movement of hydrogen ions is one means by which the pH of body fluids is balanced.
* The countercurrent mechanism concentrates the urine and reduces the volume excreted. The pituitary hormone ADH allows more water to be reabsorbed from the nephron.

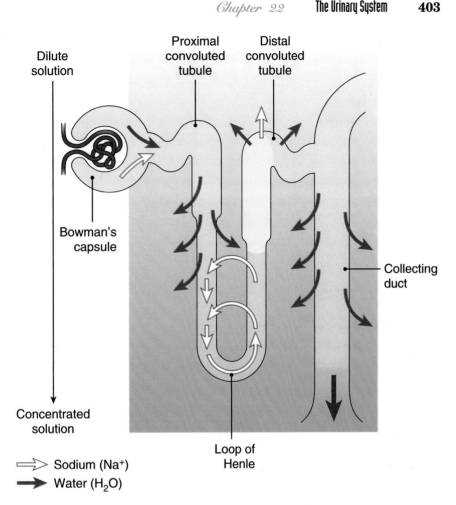

FIGURE **22•8** Loop of Henle, where the proportions of waste and water in urine are regulated according to the body's constantly changing needs. The concentration of urine is determined by means of intricate exchanges of water and salt, constituting the counter-current mechnism.

⇒ Sodium (Na⁺)

→ Water (H₂O)

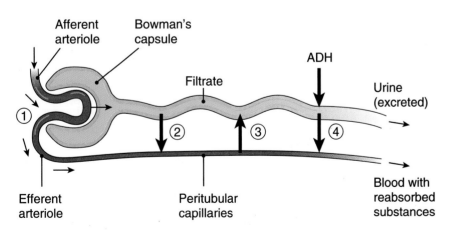

① Filtration from blood into nephron

② Reabsorption from filtrate into blood

③ Tubular secretion from blood into filtrate

④ Reabsorption of water under effects of ADH

FIGURE **22•9** Summary of urine formation in nephron.

Although this story seems complex, and there appears to be a great deal of back-and-forth exchanges, these processes together allow the kidney to "fine tune" body fluids. As the filtrate makes its slow journey through the twists and turns of the nephron, there is ample time for exchanges to take place between the kidney tubules and the circulating blood.

✓ CHECKPOINT **8**:

What are the four processes involved in the formation of urine?

THE URETERS

The two ureters are long, slender, muscular tubes that extend from the kidney down to and through the lower part of the urinary bladder (see Fig. 22-1). The ureters are entirely extraperitoneal, being located behind and, at the lower part, below the peritoneum. Their length naturally varies with the size of the individual, and they may be anywhere from 25 cm to 32 cm (10–13 inches) long. Nearly 2.5 cm (1 inch) of the lower part of the ureter enters the bladder by passing obliquely (at an angle) through the bladder wall. Because of the oblique direction taken by the ureter through the lower bladder wall, a full bladder compresses the ureter and prevents the backflow of urine.

The wall of the ureter includes a lining of epithelial cells, a relatively thick layer of involuntary muscle, and finally an outer coat of fibrous connective tissue. The lining of the ureter is continuous with that of the renal pelvis and the bladder. The muscles of the ureters are capable of the same rhythmic contraction (peristalsis) found in the digestive system. Urine is moved along the ureter from the kidneys to the bladder by gravity and by peristalsis at frequent intervals.

THE URINARY BLADDER

When it is empty, the urinary bladder (Fig. 22-10) is located below the parietal peritoneum and behind the pubic joint. When it is filled, it

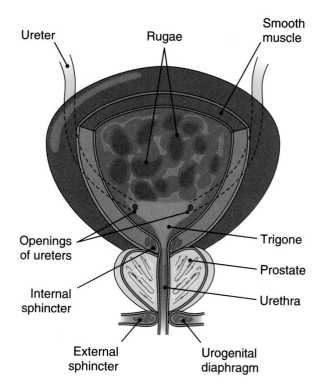

FIGURE **22•10** Interior of the urinary bladder, shown in the male. The trigone is a triangle in the floor of the bladder marked by the openings of the ureters and the urethra.

pushes the peritoneum upward and may extend well into the abdominal cavity proper. The urinary bladder is a temporary reservoir for urine, just as the gallbladder is a storage sac for bile. (See The Healthy Bladder.)

The bladder wall has many layers. It is lined with mucous membrane; the lining of the bladder, like that of the stomach, is thrown into folds called *rugae* when the organ is empty. Beneath the mucosa is a layer of connective tissue. Then follows a three-layered coat of involuntary muscle tissue that is capable of great stretching. Finally, there is an incomplete coat of peritoneum that covers only the upper portion of the bladder.

When the bladder is empty, the muscular wall becomes thick, and the entire organ feels firm. As the bladder fills, the muscular wall becomes thinner, and the organ may increase from a length of 5 cm (2 inches) up to as much as 12.5 cm (5 inches) or even more. A moderately full bladder holds about 470 mL (1 pint) of urine.

The Healthy Bladder

The bladder is a hollow muscular organ that collects and eliminates urine. While stored, urine can become a medium for bacterial growth. There are two precautions to take to help prevent bladder infections.

- Completely empty the bladder every time you urinate. Many times, in a rush, we relieve just the strong pressure and fail to empty the bladder. Partial emptying increases the chance that bacteria will remain in the bladder. The smooth muscle of the bladder wall contracts periodically, and this property can be used to empty the bladder. Urination is a spinal reflex that is controlled by centers in the brain. When a convenient time presents itself, relaxation of the external sphincter allows urine to flow. If while the sphincter is relaxed, there is enough time for a second reflex contraction to occur, the remaining urine will be voided.
- Make the urine in the bladder less suitable for bacterial growth. Certain foods, such as cranberries and blueberries, are able to change the pH of the urine so that many bacteria have a difficult time surviving. A daily dose of the juice of these fruits can reduce the likelihood of bladder infection.

In the floor of the bladder is the *trigone* (TRI-gone), a triangle formed by the openings of the two ureters and the urethra (see Fig. 22-10). As the bladder fills with urine, it expands upward, leaving the trigone at the base stationary. This stability prevents stretching of the ureteral openings and the possible back flow of urine into the ureters.

THE URETHRA

The *urethra* is the tube that extends from the bladder to the outside (see Fig. 22-1) and is the means by which the bladder is emptied. The urethra differs in men and women; in the male, it is part of both the reproductive system and the urinary system, and it is much longer than is the female urethra.

The male urethra is about 20 cm (8 inches) in length. Early in its course, it passes through the prostate gland, where it is joined by the two ducts carrying the male sex cells. From, here it leads through the **penis** (PE-nis), the male organ of copulation, to the outside. The male urethra serves the dual purpose of conveying the sex cells and draining the bladder.

The urethra in the female is a thin-walled tube about 4 cm (1.5 inches) long. It is located behind the pubic joint and is embedded in the muscle of the front wall of the vagina. The external opening, called the **urinary meatus,** is located just in front of the vaginal opening between the labia minora. The female urethra drains the bladder only and is entirely separate from the reproductive system.

Urination

The process of expelling (voiding) urine from the bladder is called **urination** or **micturition** (mik-tu-RISH-un). This process is controlled both voluntarily and involuntarily with the aid of two rings of muscle (sphincters) that surround the urethra (see Fig. 22-10). Near the outlet of the bladder is an involuntary **internal urethral sphincter** formed by a continuation of the smooth muscle of the bladder wall. Below this muscle is a voluntary **external urethral sphincter** formed by the muscles of the pelvic floor. By learning to control the voluntary sphincter, one can gain control over emptying of the bladder.

As the bladder fills with urine, stretch receptors in its wall send impulses to a center in the lower part of the spinal cord. Motor impulses from this center stimulate contraction of the bladder wall, forcing urine outward as both the internal and external sphincters are made to relax. In the infant, this emptying occurs automatically as a simple reflex. Early in life, a person learns to control urination from higher centers in the brain until the time is appropriate, a process known as *toilet training*. The impulse to urinate will override conscious controls if the bladder becomes too full.

The bladder can be emptied voluntarily by relaxing the muscles of the pelvic floor and increasing the pressure in the abdomen. The resulting increased pressure in the bladder triggers the spinal reflex that leads to urination.

✔ CHECKPOINT **9**:

What is the name of the tube that carries urine from the kidney to the bladder?

✔ CHECKPOINT **10**:

What is the name of the tube that carries urine from the bladder to the outside?

DISORDERS OF THE URINARY SYSTEM

Kidney Disorders

Kidney disorders may be acute or chronic. Acute conditions usually arise suddenly, most frequently as the result of infection with inflammation of the nephrons. These diseases commonly run a course of a few weeks and are followed by complete recovery. Chronic conditions arise slowly and are often progressive, with gradual loss of kidney function.

Acute glomerulonephritis (glo-mer-u-lo-nef-RI-tis), also known as *acute poststreptococcal glomerulonephritis,* is the most common disease of the kidneys. This condition usually occurs in children about 1 to 4 weeks after a streptococcal infection of the throat. Antibodies formed in response to the streptococci attach to the glomerular membrane and injure it. These damaged glomeruli allow protein, especially albumin, to filter into Bowman's capsule and ultimately to appear in the urine (albuminuria). They also allow red blood cells to filter into the urine (hematuria). Usually, the patient recovers without permanent kidney damage. In adult patients, the disease is more likely to become chronic, with a gradual decrease in the number of functioning nephrons, leading to chronic renal failure.

Pyelonephritis (pi-el-o-nef-RI-tis), an inflammation of the renal pelvis and the tissue of the kidney, may be either acute or chronic. In acute pyelonephritis, the inflammation results from a bacterial infection. Bacteria most commonly reach the kidney by ascending along the lining membrane from an infection in the lower part of the urinary tract (see Fig. 23-12 in Chap. 23). More rarely, bacteria are carried to the kidney by the blood.

Acute pyelonephritis is often seen in people with partial obstruction of urine flow with stagnation (urinary stasis). It is most likely to occur in pregnant women and in men with an enlarged prostate because the prostate surrounds the first portion of the urethra in males. Other causes of stasis include neurogenic bladder, which is bladder dysfunction resulting from neurologic lesions, as seen in diabetes mellitus, and structural defects in the area where the ureters enter the bladder. Pyelonephritis usually responds to the administration of antibiotics, fluid replacement, rest, and fever control.

Chronic pyelonephritis, a more serious disease, is frequently seen in patients with urinary tract stasis or backflow. It may be caused by persistent or repeated bacterial infections. Progressive damage of kidney tissue is evidenced by high blood pressure, continual loss of protein in the urine, and dilute urine.

Hydronephrosis (hi-dro-nef-RO-sis) is the distention of the renal pelvis and calyces with accumulated fluid caused by obstruction of urine flow. The obstruction may occur at any level in the urinary tract. The most common causes of obstruction, in addition to pregnancy and an enlarged prostate, are a kidney stone that has formed in the pelvis and dropped into the ureter, a tumor that presses on a ureter, and scars due to inflammation. Prompt removal of the obstruction may result in complete recovery. If the obstruction is not removed, the kidney will be permanently damaged.

A *polycystic* (pol-e-SIS-tik) *kidney* is one in which many fluid-containing sacs develop in the active tissue and gradually, by pressure, destroy the functioning parts. This disorder runs in families, and treatment has not proved very satisfactory, except for the use of dialysis machines or kidney transplantation.

Tumors of the kidneys usually grow rather slowly, but rapidly invading types are occasionally found. Blood in the urine and dull pain in the kidney region are warnings that should be heeded at once. Surgical removal of the kidney offers the best chance of cure because most renal cancers do not respond to chemotherapy or radiation.

Renal Failure

Acute renal failure may result from a medical or surgical emergency or from toxins that damage the tubules. This condition is characterized by a sudden, serious decrease in kidney function accompanied by electrolyte and acid–base imbalances. Acute renal failure occurs as a serious complication of other severe illness and may be fatal.

Chronic renal failure results from a gradual loss of nephrons. As more and more nephrons are destroyed, the kidneys gradually lose the ability to perform their normal functions. As the disease progresses, nitrogenous waste products accumulate to high levels in the blood, causing a condition known as *uremia* (u-RE-me-ah).

In many cases, there is a smaller decrease in renal function, known as **renal insufficiency**, that produces fewer symptoms.

Results of Chronic Renal Failure

A few of the characteristic signs and symptoms of chronic renal failure are the following:

- *Dehydration* (de-hi-DRA-shun). Excessive loss of body fluid may occur early in renal failure when the kidneys cannot concentrate the urine and large amounts of water are eliminated.
- *Edema* (eh-DE-mah). Accumulation of fluid in the tissue spaces may occur late in chronic renal disease when the kidneys cannot eliminate water in adequate amounts.
- **Electrolyte imbalance**, including retention of sodium and accumulation of potassium
- *Hypertension* may occur as the result of fluid overload and the increased production of renin (see Angiotensin).
- *Anemia* occurs when the kidneys cannot produce the hormone erythropoietin to activate red blood cell production in bone marrow.
- *Uremia*. If levels of nitrogenous waste products in the blood are very high, urea

Angiotensin

Angiotensin is a hormone that has a powerful effect on blood pressure. It is generated through the action of renin, an enzyme from the kidney that normally acts to keep blood pressure high enough for effective filtration. In the blood, renin promotes formation of a substance called **angiotensin I.** Under the effects of another enzyme, angiotensin I is converted to **angiotensin II.** This compound raises blood pressure by causing constriction of blood vessels. It also stimulates the release of the hormone aldosterone and antidiuretic hormone (ADH), both of which act to increase blood pressure. A class of drugs used in the treatment of hypertension are the **ACE inhibitors** (angiotensin-converting enzyme inhibitors). They control blood pressure by blocking the production of angiotensin II.

can be changed into ammonia in the stomach and intestine and cause ulcerations and bleeding.

Kidney Stones

Kidney stones, or *calculi* (KAL-ku-li), are made of substances, such as calcium salts or uric acid, that precipitate out of the urine instead of remaining in solution. They usually form in the renal pelvis, although the bladder can be another site of formation.

The causes of stone formation include dehydration, stagnation of the urine, and infection of the urinary tract. The stones may vary in size from tiny grains resembling bits of gravel up to large masses that fill the renal pelvis and extend into the calyces. The latter are described as *staghorn calculi*.

There is no way of dissolving these stones because substances that could do so would also destroy kidney tissue. Sometimes, instruments can be used to crush small stones and thus allow them to be expelled with the urine, but more often, surgical removal is required. Also in use is a device called a *lithotriptor* (LITH-o-trip-tor), literally a "stone-cracker," which employs external shock waves to shatter kidney stones. The procedure is called *lithotripsy* (LITH-o-trip-se).

✓ CHECKPOINT **11**:

What is the difference between acute and chronic kidney disorders?

Treatment of Kidney Failure

Renal Dialysis

Dialysis (di-AL-ih-sis) means "the separation of dissolved molecules based on their ability to pass through a semipermeable membrane." Molecules that can pass through the membrane move from an area of greater concentration to one of lesser concentration. In patients who have defective kidney function, the accumulation of urea and other nitrogenous waste products can be reduced by passage of the patient's blood through a dialysis machine. The principle of "molecules leaving the area of greater concentration" thus operates to remove the excess products from the blood. The fluid in the dialysis machine, the dialysate, can be adjusted to regulate the flow of substances out of the blood.

There are two methods of dialysis in use: hemodialysis (blood dialysis) and peritoneal dialysis (dialysis in the abdominal cavity). In hemodialysis, the dialysis membrane is made of cellophane or other synthetic material. In peritoneal dialysis, the surface area of the peritoneum acts as the membrane. Dialysis fluid is introduced into the peritoneal cavity and then periodically removed along with waste products.

A 1973 amendment to the Social Security Act provides federal financial assistance for people who have chronic renal disease and require dialysis. Most hemodialysis is performed in freestanding clinics. Treatment time has been reduced; a typical schedule involves 2 to 3 hours, three times a week. Access to the bloodstream has been made safer and easier through surgical establishment of a permanent exchange site (shunt). Peritoneal dialysis has been improved and simplified, so that patients are able to manage treatment at home.

Kidney Transplantation

Many hundreds of kidney transplantation procedures have been performed successfully in recent years. Kidneys have so much extra functioning tissue that the loss of one kidney normally poses no problem. Records show that the likelihood that a transplantation will be successful is greatest when a living donor who is closely related to the patient is used. Organs from deceased donors have also proved satisfactory in many cases. The problem of tissue rejection (the rejection syndrome) is discussed in Chapter 17.

Disorders of the Ureters

Abnormalities in structure of the ureter include double portions at the kidney pelvis and constricted or abnormally narrow parts, called *strictures* (STRICK-tures). Narrowing of the ureter may be caused by abnormal pressure from tumors or other masses outside the tube. Obstruction of the ureters may be due to stones from the kidneys or to kinking of the tube because of a dropping of the kidney, a condition known as *renal ptosis* (TO-sis).

Ureteral Stones

The passage of a small stone along the ureter causes excruciating pain, called *renal colic*. Relief of this pain usually requires morphine or an equally powerful drug. The first "barber surgeons," operating without benefit of anesthesia, were permitted by their patients to cut through the skin and the muscles of the back to remove stones from the ureters. "Cutting for stone" in this way was relatively successful, despite the lack of sterile technique, because the approach through the back avoided the peritoneal cavity and the serious risk of peritonitis.

Modern surgery employs a variety of instruments for removal of stones from the ureter, including endoscopes similar to those described in Chapter 19. The transurethral route through the urethra and urinary bladder and then into the ureter, as well as entrance through the skin and muscles of the back, may be used to remove calculi from the kidney pelvis or from the ureter.

> ✔ CHECKPOINT **12**:
>
> What is the scientific name for stones, as may occur in the urinary tract?

Disorders Involving the Bladder

A full (distended) bladder lies in an unprotected position in the lower abdomen, and a blow may rupture it, necessitating immediate surgical repair. Blood in the urine is a rather common symptom of infection or tumors, which may involve the bladder.

Cystitis

Inflammation of the bladder, called **cystitis** (sis-TI-tis), is 10 times as common in women as in men. This may be due at least in part to the very short urethra in the female compared with that of the male. Usually, bacteria (*e.g.,* colon bacilli) ascend from the outside through the urethra into the bladder (see Fig. 23-12 in Chap. 23). Pain, urgency to urinate, and frequency of urination are common symptoms.

Another type of cystitis, called **interstitial cystitis,** may cause pelvic pain with discomfort before and after urination. The tissues below the mucosa are involved. The disease can be diagnosed only with the use of a cystoscope (a kind of endoscope). Because no bacteria are involved, antibiotics are not effective treatment and may even be harmful.

Obstruction by an enlarged prostate gland or from a pregnancy may lead to stagnation of urine and cystitis. Reduction of a person's general resistance to infection, as in diabetes, may also lead to cystitis. The danger of cystitis is that the infection may ascend to other parts of the urinary tract.

Tumors

Tumors of the bladder, which are most prevalent in men older than 50 years of age, include benign papillomas and various kinds of cancer. About 90% of bladder tumors arise from the epithelial lining. Possible causes include toxins (particularly certain aniline dyes), chronic infestations (schistosomiasis), heavy cigarette smoking, and the presence of urinary stones, which may develop and increase in size within the bladder. Cystoscopic examinations and biopsies should be done as soon as blood in the urine (hematuria) is detected. Removal before the tumor invades the muscle wall gives the best prognosis.

> ✔ CHECKPOINT **13**:
>
> What is the term for inflammation of the bladder?

Disorders of the Urethra

Congenital anomalies (defects present at birth) involve the urethra and other parts of the urinary tract. The opening of the urethra to the outside may be too small, or the urethra itself may be narrowed. Occasionally, an abnormal valvelike structure is found at the point where the urethra enters the bladder. If it is not removed surgically, it can cause back pressure of the urine, with serious consequences. There is also a condition in the male in which the urethra opens on the undersurface of the penis instead of at the end. This is called **hypospadias** (hi-po-SPA-de-as).

Urethritis, which is characterized by inflammation of the mucous membrane and the glands of the urethra, is much more common in the male than in the female. It is often due to gonococci or chlamydia, although many other bacteria may be responsible for the infection.

"Straddle" injuries to the urethra are common in men. This type of injury occurs when, for example, a man walking along a raised beam slips and lands with the beam between his legs. Such an accident may catch the urethra between the hard surfaces of the beam and the pubic arch and rupture the urethra. In accidents in which the bones of the pelvis are fractured, rupture of the urethra is fairly common.

THE EFFECTS OF AGING

Even without kidney disease, aging causes the kidneys to lose some of their ability to concentrate urine. With aging, progressively more water is needed to excrete the same amount of waste. Older people find it necessary to drink more water than young people, and they eliminate larger amounts of urine (polyuria), even at night (nocturia).

Beginning at about 40 years of age, there is a decrease in the number and size of the nephrons. Often, more than half of them are lost before the age of 80 years. There may be an increase in blood urea nitrogen (BUN) without serious symptoms. Elderly people are more susceptible than are young people to infections of the urinary system. Childbearing may cause damage to the musculature of the pelvic floor, resulting in urinary tract problems in later years.

Enlargement of the prostate, common in older men, may cause obstruction and a back pressure in the ureters and kidneys. If this condition is untreated, it will cause permanent damage to the kidneys. Age changes may predispose to but do not cause incontinence. Most elderly people (60% in nursing homes and up to 90% living independently) have no incontinence.

THE URINE

Urine is a yellowish liquid that is about 95% water and 5% dissolved solids and gases. The pH (acidity) of freshly collected urine averages 6.0, with a range of 4.5 to 8.0. Diet may cause considerable variation in pH.

The amount of dissolved substances in urine is indicated by its *specific gravity*. The specific gravity of pure water, used as a standard, is 1.000. Because of the dissolved materials it contains, urine has a specific gravity that normally varies from 1.002 (very dilute urine) to 1.040 (very concentrated urine). When the kidneys are diseased, they lose the ability to concentrate urine, and the specific gravity no longer varies as it does when the kidneys function normally.

Normal Constituents

Some of the dissolved substances normally found in the urine are the following:

- *Nitrogenous waste products,* including urea, uric acid, and *creatinine* (kre-AT-ih-nin)
- *Electrolytes,* including sodium chloride (as in common table salt) and different kinds of sulfates and phosphates. Electrolytes are excreted in appropriate amounts to keep their blood concentration constant.
- *Yellow pigment,* which is derived from certain bile compounds. Pigments from foods and drugs also may appear in the urine.

Abnormal Constituents

Examination of urine, called a *urinalysis* (u-rin-AL-ih-sis) *(UA),* is one of the most important parts of an evaluation of a person's physical state. A routine urinalysis includes observation of color and turbidity (cloudiness) as well as measurement of pH and specific gravity. A variety of abnormal components are also tested for. Among the most significant abnormal substances found in the urine are the following:

- *Glucose* is usually an important indicator of a disease known as *diabetes mellitus,* in which blood sugar is not adequately oxidized (metabolized) in the body cells. The excess glucose, which cannot be reabsorbed, is excreted in the urine. The presence of glucose in the urine is known as *glycosuria* (gli-ko-SU-re-ah).
- *Albumin.* The presence of this protein, which is normally retained in the blood, may indicate a kidney disorder, such as glomerulonephritis. Albumin in the urine is known as *albuminuria* (al-bu-mih-NU-re-ah).
- *Blood* in the urine is usually an important indicator of urinary system disease, including nephritis. Blood in the urine is known as *hematuria* (hem-ah-TU-re-ah).
- *Ketones* (KE-tones) are produced when fats are incompletely oxidized; ketones in the urine are seen in diabetes mellitus and starvation.
- *White blood cells* (pus) are evidence of infection; they can be seen by microscopic ex-

amination of a centrifuged specimen. Pus in the urine is known as ***pyuria*** (pi-U-re-ah).

• ***Casts*** are molds formed in the microscopic kidney tubules; they usually indicate disease of the nephrons.

More extensive tests on urine may include analysis for drugs, enzymes, hormones, and other metabolites as well as cultures for microorganisms. Normal values for common urine tests are given in Appendix 3, Table 1.

Summary

I. **Urinary system**—excretory system
1. Main function is excretion—removal and elimination of waste materials from blood
   a. Other systems that eliminate waste
      (1) Digestive system—eliminates undigested food, water, salts, bile
      (2) Respiratory system—eliminates carbon dioxide, water
      (3) Skin—eliminates water, salts, nitrogen waste

II. **Organs of the urinary system**
   a. Kidneys (2)
   b. Ureters (2)
   c. Urinary bladder (1)
   d. Urethra (1)

III. **Kidneys**
   A. Location of the kidneys
      1. In upper abdomen against the back
      2. In retroperitoneal space (behind the peritoneum)
      3. Blood supply
         a. Renal artery—carries blood to kidney from aorta
         b. Renal vein—carries blood from kidney to inferior vena cava
   B. Structure of the kidney
      1. Cortex—outer portion
      2. Medulla—inner portion
      3. Pelvis

         a. Upper end of ureter
         b. Calyces—cuplike extensions that receive urine
      4. Nephron
         a. Functional unit of kidney
         b. Parts
            (1) Bowman's capsule—around glomerulus
            (2) Proximal convoluted tubule
            (3) Henle's loop
            (4) Distal convoluted tubule
      5. Blood supply to nephron
         a. Afferent arteriole—enters Bowman's capsule
         b. Glomerulus—coil of capillaries in Bowman's capsule
         c. Efferent arteriole—leaves Bowman's capsule
         d. Peritubular capillaries—surround nephron
      6. Juxtaglomerular apparatus
         a. Consists of cells in afferent arteriole and distal convoluted tubule
         b. Releases renin to regulate blood pressure
   C. Functions of the kidney
      1. Excretion of waste, excess salts, toxins
      2. Water balance
      3. Acid–base balance (pH)
      4. Regulation of blood pressure
      5. Regulation of red blood cells
         a. Releases erythropoietin (EPO)—hormone that stimulates red blood cell production
   D. Formation of urine
      1. Glomerular filtration—driven by blood pressure in glomerulus
         a. Water and soluble substances

22

forced out of blood and into Bowman's capsule

b. Blood cells and proteins remain in blood

c. Glomerular filtrate—material that leaves blood and enters the nephron

2. Tubular reabsorption

a. Most of filtrate leaves nephron by diffusion and active transport

b. Returns to blood through peritubular capillaries

3. Tubular secretion—materials moved from blood into nephron for excretion

4. Concentration of urine

a. Countercurrent mechanism—method for concentrating urine based on movement of ions out of nephron

b. ADH

(1) Hormone from posterior pituitary

(2) Promotes reabsorption of water

IV. The ureters—carry urine from the kidneys to the bladder

V. Urinary bladder

a. Stores urine until it is eliminated

b. Trigone—triangle in base of bladder; remains stable as bladder fills

VI. Urethra—carries urine out of body

1. Male urethra—20 cm long; carries both urine and semen

2. Female urethra—4 cm long; opens in front of vagina

A. Urination (micturition)

1. Both voluntary and involuntary

2. Sphincters

a. Internal urethral sphincter—involuntary (smooth muscle)

b. External urethral sphincter—voluntary (skeletal muscle)

3. Stretch receptors in bladder wall signal reflex emptying

4. Can be controlled through higher brain centers

VII. Disorders of the urinary system

A. Kidney disorders

1. Acute glomerulonephritis—damages glomeruli

2. Pyelonephritis—inflammation of kidney and renal pelvis

3. Hydronephrosis—distention with obstructed fluids

4. Polycystic kidney—fluid-containing sacs develop

5. Tumors

6. Renal failure

a. Acute—results from medical emergency or toxins

b. Chronic—signs include dehydration, electrolyte imbalance, edema, hypertension, anemia, uremia

7. Kidney stones—calculi

B. Treatment of kidney failure

1. Renal dialysis—removes unwanted substances from blood when kidneys fail

2. Kidney transplantation

C. Disorders of the ureters

1. Stricture (narrowing)

2. Stones (calculi)

D. Disorders involving the bladder

1. Cystitis—inflammation; most common in females

2. Tumors

E. Disorders of the urethra

1. Hypospadias—urethra opens on underside of penis

2. Urethritis—inflammation

VIII. Effects of aging

1. Polyuria—increased elimination of urine

2. Nocturia—urination at night

3. Incontinence

4. Increased blood urea nitrogen (BUN)

5. Prostate enlargement

IX. Urine

1. pH averages 6.0

2. Specific gravity—measures dissolved substances
A. Normal constituents—water, nitrogenous waste, electrolytes, pigments

B. Abnormal constituents—glucose, albumin, blood, ketones, white blood cells, casts

Questions for Study and Review

1. Name the body systems that have excretory functions.
2. Name the organs of the urinary system.
3. Where are the kidneys located?
4. Describe the internal structure of the kidney.
5. Describe the structure of a nephron.
6. Name and locate the blood vessels associated with the nephron.
7. Compare the afferent arteriole and the efferent arteriole in structure and function.
8. What happens to the glomerular filtrate as it passes through the nephron?
9. What is the function of the JG apparatus?
10. What results from inadequate secretion of ADH? What disease is associated with this condition?
11. What structures empty into the kidney pelvis and what drains the pelvis?
12. What is micturition? How is it controlled?
13. Compare the male urethra and female urethra in structure and function.
14. What are some of the infections that involve the kidney and what parts are most often affected?
15. What are calculi and what are some of the causes of calculi?
16. What is meant by the word *dialysis* and how is this principle used for patients with kidney failure? What kinds of membranes are used for hemodialysis? for peritoneal dialysis?
17. What types of donors are used for kidney transplantation?
18. What is inflammation of the bladder called? Why is it more common in women than in men?
19. What are some of the effects of aging on the urinary system?
20. What is urea? Where is it formed and how is it eliminated?
21. What tests are done in a routine urinalysis?
22. Tell the possible significance of six abnormal constituents of the urine.

✔ ANSWERS TO CHECKPOINTS

1. Systems other than the urinary system that eliminate waste include the digestive, respiratory, and integumentary systems.
2. The urinary system consists of two kidneys, two ureters, the bladder, and the urethra.
3. The retroperitoneal space is behind the peritoneum.
4. The renal artery supplies blood to the kidney, and the renal vein drains the kidney.
5. The functional unit of the kidney is the nephron.
6. The JG apparatus produces renin when blood pressure falls too low for effective filtration.
7. Glomerular filtration is the movement of materials under pressure from the blood into Bowman's capsule of the nephron.
8. The four processes involved in the formation of urine are glomerular filtration, tubular reabsorption, tubular secretion, and the countercurrent mechanism for concentrating the urine.
9. The ureter carries urine from the kidney to the bladder.
10. The urethra carries urine from the bladder to the outside.
11. Acute kidney disorders arise suddenly, usually as a result of infection. Chronic conditions arise slowly and are often progressive, with gradual loss of kidney functions.
12. The scientific name for stones is calculi.
13. Inflammation of the bladder is cystitis.

The last unit includes three chapters on the structures and functions related to reproduction and inheritance. The reproductive system is not necessary for the continuation of the life of the individual but rather is needed for the continuation of the human species. The germ cells and their genes have been studied intensively during recent years as part of the rapidly advancing science of genetics.

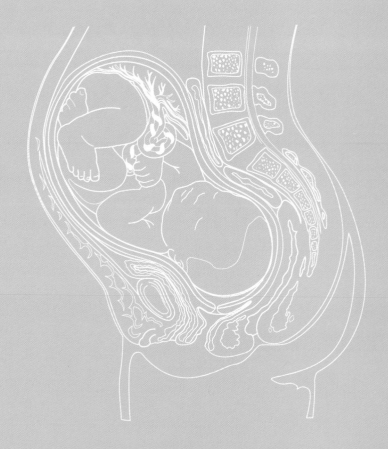

Unit VII

PERPETUATING LIFE

The Male and Female Reproductive Systems

BEHAVIORAL OBJECTIVES

After careful study of this chapter, you should be able to:

1. Name the male and female gonads and describe the function of each

2. State the purpose of meiosis

3. List the accessory organs of the male and female reproductive tracts and cite the function of each

4. Describe the composition and function of semen

5. Draw and label a spermatozoon

6. List in the correct order the hormones produced during the menstrual cycle and cite the source of each

7. Describe the functions of the main male and female sex hormones

8. Explain how negative feedback regulates reproductive function in both males and females

9. Describe the changes that occur during and after menopause

10. Define *contraception* and cite the main methods of contraception in use

11. Briefly describe the major disorders of the male and female reproductive tracts

Chapter

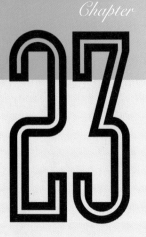

23

REPRODUCTION

The chapters in this unit deal with what is certainly one of the most interesting and mysterious attributes of life: the ability to reproduce. The simplest forms of life, one-celled organisms, usually need no partner to reproduce; they simply divide by themselves. This form of reproduction is known as *asexual* (nonsexual) reproduction.

In most animals, however, reproduction is *sexual*, meaning that there are two kinds of individuals, males and females, each of which has specialized cells designed specifically for the perpetuation of the species. These specialized sex cells are known as *germ cells,* or *gametes* (GAM-etes). In the male, they are called *spermatozoa* (sper-mah-to-ZO-ah), or simply sperm cells, and in the female, they are called *ova* (O-vah) or egg cells.

Meiosis

Germ cells are characterized by having half as many chromosomes as are found in any other cell in the body. During their formation, they go through a special process of cell division, called *meiosis* (mi-O-sis), that halves the number of chromosomes. In humans, meiosis reduces the chromosome number in a cell from 46 to 23.

Divisions of the Reproductive System

Although the male and female reproductive systems are different, the organs of both may be divided into two groups: primary and accessory.

- The primary organs are the *gonads* (GO-nads), or sex glands; they produce the germ cells and manufacture hormones. The male gonads are the *testes* (TES-teze), and the female gonads are the *ovaries* (O-vah-reze).
- The *accessory organs* include a series of ducts that provide for the transport of germ cells as well as various exocrine glands.

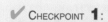

✔ CHECKPOINT **1**:

What is the process of cell division that halves the chromosome number in a cell to produce a gamete?

THE MALE REPRODUCTIVE SYSTEM

The Testes

The testes (male gonads) are located outside the body proper, suspended between the thighs in a sac called the *scrotum* (SKRO-tum) (Fig. 23-1).

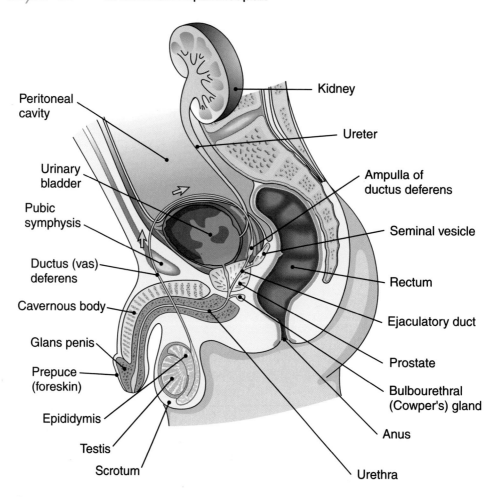

FIGURE **23•1** Male genitourinary system. The arrows indicate the course of sperm cells through the duct system.

The testes are oval organs measuring about 3.7 to 5 cm (1.5 to 2 inches) in length and about 2.5 cm (1 inch) in each of the other two dimensions. During embryonic life, each testis develops from tissue near the kidney.

A month or two before birth, the testis normally descends (moves downward) through the **inguinal** (ING-gwih-nal) **canal** in the abdominal wall into the scrotum. Each testis then remains suspended by a **spermatic cord** (Fig. 23-2) that extends through the inguinal canal. This cord contains blood vessels, lymphatic vessels, nerves, and the tube (ductus deferens) that transports spermatozoa away from the testis. The gland must descend completely if it is to function normally; to pro-duce spermatozoa, the testes must be kept at the temperature of the scrotum, which is several degrees lower than that of the abdominal cavity.

Internal Structure

Most of the specialized tissue of the testis consists of tiny coiled **seminiferous** (seh-mih-NIF-er-us) **tubules**. Cells in the walls of these tubules produce spermatozoa. Between the tubules are specialized **interstitial** (in-ter-STISH-al) **cells** that secrete the male sex hormone **testosterone** (tes-TOS-teh-rone). Figure 23-3 is a microscopic view of the testis in cross-section, showing the seminiferous tubules, interstitial cells, and developing spermatozoa.

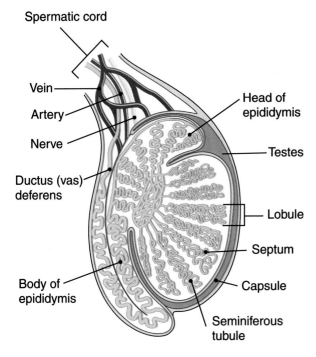

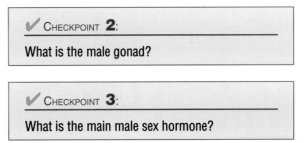

Spermatic cord

Vein

Artery

Nerve

Ductus (vas) deferens

Body of epididymis

Head of epididymis

Testes

Lobule

Septum

Capsule

Seminiferous tubule

FIGURE 23•2 Structure of the testis, also showing the epididymis and spermatic cord.

Testosterone

After being secreted by the testis, testosterone is absorbed directly into the bloodstream. This hormone has two functions:

- Maintenance of the reproductive structures, including development of the spermatozoa
- Development of **secondary sex character-**

istics, traits that characterize males and females but are not directly concerned with reproduction. In males, these traits include a deeper voice, broader shoulders, narrower hips, a greater percentage of muscle tissue, and more body hair than are found in females.

> ✔ CHECKPOINT **2**:
>
> What is the male gonad?

> ✔ CHECKPOINT **3**:
>
> What is the main male sex hormone?

The Ducts

The tubes that carry the spermatozoa begin with tubules inside the testis itself. From these tubes, the cells are collected by a greatly coiled tube called the **epididymis** (ep-ih-DID-ih-mis), which is 6 meters (20 feet) long and is located inside the scrotal sac (see Fig. 23-2). While they are temporarily stored in the epididymis, the sperm cells mature and become motile, that is, able to move, or "swim," by themselves.

The epididymis finally extends upward as the **ductus deferens** (DEF-er-enz), also called the **vas deferens**. The ductus deferens, contained in the spermatic cord, continues through the inguinal canal into the abdominal cavity. Here, it

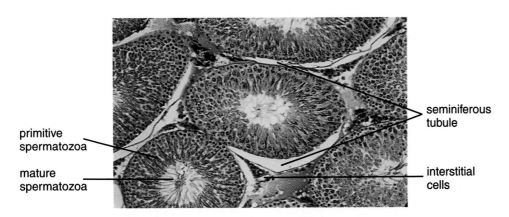

primitive spermatozoa

mature spermatozoa

seminiferous tubule

interstitial cells

FIGURE 23•3 Microscopic view of the testis. (Courtesy of Dana Morse Bittus and B. J. Cohen)

23

separates from the remainder of the spermatic cord and curves behind the urinary bladder. The ductus deferens then joins with the duct of the *seminal vesicle* (VES-ih-kl) on the same side to form the *ejaculatory* (e-JAK-u-lah-to-re) *duct*. The two ejaculatory ducts travel through the body of the prostate gland and then empty into the urethra.

> ✔ CHECKPOINT **4**:
>
> What is the order in which sperm cells travel through the ducts of the male reproductive system?

Formation of Semen

Semen (SE-men) is the mixture of sperm cells and various secretions that is expelled from the body. The secretions serve several functions:

- Nourish the spermatozoa
- Transport the spermatozoa
- Neutralize the acidity of the vaginal tract
- Lubricate the reproductive tract during sexual intercourse

The glands discussed next contribute secretions to the semen (see Fig. 23-1).

The Seminal Vesicles
The seminal vesicles are twisted muscular tubes with many small outpouchings. They are about 7.5 cm (3 inches) long and are attached to the connective tissue at the back of the urinary bladder. The glandular lining produces a thick, yellow, alkaline secretion containing large quantities of simple sugar and other substances that provide nourishment for the sperm. The seminal fluid forms a large part of the volume of the semen.

The Prostate Gland
The prostate gland lies immediately below the urinary bladder, where it surrounds the first part of the urethra. Ducts from the prostate carry its secretions into the urethra. The thin, alkaline prostatic secretion helps neutralize the acidity of the vaginal tract and enhance the motility of the

spermatozoa. The prostate gland is also supplied with muscular tissue, which, upon signal from the nervous system, contracts to aid in the expulsion of the semen from the body.

Bulbourethral Glands
The *bulbourethral* (bul-bo-u-RE-thral) *glands,* also called *Cowper's glands,* are a pair of pea-sized organs located in the pelvic floor just below the prostate gland. They secrete mucus to lubricate the urethra and tip of the penis during sexual stimulation. The ducts of these glands extend about 2.5 cm (1 inch) from each side and empty into the urethra before it extends into the penis.

Other very small glands secrete mucus into the urethra as it passes through the penis.

> ✔ CHECKPOINT **5**:
>
> What glands, aside from the testis, contribute secretions to semen?

The Urethra and Penis

The male urethra, as discussed in Chapter 22, serves the dual purpose of conveying urine from the bladder and carrying the reproductive cells and their accompanying secretions to the outside. The ejection of semen into the receiving canal (vagina) of the female is made possible by the *erection,* or stiffening and enlargement, of the penis, through which the longest part of the urethra extends. The penis is made of spongy tissue containing many blood spaces that are relatively empty when the organ is flaccid but fill with blood and distend when the penis is erect. This tissue is subdivided into three segments, each called a *corpus* (meaning "body") (Fig. 23-4). A single, ventrally located *corpus spongiosum* contains the urethra. On either side is a larger *corpus cavernosum* (pl., *corpora cavernosa*). At the distal end of the penis, the corpus spongiosum enlarges to form the *glans* penis. This enlargement is covered with a loose fold of skin, the *prepuce* (PRE-puse), commonly called the *foreskin.* It is the foreskin that is removed in a circumcision.

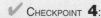

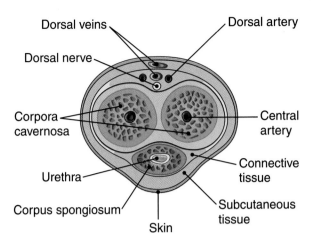

FIGURE **23•4**   Cross section of the penis.

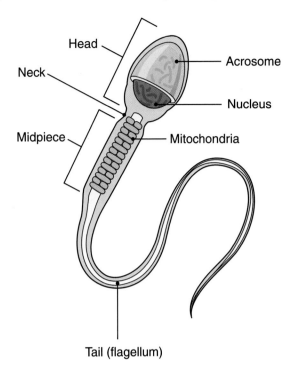

FIGURE **23•5**   Diagram of a human spermatozoon showing major structural features.

The penis and scrotum together are referred to as the *external genitalia* of the male.

Ejaculation

Ejaculation (e-jak-u-LA-shun) is the forceful expulsion of semen through the urethra to the outside. The process is initiated by reflex centers in the spinal cord that stimulate contraction of smooth muscle tissue in the prostate. This is followed by contraction of skeletal muscle in the pelvic floor, which provides the force needed for expulsion. During ejaculation, the involuntary sphincter at the base of the bladder closes to prevent the release of urine.

The Spermatozoa

Spermatozoa are tiny individual cells (Fig. 23-5). They are so small that at least 200 million are contained in the average ejaculation. Sperm cells are manufactured continuously in the testes. As they develop within the seminiferous tubules, they are nourished and protected by special cells called ***Sertoli,*** or "nurse," ***cells.***

The individual sperm cell has an oval head that is largely a nucleus containing chromosomes. Covering the head like a cap is the ***acrosome*** (AK-ro-some), which contains enzymes that help the sperm cell to penetrate the ovum.

Whiplike movements of the tail (flagellum) propel the sperm through the female reproductive system to the ovum. A middle region (midpiece) of the cell contains many mitochondria that provide energy for movement.

Out of the millions of spermatozoa in an ejaculation, only one, if any, fertilizes the ovum. The remainder of the cells live from only a few hours up to a maximum of 3 days.

✔ CHECKPOINT **6**:

What are the main subdivisions of a spermatozoon?

HORMONAL CONTROL OF MALE REPRODUCTION

The activities of the testes are under the control of two hormones produced by the anterior pituitary gland (hypophysis). These hormones are named for their activity in female reproduction, although they are chemically the same in both males and females.

- *Follicle-stimulating hormone (FSH)* stimulates the Sertoli cells and promotes the formation of spermatozoa.
- *Luteinizing hormone (LH),* called *interstitial cell–stimulating hormone (ICSH)* in males, stimulates the interstitial cells to produce testosterone, which is also needed for sperm cell development.

The pituitary gland is regulated by a region of the brain located just above it, the hypothalamus. Starting at puberty, the hypothalamus begins to secrete hormones that trigger the release of FSH and LH. These hormones are secreted continuously in the male.

The activity of the hypothalamus is in turn regulated by a negative feedback mechanism involving testosterone. As the level of testosterone in the blood increases, the hypothalamus secretes less releasing hormone; as the level of testosterone decreases, the hypothalamus secretes more releasing hormone (see Fig. 12-2 in Chap. 12).

✔ CHECKPOINT **7**:

What two pituitary hormones regulate both male and female reproduction?

The Effects of Aging on Male Reproduction

A gradual decrease in the production of testosterone and spermatozoa begins as early as 20 years of age and continues throughout life. Secretions from the prostate and seminal vesicles decrease in amount and become less viscous. In a few men (less than 10%), sperm cells remain late in life, even to 80 years of age.

DISORDERS OF THE MALE REPRODUCTIVE SYSTEM

Infertility

Infertility means significantly lower than normal ability to reproduce. If the inability is complete, the condition is termed *sterility.* The pro-

portion of infertile marriages due to defects involving the male has been estimated variously from 40% to 50%.

The tubules of the testes are sensitive to x-rays, infections, toxins, and malnutrition, all of which bring about degenerative changes. Such damage may cause a decrease in the numbers of spermatozoa produced, leading to a condition called *oligospermia* (ol-ih-go-SPER-me-ah). Adequate numbers of sperm are required to disperse the coating around the ovum, so that one sperm can fertilize it. Absence of or an inadequate number of male sex cells is a significant cause of infertility.

A male may be intentionally sterilized by an operation called a *vasectomy* (vah-SEK-to-me). In this procedure, a portion of the ductus deferens on each side is removed, and the cut end is closed to keep spermatozoa from reaching the urethra. The tiny sperm cells are simply reabsorbed. The vasectomized male retains the ability to produce hormones and all other seminal secretions as well as the ability to perform the sex act, but no fertilization can occur.

Cryptorchidism

Cryptorchidism (kript-OR-kid-izm), which means "hidden testes," is a disorder characterized by failure of the testes to descend into the scrotum. Unless corrected in childhood, this condition results in sterility. Undescended testes are also particularly subject to tumor formation. Most testes that are undescended at birth descend spontaneously by 1 year of age. Surgical correction is the usual remedy in the remaining cases.

Inguinal Hernia

Hernia (HER-ne-ah), or *rupture,* refers to the abnormal protrusion of an organ, or part of an organ, through the wall of the cavity in which it is normally contained. Hernias most often occur where there is a weak area in the abdominal wall, at the inguinal canal for example. In this region, during development, the testis pushes its way through the muscles and connective tissues of the abdominal wall, carrying with it the blood vessels and other structures that form the spermatic cord.

Normally, in the adult, the inguinal area is fairly well reinforced with connective tissue, and there is no direct connection between the abdominal cavity and the scrotal sac. As in other regions where an opening permits the passage of a structure through the abdominal wall, however, this area constitutes a weak place where a hernia may occur.

Infections

Infections of various kinds may involve the male reproductive organs, but by far the most common are chlamydial and gonococcal infections (see Preventing STDs). These sexually transmitted (venereal) diseases are manifested by a discharge from the urethra, which may be accompanied by burning and pain, especially during urination. The infection may travel along the mucous membrane into the prostate gland and into the epididymis; if both sides are affected and enough scar tissue is formed to destroy the tubules, sterility may result.

Another common sexually transmitted disease is an unpleasant, persistent infection called *genital herpes*. Caused by a virus, this disorder is characterized by fluid-filled vesicles (blisters) on and around the genital organs.

The sexually transmitted disease *syphilis* is caused by a spirochete (*Treponema pallidum*). Because syphilis spreads quickly in the bloodstream, it is regarded as a systemic disorder (see Appendix 4, Table 1). The genital ulcers caused by syphilis increase the chances of infection with the AIDS virus.

Other infectious agents that sometimes invade the reproductive organs include the tubercle bacillus and various staphylococci. The testes may be involved in mumps, with a resulting *orchitis* (or-KI-is), or inflammation of the testes, and possible sterility.

CHECKPOINT **8**:

What are some infectious diseases of the reproductive tract?

Preventing STDs

Sexually transmitted disease (STD), formerly known as venereal disease (VD), is infection spread through intimate sexual contact. Examples are gonorrhea, syphilis, human papillomavirus (HPV), genital herpes, hepatitis B, and chlamydia. These diseases can lead to sterility, cancer of the cervix, and increased susceptibility to AIDS. A trend toward participation in sex at earlier ages exposes people to more sexual contacts and an increased risk of infection.

The following techniques can prevent many cases of STD:

- Use a barrier, such as the male or female condom. The effectiveness of barriers is enhanced when one of the contraceptive foams or creams is used at the same time.
- Limit sexual activities when either partner suspects an infection. Do not engage in intimate relations until an infection has been adequately treated. Reinfection is always possible unless both partners are treated.
- Follow after-sex hygiene measures, which include cleaning the genitals after intercourse and urinating to reduce the possible ascent of organisms in the reproductive tract.

Women are more likely to contract STDs than are men. The same mechanisms that transport sperm cells through the female reproductive tract also move infectious organisms. Also, symptoms in women may be less apparent than in men.

Drugs to kill STD-causing organisms are effective in many cases. A vaccine is available for some diseases transmitted sexually, such as hepatitis B, and immunizations for other STDs are under study.

Tumors

Tumors of the Prostate

Tumors that develop in the male reproductive organs most commonly involve the prostate. The growths may be benign or malignant. Both types cause such pressure on the urethra that urination becomes difficult. Back pressure may destroy kidney tissue and may lead to stagnation of urine in the bladder with a resulting tendency to infection. The man with benign prostate enlargement may respond to medication to shrink the prostate. If kidney function is threatened, however, surgery is performed to reduce the obstruction.

Cancer of the prostate is a common disorder in men older than 50 years of age. It is frequently detected as a nodule during rectal examination. Early detection is now possible with an annual blood test for prostate-specific antigen (PSA). This protein increases in cases of prostate cancer, although it may increase in other prostate disorders as well.

Depending on the age of the patient and the nature of the cancer, the course of treatment may include surveillance, radiation therapy, or surgery.

Cancer of the Testis

Testicular cancer affects young to middle-aged adults, frequently causing death due to widespread metastasis by way of the lymphatic system. Early detection with regular self-examination allows for effective treatment and possible preservation of fertility.

Phimosis

Phimosis (fi-MO-sis) is a tightness of the foreskin (prepuce), so that it cannot be drawn back. Phimosis may be remedied by circumcision, in which part or all of the foreskin is surgically removed. Note that this operation is often performed on very young male infants as a routine measure, either for hygienic reasons or because of religious principles.

THE FEMALE REPRODUCTIVE SYSTEM

The Ovaries

In the female, the counterparts of the testes are the two **ovaries,** where the female sex cells, or **ova,** are formed (Fig. 23-6). The ovaries are small, somewhat flattened oval bodies measuring about 4 cm (1.6 inches) in length, 2 cm (0.8 inch) in width, and 1 cm (0.4 inch) in depth. Like the testes, the ovaries descend, but only as far as

the pelvic portion of the abdomen. Here, they are held in place by ligaments, including the broad ligament, the ovarian ligament, and others, that attach them to the uterus and the body wall.

The Egg Cell and Ovulation

The outer layer of the ovary is made of a single layer of epithelium. Beneath this layer, the ova (egg cells) are produced. The ovaries of a newborn female contain a large number of potential ova. Each month during the reproductive years, several ripen, but usually only one is released. The complicated process of maturation, or "ripening," of an ovum takes place in a small fluid-filled cluster of cells called the **ovarian follicle** (o-VA-re-an FOL-ih-kl) or **graafian** (GRAF-e-an) **follicle** (Fig. 23-7). As the ovum develops, the cells of the ovarian follicle wall secrete the hormone estrogen, which stimulates growth of the uterine lining. When an ovum has ripened, the ovarian follicle may rupture and discharge the egg cell from the surface of the ovary. The rupture of a follicle allowing the escape of an ovum is called **ovulation** (ov-u-LA-shun). Any developing ova that are not released simply degenerate.

After it is released, the egg cell makes its way to the nearest **oviduct** (O-vih-dukt). The oviduct is a tube that arches over the ovary and leads to the uterus.

The Corpus Luteum

After the ovum has been expelled, the remaining follicle is transformed into a solid glandular mass called the **corpus luteum** (LU-te-um), a name that means "yellow body." This structure secretes both estrogen and progesterone, another hormone needed in the reproductive cycle. Commonly, the corpus luteum shrinks and is replaced by scar tissue. When a pregnancy occurs, however, this structure remains active. (See In Vitro Fertilization.)

Sometimes, as a result of normal ovulation, the corpus luteum persists and forms a small ovarian cyst (fluid-filled sac). This condition usually resolves without treatment.

 CHECKPOINT **9**:

What is the process of releasing an egg cell from the ovary called?

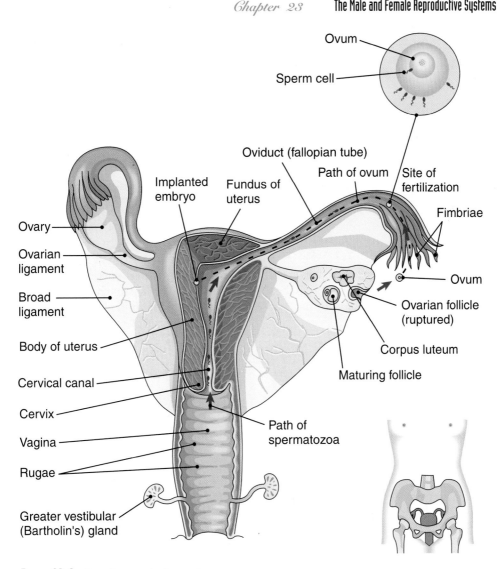

Ovum
Sperm cell
Oviduct (fallopian tube)
Path of ovum
Site of fertilization
Implanted embryo
Fundus of uterus
Fimbriae
Ovary
Ovarian ligament
Ovum
Broad ligament
Ovarian follicle (ruptured)
Body of uterus
Corpus luteum
Cervical canal
Maturing follicle
Cervix
Vagina
Rugae
Path of spermatozoa
Greater vestibular (Bartholin's) gland

FIGURE **23•6**   Female reproductive system.

The Oviducts

The tubes that transport the ova in the female reproductive system, the oviducts, are also known as *uterine* (U-ter-in) *tubes,* or *fallopian* (fah-LO-pe-an) *tubes.* Each is a small, muscular structure, nearly 12.5 cm (5 inches) long, extending from a point near the ovary to the uterus (womb). There is no direct connection between the ovary and this tube. The ovum is swept into the oviduct by a current in the peritoneal fluid produced by the small, fringe-like extensions called *fimbriae* (FIM-bre-e) that are located at the edge of the abdominal opening of the tube.

Unlike the sperm cell, the ovum cannot move by itself. Its progress through the oviduct toward the uterus depends on the sweeping action of cilia in the lining of the tube and on peristalsis of the tube. It takes about 5 days for an ovum to reach the uterus from the ovary.

The Uterus

The organ to which the oviducts lead is the *uterus* (U-ter-us), and it is within this structure that the developing fetus grows to maturity.

23

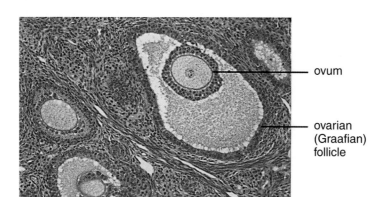

ovum

ovarian
(Graafian)
follicle

FIGURE **23•7**   Microscopic view of the ovary showing egg cells developing within ovarian follicles.
(Courtesy of Dana Morse Bittus and B. J. Cohen)

Structure of the Uterus

The uterus is a pear-shaped, muscular organ about 7.5 cm (3 inches) long, 5 cm (2 inches) wide, and 2.5 cm (1 inch) deep. The upper por-tion rests on the upper surface of the urinary bladder; the lower portion is embedded in the pelvic floor between the bladder and the rectum. The wider upper portion is called the **corpus,** or body; the lower, narrower part is the **cervix** (SER-viks), or neck. The small, rounded part above the level of the tubal entrances is known as the **fundus** (FUN-dus) (see Fig. 23-6).

The cavity inside the uterus is shaped somewhat like a capital T, but it is capable of changing shape and dilating as a fetus develops. The cervix leads to the **vagina** (vah-JI-nah), the lower part of the birth canal, which opens to the outside of the body.

The lining of the uterus is a specialized epithelium known as **endometrium** (en-do-ME-tre-um), and it is this layer that is involved in menstruation.

In Vitro Fertilization

The term *in vitro* literally means "in glass." It is used to describe tests or procedures done in the laboratory. In vitro fertilization (IVF) refers to fertilization of an egg cell outside the mother's body in a laboratory dish. The first such procedure was done successfully in 1978.

The woman participating in IVF must be given hormones to cause ovulation of several eggs. These are then withdrawn with a needle and fertilized with the father's sperm. After a few divisions, the fertilized egg is placed in the uterus for development. Additional fertilized eggs can be frozen to repeat the procedure in case of failure or for later pregnancies. Other possibilities for IVF include using donor eggs, donor sperm cells, or both, or using a surrogate mother for gestation.

Because of a lack of guidelines or restrictions in the United States in the field of assisted reproductive technology, some problems have arisen. These issues concern the use of stored embryos and gametes, the use of embryos without consent, and improper screening for disease among donors. In addition, the implantation of more than one fertilized egg has resulted in a high incidence of multiple births, even up to seven or eight offspring in a single pregnancy, a situation that imperils the survival and health of the babies.

Supporting Tissues

The **broad ligaments** support the uterus, extending from each side of the organ to the lateral body wall. Along with the uterus, these two portions of peritoneum form a partition dividing the female pelvis into anterior and posterior areas. The ovaries are suspended from the broad ligaments, and the oviducts lie within the upper borders. Blood vessels that supply these organs are found between the layers of the broad ligament (see Fig. 23-6).

✔ CHECKPOINT **10**:

In what organ does a fetus develop?

The Vagina

The vagina is a muscular tube about 7.5 cm (3 inches) long connecting the uterine cavity with the outside. At the top, it receives the cervix, which dips into the upper vagina in such a way that a circular recess known as the ***fornix*** (FOR-niks) is formed. The deepest area of the fornix, located behind the cervix, is the ***posterior fornix***

(FOR-niks) (Fig. 23-8). This recess in the posterior vagina lies adjacent to the lowest part of the peritoneal cavity, a narrow passage between the uterus and the rectum named the ***cul-de-sac*** (from a French term meaning "bottom of the sack"). This area is also known as the *rectouterine pouch* or the *pouch of Douglas*. A rather thin layer of tissue separates the posterior fornix from this region, so that abscesses or tumors in the

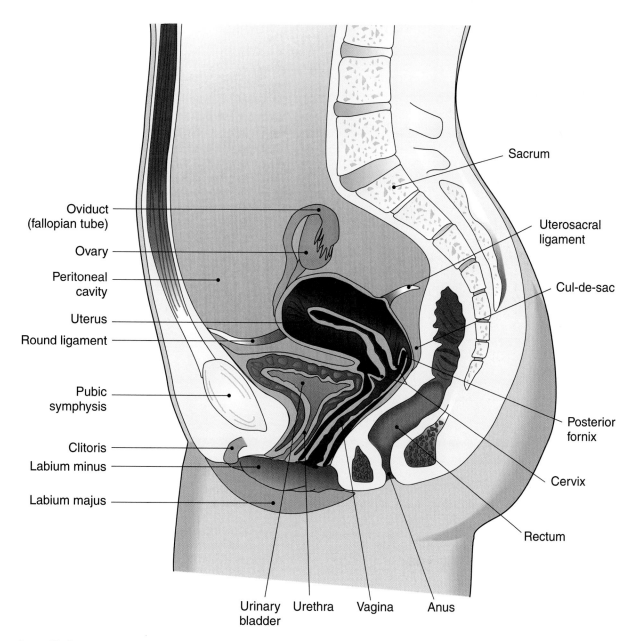

FIGURE 23•8 Female reproductive system, as seen in sagittal section.

peritoneal cavity can sometimes be detected by vaginal examination.

The lining of the vagina is a wrinkled mucous membrane something like that found in the stomach. The folds (rugae) permit enlargement so that childbirth usually does not tear the lining. In addition to being a part of the birth canal, the vagina is the organ that receives the penis during sexual intercourse. A fold of membrane called the **hymen** may sometimes be found at or near the vaginal (VAJ-ih-nal) canal opening.

The Greater Vestibular Glands

Just above and to each side of the vaginal opening are the mucus-producing **greater vestibular** (ves-TIB-u-lar), or **Bartholin's, glands**. These glands secrete into an area near the vaginal opening known as the **vestibule**. The glands may become infected, leading to painful swelling and abscess, in which case a surgical incision to promote drainage may be required.

The Vulva and the Perineum

The external parts of the female reproductive system form the **vulva** (VUL-vah), which includes two pairs of lips, or **labia** (LA-be-ah); the **clitoris** (KLIT-o-ris), which is a small organ of great sensitivity; and related structures (Fig. 23-9). Although the entire pelvic floor in both the male and female is properly called the **perineum** (per-ih-NE-um) (see Fig. 8-11 in Chap. 8), those who care for pregnant women usually refer to the limited area between the vaginal opening and the anus as the perineum.

THE MENSTRUAL CYCLE

In the female, as in the male, reproductive function is controlled by hormones from the pituitary gland as regulated by the hypothalamus. Female activity differs, however, in that it is cyclic, that is, shows regular patterns of increases and decreases in hormone levels. These changes are regulated by hormonal feedback.

The length of the menstrual cycle varies between 22 and 45 days in normal women, but 28 days is taken as an average, with the first day of menstrual flow being considered the first day of the cycle (Fig. 23-10).

Beginning of the Cycle

At the start of each cycle, under the influence of FSH produced by the pituitary, a follicle begins

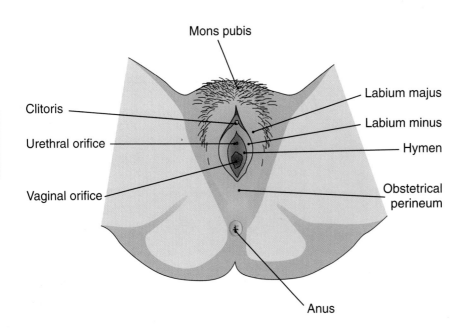

FIGURE **23•9** The external female genitalia.

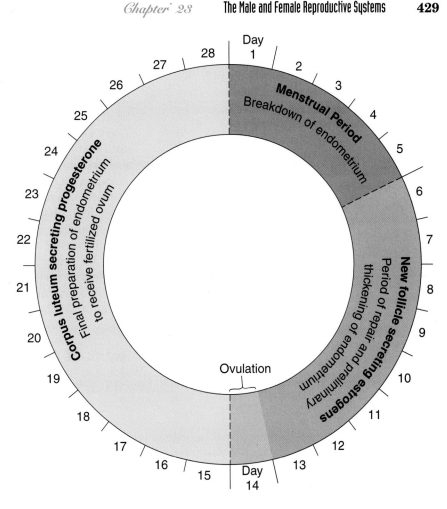

Day
1

28   2

27   3

26   Menstrual Period   4

25   Breakdown of endometrium   5

24   6

Corpus luteum secreting progesterone
Final preparation of endometrium
to receive fertilized ovum

23   7

22   **New follicle secreting estrogens**
Period of repair and preliminary
thickening of endometrium   8

21   9

20   10

19   Ovulation   11

18   12

17   13

16   Day
14

15

FIGURE **23•10** Summary of events in an average 28-day menstrual cycle.

to develop in the ovary. This follicle produces increasing amounts of ***estrogen*** as the ovum matures. (*Estrogen* is the term used for a group of related hormones, the most active of which is estradiol.) The estrogen is carried in the bloodstream to the uterus, where it starts preparing the endometrium for a possible pregnancy. This preparation includes thickening of the endometrium and elongation of the glands that produce the uterine secretion. Estrogen in the blood also acts as a feedback messenger to inhibit the release of FSH and stimulate the release of LH from the pituitary (see Fig. 12-2 in Chap. 12).

Ovulation

About 1 day before ovulation, there is an ***LH surge,*** a sharp rise in LH. This hormone causes ovulation and transforms the ruptured follicle

into the corpus luteum. The corpus luteum produces some estrogen and large amounts of ***progesterone***. Under the influence of these hormones, the endometrium continues to thicken, and the glands and blood vessels increase in size. The rising levels of estrogen and progesterone feed back to inhibit the release of FSH and LH from the pituitary (Fig. 23-11). During this time, the ovum makes its journey to the uterus by way of the oviduct. If the ovum is not fertilized while passing through the uterine tube, it dies within 2 to 3 days and then disintegrates.

Menstrual Flow

If fertilization does not occur, the corpus luteum degenerates, and the levels of estrogen and progesterone decrease. Without the hormones

23

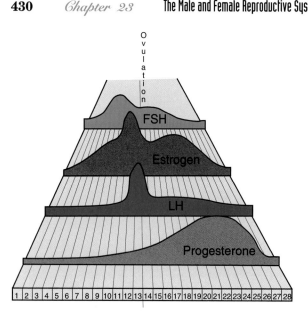

FIGURE **23•11** Hormones in the menstrual cycle. (Redrawn from Djerassi C.: Fertility awareness: Jet-age rhythm method? Science 1990;248: 1061)

to support growth, the endometrium degenerates. Small hemorrhages appear in this lining, producing the bleeding known as ***menstrual flow,*** or ***menses*** (MEN-seze). Bits of endometrium break away and accompany the flow of blood. The average duration of this discharge is 2 to 6 days.

Before the flow ceases, the endometrium begins to repair itself through the growth of new cells. The low levels of estrogen and progesterone allow the release of FSH from the anterior pituitary. FSH causes a new ovum to begin to ripen within the ovaries, and the cycle begins anew.

The activity of ovarian hormones as negative feedback messengers is the basis of hormonal methods of contraception (birth control). Estrogen and progesterone act to inhibit the release of FSH and LH from the pituitary, resulting in a menstrual period but no ovulation.

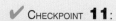

✔ CHECKPOINT **11**:

What are the two hormones produced in the ovaries?

MENOPAUSE

Menopause (MEN-o-pawz) is the period during which menstruation ceases altogether. It ordinarily occurs between the ages of 45 and 55 years and is caused by a normal decline in ovarian function. The ovary becomes chiefly scar tissue and no longer produces ova or appreciable amounts of estrogen. Eventually, the uterus, oviducts, vagina, and vulva all become somewhat atrophied.

Menopause is an entirely normal condition, but its onset sometimes brings about effects that are temporarily disturbing. The decrease in estrogen levels can cause such nervous symptoms as irritability, "hot flashes," and dizzy spells.

Hormone Replacement Therapy

Although still a subject of controversy, the use of estrogen replacement therapy generally is considered to be of overall benefit for menopausal and postmenopausal women. Estrogen therapy, also called hormone replacement therapy (HRT), has proved effective in alleviating hot flashes and the sensitivity of a thinning vaginal mucosa. Some women may require hormone therapy to prevent or halt osteoporosis (bone weakening). It has also been found to reduce the risk of heart attacks, which increase among women after menopause.

Risks of HRT
Hormone replacement therapy has some potential side effects, and each woman should weigh the pros and cons with her physician before beginning treatment. Cancer of the uterine lining (endometrial cancer) is one possible risk, and the longer the duration of hormone treatment, the greater the risk. Reducing the dosages and the duration of the therapy lessens this danger, as does giving the estrogen in combination with progesterone (progestin) to prevent overgrowth of the endometrium.

Other factors that must be considered involve the risk for thrombosis and embolism, which is highest among women who smoke. Some studies have also shown an increased risk for breast cancer in the wake of long-term estrogen therapy. A woman who has a family history of cancer of the breast or of the uterus should avoid such treatment (see News on Breast Cancer).

News on Breast Cancer

The incidence of breast cancer increased considerably in the Untied States from 1970 to 1990 and then leveled off. The rise was partly due to the use of mammograms to detect the disease at an early stage and partly due to aging of the population. Some of the risk factors for breast cancer include the following:

- High levels of exposure to estrogen. Estrogen stimulates the growth of breast cells, increasing the chances for harmful mutations. Circumstances that lead to estrogen exposure are early onset of menstruation, menopause after 50 years of age, obesity (fat cells produce estrogen), and long-term postmenopausal hormone replacement therapy (HRT).
- Having no children or having children late in life. Pregnancy and lactation cause breast cells to specialize, making them less likely to undergo cancerous changes.
- Genetics. Genes have been identified that correlate with the increased incidence of breast cancer within families. Mutations in these genes, BRCA-1 and BRCA-2, are, however, thought to be responsible for only about 7% of cases of breast cancer.

Beyond the typical recommendations for healthy living to prevent breast cancer, women at high risk may consider preventive chemotherapy with drugs that have been shown to lower cancer rates. Some women with strong evidence of hereditary breast cancer are opting for surgical removal of their breasts. Breast self-examination and regular mammograms remain important. Although mammograms are believed to be responsible for the higher reports of breast cancer through the second half of the 20th century, they have also, along with improved methods of treatment, contributed to a recent decrease in the death rate from breast cancer.

✔ CHECKPOINT **12**:

What is the definition of menopause?

CONTRACEPTION

Contraception is defined as the use of artificial methods to prevent fertilization of the ovum or implantation of the fertilized ovum. Table 23-1 presents a brief description of the main contraceptive methods currently in use along with some advantages and disadvantages of each. The list is given in rough order of decreasing effectiveness.

The spread of AIDS and other sexually transmitted diseases has stimulated interest in the development of better condoms, including a female condom, because these not only prevent conception but also reduce the chances of infection.

Most other advances involve new methods for administering birth control hormones. Capsules of synthetic progesterone implanted under the skin are effective for 5 years and avoid the side effects of estrogen. This same drug may be given by injection at 3-month intervals.

Although not strictly a contraceptive, the drug **RU 486** is taken after conception to terminate an early pregnancy. It blocks the action of progesterone, causing the uterus to shed its lining and release the fertilized egg. It must be combined with administration of prostaglandins to expel the uterine tissue.

Other drugs for producing medical abortions are also being tested.

✔ CHECKPOINT **13**:

What is the definition of contraception?

DISORDERS OF THE FEMALE REPRODUCTIVE SYSTEM

Menstrual Disorders

Absence of menstrual flow is known as *amenorrhea* (ah-men-o-RE-ah). This condition can be symptomatic of such a disorder as insufficient

Table 23•1	Main Methods of Contraception Currently in Use		
METHOD	DESCRIPTION	ADVANTAGES	DISADVANTAGES
Surgical			
Vasectomy/tubal ligation	Cutting and tying of tubes carrying gametes	Nearly 100% effective; involves no chemical or mechanical devices	Not usually reversible: rare surgical complications
Hormonal			
Birth control pills	Estrogen and progesterone or progesterone alone taken orally to prevent ovulation	Highly effective; requires no last-minute preparation	Alters physiology; possible serious side effects
Birth control shot	Injection of synthetic progesterone every 3 months to prevent ovulation	Highly effective; lasts for 3 to 4 months	Alters physiology; possible side effects include menstrual irregularity, amenorrhea
Birth control implants	Devices containing synthetic progesterone implanted under skin to prevent ovulation	Highly effective; lasts for 5 years	Alters physiology; possible side effects include menstrual irregularity, amenorrhea; expensive
Barrier			
Male condom	Sheath that fits over erect penis and prevents release of semen	Easily available; does not affect physiology; protects against sexually transmitted disease (STD)	Must be applied just before intercourse; may slip or tear
Female condom	Sheath that fits in vagina, held in place with rings	Easily available; protects against STD	More expensive than male condom; must be applied before intercourse
Diaphragm (with spermicide)	Rubber cap that fits over cervix and prevents entrance of sperm	Does not affect physiology; some protection against STD	Must be inserted before intercourse; requires fitting by physician
Other			
Spermicide	Chemicals used to kill sperm; best when used in combination with a barrier method	Easily available; does not affect physiology; some protection against STD	Local irritation; must be used just before intercourse
Fertility awareness	Abstinence during fertile part of cycle as determined by menstrual history, basal body temperature, or quality of cervical mucus	Does not affect physiology; accepted by certain religions	High failure rate; requires careful record keeping

hormone secretion or congenital abnormality of the reproductive organs. Stress and other psychological factors often play a part in cessation of the menstrual flow. For example, any significant change in a woman's general state of health or change in her living habits, such as a shift in working hours, can interfere with menstruation.

Dysmenorrhea (dis-men-o-RE-ah) means painful or difficult menstruation. In young women, this may be due to immaturity of the uterus. Dysmenorrhea is frequently associated with cycles in which ovulation has occurred. Often, the pain can be relieved by drugs that block prostaglandins because some prostaglandins are known to cause painful uterine contractions.

In many cases, women have been completely relieved of menstrual cramps by their first pregnancies. Apparently, enlargement of the cervical opening remedies the condition. Artificial dilation of the cervical opening may alleviate dysmenorrhea for several months. Often, such health measures as sufficient rest, a well-balanced diet, and appropriate exercises remedy the disorder. In cases of dysmenorrhea, the application of heat over the abdomen usually relieves the pain, just as it may ease other types of muscular cramps.

Premenstrual syndrome (PMS), also called ***premenstrual tension,*** is a condition in which nervousness, irritability, and depression precede the menstrual period. It is thought to be due to fluid retention in various tissues, including the brain. Sometimes, a low-salt diet and appropriate medication for 2 weeks before the menses prevent this disorder. This treatment may also avert dysmenorrhea. PMS treatment centers in some areas of the United States are proving helpful for many women.

Abnormal uterine bleeding includes excessive menstrual flow, too-frequent menstruation, and nonmenstrual bleeding. Any of these may cause serious anemias and deserve careful medical attention. Nonmenstrual bleeding may be an indication of a tumor, possibly cancer.

Benign Tumors

Fibroids, which are more correctly called *myomas,* are common tumors of the uterus. Studies indicate that about 50% of women who reach the age of 50 have one or more of these growths in the walls of the uterus. Often, these tumors are small, and usually they remain benign and produce no symptoms. They develop between puberty and menopause and ordinarily stop growing after a woman has reached the age of 50 years. In some cases, these growths interfere with pregnancy, and in a patient younger than 40 years of age, a surgeon may simply remove the tumor and leave the uterus fairly intact. Normal pregnancies have occurred after such surgery.

Fibroids may become so large that pressure on adjacent structures causes grave disorders. In some cases, invasion of blood vessels near the uterine cavity causes serious hemorrhages. For these and other reasons, it may be necessary to remove the entire uterus or a large part of it. Surgical removal of the uterus is called a ***hysterectomy*** (his-ter-EK-to-me).

Malignant Tumors

Breast Cancer

Cancer of the breast is the most commonly occurring malignant disease in women. The tumor is usually a painless, movable mass that is often noticed by a woman and all too frequently ignored. In recent years, however, there has been increasing emphasis on the importance of regular self-examination of the breasts. Most breast lumps are discovered by women themselves. Any lump, no matter how small, should be reported to a physician immediately. The ***mammogram,*** a radiographic study of the breast, has improved the detection of early breast cancer. Regular mammograms are recommended after the age of 40 years unless there is a history of breast cancer in the family, in which case earlier studies are recommended.

The treatment of breast cancer consists of surgery with follow-up therapy of radiation or chemotherapy or both of these. Surgical treatment by removal of the lump or a segment of the breast is most common. Removal of the entire breast and dissection of the lymph nodes in the axilla (armpit) is called ***modified radical mastectomy*** (mas-TEK-to-me). Studies are underway to determine which combinations of therapy are most effective in each stage.

Endometrial Cancer

The most common cancer of the female reproductive tract is cancer of the endometrium (the lining of the uterus). This type of cancer usually affects women during or after menopause. It is seen most frequently in women who have had few pregnancies, abnormal bleeding, or cycles in which ovulation did not occur. Symptoms include an abnormal discharge or irregular bleeding. The usual methods of treatment include surgery and irradiation. Early, aggressive treatment of this, as of all cancers, can save the patient's life.

Ovarian Cancer

Ovarian cancer is a leading cause of cancer deaths in women. Although most ovarian cysts are not malignant, they should always be investigated for possible malignant change. Ovarian malignancies tend to progress rapidly, so that careful staging (see Chap. 4) is important if a patient's life is to be saved. Ovarian cancer is the second most common reproductive tract cancer in the female, usually occurring in women between the ages of 40 and 65 years. Early surgery, irradiation, and especially chemotherapy have proved to be effective in many cases.

Cervical Cancer

Cancer of the cervix, the third most common cancer of the female reproductive tract, is most frequent in women from 30 to 50 years of age. Appropriate screening allows the discovery and treatment of many early cases. Although no specific cause has been identified, statistics in-dicate that the risk of development of cervical cancer is strongly increased by factors such as first sexual intercourse at an early age, many sexual partners, and infection, as with genital herpes or a virus that causes genital warts.

The decline in the death rate from this type of cancer is directly related to use of the ***Papanicolaou*** (pap-ah-nik-o-LAH-o) ***test,*** also known as the *Pap test* or *Pap smear.* The Pap smear is a microscopic examination of cells obtained

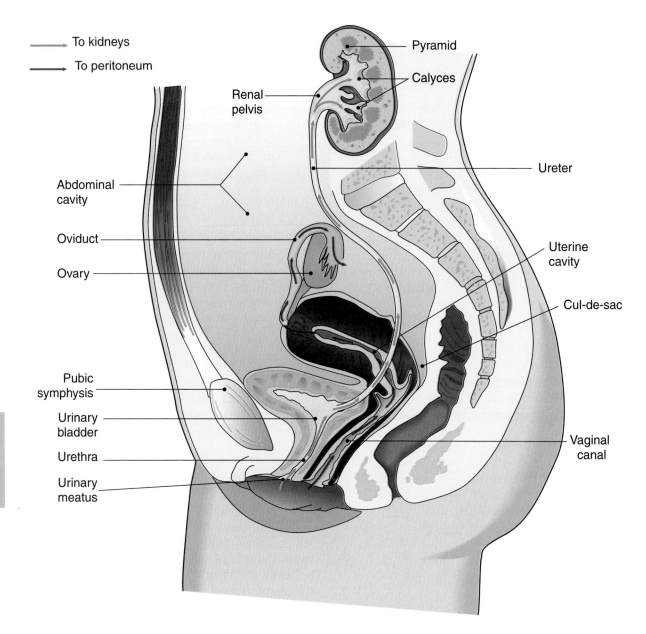

To kidneys

To peritoneum

FIGURE **23•12** Pathway of infection from outside to the peritoneum and into the urinary system.

from scrapings of the cervix and swabs of the cervical canal. All women should be encouraged to have this test every year. Even girls younger than 18 years of age should be tested if they are sexually active.

The incidence of the various types of cancer should not be confused with the death rates for each type. Owing to education of the public and increasingly better methods of diagnosis and treatment, some forms of cancer have a higher cure rate than others. For example, cancer of the breast appears much more often in women than does cancer of the lung, but more women now die each year from lung cancer than from breast cancer.

Infections

The sexually transmitted diseases that involve the male reproductive system also attack the female genital organs (Fig. 23-12); the most common are chlamydial infections, gonorrhea, and genital herpes. Syphilis also occurs in women and can be passed through the placenta from mother to child. The fetus of an untreated syphilitic mother may be stillborn; an infant born alive may have highly infectious lesions of the palms or the soles as well as other manifestations of the disease.

The incidence of *genital warts,* caused by human papillomavirus, has increased in recent years. These infections have been linked to cancer of the reproductive tract, especially cancer of the uterine cervix.

Salpingitis (sal-pin-JI-tis) means "inflammation of a tube." However, the term is used most often to refer to disease of the uterine tubes. Most cases of infection of the uterine tubes are caused by gonococci or by the bacterium *Chlamydia trachomatis,* but other bacteria may be the cause. Salpingitis may cause sterility by obstructing the tubes, thus preventing the passage of ova.

Pelvic inflammatory disease (PID) is due to extension of infections from the reproductive organs into the pelvic cavity, and it often involves the peritoneum. (See the red arrow pathway in Fig. 23-12.) Gonococci or chlamydia are usually the initial cause of infection, but most cases of PID involve multiple organisms.

Infertility

Infertility is much more difficult to diagnose and evaluate in the female than in the male. Whereas a microscopic examination of properly collected semen may be all that is required to determine the presence of abnormal or too few sperm cells in the male, no such simple study can be made in the female. Infertility in women, as in men, may be relative or absolute. Causes of female infertility include infections, endocrine disorders, psychogenic factors, and abnormalities in the structure and function of the reproductive organs themselves. In all cases of apparent infertility, the male partner should be investigated first because the procedures for determining lack of fertility in the male are much simpler and less costly than those in the female, as well as being essential for the evaluation.

Summary

I. Reproduction
  A. Meiosis—reduces chromosome number from 46 to 23
    1. Gametes (sex cells)
      a. Spermatozoa—male
      b. Ova—female

  B. Divisions of the reproductive system
    1. Gonads
      a. Testes—male
      b. Ovaries—female
    2. Accessory organs
      a. Ducts
      b. Endocrine glands

II. Male reproductive system
  A. Testes

1. Scrotum—sac that holds the testes
2. Inguinal canal—channel through which testis descends
3. Internal structure
   a. Seminiferous tubules—tubes in which sperm cells are produced
   b. Interstitial cells—secrete hormones
      (1) Testosterone
         (a) Maintains reproductive structures
         (b) Promotes development of secondary sex characteristics
B. Ducts
   1. Epididymis—stores spermatozoa until ejaculation
   2. Ductus (vas) deferens—conducts sperm cells through spermatic cord
   3. Ejaculatory duct—empties into urethra
C. Formation of semen
   1. Functions of semen
      a. Nourish spermatozoa
      b. Transport spermatozoa
      c. Neutralize vaginal tract
      d. Lubricate reproductive tract during intercourse
   2. Glands
      a. Seminal vesicles
      b. Prostate—around first portion of urethra
      c. Bulbourethral (Cowper's) glands
D. Urethra and penis
   1. Urethra
      a. Conveys urine and semen through penis
   2. Penis
      a. Structure
         1. Corpus spongiosum—central
         2. Corpora cavernosa—lateral
         3. Glans—distal enlargement of corpus spongiosum
         4. Prepuce—foreskin
      b. Erection—stiffening and enlargement of penis
      c. Ejaculation—forceful expulsion of semen

E. Spermatozoa (sperm cells)
   1. Sertoli (nurse) cells—nourish and protect spermatozoa
   2. Parts of sperm cell
      a. Head—contains chromosomes
      b. Acrosome—covers head; has enzymes to help penetration of ovum
      c. Midpiece—contains mitochondria
      d. Tail (flagellum)—propels sperm

III. **Hormonal control of male reproduction**
   1. Pituitary hormones
      a. FSH (follicle stimulating hormone)
         (1) Stimulates Sertoli cells
         (2) Promotes formation of spermatozoa
      b. LH (luteinizing hormone)
         (1) Also called ICSH (interstitial cell–stimulating hormone)
         (2) Stimulates interstitial cells to produce testosterone
   B. Effects of aging on male reproduction
      1. Decline in testosterone, spermatozoa, and semen

IV. **Disorders of the male reproductive system**
   A. Infertility—lower than normal ability to reproduce
   B. Cryptorchidism—failure of testis to descend
   C. Inguinal hernia
   D. Infections
      1. Orchitis—inflammation of the testis
   E. Tumors
      1. Tumors of the prostate
      2. Cancer of the testis
   F. Phimosis—tightness of the foreskin

V. **Female reproductive system**
   A. Ovaries—glands in which ova (egg cells) form
      1. Egg cell and ovulation
         a. Egg ripens in graafian follicle

      b. Ovulation—release of ovum from ovary

    2. Corpus luteum

      a. Remainder of follicle in ovary

      b. Continues to function if egg fertilized

      c. Disintegrates if egg not fertilized

B. Oviducts (uterine tubes, fallopian tubes)

    1. Fimbriae—fringelike extensions that sweep egg into oviduct

C. Uterus

    1. Holds developing fetus

    2. Endometrium—lining of uterus

    3. Cervix—narrow, lower part

D. Vagina

    1. Tube connecting uterus to outside

    2. Hymen—fold of membrane over vaginal opening

    3. Greater vestibular glands- secrete mucus

E. Vulva and perineum

    1. Vulva—external genitalia

      a. Labia—two sets of folds (major, minor)

      b. Clitoris—organ of great sensitivity

    2. Perineum—pelvic floor

      a. In obstetrics—area between vagina and anus

VI. Menstrual cycle—average 28 days

A. Beginning of the cycle

    1. FSH stimulates follicle

    2. Follicle secretes estrogen

    3. Estrogen thickens lining of uterus

B. Ovulation

    1. LH surge 1 day before

    2. Corpus luteum produces progesterone

    3. Progesterone continues growth of endometrium

    4. Ovum disintegrates if not fertilized

C. Menstrual flow (menses)

    1. If egg not fertilized, corpus luteum degenerates

    2. Lining of uterus breaks down

VII. Menopause—period during which menstruation stops

A. Hormone replacement therapy (HRT)

    1. Reduces symptoms of menopause; other beneficial effects

      a. Risks of HRT—endometrial cancer, thrombosis, embolism, breast cancer

VIII. Contraception—use of artificial methods to prevent fertilization

IX. Disorders of the female reproductive system

A. Menstrual disorders

    1. Amenorrhea—absence of menstrual flow

    2. Dysmenorrhea—painful or difficult menstruation

    3. Premenstrual syndrome

    4. Abnormal uterine bleeding

B. Benign tumors

    1. Fibroids (myomas)—common tumors of uterus

C. Malignant tumors

    1. Breast cancer

      a. Mammogram—radiographic study of the breast

      b. Mastectomy—removal of breast or breast tissue

    2. Endometrial cancer—cancer of uterine lining

    3. Ovarian cancer

    4. Cervical cancer

      a. Pap test (smear) for cervical cancer

D. Infections

    1. Sexually transmitted diseases

    2. Genital warts—caused by papillomavirus

    3. Salpingitis—inflammation of uterine tubes

    4. Pelvic inflammatory disease (PID)

E. Infertility

23

Questions for Study and Review

1. In what fundamental respect does reproduction in some single-celled animals, such as the ameba, differ from that in most animals?
2. Name the sex cells of both the male and the female.
3. Name all the parts of the male reproductive system and describe the function of each.
4. List the functions of semen.
5. Name and locate the glands that contribute to semen.
6. Draw and label the parts of a sperm cell.
7. Name the hormones that regulate male reproductive activity.
8. What changes occur in the male reproductive system with age?
9. What is cryptorchidism? Why does this condition cause sterility?
10. Name several sexually transmitted diseases.
11. What organ is a common site for tumors in men older than 50 years of age?
12. Name the principal parts of the female reproductive system and describe the function of each.
13. Beginning with the first day of the menstrual flow, describe the events of one complete cycle, including the role of the various hormones.
14. Describe the process of ovulation.
15. What is menopause? What causes it? What are some of the changes that take place in the body as a result?
16. What are the values of hormone replacement therapy after menopause? What are some of the dangers of such therapy?
17. Define *contraception*. Describe methods of contraception that involve (1) barriers; (2) chemicals; (3) hormones; (4) prevention of implantation.
18. Distinguish between dysmenorrhea and amenorrhea.
19. What is the most common malignant disease in women? For early detection, what should a woman do at regular intervals?
20. What are the two most common cancers of the uterus?
21. What is a Pap test? Why is it important?
22. What are some causes of infertility in both males and females?

✔ ANSWERS TO CHECKPOINTS

1. Meiosis is the process of cell division that halves the chromosome number in a cell to produce a gamete.
2. The testis is the male gonad.
3. Testosterone is the main male sex hormone.
4. Sperm cells leave the ducts within the testis and then travel through the epididymis, ductus (vas) deferens, ejaculatory duct, and urethra.
5. Glands that contribute secretions to the semen are the seminal vesicles, prostate, and bulbourethral glands.
6. The main subdivisions of the sperm cell are the head, midpiece, and tail (flagellum).
7. Follicle-stimulating hormone (FSH) and luteinizing hormone (LH), also called ICSH, are the pituitary hormones that regulate male and female reproduction.
8. Infectious diseases of the reproductive tract include chlamydial and gonococcal infections, genital herpes, syphilis, tuberculosis, and staphylococcal infections.
9. Ovulation is the process of releasing an egg cell from the ovary.
10. The fetus develops in the uterus.
11. The two hormones produced in the ovaries are estrogen and progesterone.
12. Menopause is the period during which menstruation ceases.
13. Contraception is the use of artificial methods to prevent fertilization of the ovum or implantation of the fertilized ovum.

Development and Birth

BEHAVIORAL OBJECTIVES

After careful study of this chapter, you should be able to:

1. Describe fertilization and the early development of the fertilized egg

2. Describe the structure and function of the placenta

3. Briefly describe changes that occur in the fetus and the mother during pregnancy

4. Briefly describe the four stages of labor

5. Compare fraternal and identical twins

6. Cite the advantages of breastfeeding

7. Describe several disorders associated with pregnancy, childbirth, and lactation

Chapter

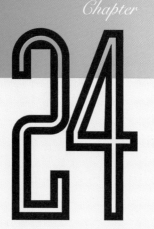

24

PREGNANCY

Pregnancy begins with fertilization of an ovum and ends with delivery of the fetus and afterbirth. During this 38-week period of development, known as *gestation* (jes-TA-shun), all body tissues differentiate from a single fertilized egg. Along the way, many changes occur in both the mother and the growing offspring.

Fertilization and the Start of Pregnancy

When semen is deposited in the vagina, the many spermatozoa immediately wriggle about in all directions, some traveling into the uterus and oviducts (see Fig. 23-6 in Chap. 23). If an egg cell is present in the oviduct, many spermatozoa cluster around it. Using enzymes, they dissolve the coating around the ovum, so that eventually one sperm cell can penetrate the cell membrane of the egg. The nuclei of the sperm and egg then combine.

The result of this union is a single cell with the full human chromosome number of 46. This new cell, called a *zygote* (ZI-gote), can divide and grow into a new individual. The zygote divides rapidly into two cells and then four cells, and soon a ball of cells is formed. During this time, the cell cluster is traveling toward the uterine cavity, pushed along by cilia lining the oviduct and by peristalsis (contractions) of the tube. After reaching the uterus, the little ball of cells burrows into the greatly thickened uterine lining, where it is soon completely covered and implanted.

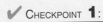

✔ CHECKPOINT **1**:

What structure is formed by the union of an ovum and a spermatozoon?

Development and Functions of the Placenta

After *implantation* in the lining of the uterus, a group of cells within the developing ball of cells becomes an *embryo* (EM-bre-o), the future offspring. The outer cells of the cluster form projections, called *villi,* that invade the uterine wall and maternal blood channels (venous sinuses). This tissue eventually forms the *placenta* (plah-SEN-tah), a flat, circular organ that consists of a spongy network of blood-filled lakes and capillary-containing villi (Fig. 24-1). The placenta serves as the organ of nutrition, respiration, and excretion for the embryo by means of exchanges that occur between the blood of the embryo and the blood of the mother through the capillaries of the placental villi.

The Umbilical Cord

The embryo, later called the *fetus* (FE-tus), is connected to the developing placenta by a stalk of tissue that eventually becomes the *umbilical* (um-BIL-ih-kal) *cord*. This cord carries blood to and from the fetus. It encloses two arteries that carry blood from the fetus to the placenta and one vein that carries blood from the placenta to the fetus (see Fig. 24-1). The fetus has special features of the circulation to carry blood to and from the umbilical cord and to bypass the lungs (see Fetal Circulation).

Placental Hormones

In addition to maintaining the fetus, the placenta serves as an endocrine organ. Beginning soon after implantation, some of the embryonic cells produce a hormone called *human chorionic gonadotropin* (ko-re-ON-ik gon-ah-do-TRO-pin) *(hCG).* This hormone stimulates the corpus luteum of the ovary, prolonging its lifespan (to 11 or 12 weeks) and causing it to secrete increasing amounts of progesterone and estrogen.

Progesterone is essential for the maintenance of pregnancy. It promotes endometrial secretion to nourish the embryo, and it decreases the ability of the uterine muscle to contract, thus preventing the embryo from being expelled from the body. During pregnancy, progesterone also helps prepare the breasts for the secretion of milk.

Estrogen promotes enlargement of the uterus and breasts. By the 11th or 12th week of pregnancy, the corpus luteum is no longer needed; by this time, the placenta itself can secrete adequate amounts of progesterone and estrogen, and the corpus luteum disintegrates. Miscarriages (loss of an embryo or fetus) frequently occur during this critical time when hormone secretion is shifting from the corpus luteum to the placenta.

Fetal Circulation

The developing fetus has several adaptations in the cardiovascular system that change at birth. These adaptations serve to bypass the lungs, which are not functional. Fetal blood is oxygenated instead by the placenta (see Fig. 24-1).

Blood comes from the placenta to the fetus in the umbilical vein, which is contained in the umbilical cord. Most of this blood joins the inferior vena cava by way of a small vessel, the ductus venosus, and is carried to the heart. Once in the right atrium, a portion of the blood flows directly into the left atrium through a hole in the septum called the foramen ovale. This blood bypasses the pulmonary circuit.

Blood that does enter the right ventricle is pumped into the pulmonary artery. However, most of this blood shunts directly into the systemic circulation through a small vessel, the ductus arteriosus, that connects the pulmonary artery to the aorta. Blood returns to the placenta through two umbilical arteries.

Most of these adaptations close at birth, when the lungs begin to function. The foramen ovale seals to become a depression in the septum between the atria. The various vessels constrict into fibrous cords. Only the proximal parts of the umbilical arteries persist as arteries to the urinary bladder.

Development of the Embryo

For the first 8 weeks of life, the developing offspring is referred to as an *embryo* (Fig. 24-2). The beginnings of all body systems are established during this period. The heart and the brain are among the first organs to develop. A primitive nervous system begins to form in the third week. The heart and blood vessels originate during the second week, and the first heartbeat appears during week 4, at the same time that other muscles begin to develop.

By the end of the first month, the embryo is about 0.62 cm (0.25 inches) long, with four small swellings at the sides called *limb buds,* which will develop into the four extremities. At

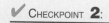

CHECKPOINT **2**:

What organ nourishes the developing fetus?

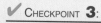

CHECKPOINT **3**:

What is the function of the umbilical cord?

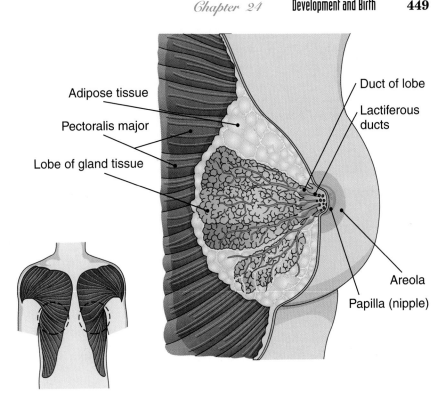

FIGURE **24•4** Section of the breast.

- The proportions of various nutrients and other substances in human milk are perfectly suited to the human infant. Substitutes are not exact imitations of human milk. Nutrients are present in more desirable amounts if the mother's diet is well balanced.
- The psychological and emotional benefits of nursing are of infinite value to both the mother and the infant.

✔ CHECKPOINT **8**:

What is lactation?

DISORDERS OF PREGNANCY, CHILDBIRTH, AND LACTATION

Ectopic Pregnancy

A pregnancy that develops in a location outside the uterine cavity is said to be an ***ectopic*** (ek-TOP-ik) ***pregnancy,*** *ectopic* meaning "out of normal place." The most common type is the ***tubal ectopic pregnancy,*** in which the embryo grows in the oviduct. This structure, which is not designed by nature for pregnancy, is not able to expand to contain the growing embryo and may rupture. Ectopic pregnancy may threaten the mother's life if it does not receive prompt surgical treatment.

Placenta Previa

The placenta is usually attached to the upper part of the uterus. In ***placenta previa*** (PRE-ve-ah), the placenta becomes attached at or near the internal opening of the cervix. The normal softening and dilation of the cervix that occur in later pregnancy separate part of the placenta from its attachment. The result is painless bleeding and interference with the fetal oxygen supply.

Placental Abruption

The placenta sometimes separates from the wall of the uterus prematurely, often after the 20th week of pregnancy, causing hemorrhage.

This disorder, known as ***abruptio placentae*** (ab-RUP-she-o plah-SEN-te), occurs most often in women older than 35 years of age who have had several pregnancies (multigravidas). This is a common cause of bleeding during the second half of pregnancy and may require the termination of pregnancy to save the mother's life.

Pregnancy-Induced Hypertension

A serious disorder that can develop in the latter part of pregnancy is ***preeclampsia*** (pre-eh-KLAMP-se-ah), also called *toxemia of pregnancy*. Symptoms include hypertension, protein in the urine (proteinuria), general edema, and sudden weight gain. The causes of this disorder are unknown. However, it is most common in women whose nutritional state is poor and who have received little or no health care during pregnancy. If the condition remains untreated, it may lead to ***eclampsia*** (eh-KLAMP-se-ah) with the onset of kidney failure, convulsions, and coma during pregnancy or after delivery. The result may be the death of both the mother and the infant.

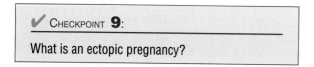

✔ CHECKPOINT **9**:

What is an ectopic pregnancy?

Postpartum Disorders

Puerperal Infection

Childbirth-related deaths are often due to infections. ***Puerperal*** (pu-ER-per-al) ***infections*** (those related to childbirth) were once the cause of death in as many as 10% to 12% of women going through labor. Cleanliness and sterile

techniques have improved the chances of avoiding such outcomes of pregnancies. Nevertheless, in the United States, puerperal infection still develops in about 6% of maternity patients. Antibiotics have dramatically improved the chances of recovery of both the mother and the child.

Choriocarcinoma

A very malignant tumor that is made of placental tissue is ***choriocarcinoma*** (ko-re-o-kar-sih-NO-mah). This tumor spreads rapidly, and if the mother is not treated, it may be fatal within 3 to 12 months. With the use of modern chemotherapy, the outlook for cure is very good. If metastases have developed, irradiation and other forms of treatment may be necessary.

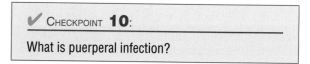

✔ CHECKPOINT **10**:

What is puerperal infection?

Lactation Disturbances

Disturbances in lactation may have a variety of causes, including the following:

- Malnutrition or anemia, which may prevent lactation entirely
- Emotional disturbances, which may affect lactation (as they may affect other glandular activities)
- Abnormalities of parts of the mammary glands or injuries to these organs, which may cause interference with their functioning
- ***Mastitis*** (mas-TI-tis), which means "inflammation of the breast," and is due to infection. Antibiotic treatment usually allows for the continuation of nursing.

24

Summary

I. Pregnancy (gestation)—lasts 38 weeks

A. Fertilization and the start of pregnancy
1. Fertilization occurs in oviduct
2. Zygote (fertilized egg)—formed by fusion of egg and sperm nuclei
   a. Divides rapidly
   b. Travels to uterus
   c. Implants in lining

B. Development and functions of the placenta
1. Formed by cells around embryo and lining of uterus
2. Umbilical cord—connects fetus to placenta
3. Functions
   a. Provision of nourishment to embryo
   b. Gas exchange with embryo
   c. Removal of waste from embryo
   d. Production of human chorionic gonadotropin (hCG)—maintains corpus luteum until 11 to 12 weeks of pregnancy

C. Development of the embryo
1. First 8 weeks
2. All body systems begin to develop

D. The fetus
1. Third month to birth
2. Amniotic sac
   a. Surrounds fetus
   b. Contains fluid to cushion and protect fetus

E. The mother
1. Increased demands on heart, lungs, kidneys
2. Increased nutritional needs
3. Ultrasound used to monitor pregnancy and delivery

II. Childbirth

A. Four stages of labor
1. Contractions
2. Delivery of baby
3. Expulsion of afterbirth
4. Contraction of uterus

B. Cesarean section
1. Incision to remove fetus

C. Multiple births
1. Fraternal twins formed from two different ova
2. Identical twins develop from a single zygote
3. Larger multiples follow either pattern or a combination
4. Increased by fertility drugs

D. Termination of pregnancy
1. Immature (premature) infant—born before organ system mature
2. Preterm—born before 37th week or weighing less than 2500 grams
3. Abortion—loss of fetus before 20th week or weighing less than 500 grams
4. Fetal death—loss of fetus after 8 weeks of pregnancy

III. Mammary glands and lactation

1. Lactation—secretion of milk
   a. Colostrum—first mammary secretion
2. Hormones
   a. Prolactin—stimulates secretory cells
   b. Oxytocin—promotes letdown (ejection) of milk
3. Advantages of breastfeeding
   a. Reduces infections
   b. Transfers antibodies
   c. Provides best form of nutrition
   d. Emotional satisfaction

IV. Disorders of pregnancy, childbirth, and lactation

A. Ectopic pregnancy—pregnancy outside of uterus; commonly in oviduct

B. Placenta previa—improper attachment of placenta to uterus

C. Placental abruption—separation of placenta from uterus

D. Pregnancy-induced hypertension
1. Preeclampsia (toxemia of pregnancy)
2. Eclampsia—results from untreated preeclampsia

E. Postpartum disorders
1. Puerperal infection

24

2. Choriocarcinoma—malignant tumor of placental tissue
F. Lactation disturbances
   1. Possible causes
      a. Malnutrition
      b. Emotional disturbances
      c. Abnormalities of mammary glands
      d. Mastitis—inflammation of the breast

Questions for Study and Review

1. Distinguish among the following: zygote, embryo, fetus.
2. Describe events between fertilization of an ovum and the start of its growth within the uterus.
3. List hormones specifically involved in pregnancy and cite the functions of each.
4. Explain the role of the placenta in fetal development.
5. Describe the amniotic sac and explain its role in development.
6. Is blood in the umbilical arteries relatively low or high in oxygen? in the umbilical vein?
7. Describe some of the changes that take place in the mother's body during pregnancy.
8. What is the major event of each of the four stages of labor and delivery?
9. What is an episiotomy? Why is it done?
10. Distinguish between fraternal and identical twins.
11. Define *abortion; premature infant; preterm infant.*
12. Name two hormones involved in lactation. Where do they originate and what do they do?
13. List some of the advantages associated with breastfeeding a baby.
14. Define *ectopic pregnancy; placenta previa; preeclampsia.*

✔ ANSWERS TO CHECKPOINTS

1. A zygote is formed by the union of an ovum and a spermatozoon.
2. The placenta nourishes the developing fetus.
3. The umbilical cord carries blood between the fetus and the placenta.
4. The heartbeat first appears during the fourth week of embryonic development.
5. The amniotic sac is the fluid-filled sac that holds the fetus.
6. Parturition is the process of labor and delivery.
7. A cesarean section is an incision made in the abdominal wall and the wall of the uterus for delivery of a fetus.
8. Lactation is the secretion of milk from the mammary glands.
9. An ectopic pregnancy is one that develops in a location outside the uterine cavity.
10. Puerperal infection is an infection that is related to childbirth.

Heredity and Hereditary Diseases

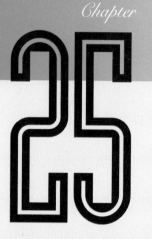

Chapter

25

BEHAVIORAL OBJECTIVES

After careful study of this chapter, you should be able to:

1. Briefly describe the mechanism of gene function

2. Explain the difference between dominant and recessive genes

3. Describe what is meant by a *carrier* of a genetic trait

4. Define *meiosis* and explain the function of meiosis in reproduction

5. Explain how sex is determined in humans

6. Describe what is meant by the term *sex linked* and list several sex-linked traits

7. List several factors that may influence the expression of a gene

8. Define *mutation*

9. Differentiate among congenital, genetic, and hereditary disorders and give several examples of each

10. List several factors that may produce genetic disorders

11. Define *karyotype* and explain how karyotypes are used in genetic counseling

12. Briefly describe several methods used to treat genetic disorders

We are often struck by the resemblance of a baby to one or both of its parents, yet rarely do we stop to consider *how* various traits are transmitted from parents to offspring. This subject—heredity—has fascinated humans for thousands of years; the *Old Testament* contains numerous references to heredity (although, of course, the word was unknown in biblical times). It was not until the 19th century, however, that methodical investigation into heredity was begun. At that time, an Austrian monk, Gregor Mendel, discovered through his experiments with garden peas that there was a precise pattern in the appearance of differences among parents and their progeny. Mendel's most important contribution to the understanding of heredity was the demonstration that there are independent units of heredity in the cells. Later, these independent units were given the name *genes* (see The Human Genome Project).

GENES AND CHROMOSOMES

Genes are actually segments of DNA (deoxyribonucleic acid) contained in the threadlike chromosomes within the nucleus of each cell. Genes act by controlling the manufacture of enzymes, which are necessary for all the chemical reactions that occur within the cell.

When body cells divide by the process of mitosis, the DNA that makes up the chromosomes is duplicated and distributed to the daughter cells, so that each daughter cell gets exactly the same kind and number of chromosomes as were in the original cell. Each chromosome (aside from the Y chromosome, which determines sex) may carry thousands of genes, and each gene carries the code for a specific trait (characteristic). These traits constitute the physical, biochemical, and physiologic makeup of every cell in the body.

In humans, every cell except the sex cells contains 46 chromosomes. These chromosomes exist in pairs. One member of each pair was received at the time of fertilization from the father of the offspring, and one was received from the mother. These paired chromosomes, except for the pair that determines sex, are alike in size and appearance and carry genes for the same traits. Thus, the genes for each trait exist in pairs.

> ✔ CHECKPOINT **1**:
>
> What is a gene?

Dominant and Recessive Genes

Another of Mendel's discoveries was that genes can be either dominant or recessive. A ***dominant*** gene is one that expresses its effect in the

The Human Genome Project

The goal of the Human Genome Project is to produce a complete map of the human chromosomes. By the end of the project, the exact location and the chemical code of all 100,000 human genes will be known. Scientists from around the world have been working since the late 1980s to meet an original target date of 2005. Improved methods for identifying the chemical pattern (sequence) of individual genes has advanced this date to 2003, or even earlier.

So far, about one third of the total human genes have been located (mapped) on the chromosomes, including more than 200 genes associated with genetic diseases. More than 10% of all the genes have been completely analyzed. Along the way, the total genomes of several microorganisms and a small worm have been described. Those of the fruit fly and the mouse are under study.

The information obtained from the Human Genome Project will form a fundamental core of knowledge for all biologic researchers and clinicians.

✔ CHECKPOINT **2**:

What is the difference between a dominant and a recessive gene?

Distribution of Chromosomes to Offspring

The reproductive cells (ova and spermatozoa) are produced by a special process of cell division called *meiosis* (mi-O-sis). This process divides the chromosome number in half, so that each reproductive cell has 23 chromosomes. Moreover, the division occurs in such a way that each cell receives one member of each chromosome pair that was present in the original cell. The separation occurs at random, meaning that either member of the original pair may be included in a given germ cell. Thus, the maternal and paternal sets of chromosomes get mixed up and redistributed at this time, leading to increased variety within the population.

✔ CHECKPOINT **3**:

What is the process of cell division that forms the gametes?

---

cell regardless of whether the gene at the same site on the matching chromosome is the same as or different from the dominant gene. The gene need be received from only one parent to be expressed in the offspring.

The effect of a *recessive* gene is not evident unless the gene at that site in the matching chromosome of the pair is also recessive. Thus, a recessive trait appears only if the recessive genes for that trait are received from both parents. For example, genes for dark eyes are dominant, whereas genes for light eyes are recessive. Light eyes appear in the offspring only if genes for light eyes are received from both parents.

A recessive gene is not expressed if it is present in the cell together with a dominant gene. However, the recessive gene can be passed on to offspring and may thus appear in future generations. An individual who shows no evidence of a trait but has a recessive gene for that trait is described as a *carrier* of the gene.

Sex Determination

The two chromosomes that determine the sex of the offspring, unlike the other 22 pairs of chromosomes, are not matched in size and appearance. The female X chromosome is larger than most other chromosomes and carries genes for other characteristics in addition to that for sex. The male Y chromosome is smaller than other chromosomes and mainly determines sex. A female has two X chromosomes in each body cell; a male has one X and one Y.

By the process of meiosis, each male sperm cell receives either an X or a Y chromosome, whereas every egg cell receives only an X chromosome (Fig. 25-1). If a sperm cell with an X chromosome fertilizes an ovum, the resulting infant will be female; if a sperm with a Y chromosome fertilizes an ovum, the resulting infant will be male (see Fig. 25-1).

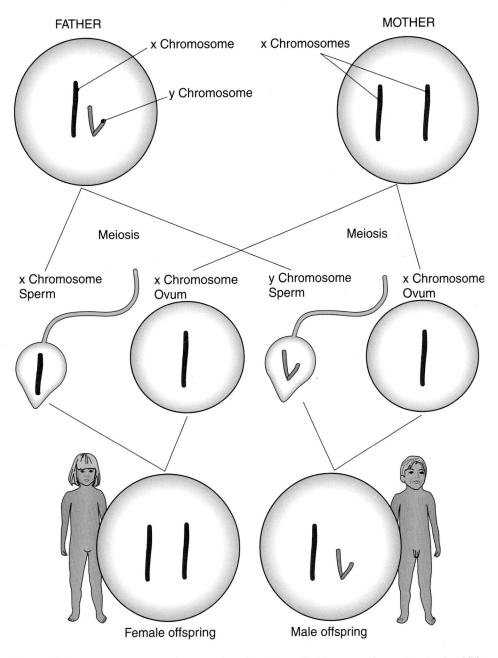

FATHER

x Chromosome

y Chromosome

MOTHER

x Chromosomes

Meiosis

Meiosis

x Chromosome
Sperm

x Chromosome
Ovum

y Chromosome
Sperm

x Chromosome
Ovum

Female offspring

Male offspring

Figure **25•1** If an X chromosome from a male unites with an X chromosome from a female, the child is female; if a Y chromosome from a male unites with an X chromosome from a female, the child is male.

Sex-Linked Traits

Any trait that is carried on a sex chromosome is said to be **sex linked.** Because the Y chromosome carries few traits aside from sex determination, most sex-linked traits are carried on the X chromosome and are described as *X linked.*

Examples are hemophilia, certain forms of baldness, and red-green color blindness.

Sex-linked traits appear almost exclusively in males. The reason for this is that most of these traits are recessive, and if a recessive gene is located on the X chromosome in a male it cannot be masked by a matching dominant gene.

(Remember that the Y chromosome with which the X chromosome pairs is very small and carries few genes.) Thus, a male who has only one recessive gene for a trait will exhibit that characteristic, whereas a female must have two recessive genes to show the trait.

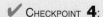

✔ CHECKPOINT **4**:

What sex chromosome combination determines a female? a male?

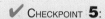

✔ CHECKPOINT **5**:

What term is used to describe a trait carried on a sex chromosome?

HEREDITARY TRAITS

Some observable hereditary traits are skin, eye, and hair color and facial features. Also influenced by genetics are less clearly defined traits, such as weight, body build, life-span, and susceptibility to disease.

Some human traits, including the traits involved in many genetic diseases, are determined by a single pair of genes; most, however, are the result of two or more gene pairs acting together in what is termed ***multifactorial inheritance.*** This type of inheritance accounts for the wide range of variations within populations in such characteristics as coloration, height, and weight, all of which are determined by more than one pair of genes.

Gene Expression

The effect or expression of a gene may be influenced by a variety of factors, including the sex of the individual and the presence of other genes. For example, the genes for certain types of baldness and certain types of color blindness may be inherited by either males or females, but the traits appear mostly in males under the effects of male sex hormone.

Environment also plays a part in the expression of genes. One inherits a potential for a

given size, for example, but one's actual size is additionally influenced by such factors as nutrition, development, and general state of health. The same is true of life-span and susceptibility to diseases.

Genetic Mutation

As a rule, chromosomes replicate exactly during cell division. Occasionally, however, for reasons not yet totally understood, the genes or chromosomes change. This change may involve a single gene or whole chromosomes. Alternatively, it may consist of chromosomal breakage, in which there is loss or rearrangement of gene fragments. Such changes are termed genetic ***mutations***. Mutations may occur spontaneously or may be induced by some agent, such as ionizing radiation or chemicals, described as a ***mutagenic agent***.

If the mutation occurs in an ovum or a sperm cell involved in reproduction, the altered trait will be inherited by the offspring. The vast majority of harmful mutations never are expressed because the affected fetus dies and is spontaneously aborted. Most remaining mutations are so inconsequential that they have no visible effect. Beneficial mutations, on the other hand, tend to survive and increase as a population evolves.

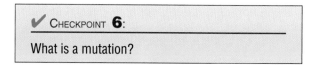

✔ CHECKPOINT **6**:

What is a mutation?

GENETIC DISEASES

Any disorders that involve the genes may be said to be genetic, but they are not always hereditary, that is, passed from parent to offspring in the reproductive cells. Noninherited genetic disorders may begin during maturation of the sex cells or even during development of the embryo.

Advances in genetic research have made it possible to identify the causes of many hereditary disorders and to develop methods of genetic screening. People who are "at risk" for having a child with a genetic disorder, as well as fetuses and newborns in whom the presence of an abnormality may be suspected, can have chromosome studies done to identify genetic abnormalities (see Mitochondrial DNA and Disease).

Congenital Versus Hereditary Diseases

Before we discuss hereditary diseases, we need to distinguish them from other congenital diseases. To illustrate, let us assume that two infants are born within seconds in adjoining delivery rooms of the same hospital. It is noted that one infant has a clubfoot, a condition called *talipes* (TAL-ih-pes); the second infant has a rudimentary extra finger attached to the fifth finger of each hand, a condition called *polydactyly* (pol-e-DAK-til-e). Are both conditions hereditary? both congenital? Is either hereditary? We

can answer these questions by defining the key terms, *congenital* and *hereditary*. *Congenital* means present at the time of birth; *hereditary* means genetically transmitted or transmissible. Thus, one condition may be both congenital and hereditary; another, congenital yet not hereditary.

Hereditary conditions are usually evident at birth or soon thereafter. However, certain inherited disorders, such as adult polycystic kidney disease and Huntington's disease, a nervous disorder, do not manifest themselves until about midlife (40 to 50 years of age). In the case of our earlier examples, the clubfoot is congenital, but not hereditary, having resulted from severe distortion of the developing extremities during intrauterine growth; the extra fingers are hereditary, a familial trait that appears in another relative, a grandparent perhaps, or a parent, and that is evident at the time of birth.

Causes of Congenital Disorders

Although causes of congenital deformities and birth defects often are not known, in some cases, they are known and can be avoided. For example, certain infections and toxins may be transmitted from the mother's blood by way of the placenta to the circulation of the fetus. Some of these cause serious developmental disorders in affected babies.

German measles (rubella) is a contagious viral infection that is ordinarily a mild disease, but if maternal infection occurs during the first 3 or 4 months of pregnancy, the fetus has a 40% chance of developing defects of the eye (cataracts), of the ear (deafness), and of the brain and heart. Infection can be prevented by appropriate immunizations.

Ionizing radiation and various toxins may damage the genes, and the disorders they produce are sometimes transmissible. Environmental agents, such as mercury and some chemicals used in industry (*e.g.,* certain phenols and PCB), as well as some drugs, notably LSD, are known to disrupt genetic organization.

Intake of alcohol and cigarette smoking by a pregnant woman often cause growth retardation and low birthweight in her infant. Smaller than normal infants do not do as well as babies of average weight. Some congenital heart defects have been associated with a condition

Mitochondrial DNA and Disease

Mitochondria are the little powerhouse organelles of cells. They are responsible for converting the energy in nutrients into the ATP needed for cell activities. Because they may have evolved as separate organisms early in the history of life on earth, they exist almost as special entities within the cell. They have their own DNA and multiply at their own pace, independent of the cell's pattern.

It has been discovered that genetic defects can involve mitochondrial DNA. Such diseases are believed to affect several thousand children in the United States. The disorders may interfere with the nervous system or overall metabolism, causing a variety of symptoms that have been confused with epilepsy, cerebral palsy, and multiple sclerosis.

If a mitochondrial defect is programmed in the nuclear DNA, it could be inherited from either parent. If, however, it is carried in the mitochondrion itself, it would be passed only from a mother to her offspring. The mitochondria in the zygote (fertilized egg) come only from the ovum; sperm cells, which are much smaller, do not carry any mitochondria.

called *fetal alcohol syndrome.* Total abstinence from alcohol and cigarettes is strongly recommended during pregnancy.

✔ CHECKPOINT **7**:

Can a disorder be congenital but not hereditary? Explain.

See Preventing Genetic Damage.

Examples of Genetic Diseases

The best known example of a genetic disorder that is not hereditary is the most common form of **Down syndrome,** which results from the presence of an extra chromosome per cell. This abnormality arises during formation of a sex cell. The disorder is usually recognizable at birth by the afflicted child's distinctive facial features. The face is round, with close-set eyes that slant upward at the outside. The head is small and grows at an unusually slow rate. The nose is flat, the tongue is large and protruding, and the muscles and joints are lax. Intellectual function is impaired in Down children; however, the amount of skill they can gain depends on the severity of the disease and their family and school environments. Down syndrome is usually not inherited, although there is a hereditary form of the disorder. In most cases, both parents are normal, as are the child's siblings. The likelihood of having a baby with Down syndrome increases dramatically in women past the age of 35 years and may be the result of defects in the germ cells, either male or female, due to age.

Most genetic diseases are *familial* or *hereditary;* that is, they are passed on from parent to child by way of the egg or sperm. In the case of a disorder carried by a dominant gene, one parent usually carries the abnormal gene that gives rise to the disease, as is the case in **Huntington's disease**. The disturbance appears in one parent and any of the offspring who receive the defective gene.

If the trait is a recessive one, as is the case in most inheritable disorders, a defective gene must come from each parent. Important inheri-

Preventing Genetic Damage

Many problems are encountered in trying to find out whether an observed genetic defect is a spontaneous random occurrence or is related to exposure of a germ cell to some toxic event in the environment. The reproductive cells in the male and female are present at birth but do not become active until the reproductive years. This leaves a long time span during which toxic exposure can occur.

Most of what we know about chemicals that cause mutations has been learned from environmental accidents. Some examples are:

- Mercury compounds have found their way into the food chain, causing damage to children of parents who consumed foods containing mercury.

- Lead is toxic when ingested, either from air or water pollution. Lead has been implicated in sperm cell abnormalities and in reduced sperm counts.

- Radiation accidents have been linked to increased susceptibility to certain cancers in children born after these accidents.

Meiosis, the process by which the number of chromosomes is reduced by half, is the step most prone to errors. This process is studied more in the male due to the availability of specimens from testicular biopsy. There is also an ongoing production of sperm in the male, samples of which can be obtained and studied for visible defects.

Advancing age in both the father and the mother is known to increase errors in meiosis. Males between 20 and 45 years of age carry the least risk of transmitting a genetic error. For females, the least risk is between ages 15 to 35 years. Because new sperm cells are produced on a 64-day cycle, men are advised to avoid conception for a few months after exposure to x-rays, cancer chemotherapy, or other chemicals capable of causing mutations.

table diseases that are carried as recessive traits include diabetes mellitus, cystic fibrosis, and sickle cell anemia.

As stated earlier, genes control the production of specific enzymes. In the case of **PKU,** or **phenylketonuria** (fen-il-ke-to-NU-re-ah), the lack of a certain enzyme prevents the proper metabolism of **phenylalanine** (fen-il-AL-ah-nin), one of the common amino acids. As a result, phenylalanine accumulates in the infant's blood. If the condition remains untreated, it leads to mental retardation before the age of 2 years. Newborn infants are routinely screened for PKU.

Sickle cell disease is described in Chapter 13, where it is stated that the disease is found almost exclusively among blacks. By contrast, **cystic fibrosis** is most common in white populations; in fact, it is the most frequently inherited disease among whites. Cystic fibrosis is characterized by excessively thickened secretions of the linings of the bronchi, the intestine, and the ducts of the pancreas. Such secretions in the pancreatic ducts prevent the flow of pancreatic juice to the small intestine. Obstruction and blockage of these vital organs follows, in association with frequent respiratory infections, with uncontrollable intestinal losses, particularly of fats (and the vitamins these fats carry), as well as massive salt loss. Treatment includes oral administration of pancreatic enzymes and special pulmonary exercises. Cystic fibrosis was once fatal by the time of adolescence, but now, with appropriate care, life expectancies are extending into the third decade. The gene responsible for the disease has been identified, raising hope of better diagnosis, treatment, and perhaps even correction of the defective gene that causes the disorder.

Another group of heritable muscle disorders is known collectively as the **progressive muscular atrophies**. Atrophy (AT-ro-fe) means wasting due to decrease in the size of a normally developed part. The absence of normal muscle movement in the infant proceeds within a few months to extreme weakness of the respiratory muscles, until ultimately the infant is unable to breathe adequately. Most afflicted babies die within several months. The name *floppy baby syndrome,* as the disease is commonly called, provides a vivid description of its effects.

Albinism is an inherited disorder that is carried by recessive genes. It is of particular interest because of the easily recognizable appearance it lends to the affected person. The skin

and hair color are strikingly white and do not darken with age. The skin is abnormally sensitive to sunlight and may appear wrinkled. People with albinism are especially susceptible to skin cancer and to some severe visual disturbances, such as myopia (nearsightedness) and abnormal sensitivity to light (photophobia).

Other inherited disorders include **osteogenesis** (os-te-o-JEN-eh-sis) **imperfecta,** or *brittle bones,* in which multiple fractures may occur during and shortly after fetal life, and a disorder of skin, muscles, and bones called **neurofibromatosis** (nu-ro-fi-bro-mah-TO-sis). In the latter condition, multiple masses, often on stalks (pedunculated), grow along nerves all over the body.

More than 20 different cancers have been linked to mutations in specific genes. These include cancers of the breast, ovary, and colon as well as some forms of leukemia. Note, however, that hereditary forms of cancer account for only about 1% of all cancers and that the development of cancer is complex, involving not only specific genes but also gene interactions and environmental factors.

Genetic components have been suggested in some other diseases as well, including certain forms of heart disease, types of cleft lip and cleft palate, and perhaps Parkinson's and Alzheimer's disease.

✔ CHECKPOINT **8**:

What causes phenylketonuria?

TREATMENT AND PREVENTION OF GENETIC DISEASES

The list of genetic diseases is so lengthy (more than 4000) that many pages of this book would be needed simply to enumerate them. Moreover, the list continues to grow as sophisticated research techniques and advances in biology make it clear that various diseases of previously unknown origin are genetic—some hereditary, others not. Can we identify which are inherited genetic disorders and which are due to environmental factors? Can we prevent the occurrence of any of them?

Genetic Counseling

It is possible to prevent genetic disorders in many cases and even to treat some of them. The most effective method of preventing genetic disease is through genetic counseling, a specialized field of health care. Genetic counseling centers use a team approach of medical, nursing, laboratory, and social service professionals to advise and care for the clients.

The Family History

An accurate and complete family history of both prospective parents is necessary for genetic counseling. This history should include information about relatives with respect to age, onset of a specific disease, health status, and cause of death. The families' ethnic origins may be relevant because some genetic diseases predominate in certain ethnic groups. Hospital and physician records are studied, as are photographs of family members. The ages of the prospective parents are factors, as is parental or ancestral relationship (*e.g.,* marriage between first cousins). The complete, detailed family history, or tree, is called a *pedigree*. Pedigrees are used to determine the pattern of inheritance of a genetic disease within a family. They may also indicate whether a given member of the family is a carrier of the disease.

Laboratory Studies

Amniocentesis

A technique that enables the geneticist to study an unborn fetus is *amniocentesis* (am-ne-o-sen-TE-sis). During this procedure, a small amount of the amniotic fluid that surrounds the fetus is withdrawn. Fetal skin cells in the amniotic fluid are removed, grown (cultured), and separated for study. The chromosomes are examined. The amniotic fluid is also analyzed for biochemical abnormalities. With these methods, almost 200 genetic diseases can be detected before birth.

Chorionic Villus Sampling

A newer method for obtaining fetal cells for study involves sampling of the chorionic villi through the cervix. The chorionic villi are hair-like projections of the membrane that surrounds the embryo in early pregnancy. The method is called *chorionic villus sampling (CVS).* Samples may be taken between 8 and 10 weeks of pregnancy, and the cells obtained may be analyzed immediately. In contrast, amniocentesis cannot be done before the 14th to 16th week of pregnancy, and test results are not available for about 2 weeks.

Karyotype

Abnormalities in the number of chromosomes and some abnormalities within the chromosomes can be detected by analysis of the *karyotype* (KAR-e-o-tipe), a name derived from *karyon,* which means "nucleus." A karyotype is produced by growing cells obtained by amniocentesis or CVS in a special medium and arresting cell division at the metaphase stage. The chromosomes, visible under the microscope, are then photographed, and the photographs are cut out and arranged in groups according to their size and form (Fig. 25-2). Abnormalities in the number and structure of chromosomes—called *chromosomal errors*—can thereby be detected. Special stains are used to reveal certain changes in fine structure within the chromosomes.

Counseling the Prospective Parents

Armed with all the available pertinent facts, as well as with knowledge of the risk of recurrence, the counselor is equipped to inform the prospective parents of the possibility of their having genetically abnormal offspring. The couple may then elect to have no children, to have an adoptive family, to consider artificial insemination, to terminate the pregnancy, or to accept the risk.

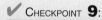

✔ CHECKPOINT **9**:

What is a pedigree and how is a pedigree used in genetic counseling?

Progress in Medical Treatment

The mental and physical ravages of many genetic diseases are largely preventable, provided the diseases are diagnosed and treated early in the individual's life. Some of these diseases respond well to dietary control. One such disease, called

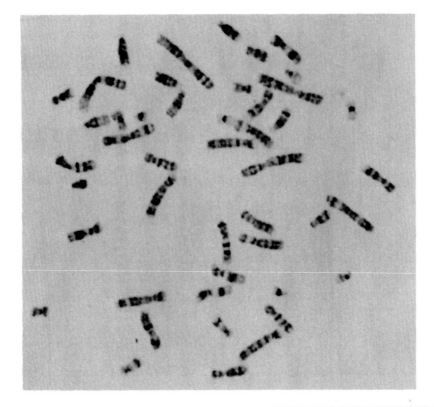

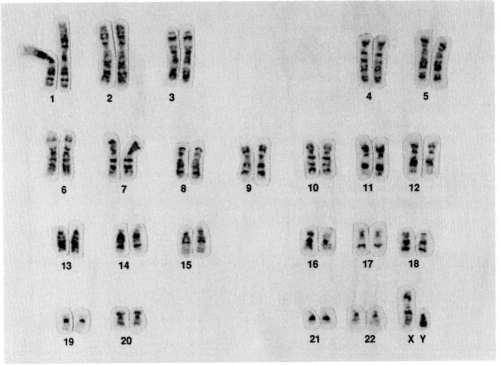

FIGURE **25•2** (*Top*) Metaphase spread of normal male chromosomes. The chromosomes have doubled and are ready to divide. The bands are produced by staining. (*Bottom*) Karyotype. The chromosomes are arranged in matching pairs according to size and other characteristics. (Courtesy of Wenda S. Long, Thomas Jefferson University, Philadelphia)

maple syrup urine disease, responds to very large doses of thiamine along with control of the intake of certain amino acids. The disastrous effects of Wilson's disease, in which abnormal accumulations of copper in the tissue cause tremor, rigidity, uncontrollable stagger, and finally extensive liver damage, can be prevented by a combination of dietary and drug therapy.

Phenylketonuria is perhaps the best-known example of dietary management of inherited disease. If the disorder is undiagnosed and untreated, 98% of affected patients will be severely mentally retarded by 10 years of age; in contrast, if the condition is diagnosed and treated before the baby reaches the age of 6 months, and treatment is maintained until the age of 10 years, mental deficiency will be prevented or at least minimized. A simple blood test for PKU is now done routinely in hospitals throughout the United States. The test is done immediately after birth and should be repeated 24 to 48 hours after the infant has received protein.

Klinefelter's (KLINE-fel-terz) ***syndrome,*** which occurs in about 1 in 600 males, is a common cause of underdevelopment of the gonads with resulting infertility. Victims of this disorder have abnormal sex chromosome patterns, usually an extra X chromosome. Instead of the typical male XY pattern, the cells contain an XXY combination owing to failure of the sex chromosomes to separate during cell division. Treatment of this disorder includes the use of hormones and psychotherapy.

In the future, we can anticipate greatly improved methods of screening, diagnosis, and treatment of genetic diseases. There have been reports of fetuses being treated with vitamins or hormones after prenatal diagnosis of a genetic disorder. Ahead lies the possibility of treating or correcting genetic disorders through genetic engineering—introducing genetically altered cells to produce missing factors, such as enzymes or hormones, or even correcting faulty genes in the victim's cells. Some attempts have already been made to supplement failed genes with healthy ones.

For the present, it is important to educate the public about the availability of screening methods for both parents and offspring. People should also be made aware of the damaging effects of radiation, drugs, and other toxic substances on the genes.

Summary

I. Genes and chromosomes
1. Genes
   a. Hereditary units
   b. Segments of DNA
   c. Control manufacture of enzymes
2. Chromosomes
   a. Threadlike bodies in nucleus
   b. Composed of genes
   c. Exist in matched pairs
   d. Human cells (except sex cells) have 46

A. Dominant and recessive genes
   1. Dominant gene—always expressed
   2. Recessive gene—expressed only if gene received from both parents
      a. Carrier—person with recessive gene that is not apparent but can be passed to offspring

B. Distribution of chromosomes to offspring
   1. Meiosis
      a. Cell division that forms sex cells
      b. Divides chromosomes number in half (23)
      c. Each cell receives one of each chromosome pair

C. Sex determination
   1. Sex chromosomes not matched in size and appearance
   2. X larger and carries other traits
   3. Y smaller and carries mainly gene for sex determination
   4. Female cells have XX; male cells have XY

D. Sex-linked traits
1. Traits carried on sex chromosome (usually X)
2. Sex-linked traits appear mostly in males
   a. Passed from mother to son on X chromosome
   b. If recessive, not masked by dominant gene on Y
   c. Examples—hemophilia, baldness, red-green color blindness

II. Hereditary traits
1. Genes determine physical, biochemical, and physiologic characteristics of every cell
2. Some traits determined by single gene pairs
3. Most determined by multifactorial inheritance
   a. Involves multiple gene pairs
   b. Produces a range of variations in a population
   c. Examples—height, weight, coloration, susceptibility to disease
A. Gene expression
1. Factors
   a. Sex
   b. Presence of other genes
   c. Environment
B. Genetic mutation
1. Change in genes or chromosomes
2. May be passed to offspring if occurs in germ cells
3. Mutagenic agents
   a. Factors causing mutation
   b. Examples—ionizing radiation, chemicals

III. Genetic diseases—disorders involving genes
A. Congenital versus hereditary diseases
1. Congenital disorders

a. Present at birth
b. May or may not be hereditary
c. Causes: infections, toxins, ionizing radiation, alcohol, smoking
2. Hereditary (familial) disorders
   a. Passed from parent to offspring in sex cells
B. Examples of genetic diseases
1. Down syndrome—results from extra chromosome
2. PKU (phenylketonuria)—inability to metabolize phenylalanine
3. Cystic fibrosis—common in white populations
4. Progressive muscular atrophies
5. Albinism—lack of pigment
6. Others: Huntington's disease, sickle cell anemia, osteogenesis imperfecta, neurofibromatosis, cancer

IV. Treatment and prevention of genetic diseases
A. Genetic counseling
1. Family history to establish pedigree
2. Laboratory studies
   a. Amniocentesis—withdrawal of amniotic fluid for study at 14 to 16 weeks of pregnancy
   b. Chorionic villus sampling—done at 8 to 10 weeks of pregnancy
   c. Karyotype—analysis of chromosomes
3. Counseling the prospective parents
B. Progress in medical treatment
1. Dietary control—maple syrup urine disease, Wilson's disease, PKU
2. Hormone therapy—Klinefelter's disease
3. Fetal therapy
4. Correction of faulty genes—experimental

25

Questions for Study and Review

1. Explain the relationship between genes and chromosomes.
2. How many chromosomes are there in a human body cell? in a human sex cell?
3. What process results in the distribution of chromosomes to the offspring?
4. Under what circumstances are dominant genes expressed? Recessive genes?
5. What sex chromosomes are present in a male? in a female?
6. From which parent does a male child receive an X-linked gene?
7. Explain how two normal parents can give birth to a child with a recessive hereditary disease.
8. Explain the great variation in the color of skin, hair, and eyes in humans.
9. Explain how a hereditary disease can suddenly appear in a family with no history of the disease.
10. A baby is born with syphilis. Is this congenital or hereditary? Explain.
11. What is a mutation?
12. List several mutagenic agents.
13. What is a pedigree and how is a pedigree used in genetic counseling?
14. How is an amniocentesis performed and what can be learned from it?
15. Could a karyotype be used to diagnose Down syndrome? Klinefelter's syndrome?
16. What is PKU and how should this disease be treated?
17. What are some characteristics of albinism and what are the risks associated with this disorder?
18. What inheritable disorder is most common among black people and how does it manifest itself?
19. What is the most common heritable disease among white people and what are some of its symptoms?

✔ ANSWERS TO CHECKPOINTS

1. A gene is an independent unit of heredity. Each is a segment of DNA contained in a chromosome.
2. A dominant gene is always expressed, regardless of the gene on the matching chromosome. A recessive gene is only expressed if the gene on the matching chromosome is also recessive.
3. Meiosis is the process of cell division that forms the gametes.
4. The sex chromosome combination that determines a female is XX; a male is XY.
5. A trait carried on a sex chromosome is described as sex linked.
6. A mutation is a change in the genetic material (a gene or chromosome) of a cell.
7. A congenital disease is present at birth. A hereditary disease is genetically transmitted or transmissible. A disorder may occur during development and be present at birth but not be inherited through the genes.
8. Phenylketonuria is caused by a hereditary lack of an enzyme needed for the metabolism of phenylalanine.
9. A pedigree is a complete, detailed family history. It is used to determine the pattern of inheritance of a genetic disease within a family.

Suggestions for Further Study

Agur A: Grant's Atlas of Anatomy, 10th ed. Baltimore, Williams & Wilkins, 1999

Anne EA: Clinical Hematology, 2nd ed. Philadelphia, Lippincott-Raven, 1998

Bishop ML, et al: Clinical Chemistry: Principles, Procedures, Correlations, 3rd ed. Philadelphia, Lippincott-Raven, 1996

Black JG: Microbiology, 4th ed. Upper Saddle River, NJ, Prentice-Hall, 1999

Clemente CD: Gray's Anatomy of the Human Body, 13th ed. Baltimore, Williams & Wilkins, 1985

Clinical Laboratory Tests, 2nd ed. Springhouse, PA, Springhouse Corp, 1995

Cormack DH: Clinically Integrated Histology. Philadelphia, Lippincott-Raven, 1998

DeMyer W: Neuroanatomy, 2nd ed. Baltimore, Williams & Wilkins, 1997

Diseases, 6th ed. Springhouse, PA, Springhouse Corp, 1998

Dorland's Illustrated Medical Dictionary, 28th ed. Philadelphia, WB Saunders, 1994

Escott-Stump S: Nutrition and Diagnosis Related Care, 4th ed. Baltimore, Williams & Wilkins, 1997

Fischbach FT: Nurses' Quick Reference to Common Laboratory and Diagnostic Tests, 2nd ed. Philadelphia, Lippincott-Raven, 1997

Foley, JF, et al: Current Therapy in Cancer. Philadelphia, WB Saunders, 1999

Friedman JM: Genetics, 2nd ed. Baltimore, Williams & Wilkins, 1996

Ganong WF: Review of Medical Physiology, 18th ed. Stamford, CT, Appleton & Lange, 1997

Gartner LP, Hiatt JL: Color Atlas of Histology, 2nd ed. Baltimore, Williams & Wilkins, 1994

Guyton AC, Hall JE: Textbook of Medical Physiology, 9th ed. Philadelphia, WB Saunders, 1996

Innerarity SA: Fluids and Electrolytes, 3rd ed. Springhouse, PA, Springhouse Corp, 1997

Jean AT, et al: Bowes and Church's Food Values of Portions Commonly Used, 17th ed. Philadelphia, Lippincott-Raven, 1997

Junqueira LC, et al: Basic Histology, 9th ed. Englewood Cliffs, NJ, Prentice Hall, 1998

Martini F: Fundamentals of Anatomy and Physiology, 4th ed. Upper Saddle River, NJ, Prentice Hall, 1998

Medical Emergencies. Springhouse, PA, Springhouse Corp, 1998

Moore KL: Clinically Oriented Anatomy, 4th ed. Baltimore, Williams & Wilkins, 1998

Moore KI, et al: Before We Are Born: Essentials of Embryology and Birth Defects, 5th ed. Philadelphia, WB Saunders, 1998

Rakel RE: Conn's Current Therapy. Philadelphia, WB Saunders, 1999 (published yearly)

Rakel RE: Essentials of Family Practice, 2nd ed. Philadelphia, WB Saunders, 1998

Schull PD: Nursing Procedures. Springhouse, PA, Springhouse Corp, 1996

Schull PD: Assessment Made Incredibly Easy. Springhouse, PA, Springhouse Corp, 1997

Shier D, et al: Hole's Human Anatomy and Physiology, 7th ed. New York, McGraw-Hill, 1996

Signs and Symptoms, 2nd ed. Springhouse, PA, Springhouse Corp, 1997

Shaw P: Fluids and Electrolytes. Springhouse, PA, Springhouse Corp, 1997

Tortora GJ, Grabowski SR: Principles of Anatomy and Physiology, 8th ed. Menlo Park, CA, Addison-Wesley, 1999

Tortora GJ, et al: Microbiology, 6th ed. Menlo Park, CA, Addison Wesley, 1997

Whitney EN, Rolfes SR: Understanding Nutrition, 8th ed. Belmont, CA, West/Wadsworth, 1999

Willis MC: Medical Terminology. Baltimore, Williams & Wilkins, 1996

Glossary

Abduction (ab-DUK-shun) Movement away from the midline

Abortion (ah-BOR-shun) Loss of an embryo or fetus before the 20th week of pregnancy

Abscess (AB-ses) Area of tissue breakdown; a localized space in the body containing pus and liquefied tissue

Absorption (ab-SORP-shun) Transfer of digested nutrients from the digestive tract into the circulation

Accommodation (ah-kom-o-DA-shun) Coordinated changes in the eye that enable one to focus on near and far objects

Acetylcholine (as-e-til-KO-lene) **(ACh)** Neurotransmitter; released at synapses within the nervous system and at the neuromuscular junction

Acid (AH-sid) Substance that can donate a hydrogen ion to another substance

Acidosis (as-ih-DO-sis) Condition that results from a decrease in the pH of body fluids

Acquired immunodeficiency syndrome (AIDS) Viral disease that attacks the immune system, specifically the T-helper lymphocytes with CD4 receptors

Acrosome (AK-ro-some) Caplike structure over the head of the sperm cell that helps the sperm to penetrate the ovum

ACTH See Adrenocorticotropic hormone

Actin (AK-tin) One of the two contractile proteins in muscle cells, the other being myosin

Action potential Sudden change in the electric charge on a cell membrane, which then spreads along the membrane; nerve impulse

Active transport Movement of a substance into or out of a cell in a direction opposite that in which it would normally flow by diffusion

Acute (ah-KUTE) Referring to a severe but short-lived disease or condition

Adduction (ad-DUK-shun) Movement toward the midline

Adenosine triphosphate (ah-DEN-o-sene tri-FOS-fate) **(ATP)** Energy-storing compound found in all cells

ADH See Antidiuretic hormone

Adhesion (ad-HE-zhun) Holding together of two surfaces or parts; band of connective tissue between parts that are normally separate; molecular attraction between contacting bodies

Adipose (AD-ih-pose) Referring to a type of connective tissue that stores fat

Adrenal (ah-DRE-nal) Endocrine gland located above the kidney; suprarenal gland

Adrenaline (ah-DREN-ah-lin) See Epinephrine

Adrenocorticotropic (ah-dre-no-kor-tih-ko-TRO-pik) **hormone (ACTH)** Hormone produced by the pituitary that stimulates the adrenal cortex

Aerobic (air-O-bik) Requiring oxygen

Afferent (AF-fer-ent) Carrying toward a given point, such as a sensory neuron that carries nerve impulses toward the central nervous system

Agglutination (ah-glu-tih-NA-shun) Clumping of cells due to an antigen–antibody reaction

AIDS See Acquired immunodeficiency syndrome

Albumin (al-BU-min) Protein in blood plasma and other body fluids; helps maintain the osmotic pressure of the blood

Albuminuria (al-bu-mih-NU-re-ah) Presence of albumin in the urine, usually as a result of a kidney disorder

468

Aldosterone (al-DOS-ter-one) Hormone released by the adrenal cortex that promotes the reabsorption of sodium and water in the kidneys

Alkalosis (al-kah-LO-sis) Condition that results from an increase in the pH of body fluids

Allergen (AL-er-jen) Substance that causes hypersensitivity; substance that induces allergy

Allergy (AL-er-je) Tendency to react unfavorably to a certain substance that is normally harmless to most people; hypersensitivity

Alveolus (al-VE-o-lus) Small sac or pouch; usually a tiny air sac in the lungs through which gases are exchanged between the outside air and the blood; tooth socket; pl., alveoli

Amino (ah-ME-no) **acid** Building block of protein

Amniocentesis (am-ne-o-sen-TE-sis) Removal of fluid and cells from the amniotic sac for prenatal diagnostic tests

Amniotic (am-ne-OT-ik) **sac** Fluid-filled sac that surrounds and cushions the developing fetus

Amphiarthrosis (am-fe-ar-THRO-sis) Slightly movable joint

Anabolism (ah-NAB-o-lizm) Metabolic building of simple compounds into more complex substances needed by the body

Anaerobic (an-air-O-bik) Not requiring oxygen

Analgesic (an-al-JE-zik) Relieving pain; a pain-relieving agent that does not cause loss of consciousness

Anastomosis (ah-nas-to-MO-sis) Communication between two structures, such as blood vessels

Anatomy (ah-NAT-o-me) Study of body structure

Anemia (ah-NE-me-ah) Abnormally low level of hemoglobin or red cells in the blood, resulting in inadequate delivery of oxygen to the tissues

Anesthesia (an-es-THE-ze-ah) Loss of sensation, particularly of pain

Aneurysm (AN-u-rizm) Bulging sac in the wall of a vessel

Angiotensin (an-je-o-TEN-sin) Substance formed in the blood by the action of the enzyme renin from the kidneys. It increases blood pressure by causing constriction of the blood vessels and stimulating the release of aldosterone from the adrenal cortex.

Angina (an-JI-nah) Severe choking pain; disease or condition producing such pain. Angina pectoris is suffocating pain in the chest, usually caused by lack of oxygen supply to the heart muscle

Anion (AN-i-on) Negatively charged particle (ion)

Anorexia (an-o-REK-se-ah) Loss of appetite. Anorexia nervosa is a psychological condition in which a person may become seriously, even fatally, weakened from lack of food.

Anoxia (ah-NOK-se-ah) See Hypoxia

ANS See Autonomic nervous system

Antagonist (an-TAG-o-nist) Muscle that has an action opposite that of a given movement; substance that opposes the action of another substance

Anterior (an-TE-re-or) Toward the front or belly surface; ventral

Antibody (AN-te-bod-e) Substance produced in response to a specific antigen

Antidiuretic (an-ti-di-u-RET-ik) **hormone (ADH)** Hormone released from the posterior pituitary gland that increases the reabsorption of water in the kidneys, thus decreasing the volume of urine excreted

Antigen (AN-te-jen) **(Ag)** Foreign substance that produces an immune response

Antiserum (an-te-SE-rum) Serum containing antibodies; may be given for the purpose of providing passive immunity

Aorta (a-OR-tah) Large artery that carries blood out of the left ventricle of the heart

Apex (A-peks) The pointed region of a cone-shaped structure

Aphasia (ah-FA-ze-ah) Loss or defect in language communication. Loss of the ability to speak or write is expressive aphasia; loss of understanding of written or spoken language is receptive aphasia.

Aponeurosis (ap-o-nu-RO-sis) Broad sheet of fibrous connective tissue that attaches muscle to bone or to other muscle

Appendicular (ap-en-DIK-u-lar) **skeleton** Part of the skeleton that includes the bones of the upper extremities, lower extremities, shoulder girdle, and hips

Arachnoid (ah-RAK-noyd) Middle layer of the meninges

Areolar (ah-RE-o-lar) Referring to loose connective tissue

Arrhythmia (ah-RITH-me-ah) Abnormal rhythm of the heartbeat

Arteriole (ar-TE-re-ole) Vessel between a small artery and a capillary

Arteriosclerosis (ar-te-re-o-skle-RO-sis) Hardening of the arteries

Artery (AR-ter-e) Vessel that carries blood away from the heart

Arthritis (arth-RI-tis) Inflammation of the joints

Arthrocentesis (ar-thro-sen-TE-sis) Puncture of a joint to withdraw fluid

Ascites (ah-SI-teze) Abnormal collection of fluid in the abdominal cavity

Asepsis (a-SEP-sis) Condition in which no pathogens are present; adj., aseptic

Astigmatism (ah-STIG-mah-tizm) Visual defect due to an irregularity in the curvature of the cornea or the lens

Ataxia (ah-TAK-se-ah) Lack of muscular coordination; irregular muscular action

Atherosclerosis (ath-er-o-skle-RO-sis) Hardening of the arteries due to the deposit of yellowish, fatlike material in the lining of these vessels

Atom (AT-om) Fundamental unit of a chemical element

Atopic dermatitis (ah-TOP-ik der-mah-TI-tis) Skin condition that may involve redness, blisters, pimples, scaling, and crusting; eczema

ATP See Adenosine triphosphate

Atrioventricular (a-tre-o-ven-TRIK-u-lar) **(AV) node** Part of the conduction system of the heart

Atrium (A-tre-um) One of the two upper chambers of the heart; adj., atrial

Atrophy (AT-ro-fe) Wasting or decrease in size of a part

Attenuated (ah-TEN-u-a-ted) Weakened

Autoimmunity (aw-to-ih-MU-nih-te) Abnormal reactivity to one's own tissues

Autonomic (aw-to-NOM-ik) **nervous system (ANS)** The part of the nervous system that controls smooth muscle, cardiac muscle, and glands; motor portion of the visceral or involuntary nervous system

AV node See Atrioventricular node

Axial (AK-se-al) **skeleton** The part of the skeleton that includes the skull, spinal column, ribs, and sternum

Axilla (ak-SIL-ah) Hollow beneath the arm where it joins the body; armpit

Axon (AK-son) Fiber of a neuron that conducts impulses away from the cell body

Bacillus (bah-SIL-us) Rod-shaped bacterium; pl., bacilli (bah-SIL-i)

Bacterium (bak-TE-re-um) Type of microorganism; pl., bacteria (bak-TE-re-ah)

Bacteriostasis (bak-te-re-o-STA-sis) Condition in which bacterial growth is inhibited but the organisms are not killed

Basal ganglia (BA-sal GANG-le-ah) Gray masses in the lower part of the forebrain that aid in muscle coordination

Base Substance that can accept a hydrogen ion (H^+); substance that donates a hydroxide ion (OH^-)

Basophil (BA-so-fil) Granular white blood cell that shows large, dark blue cytoplasmic granules when stained with basic stain

B cell Agranular white blood cell that produces antibodies in response to an antigen; B lymphocyte

Benign (be-NINE) Describing a tumor that does not spread; not recurrent nor becoming worse

Bile Substance produced in the liver that emulsifies fats

Biopsy (BI-op-se) Removal of tissue or other material from the living body for examination, usually under the microscope

Blood urea nitrogen (BUN) Amount of nitrogen from urea in the blood; test to evaluate kidney function

Bradycardia (brad-e-KAR-de-ah) Heart rate of less than 60 beats per minute

Brain stem Portion of the brain that connects the cerebrum with the spinal cord; contains the midbrain, pons, and medulla oblongata

Bronchiole (BRONG-ke-ole) Microscopic terminal branch of a bronchus

Bronchus (BRONG-kus) Large air passageway in the lung; pl., bronchi (BRONG-ki)

Buffer (BUF-er) Substance that prevents sharp changes in the pH of a solution

BUN See Blood urea nitrogen

Bursa (BER-sah) Small, fluid-filled sac found in an area subject to stress around bones and joints; pl., bursae (BER-se)

Bursitis (ber-SI-tis) Inflammation of a bursa

Cancer (KAN-ser) Tumor that spreads to other tissues; a malignant neoplasm

Capillary (CAP-ih-lar-e) Microscopic vessel through which exchanges take place between the blood and the tissues

Carbohydrate (kar-bo-HI-drate) Simple sugar or compound made from simple sugars linked together, such as starch or glycogen

Carbon dioxide (di-OX-ide) (CO_2) The gaseous waste product of cellular metabolism

Carcinogen (kar-SIN-o-jen) Cancer-causing substance

Carcinoma (kar-sih-NO-mah) Malignant growth of epithelial cells; a form of cancer

Cardiopulmonary resuscitation (CPR) Method to restore heartbeat and breathing by mouth-to-mouth resuscitation and closed chest cardiac massage

Caries (KA-reze) Tooth decay

Carrier Individual who has a gene that is not expressed but that can be passed to offspring

Cartilage (KAR-tih-lij) Type of hard connective tissue

CAT See Computed tomography

Catabolism (kah-TAB-o-lizm) Metabolic breakdown of substances into simpler substances; includes the digestion of food and the oxidation of nutrient molecules for energy

Cataract (KAT-ah-rakt) Opacity of the eye lens or lens capsule

Catheter (KATH-eh-ter) Tube that can be inserted into a vessel or cavity; may be used to remove fluid, such as urine or blood; v., catheterize

Cation (KAT-i-on) Positively charged particle (ion)

Cecum (SE-kum) Small pouch at the beginning of the large intestine

Cell Basic unit of life

Cell membrane Outer covering of a cell; regulates what enters and leaves cell; plasma membrane

Cellular respiration Series of reactions by which nutrients are oxidized for energy within the cell

Central nervous system (CNS) Part of the nervous system that includes the brain and spinal cord

Centrifuge (SEN-trih-fuje) An instrument that separates materials in a mixture based on density

Centriole (SEN-tre-ole) Rod-shaped body near the nucleus of a cell; functions in cell division

Cerebellum (ser-eh-BEL-um) Small section of the brain located under the cerebral hemispheres; functions in coordination, balance, and muscle tone

Cerebral (SER-e-bral) **cortex** The very thin outer layer of gray matter on the surface of the cerebral hemispheres

Cerebrospinal (ser-e-bro-SPI-nal) **fluid (CSF)** Fluid that circulates in and around the brain and spinal cord

Cerebrovascular (ser-e-bro-VAS-ku-lar) **accident** (CVA) Condition involving obstruction of blood flow to brain tissue or bleeding into brain tissue, usually as a result of hypertension or atherosclerosis; stroke

Cerebrum (SER-e-brum) Largest part of the brain; composed of the cerebral hemispheres

Cerumen (seh-RU-men) Earwax; adj., ceruminous (seh-RU-min-us)

Cervix (SER-vix) Constricted portion of an organ or part, such as the lower portion of the uterus; neck.; adj., cervical

Chemoreceptor (ke-mo-re-SEP-tor) Receptor that detects chemical changes

Chemotherapy (ke-mo-THER-ah-pe) Treatment of a disease by administration of a chemical agent

Chlamydia (klah-MID-e-ah) A type of very small bacterium that can exist only within a living cell; members of this group cause inclusion conjunctivitis, trachoma, sexually transmitted diseases, and respiratory diseases

Cholesterol (ko-LES-ter-ol) An organic fatlike compound found in animal fat, bile, blood, myelin, liver, and other parts of the body

Choroid (KO-royd) Pigmented middle layer of the eye

Chromosome (KRO-mo-some) Dark-staining, threadlike body in the nucleus of a cell; contains genes that determine hereditary traits

Chronic (KRON-ik) Referring to a disease that develops slowly, persists over a long time, or is recurring

Chyle (kile) Milky-appearing fluid absorbed into the lymphatic system from the small intestine. It consists of lymph and droplets of digested fat.

Chyme (kime) Mixture of partially digested food, water, and digestive juices that forms in the stomach

Cilia (SIL-e-ah) Hairs or hairlike processes, such as eyelashes or microscopic extensions from the surface of a cell; sing., cilium

Circumduction (ser-kum-DUK-shun) Circular movement at a joint

Cirrhosis (sih-RO-sis) Chronic disease, usually of the liver, in which active cells are replaced by inactive scar tissue

CNS See Central nervous system

Coagulation (ko-ag-u-LA-shun) Clotting, as of blood

Coccus (KOK-us) A round bacterium; pl., cocci (KOK-si)

Cochlea (KOK-le-ah) Coiled portion of the inner ear that contains the organ of hearing

Collagen (KOL-ah-jen) Flexible white protein that gives strength and resilience to connective tissue, such as bone and cartilage

Colloidal (kol-OYD-al) **suspension** Mixture in which suspended particles do not dissolve but remain distributed in the solvent because of their small size (*e.g.*, cytoplasm); colloid

Colon (KO-lon) Main portion of the large intestine

Complement (KOM-ple-ment) Group of blood proteins that helps antibodies to destroy foreign cells

Compliance (kom-PLI-ans) The ease with which the lungs and thorax can be expanded

Compound Substance composed of two or more chemical elements

Computed tomography (to-MOG-rah-fe) **(CT)** Imaging method in which multiple radiographic views taken from different angles are analyzed by computer to show a cross-section of an area; used to detect tumors and other abnormalities; also called computed axial tomography (CAT)

Congenital (con-JEN-ih-tal) Present at birth

Conjunctiva (kon-junk-TI-vah) Membrane that lines the eyelid and covers the anterior part of the sclera (white of the eye)

Contraception (con-trah-SEP-shun) Prevention of fertilization of an ovum or implantation of a fertilized ovum; birth control

Convergence (kon-VER-jens) The centering of both eyes on the same visual field

Cornea (KOR-ne-ah) Clear portion of the sclera that covers the front of the eye

Coronary (KOR-on-ar-e) Referring to the heart or to the arteries supplying blood to the heart

Corpus callosum (kal-O-sum) Thick bundle of myelinated nerve cell fibers, deep within the brain, that carries nerve impulses from one cerebral hemisphere to the other

Corpus luteum (LU-te-um) Yellow body formed from ovarian follicle after ovulation; produces progesterone

Cortex (KOR-tex) Outer layer of an organ, such as the brain, kidney, or adrenal gland

Covalent (KO-va-lent) **bond** Chemical bond formed by the sharing of electrons between atoms

CPR See Cardiopulmonary resuscitation

CSF See Cerebrospinal fluid

CT See Computed tomography

Cutaneous (ku-TA-ne-us) Referring to the skin

Cyanosis (si-ah-NO-sis) Bluish discoloration of the skin and mucous membranes resulting from insufficient oxygen in the blood

Cystitis (sis-TI-tis) Inflammation of the urinary bladder

Cytology (si-TOL-o-je) Study of cells

Cytoplasm (SI-to-plazm) Substance that fills the cell and holds the organelles

Defecation (def-e-KA-shun) Act of eliminating undigested waste from the digestive tract

Degeneration (de-jen-er-A-shun) Breakdown, as from age, injury, or disease

Deglutition (deg-lu-TISH-un) Act of swallowing

Dehydration (de-hi-DRA-shun) Excessive loss of body fluid

Dendrite (DEN-drite) Fiber of a neuron that conducts impulses toward the cell body

Deoxyribonucleic (de-OK-se-ri-bo-nu-kle-ik) **acid (DNA)** Genetic material of the cell; makes up the chromosomes in the nucleus of the cell

Dermatitis (der-mah-TI-tis) Inflammation of the skin

Dermis (DER-mis) True skin; deeper part of the skin

Dextrose (DEK-strose) Glucose; simple sugar

Diabetes mellitus (di-ah-BE-teze mel-LI-tus) Disease of insufficient insulin in which excess glucose is found in blood and urine; characterized by abnormal metabolism of glucose, protein, and fat

Diagnosis (di-ag-NO-sis) Identification of an illness

Dialysis (di-AL-ih-sis) Method for separating molecules in solution based on differences in their ability to pass through a semipermeable membrane; method for removing nitrogen waste products from the body, as by hemodialysis or peritoneal dialysis

Diaphragm (DI-ah-fram) Dome-shaped muscle under the lungs that flattens during inhalation; separating membrane or structure

Diaphysis (di-AF-ih-sis) Shaft of a long bone

Diarthrosis (di-ar-THRO-sis) Freely movable joint; synovial joint

Diastole (di-AS-to-le) Relaxation phase of the cardiac cycle; adj., diastolic (di-as-TOL-ik)

Diencephalon (di-en-SEF-ah-lon) Region of the brain between the cerebral hemispheres and the midbrain; contains the thalamus, hypothalamus, and pituitary gland

Diffusion (dih-FU-zhun) Movement of molecules from a region where they are in higher concentration to a region where they are in lower concentration

Digestion (di-JEST-yun) Process of breaking down food into absorbable particles

Dilation (di-LA-shun) Widening of a part, such as the pupil of the eye, a blood vessel, or the uterine cervix; dilatation

Disease Illness; abnormal state in which part or all of the body does not function properly

Distal (DIS-tal) Farther from the origin of a structure or from a given reference point

DNA See Deoxyribonucleic acid

Dominant (DOM-ih-nant) Referring to a gene that is always expressed if present

Dorsal (DOR-sal) Toward the back; posterior

Duct Tube or vessel

Ductus deferens (DEF-er-enz) Tube that carries sperm cells from the testis to the urethra; vas deferens

Duodenum (du-o-DE-num) First portion of the small intestine

Dura mater (DU-rah MA-ter) Outermost layer of the meninges

Dyspnea (disp-NE-ah) Difficult or labored breathing

ECG See Electrocardiograph

Echocardiograph (ek-o-KAR-de-o-graf) Instrument to study the heart by means of ultrasound; the record produced is an echocardiogram

Eclampsia (eh-KLAMP-se-ah) Serious and sometimes fatal condition involving convulsions, liver damage, and kidney failure that can develop from preeclampsia (toxemia of pregnancy)

Eczema (EK-ze-mah) See atopic dermatitis

Edema (eh-DE-mah) Accumulation of fluid in the tissue spaces

EEG See Electroencephalograph

Effector (ef-FEK-tor) Muscle or gland that responds to a stimulus; effector organ

Efferent (EF-fer-ent) Carrying away from a given point, such as a motor neuron that carries nerve impulses away from the central nervous system

Effusion (eh-FU-zhun) Escape of fluid into a cavity or space; the fluid itself

Ejaculation (e-jak-u-LA-shun) Expulsion of semen through the urethra

EKG See Electrocardiograph

Electrocardiograph (e-lek-tro-KAR-de-o-graf) **(ECG, EKG)** Instrument to study the electrical activity of the heart; record made is an electrocardiogram

Electroencephalograph (e-lek-tro-en-SEF-ah-lo-graf) **(EEG)** Instrument used to study electrical activity of the brain; record made is an electroencephalogram

Electrolyte (e-LEK-tro-lite) Compound that forms ions in solution; substance that conducts an electric current in solution

Electron (e-LEK-tron) Negatively charged particle located in an orbital outside the nucleus of an atom

Element (EL-eh-ment) One of the substances from which all matter is made; substance that cannot be decomposed into a simpler substance

Embolism (EM-bo-lizm) The condition of having an embolus

Embolus (EM-bo-lus) Blood clot or other obstruction in the circulation

Embryo (EM-bre-o) Developing offspring during the first 2 months of pregnancy

Emesis (EM-eh-sis) Vomiting

Emphysema (em-fih-SE-mah) Pulmonary disease characterized by dilation and destruction of the alveoli

Emulsify (e-MUL-sih-fi) To break up fats into small particles; n., emulsification

Endocardium (en-do-KAR-de-um) Membrane that lines the heart chambers and covers the valves

Endocrine (EN-do-krin) Referring to a gland that secretes directly into the bloodstream

Endometrium (en-do-ME-tre-um) Lining of the uterus

Endoplasmic reticulum (en-do-PLAS-mik re-TIK-u-lum) **(ER)** Network of membranes in the cytoplasm of a cell

Endosteum (en-DOS-te-um) Thin membrane that lines the marrow cavity of a bone

Endothelium (en-do-THE-le-um) Epithelium that lines the heart, blood vessels, and lymphatic vessels

Enzyme (EN-zime) Organic catalyst; speeds the rate of a reaction but is not changed in the reaction

Eosinophil (e-o-SIN-o-fil) Granular white blood cell that shows beadlike, bright pink cytoplasmic granules when stained with acid stain; acidophil

Epicardium (ep-ih-KAR-de-um) Membrane that forms the outermost layer of the heart wall and is continuous with the lining of the pericardium; visceral pericardium

Epidemic (ep-ih-DEM-ik) Occurrence of a disease among many people in a given region at the same time

Epidermis (ep-ih-DER-mis) Outermost layer of the skin

Epiglottis (ep-e-GLOT-is) Leaf-shaped cartilage that covers the larynx during swallowing

Epilepsy (EP-ih-lep-se) Chronic disorder of the nervous system involving abnormal electrical activity of the brain; characterized by seizures of varying severity

Epimysium (ep-ih-MIS-e-um) Sheath of fibrous connective tissue that encloses a muscle

Epinephrine (ep-ih-NEF-rin) Neurotransmitter and hormone; released from neurons of the sympathetic nervous system and from the adrenal medulla; adrenaline

Epiphysis (eh-PIF-ih-sis) End of a long bone

Episiotomy (eh-piz-e-OT-o-me) Cutting of the perineum between the vaginal opening and the anus to reduce the tearing of tissue in childbirth

Epithelium (ep-ih-THE-le-um) One of the four main types of tissue; forms glands, covers surfaces, and lines cavities; adj., epithelial

ER See Endoplasmic reticulum

Eruption (e-RUP-shun) Raised skin lesion; rash

Erythema (er-eh-THE-mah) Redness of the skin

Erythrocyte (eh-RITH-ro-site) Red blood cell

Erythropoietin (EPO) (eh-rith-ro-POY-eh-tin) Hormone released from the kidney that stimulates the production of red blood cells in the bone marrow

Esophagus (eh-SOF-ah-gus) Tube that carries food from the throat to the stomach

Estrogen (ES-tro-jen) Group of female sex hormones that promotes development of the uterine lining and maintains secondary sex characteristics

Etiology (e-te-OL-o-je) Study of the cause of a disease or the theory of its origin

Eustachian (u-STA-shun) **tube** Tube that connects the middle ear cavity to the throat; auditory tube

Eversion (e-VER-zhun) Turning outward, with reference to movement of the foot

Excretion (eks-KRE-shun) Removal and elimination of metabolic waste products from the blood

Exocrine (EK-so-krin) Referring to a gland that secretes through a duct

Extracellular (EK-strah-sel-u-lar) Outside the cell

Fascia (FASH-e-ah) Band or sheet of fibrous connective tissue

Fascicle (FAS-ih-kl) Small bundle, as of muscle cells or nerve cell fibers

Feces (FE-seze) Waste material discharged from the large intestine; excrement; stool

Feedback Return of information into a system, so that it can be used to regulate that system

Fertilization (fer-til-ih-ZA-shun) Union of an ovum and a spermatozoon

Fetus (FE-tus) Developing offspring from the third month of pregnancy until birth

Fever (FE-ver) Abnormally high body temperature

Fibrin (FI-brin) Blood protein that forms a blood clot

Filtration (fil-TRA-shun) Movement of material through a semipermeable membrane under mechanical force

Fissure (FISH-ure) Deep groove

Flaccid (FLAK-sid) Flabby, limp, soft

Flagellum (flah-JEL-lum) Long whiplike extension from a cell used for locomotion; pl., flagella

Flatus (FLA-tus) Gas in the digestive tract

Flexion (FLEK-shun) Bending motion that decreases the angle between bones at a joint

Follicle (FOL-lih-kl) Sac or cavity, such as the ovarian follicle or hair follicle

Follicle-stimulating hormone (FSH) Hormone produced by the anterior pituitary that stimulates development of ova in the ovary and spermatozoa in the testes

Fontanelle (fon-tah-NEL) Area in the infant skull where bone formation has not yet occurred; "soft spot"

Foramen (fo-RA-men) Opening or passageway, as into or through a bone; pl., foramina (fo-RAM-in-ah)

Fornix (FOR-niks) A recess or archlike structure

Fossa (FOS-sah) Hollow or depression, as in a bone; pl., fossae (FOS-se)

Fovea (FO-ve-ah) Small pit or cup-shaped depression in a surface; the fovea centralis near the center of the retina is the point of sharpest vision

FSH See Follicle-stimulating hormone

Fungus (FUN-gus) Type of plantlike microorganism; yeast or mold; pl., fungi (FUN-ji)

Gamete (GAM-ete) Reproductive cell; ovum or spermatozoon

Gamma globulin (GLOB-u-lin) Protein fraction in the blood plasma that contains antibodies

Ganglion (GANG-le-on) Collection of nerve cell bodies located outside the central nervous system

Gangrene (GANG-grene) Death of tissue accompanied by bacterial invasion and putrefaction

Gastrointestinal (gas-tro-in-TES-tih-nal) **(GI)** Pertaining to the stomach and intestine or the digestive tract as a whole

Gene Hereditary unit; portion of the DNA on a chromosome

Genetic (jeh-NET-ik) Pertaining to the genes or heredity

Gestation (jes-TA-shun) Period of development from conception to birth

GH See Growth hormone

GI See Gastrointestinal

Gingiva (JIN-jih-vah) Tissue around the teeth; gum

Glaucoma (glaw-KO-mah) Disorder involving increased fluid pressure within the eye

Glial cells (GLI-al) The connective tissue cells of the nervous system; neuroglia

Glomerular (glo-MER-u-lar) **filtrate** Fluid and dissolved materials that leave the blood and enter the kidney nephron through Bowman's capsule

Glomerulonephritis (glo-mer-u-lo-nef-RI-tis) Kidney disease often resulting from antibodies to a streptococcal infection

Glomerulus (glo-MER-u-lus) Cluster of capillaries in Bowman's capsule of the nephron

Glucose (GLU-kose) Simple sugar; main energy source for the cells; dextrose

Glycogen (GLI-ko-jen) Compound built from glucose molecules that is stored for energy in liver and muscles

Golgi (GOL-je) **apparatus** System of membranes in the cell that formulates special substances

Gonad (GO-nad) Sex gland; ovary or testis

Gonadotropin (gon-ah-do-TRO-pin) Hormone that acts on a reproductive gland (ovary or testis) *e.g.,* FSH, LH

Gram (g) Basic unit of weight in the metric system

Gray matter Nervous tissue composed of unmyelinated fibers and cell bodies

Growth hormone (GH) Hormone produced by anterior pituitary that promotes growth of tissues; somatotropin

Gustatory (GUS-tah-to-re) Pertaining to the sense of taste (gustation)

Gyrus (JI-rus) Raised area of the cerebral cortex; pl., gyri (JI-ri)

Helminth (HEL-minth) Worm

Hematocrit (he-MAT-o-krit) **(Hct)** Volume percentage of red blood cells in whole blood; packed cell volume

Hematoma (he-mah-TO-mah) Tumor or swelling filled with blood

Hematuria (hem-ah-TU-re-ah) Blood in the urine

Hemodialysis (he-mo-di-AL-ih-sis) Removal of impurities from the blood by their passage through a semipermeable membrane in a fluid bath

Hemoglobin (he-mo-GLO-bin) **(Hb)** Iron-containing protein in red blood cells that transports oxygen

Hemolysis (he-MOL-ih-sis) Rupture of red blood cells; v., hemolyze (HE-mo-lize)

Hemopoiesis (he-mo-poy-E-sis) Production of blood cells; hematopoiesis

Hemorrhage (HEM-eh-rij) Loss of blood

Hemostasis (he-mo-STA-sis) Stoppage of bleeding

Heparin (HEP-ah-rin) Substance that prevents blood clotting; anticoagulant

Hepatitis (hep-ah-TI-tis) Inflammation of the liver

Heredity (he-RED-ih-te) Transmission of characteristics from parent to offspring by means of the genes; the genetic makeup of the individual

Hernia (HER-ne-ah) Protrusion of an organ or tissue through the wall of the cavity in which it is normally enclosed

Hilum (HI-lum) See hilus

Hilus (HI-lus) Area where vessels and nerves enter or leave an organ

Histamine (HIS-tah-mene) Substance released from tissues during an antigen–antibody reaction

Histology (his-TOL-o-je) Study of tissues

HIV See Human immunodeficiency virus

Homeostasis (ho-me-o-STA-sis) State of balance within the body; maintenance of body conditions within set limits

Hormone Secretion of an endocrine gland; chemical messenger that has specific regulatory effects on certain other cells

Human immunodeficiency virus (HIV) The virus that causes AIDS

Hydrolysis (hi-DROL-ih-sis) Splitting of large molecules by the addition of water, as in digestion

Hydroxycholecalciferol (hy-drok-se-ko-le-kal-SIF-eh-rol) The active form of vitamin D; promotes absorption of calcium in the small intestine to increase blood calcium levels

Hyperglycemia (hi-per-gli-SE-me-ah) Abnormal increase in the amount of glucose in the blood

Hypersensitivity (hi-per-SEN-sih-tiv-ih-te) Exaggerated reaction of the immune system to a substance that is normally harmless to most people; allergy

Hypertension (hi-per-TEN-shun) High blood pressure

Hypertonic (hi-per-TON-ik) Describing a solution that is more concentrated than the fluids within a cell

Hypertrophy (hy-PER-tro-fe) Enlargement or overgrowth of an organ or part

Hypoglycemia (hi-po-gli-SE-me-ah) Abnormal decrease in the amount of glucose in the blood

Hypophysis (hi-POF-ih-sis) Pituitary gland

Hypotension (hi-po-TEN-shun) Low blood pressure

Hypothalamus (hi-po-THAL-ah-mus) Region of the brain that controls the pituitary and maintains homeostasis

Hypothermia (hi-po-THER-me-ah) Abnormally low body temperature

Hypotonic (hi-po-TON-ik) Describing a solution that is less concentrated than the fluids within a cell

Hypoxemia (hi-pok-SE-me-ah) Lower than normal concentration of oxygen in arterial blood

Hypoxia (hi-POK-se-ah) Lower than normal level of oxygen in the tissues

ICSH See Interstitial cell-stimulating hormone

Ileum (IL-e-um) The last portion of the small intestine

Immunity (ih-MU-nih-te) Power of an individual to resist or overcome the effects of a particular disease or other harmful agent

Immunization (ih-mu-nih-ZA-shun) Use of a vaccine to produce immunity

Immunodeficiency (im-u-no-de-FISH-en-se) Any failure of the immune system

Implantation (im-plan-TA-shun) The embedding of the fertilized egg into the lining of the uterus

Infarct (IN-farkt) Area of tissue damaged from lack of blood supply caused by blockage of a vessel

Inferior (in-FE-re-or) Below or lower

Inferior vena cava (VE-nah KA-vah) Large vein that drains the lower part of the body and empties into the right atrium of the heart

Infertility (in-fer-TIL-ih-te) Decreased ability to reproduce

Inflammation (in-flah-MA-shun) Response of tissues to injury; characterized by heat, redness, swelling, and pain

Insertion (in-SER-shun) End of a muscle attached to a movable part

Integument (in-TEG-u-ment) Skin; adj., integumentary

Intercellular (in-ter-SEL-u-lar) Between cells

Interleukin (in-ter-LU-kin) A substance released by a T cell or macrophage that stimulates other cells of the immune system

Interneuron (in-ter-NU-ron) A nerve cell that transmits impulses within the central nervous system

Interstitial (in-ter-STISH-al) Between; pertaining to spaces or structures in an organ between active tissues

Interstitial cell–stimulating hormone (ICSH) See Luteinizing hormone

Intracellular (in-trah-SEL-u-lar) Within a cell

Inversion (in-VER-zhun) Turning inward, with reference to movement of the foot

Ion (I-on) Charged particle formed when an electrolyte goes into solution

Iris (I-ris) Circular colored region of the eye around the pupil

Ischemia (is-KE-me-ah) Lack of blood supply to an area

Islets (I-lets) Groups of cells in the pancreas that produce hormones; islets of Langerhans (LAHNG-er-hanz)

Isometric (i-so-MET-rik) **contraction** Muscle contraction in which there is no change in muscle length but an increase in muscle tension, as in pushing against an immovable force

Isotonic (i-so-TON-ik) Describing a solution that has the same concentration as the fluid within a cell

Isotonic contraction Muscle contraction in which the tone within the muscle remains the same but the muscle shortens to produce movement

Isotope (I-so-tope) Form of an element that has the same atomic number as another but a different atomic weight

Jaundice (JAWN-dis) Yellowish discoloration of the skin that is usually due to the presence of bile in the blood

Jejunum (je-JU-num) Second portion of the small intestine

Joint Area of junction between two or more bones; articulation

Juxtaglomerular (juks-tah-glo-MER-u-lar) **(JG) apparatus** Structure in the kidney composed of cells of the afferent arteriole and distal convoluted tubule that secretes the enzyme renin when blood pressure decreases below a certain level

Karyotype (KAR-e-o-type) Picture of the chromosomes arranged according to size and form

Keratin (KER-ah-tin) Protein that thickens and protects the skin; makes up hair and nails

Kidney (KID-ne) Organ of excretion

Kilocalorie (kil-o-KAL-o-re) A measure of the energy content of food. Technically, the amount of heat needed to raise l kg of water 1° centigrade

Lacrimal (LAK-rih-mal) Referring to tears or the tear glands

Lactation (lak-TA-shun) Secretion of milk

Lacteal (LAK-te-al) Capillary of the lymphatic system; drains digested fats from the villi of the small intestine

Lactic (LAK-tik) **acid** Organic acid that accumulates in muscle cells functioning without oxygen

Larynx (LAR-inks) Structure between the pharynx and trachea that contains the vocal cords; voice box

Laser (LA-zer) Device that produces a very intense beam of light

Lateral (LAT-er-al) Farther from the midline; toward the side

Lens Biconvex structure of the eye that changes in thickness to accommodate for near and far vision; crystalline lens

Lesion (LE-zhun) Wound or local injury

Leukemia (lu-KE-me-ah) Malignant blood disease characterized by abnormal development of white blood cells

Leukocyte (LU-ko-site) White blood cell

LH See Luteinizing hormone

Ligament (LIG-ah-ment) Band of connective tissue that connects a bone to another bone; thickened portion or fold of the peritoneum that supports an organ or attaches it to another organ

Lipid (LIP-id) Type of organic compound, one example of which is a fat

Liter (LE-ter) **(L)** Basic unit of volume in the metric system.

Lumen (LU-men) Central opening of an organ or vessel

Lung Organ of respiration

Luteinizing (LU-te-in-i-zing) **hormone** Hormone produced by the anterior pituitary that induces ovulation and formation of the corpus luteum in females; in males, it stimulates cells in the testes to produce testosterone and is called *interstitial cell–stimulating hormone (ICSH)*

Lymph (limf) Fluid in the lymphatic system

Lymphadenitis (lim-fad-en-I-tis) Inflammation of the lymph nodes

Lymphadenopathy (lim-fad-en-OP-ah-the) Any disorder of the lymph nodes

Lymphangitis (lim-fan-JI-tis) Inflammation of the lymphatic vessels

Lymphatic duct Vessel of the lymphatic system

Lymph node Mass of lymphoid tissue along the path of a lymphatic vessel that filters lymph and harbors white blood cells active in immunity

Lymphocyte (LIM-fo-site) Agranular white blood cell that functions in immunity

Lysosome (LI-so-some) Cell organelle that contains digestive enzymes

Macrophage (MAK-ro-faj) Large phagocytic cell that develops from a monocyte

Macula (MAK-u-lah) Spot; flat, discolored spot on the skin, such as a freckle or measles lesion; small yellow spot in the retina of the eye that contains the fovea, the point of sharpest vision; also called macule

Magnetic resonance imaging (MRI) Method for studying tissue based on nuclear movement after exposure to radio waves in a powerful magnetic field

Major histocompatibility complex Group of genes that codes for specific proteins (antigens) on the surface of cells. These antigens are important in cross-matching for tissue transplantation. They are also important in immune reactions.

Malignant (mah-LIG-nant) Describing a tumor that spreads; describing a disorder that tends to become worse and cause death

Malnutrition (mal-nu-TRISH-un) State resulting from lack of food, lack of an essential component of the diet, or faulty use of food in the diet

Mastectomy (mas-TEK-to-me) Removal of the breast; mammectomy

Mastication (mas-tih-KA-shun) Act of chewing

Matrix (MA-triks) The nonliving background material in a tissue; the intercellular material

Medial (ME-de-al) Nearer the midline of the body

Mediastinum (me-de-as-TI-num) Region between the lungs and the organs and vessels it contains

Medulla (meh-DUL-lah) Inner region of an organ; marrow

Medulla oblongata (ob-long-GAH-tah) Part of the brain stem that connects the brain to the spinal cord

Megakaryocyte (meg-ah-KAR-e-o-site) Very large cell that gives rise to blood platelets

Meiosis (mi-O-sis) Process of cell division that halves the chromosome number in the formation of the reproductive cells

Melanin (MEL-ah-nin) Dark pigment found in skin, hair, parts of the eye, and certain parts of the brain

Membrane Thin sheet of tissue

Mendelian (men-DE-le-en) **laws** Principles of heredity discovered by an Austrian monk named Gregor Mendel

Meninges (men-IN-jeze) Three layers of fibrous membranes that cover the brain and spinal cord

Menopause (MEN-o-pawz) Time at which menstruation ceases

Menses (MEN-seze) Monthly flow of blood from the female reproductive tract

Mesentery (MES-en-ter-e) Membranous peritoneal ligament that attaches the small intestine to the dorsal abdominal wall

Mesocolon (mes-o-KO-lon) Peritoneal ligament that attaches the colon to the dorsal abdominal wall

Metabolic rate Rate at which energy is released from nutrients in the cells

Metabolism (meh-TAB-o-lizm) Physical and chemical processes by which an organism is maintained

Metastasis (meh-TAS-tah-sis) Spread of tumor cells; pl., metastases (meh-TAS-tah-seze)

Meter (ME-ter) **(m)** Basic unit of length in the metric system

MHC See Major histocompatibility complex

Microbiology (mi-kro-bi-OL-o-je) Study of microscopic organisms

Micrometer (MI-kro-me-ter) **(μm)** 1/1000th of a millimeter; micron; also an instrument for measuring through a microscope (pronounced mi-KROM-eh-ter)

Microorganism (mi-kro-OR-gan-izm) Microscopic organism

Micturition (mik-tu-RISH-un) Act of urination; voiding of the urinary bladder

Midbrain Upper portion of the brainstem

Mineral (MIN-er-al) Inorganic substance; in the diet, an element needed in small amounts for health

Mitochondria (mi-to-KON-dre-ah) Cell organelles that manufacture ATP with the energy released from the oxidation of nutrients; sing., mitochondrion

Mitosis (mi-TO-sis) Type of cell division that produces two daughter cells exactly like the parent cell

Mitral (MI-tral) **valve** Valve between the left atrium and left ventricle of the heart; bicuspid valve

Mixture Blend of two or more substances

Molecule (MOL-eh-kule) Particle formed by chemical bonding of two or more atoms; smallest subunit of a compound

Monocyte (MON-o-site) Agranular white blood cell active in phagocytosis

Motor (MO-tor) Describing structures or activities involved in transmitting impulses away from the central nervous system; efferent

MRI See Magnetic resonance imaging

Mucosa (mu-KO-sah) Lining membrane that produces mucus; mucous membrane

Mucus (MU-kus) Thick protective fluid secreted by mucous membranes and glands; adj., mucous

Murmur Abnormal heart sound

Mutagenic (mu-tah-JEN-ik) Causing mutation

Mutation (mu-TA-shun) Change in a gene or a chromosome

Myalgia (mi-AL-je-ah) Muscular pain

Myelin (MI-el-in) Fatty material that covers and insulates the axons of some neurons

Myocardium (mi-o-KAR-de-um) Middle layer of the heart wall; heart muscle

Myoglobin (MI-o-glo-bin) Compound that stores oxygen in muscle cells

Myometrium (mi-o-ME-tre-um) The muscular layer of the uterus

Myopia (mi-O-pe-ah) Nearsightedness

Myosin (MI-o-sin) One of the two contractile proteins in muscle cells, the other being actin

Necrosis (neh-KRO-sis) Tissue death

Negative feedback Self-regulating system in which the result of an action is the control over that action; a method for keeping body conditions within a normal range and maintaining homeostasis

Neoplasm (NE-o-plazm) Abnormal growth of cells; tumor; adj., neoplastic

Nephron (NEF-ron) Microscopic functional unit of the kidney

Nerve Bundle of neuron fibers outside the central nervous system

Nerve impulse Electrical charge that spreads along the membrane of a neuron; action potential

Neuralgia (nu-RAL-je-ah) Pain in a nerve

Neurilemma (nu-rih-LEM-mah) Thin sheath that covers certain peripheral axons; aids in regeneration of the axon

Neuroglia (nu-ROG-le-ah) Supporting and protective cells of the central nervous system; glial cells

Neuromuscular junction Point at which a nerve fiber contacts a muscle cell

Neuron (NU-ron) Conducting cell of the nervous system

Neurotransmitter (nu-ro-TRANS-mit-er) Chemical released from the ending of an axon that enables a nerve impulse to cross a synapse

Neutrophil (NU-tro-fil) Phagocytic granular white blood cell; polymorph; poly; PMN; seg

Node Small mass of tissue, such as a lymph node; space between cells in the myelin sheath

Norepinephrine (nor-epi-ih-NEF-rin) Neurotransmitter similar to epinephrine; noradrenaline

Nucleotide (NU-kle-o-tide) Building block of DNA and RNA

Nucleus (NU-kle-us) Largest organelle in the cell, containing the DNA, which directs all cell activities; group of neurons in the central nervous system; in chemistry, the central part of an atom

Olfactory (ol-FAK-to-re) Pertaining to the sense of smell (olfaction)

Oncology (on-KOL-o-je) Study of tumors

Ophthalmic (of-THAL-mik) Pertaining to the eye

Organ (OR-gan) Body part containing two or more tissues functioning together for specific purposes

Organelle (or-gan-EL) Specialized subdivision within a cell

Organic (or-GAN-ik) Referring to compounds found in living things and containing carbon, hydrogen, and oxygen

Organism (OR-gan-izm) Individual plant or animal; any organized living thing

Organ of Corti (KOR-te) Receptor for hearing located in the cochlea of the internal ear

Origin (OR-ih-jin) Source; beginning; end of a muscle attached to a nonmoving part

Osmosis (os-MO-sis) Movement of water through a semipermeable membrane

Osmotic (os-MOT-ik) **pressure** Tendency of a solution to draw water into it; is directly related to the concentration of the solution

Ossicle (OS-ih-kl) One of three small bones of the middle ear: malleus, incus, or stapes

Ossification (os-ih-fih-KA-shun) Process of bone formation

Osteoblast (OS-te-o-blast) Bone-forming cell

Osteoclast (OS-te-o-clast) Cell that breaks down bone

Osteocyte (OS-te-o-site) Mature bone cell; maintains bone but does not divide

Osteoporosis (os-te-o-po-RO-sis) Abnormal loss of bone tissue with tendency to fracture

Ovary (O-vah-re) Female reproductive gland

Ovulation (ov-u-LA-shun) Release of a mature ovum from a follicle in the ovary

Ovum (O-vum) Female reproductive cell or gamete; pl., ova

Oxidation (ok-sih-DA-shun) Chemical breakdown of nutrients for energy

Oxygen (OK-sih-jen) **(O_2)** The gas needed to break down nutrients completely for energy within the cell

Oxygen debt Amount of oxygen needed to reverse the effects produced in muscles functioning without oxygen

Pacemaker Sinoatrial (SA) node of the heart; group of cells or artificial device that sets the rate of heart contractions

Pancreas (PAN-kre-as) Large, elongated gland behind the stomach; produces digestive enzymes and hormones (*e.g.,* insulin)

Papilla (pah-PIL-ah) Small nipplelike projection or elevation

Paracentesis (par-eh-sen-TE-sis) Puncture of the abdominal cavity, usually to remove a fluid accumulation, such as ascites; abdominocentesis

Parasite (PAR-ah-site) Organism that lives on or within another (the host) at the other's expense

Parasympathetic nervous system Craniosacral division of the autonomic nervous system

Parathyroid (par-ah-THI-royd) Any of four small glands embedded in the capsule enclosing the thyroid gland; produces hormone that regulates calcium in the blood

Parietal (pah-RI-eh-tal) Pertaining to the wall of a space or cavity

Parturition (par-tu-RISH-un) Childbirth; labor

Pathogen (PATH-o-jen) Disease-causing organism; adj., pathogenic (path-o-JEN-ik)

Pathology (pah-THOL-o-je) Study of disease

Pathophysiology (path-o-fiz-e-OL-o-je) Study of the physiologic basis of disease

Pedigree (PED-ih-gre) Family history; used in the study of heredity

Pelvic inflammatory disease (PID) Ascending infection that involves the pelvic organs; common causes are gonorrhea and chlamydia

Pelvis (PEL-vis) Basinlike structure, such as the lower portion of the abdomen or the upper flared portion of the ureter (renal pelvis)

Penis (PE-nis) Male organ of urination and sexual intercourse

Pericardium (per-ih-KAR-de-um) Fibrous sac lined with serous membrane that encloses the heart

Perichondrium (per-ih-KON-dre-um) Layer of connective tissue that covers cartilage

Perineum (per-ih-NE-um) Pelvic floor; external region between the anus and genital organs

Periosteum (per-e-OS-te-um) Connective tissue membrane covering a bone

Peripheral (peh-RIF-er-al) Located away from a center or central structure

Peripheral nervous system (PNS) All the nerves and nervous tissue outside the central nervous system

Peristalsis (per-ih-STAL-sis) Wavelike movements in the wall of an organ or duct that propel its contents forward

Peritoneum (per-ih-to-NE-um) Serous membrane that lines the abdominal cavity and forms outer layer of abdominal organs; forms supporting ligaments for some organs

pH Symbol indicating hydrogen ion (H^+) concentration; scale that measures the relative acidity and alkalinity (basicity) of a solution

Phagocytosis (fag-o-si-TO-sis) Engulfing of large particles through the cell membrane

Pharynx (FAR-inks) Throat; passageway between the mouth and esophagus

Phlebitis (fleh-BI-tis) Inflammation of a vein

Physiology (fiz-e-OL-o-je) Study of the function of living organisms

Pia mater (PI-ah MA-ter) Innermost layer of the meninges

PID See Pelvic inflammatory disease

Pineal (PIN-e-al) Gland in the brain that is regulated by light; involved in sleep–wake cycles

Pinocytosis (pi-no-si-TO-sis) Intake of small particles and droplets by the cell membrane

Pituitary (pih-TU-ih-tar-e) **gland** Endocrine gland located under and controlled by the hypothalamus; releases hormones that control other glands; hypophysis

Placenta (plah-SEN-tah) Structure that nourishes and maintains the developing individual during pregnancy

Plasma (PLAZ-mah) Liquid portion of the blood

Plasma cell Cell that produces antibodies; derived from a B cell

Plasma membrane Outer covering of a cell; regulates what enters and leaves cell; cell membrane

Platelet (PLATE-let) Cell fragment that forms a plug to stop bleeding and acts in blood clotting; thrombocyte

Pleura (PLU-rah) Serous membrane that lines the chest cavity and covers the lungs

Plexus (PLEK-sus) Network of vessels or nerves

Pneumothorax (nu-mo-THO-raks) Accumulation of air in the pleural space

PNS See Peripheral nervous system

Polyp (POL-ip) Protruding growth, often grapelike, from a mucous membrane

Pons (ponz) Area of the brain between the midbrain and medulla; connects the cerebellum with the rest of the central nervous system

Portal system Venous system that carries blood to a second capillary bed before it returns to the heart

Posterior (pos-TE-re-or) Toward the back; dorsal

Preeclampsia (pre-eh-KLAMP-se-ah) Disorder of unknown cause that develops late in pregnancy, with hypertension, proteinuria, general edema, and sudden weight gain; if untreated, it may lead to eclampsia; toxemia of pregnancy; pregnancy-induced hypertension

Prime mover Muscle that performs a given movement; agonist

Progeny (PROJ-eh-ne) Offspring

Progesterone (pro-JES-ter-one) Hormone produced by the corpus luteum and placenta; maintains the lining of the uterus for pregnancy

Prognosis (prog-NO-sis) Prediction of the probable outcome of a disease based on the condition of the patient and knowledge about the disease

Prophylaxis (pro-fih-LAK-sis) Prevention of disease

Proprioceptor (pro-pre-o-SEP-tor) Sensory receptor that aids in judging body position and changes in position; located in muscles, tendons, and joints

Prostaglandins (pros-tah-GLAN-dinz) Group of hormones produced by many cells; these hormones have a variety of effects

Protein (PRO-tene) Organic compound made of amino acids; contains nitrogen in addition to carbon, hydrogen, and oxygen (some contain sulfur or phosphorus)

Prothrombin (pro-THROM-bin) Clotting factor; converted to thrombin during blood clotting

Proton (PRO-ton) Positively charged particle in the nucleus of an atom

Protozoon (pro-to-ZO-on) Animal-like microorganism; pl., protozoa

Proximal (PROK-sih-mal) Nearer to point of origin or to a reference point

Pulse Wave of increased pressure in the vessels produced by contraction of the heart

Pupil (PU-pil) Opening in the center of the eye through which light enters

Pyrogen (PI-ro-jen) Substance that produces fever

Radiograph (RA-de-o-graf) Image produced by passage of x-rays through the body onto sensitized film

Receptor (re-SEP-tor) Specialized cell or ending of a sensory neuron that can be excited by a stimulus; also, a site in the cell membrane to which a special substance (*e.g.*, hormone, antibody) may attach

Recessive (re-SES-iv) Referring to a gene that is not expressed if a dominant gene for the same trait is present

Reflex (RE-flex) Simple, rapid, automatic response involving few neurons

Reflex arc (ark) A pathway through the nervous system from stimulus to response; commonly involves a receptor, sensory neuron, central neuron(s), motor neuron, and effector

Refraction (re-FRAK-shun) Bending of light rays as they pass from one medium to another of a different density

Renin (RE-nin) Enzyme released from the juxtaglomerular apparatus of the kidneys that indirectly increases blood pressure by activating angiotensin

Resorption (re-SORP-shun) Loss of substance, such as that of bone or a tooth

Respiration (res-pih-RA-shun) Exchange of oxygen and carbon dioxide between the outside air and body cells

Reticuloendothelial (reh-tik-u-lo-en-do-THE-le-al) **system** Protective system consisting of highly phagocytic cells in body fluids and tissues, such as the spleen, lymph nodes, bone marrow, and liver

Retina (RET-ih-nah) Innermost layer of the eye; contains light-sensitive cells (rods and cones)

Retroperitoneal (ret-ro-per-ih-to-NE-al) Behind the peritoneum, as are the kidneys, pancreas, and abdominal aorta

Ribonucleic (RI-bo-nu-kle-ik) **acid (RNA)** Substance needed for protein manufacture in the cell

Ribosome (RI-bo-some) Small body in the cytoplasm of a cell that is a site of protein manufacture

Rickettsia (rih-KET-se-ah) Extremely small oval to rod-shaped bacterium that can grow only within a living cell

RNA See Ribonucleic acid

Roentgenogram (rent-GEN-o-gram) Image produced by means of x-rays; radiograph

Rugae (RU-je) Folds in the lining of an organ, such as the stomach or urinary bladder; sing., ruga (RU-gah)

Saliva (sah-LI-vah) Secretion of the salivary glands; moistens food and contains an enzyme that digests starch

SA node See Sinoatrial node

Sarcoma (sar-KO-mah) Malignant tumor of connective tissue; a form of cancer

Schwann cell (shvahn) Cell in the nervous system that produces the myelin sheath around peripheral axons

Sclera (SKLE-rah) Outermost layer of the eye; made of tough connective tissue; "white" of the eye

Scrotum (SKRO-tum) Sac in which testes are suspended

Sebum (SE-bum) Oily secretion that lubricates the skin; adj., sebaceous (se-BA-shus)

Semen (SE-men) Mixture of sperm cells and secretions from several glands of the male reproductive tract

Semicircular canal Bony canal in the internal ear that contains receptors for the sense of dynamic equilibrium; there are three semicircular canals in each ear

Sensory (SEN-so-re) Describing cells or activities involved in transmitting impulses toward the central nervous system; afferent

Sensory adaptation Gradual loss of sensation when sensory receptors are exposed to continuous stimulation

Sepsis (SEP-sis) Presence of pathogenic microorganisms or their toxins in the bloodstream or other tissues; adj., septic

Septicemia (sep-tih-SE-me-ah) Presence of pathogenic organisms or their toxins in the bloodstream; blood poisoning

Septum (SEP-tum) Dividing wall, as between the chambers of the heart or the nasal cavities

Serosa (se-RO-sah) Serous membrane; epithelial membrane that secretes a thin, watery fluid

Serum (SE-rum) Liquid portion of blood without clotting factors; thin, watery fluid; adj., serous (SE-rus)

Sex-linked Referring to a gene carried on a sex chromosome, usually the X chromosome

Sexually transmitted disease (STD) Disease acquired through sexual relations; venereal disease (VD)

Shock Pertaining to the circulation: inadequate output of blood by the heart

Sign Manifestation of a disease as noted by an observer

Sinoatrial (si-no-A-tre-al) **(SA) node** Tissue in the upper wall of the right atrium that sets the rate of heart contractions; pacemaker of the heart

Sinusoid (SI-nus-oyd) Enlarged capillary that serves as a blood channel

Solute (SOL-ute) Substance that is dissolved in another substance (the solvent)

Solution (so-LU-shun) Mixture, the components of which are evenly distributed

Solvent (SOL-vent) Substance in which another substance (the solute) is dissolved

Somatic nervous system The division of the nervous system that controls voluntary activities and stimulates skeletal muscle

Spermatozoon (sper-mah-to-ZO-on) Male reproductive cell or gamete; pl., spermatozoa

Sphincter (SFINK-ter) Muscular ring that regulates the size of an opening

Sphygmomanometer (sfig-mo-mah-NOM-eh-ter) Device used to measure blood pressure

Spirillum (spi-RIL-um) Corkscrew or spiral-shaped bacterium; pl., spirilla

Spirochete (SPI-ro-kete) Spiral-shaped microorganism that moves in a waving and twisting motion

Spleen Lymphoid organ in the upper left region of the abdomen

Spore Resistant form of bacterium; reproductive cell in lower plants

Staphylococcus (staf-ih-lo-KOK-us) Round bac-

terium found in a cluster resembling a bunch of grapes; pl., staphylococci (staf-ih-lo-KOK-si)

Stasis (STA-sis) Stoppage in the normal flow of fluids, such as blood, lymph, urine, or contents of the digestive tract

STD See Sexually transmitted disease

Stenosis (sten-O-sis) Narrowing of a duct or canal

Sterilization (ster-ih-li-ZA-shun) Process of killing every living microorganism on or in an object; procedure that makes an individual incapable of reproduction

Steroid (STE-royd) Category of lipids that includes the hormones of the sex glands and the adrenal cortex

Stethoscope (STETH-o-skope) Instrument for conveying sounds from the patient's body to the examiner's ears

Stimulus (STIM-u-lus) Change in the external or internal environment that produces a response

Subcutaneous (sub-ku-TA-ne-us) Under the skin

Sudoriferous (su-do-RIF-er-us) Producing sweat; referring to the sweat glands

Sulcus (SUL-kus) Shallow groove, as between convolutions of the cerebral cortex; pl., sulci (SUL-si)

Superior (su-PE-re-or) Above; in a higher position

Superior vena cava (VE-nah KA-vah) Large vein that drains the upper part of the body and empties into the right atrium of the heart

Surfactant (sur-FAK-tant) Substance in the alveoli that prevents their collapse by reducing surface tension of the fluids within

Suspension (sus-PEN-shun) Mixture that will separate unless shaken

Suture (SU-chur) Type of joint in which bone surfaces are closely united, as in the skull; stitch used in surgery to bring parts together or to stitch parts together in surgery

Sympathetic nervous system Thoracolumbar division of the autonomic nervous system

Symptom (SIMP-tom) Evidence of disease noted by the patient; such evidence noted by an examiner is called a sign or an objective symptom

Synapse (SIN-aps) Junction between two neurons or between a neuron and an effector

Synarthrosis (sin-ar-THRO-sis) Immovable joint

Syndrome (SIN-drome) Group of symptoms characteristic of a disorder

Synovial (sin-O-ve-al) Pertaining to a thick lubricating fluid found in joints, bursae, and tendon sheaths; pertaining to a freely movable (di-arthrotic) joint

System (SIS-tem) Group of organs functioning together for the same general purposes

Systemic (sis-TEM-ik) Referring to a generalized infection or condition

Systole (SIS-to-le) Contraction phase of the cardiac cycle; adj., systolic (sis-TOL-ik)

Tachycardia (tak-e-KAR-de-ah) Heart rate more than 100 beats per minute

Tachypnea (tak-IP-ne-ah) Excessive rate of respiration

Target tissue Tissue that is capable of responding to a specific hormone

T cell Lymphocyte active in immunity that matures in the thymus gland; destroys foreign cells directly; T lymphocyte

Tendinitis (ten-din-I-tis) Inflammation of a tendon

Tendon (TEN-don) Cord of fibrous connective tissue that attaches a muscle to a bone

Testis (TES-tis) Male reproductive gland; pl., testes (TES-teze)

Testosterone (tes-TOS-ter-one) Male sex hormone produced in the testes; promotes the development of sperm cells and maintains secondary sex characteristics

Tetanus (TET-an-us) Constant contraction of a muscle; infectious disease caused by a bacterium (*Clostridium tetani*); lockjaw

Tetany (TET-an-e) Muscle spasms due to abnormal calcium metabolism, as in parathyroid deficiency

Thalamus (THAL-ah-mus) Region of the brain located in the diencephalon; chief relay center for sensory impulses traveling to the cerebral cortex

Thoracentesis (thor-a-sen-TE-sis) Puncture of the chest for aspiration of fluid in the pleural space

Thorax (THO-raks) Chest; adj., thoracic (tho-RAS-ik)

Thrombocyte (THROM-bo-site) Blood platelet; cell fragment that participates in clotting

Thrombocytopenia (throm-bo-si-to-PE-ne-ah) Deficiency of platelets in the blood

Thrombosis (throm-BO-sis) Condition of having a thrombus

Thrombus (THROM-bus) Blood clot within a vessel

Thymus (THI-mus) Endocrine gland in the upper portion of the chest; stimulates development of T cells

Thyroid (THI-royd) Endocrine gland in the neck

Thyroid-stimulating hormone (TSH) Hormone produced by the anterior pituitary that stimulates the thyroid gland

Thyroxine (thi-ROK-sin) Hormone produced by the thyroid gland; increases metabolic rate and needed for normal growth; T_4

Tissue Group of similar cells that performs a specialized function

Tonsil (TON-sil) Mass of lymphoid tissue in the region of the pharynx

Tonus (TO-nus) Partially contracted state of muscle; also, tone

Toxemia (tok-SE-me-ah) General toxic condition in which poisonous bacterial substances are absorbed into the bloodstream; condition caused by abnormal metabolism

Toxin (TOK-sin) Poison

Toxoid (TOK-soyd) Altered toxin used to produce active immunity

Trachea (TRA-ke-ah) Tube that extends from the larynx to the bronchi; windpipe

Tracheostomy (tra-ke-OS-to-me) Surgical opening into the trachea for the introduction of a tube through which a person may breathe

Tract Bundle of neuron fibers within the central nervous system

Trait Characteristic

Transplantation (trans-plan-TA-shun) The grafting to a recipient of an organ or tissue from an animal or other human to replace an injured or incompetent part of the body

Trauma (TRAW-mah) Injury or wound

Tricuspid (tri-KUS-pid) **valve** Valve between the right atrium and right ventricle of the heart

Triiodothyronine (tri-i-o-do-THI-ro-nin) Thyroid hormone that functions with thyroxine to raise cellular metabolism; T_3

TSH See Thyroid-stimulating hormone

Tympanic (tim-PAN-ik) **membrane** Membrane between the external and middle ear that transmits sound waves to the bones of the middle ear; eardrum

Ulcer (UL-ser) Sore or lesion associated with death and disintegration of tissue

Umbilical (um-BIL-ih-kal) **cord** Structure that connects the fetus with the placenta; contains vessels that carry blood between the fetus and placenta

Umbilicus (um-BIL-ih-kus) Small scar on the abdomen that marks the former attachment of the umbilical cord to the fetus; navel

Urea (u-RE-ah) Nitrogen waste product excreted in the urine; end product of protein metabolism

Ureter (U-re-ter) Tube that carries urine from the kidney to the urinary bladder

Urethra (u-RE-thrah) Tube that carries urine from the urinary bladder to the outside of the body

Urinalysis (u-rin-AL-ih-sis) Laboratory examination of the physical and chemical properties of urine

Urinary bladder Hollow organ that stores urine until it is eliminated

Urine (U-rin) Liquid waste excreted by the kidneys

Uterus (U-ter-us) Muscular, pear-shaped organ in the female pelvis within which the fetus develops during pregnancy

Uvea (U-ve-ah) Middle coat of the eye, including the choroid, iris, and ciliary body; vascular and pigmented structures of the eye

Uvula (U-vu-lah) Soft, fleshy, V-shaped mass that hangs from the soft palate

Vaccine (vak-SENE) Substance used to produce active immunity; usually, a suspension of attenuated or killed pathogens given by inoculation to prevent a specific disease

Vagina (vah-JI-nah) Lower part of the birth canal that opens to the outside of the body; female organ of sexual intercourse

Valve Structure that prevents fluid from flowing backward, as in the heart, veins, and lymphatic vessels

Varicose (VAR-ih-kose) Pertaining to an enlarged and twisted vessel, as in varicose vein

Vas deferens (DEF-er-enz) Tube that carries sperm cells from the testis to the urethra; ductus deferens

Vasectomy (vah-SEK-to-me) Surgical removal of part or all of the ductus (vas) deferens; usually done on both sides to produce sterility

Vasoconstriction (vas-o-kon-STRIK-shun) Decrease in the diameter of a blood vessel

Vasodilation (vas-o-di-LA-shun) Increase in the diameter of a blood vessel

VD Venereal disease; see Sexually transmitted disease

Vector (VEK-tor) An insect or other animal that transmits a disease-causing organism from one host to another

Vein (vane) Vessel that carries blood toward the heart

Vena cava (VE-nah KA-vah) A large vein that carries blood into the right atrium of the heart; superior vena cava or inferior vena cava

Venereal (ve-NE-re-al) **disease (VD)** Disease acquired through sexual activity; sexually transmitted disease (STD)

Venous sinus (VE-nus SI-nus) Large channel that drains deoxygenated blood

Ventilation (ven-tih-LA-shun) Movement of air into and out of the lungs

Ventral (VEN-tral) Toward the front or belly surface; anterior

Ventricle (VEN-trih-kl) Cavity or chamber; one of the two lower chambers of the heart; one of the four chambers in the brain in which cerebrospinal fluid is produced; adj., ventricular (ven-TRIK-u-lar)

Venule (VEN-ule) Very small vein that collects blood from the capillaries

Vertebra (VER-teh-brah) A bone of the spinal column; pl., vertebrae (VER-teh-bre)

Vesicle (VES-ih-kl) Small sac or blister filled with fluid

Vestibule (VES-tih-bule) Part of the internal ear that contains receptors for the sense of equilibrium; any space at the entrance to a canal or organ

Vibrio (VIB-re-o) Slight curved or comma-shaped bacterium; pl., vibrios

Villi (VIL-li) Small fingerlike projections from the surface of a membrane; projections in the lining of the small intestine through which digested food is absorbed; sing., villus

Virulence (VIR-u-lens) Power of an organism to overcome defenses of the host

Virus (VI-rus) Extremely small microorganism that can reproduce only within a living cell

Viscera (VIS-er-ah) Organs in the ventral body cavities, especially the abdominal organs

Vitamin (VI-tah-min) Organic compound needed in small amounts for health

Vitreous (VIT-re-us) **body** Soft, jellylike substance that fills the eyeball and holds the shape of the eye; vitreous humor

White matter Nervous tissue composed of myelinated fibers

X-ray Ray or radiation of extremely short wavelength that can penetrate opaque substances and affect photographic plates and fluorescent screens

Zygote (ZI-gote) Fertilized ovum; cell formed by the union of a sperm and an egg

Medical Terminology

Medical terminology, the special language of the health occupations, is based on an understanding of a relatively few basic elements. These elements—roots, prefixes, and suffixes—form the foundation of almost all medical terms. A useful way to familiarize yourself with each term is to learn to pronounce it correctly and say it aloud several times. Soon it will become an integral part of your vocabulary.

The foundation of a word is the word root. Examples of word roots are *abdomin-,* referring to the belly region; and *aden-,* pertaining to a gland. A word root is often followed by a vowel to facilitate pronunciation, as in *abdomino-* and *adeno-.* We then refer to it as a "combining form." The hyphen appended to a combining form indicates that it is not a complete word; if the hyphen precedes the combining form, then it commonly appears as the terminal element of the word, as in *-algia,* meaning "a painful condition."

A prefix is a part of a word that precedes the word root and changes its meaning. For example, the prefix *mal-* in *malunion* means "abnormal." A suffix, or word ending, is a part that follows the word root and adds to or changes its meaning. The suffix *-rhea* means "profuse flow" or "discharge," as in *diarrhea,* a condition characterized by excessive discharge of liquid stools.

Many medical words are compound words; that is, they are made up of more than one root or combining form. Examples of such compound words are *erythrocyte* (red blood cell) and *hydrocele* (fluid-containing sac), and many more difficult words, such as *sternoclavicular* (indicating relations to both the sternum and the clavicle).

A general knowledge of language structure and spelling rules is also helpful in mastering medical terminology. For example, adjectives include words that end in *-al,* as in *sternal* (the noun is *sternum*), and words that end in *-ous,* as in *mucous* (the noun is *mucus*).

The following list includes some of the most commonly used word roots, combining forms, prefixes, and suffixes, as well as examples of their use.

a-, an- absent, deficient, lack of: *atrophy, anemia, anuria*

ab- away from: *abduction, aboral*

abdomin-, abdomino- belly or abdominal area: *abdominocentesis, abdominoscopy*

acou- hearing, sound: *acoustic*

acr-, acro- extreme ends of a part, especially of the extremities: *acromegaly, acromion*

actin-, actini-, actino- relation to raylike structures or, more commonly, to light or roentgen (x-) rays, or some other type of radiation: *actiniform, actinodermatitis*

ad- (sometimes converted to *ac-, af-, ag-, ap-, as-, at-,*) toward, added to, near: *adrenal, accretion, agglomerated, afferent*

aden-, adeno, gland: *adenectomy, adenitis, adenocarcinoma*

-agogue inducing, leading, stimulating: *cholagogue, galactagogue*

alge-, algo-, algesi- pain: *algetic, algophobia, analgesic*

-algia pain, painful condition: *myalgia, neuralgia*

amb-, ambi-, ambo- both, on two sides: *ambidexterity, ambivalent*

ambly- dimness, dullness: *amblyopia*

angio- vessel: *angiogram, angiotensin*

ant-, anti- against; to prevent, suppress, or destroy: *antarthritic, antibiotic, anticoagulant*

ante-   before, ahead of: *antenatal, antepartum*

antero-   position ahead of or in front of (*i.e.,* anterior to) another part: *anterolateral, anteroventral*

arthr-, arthro-   joint or articulation: *arthrolysis, arthrostomy, arthritis*

-ase   enzyme: *lipase, protease*

-asis   *see* -sis.

audio-   sound, hearing: *audiogenic, audiometry, audiovisual*

aur-   ear: *aural, auricle*

aut-, auto-   self: *autistic, autodigestion, autoimmune*

bi-   two, twice: *bifurcate, bisexual*

bio-   life, living organism: *biopsy, antibiotic*

blast-, blasto-, -blast   early stage, immature cell or bud: *blastula, blastophore, erythroblast*

bleph-, blephar-, blepharo-   eyelid, eyelash: *blepharism, blepharitis, blepharospasm*

brachi-   arm: *brachial, brachiocephalic, brachiotomy*

brachy-   short: *brachydactylia, brachyesophagus*

brady-   slow: *bradycardia*

bronch-, broncho-, bronchi-   windpipe or other air tubes: *bronchiectasis, bronchoscope*

bucc-   cheek: *buccal*

carcin-   cancer: *carcinogenic, carcinoma*

cardi-, cardia-, cardio-   heart: *carditis, cardiac, cardiologist*

-cele   swelling; enlarged space or cavity: *cystocele, meningocele, rectocele*

centi-   relating to 100 (used in naming units of measurements): *centigrade, centimeter*

-centesis   perforation, tapping: *aminocentesis, paracentesis*

cephal-, cephalo-   head: *cephalalgia, cephalopelvic*

cerebro-   brain: *cerobrospinal, cerebrum*

cervi-   neck: *cervical, cervix*

cheil-, cheilo-,   lips; brim or edge: *cheilitis, cheilosis*

cheir-, cheiro-   (also written **chir-, chiro-**) hand: *cheiralgia, cheiromegaly, chiropractic*

chol-, chole-, cholo-   bile, gall: *chologogue, cholecyst, cholecystitis, cholecystokinin*

chondr-, chondri-, chondrio-   cartilage: *chondric, chondrocyte, chondroma*

-cid, -cide   to cut, kill or destroy: *bactericidal, germicide, suicide*

circum-   around, surrounding: *circumorbital, circumrenal, circumduction*

-clast   break: *osteoclast*

colp-, colpo-   vagina: *colpectasia, colposcope, colpotomy*

contra-   opposed, against: *contraindication, contralateral*

cost-, costa-, costo-   ribs: *intercostal, costosternal*

counter-   against, opposite to: *counteract, counterirritation, countertraction*

crani-, cranio-   skull: *cranium, craniotomy*

cry-, cryo-   cold: *cryalgesia, cryogenic, cryotherapy*

crypt-, crypto-   hidden, concealed: *cryptic, cryptogenic, cryptorchidism*

cut-   skin: *subcutaneous*

cysti-, cysto-   sac, bladder: *cystitis, cystoscope*

cyt-, cyto-, -cyte   cell: *cytology, cytoplasm, osteocyte*

dactyl-, dactylo-   digits (usually fingers, but sometimes toes): *dactylitis, polydactyly*

de-   remove: *detoxify, dehydration*

dendr-   tree: *dendrite*

dento-, dent-, denti-   tooth: *dentition, dentin, dentifrice*

derm-, derma-, dermo-, dermat-, dermato-   skin: *dermatitis, dermatology, dermatosis*

di-, diplo-   twice, double: *dimorphism, diplopia*

dia-   through, between, across, apart: *diaphragm, diaphysis*

dis-   apart, away from: *disarticulation, distal*

dors-, dorsi-, dorso-   back (in the human, this combining form refers to the same regions as postero-): *dorsal, dorsiflexion, dorsonuchal*

-dynia   pain, tenderness: *myodynia, neurodynia*

dys-   disordered, difficult, painful: *dysentery, dysphagia, dyspnea*

-ectasis   expansion, dilation, stretching: *angiectasis, bronchiectasis*

ecto-   outside, external: *ectoderm, ectogenous*

-ectomy   surgical removal or destruction by other means: *appendectomy, thyroidectomy*

edem-   swelling: *edema*

-emia   blood: *glycemia, hyperemia*

encephal-, encephalo-   brain: *encephalitis, encephalogram*

end-, endo-   within, innermost: *endarterial, endocardium, endothelium*

enter-, entero-   intestine: *enteritis, enterocolitis*

epi-   on, upon: *epicardium, epidermis*

eryth-, erythro-   red: *erythema, erythrocyte*

-esthesia   sensation: *anesthesia, paresthesia*

eu-   well, normal, good: *euphoria, eupnea*

ex-, exo-   outside, out of, away from: *excretion, exocrine, exophthalmic*

extra-   beyond, outside of, in addition to: *extracellular, extrasystole, extravasation*

fasci- fibrous connective tissue layers: *fascia, fascitis, fascicle*

-ferent to bear, to carry: *afferent, efferent*

fibr-, fibro- threadlike structures, fibers: *fibrillation, fibroblast, fibrositis*

galact-, galacta-, galacto- milk: *galactemia, galactagogue, galactocele*

gastr-, gastro- stomach: *gastritis, gastroenterostomy*

-gen an agent that produces or originates: *allergen, pathogen, fibrinogen*

-genic produced from, producing: *neurogenic, pyogenic, psychogenic*

genito- organs of reproduction: *genitoplasty, genitourinary*

gen-, geno- a relationship to reproduction or sex: *genealogy, generate, genetic, genotype*

-geny manner of origin, development or production: *ontogeny, progeny*

glio-, glia gluey material; specifically, the connective tissue of the central nervous system: *glioma, neuroglia*

gloss-, glosso- tongue: *glossitis, glossopharyngeal*

gly-, glyco- sweet, relating to sugar: *glycemia, glycosuria*

gnath, gnatho- related to the jaw: *prognathic, gnathoplasty*

gon- seed, knee: *gonad, gonarthritis*

-gram record, that which is recorded: *electrocardiogram, electroencephalogram*

-graph instrument for recording: *electrocardiograph, electroencephalograph*

gyn-, gyne-, gyneco-, gyno- female, woman: *gynecology, gynecomastia, gynoplasty*

hem-, hema-, hemato-, hemo- blood: *hematoma, hematuria, hemorrhage*

hemi- one half: *hemisphere, heminephrectomy, hemiplegia*

hepat-, hepato- liver: *hepatitis, hepatogenous*

heter-, hetero- other, different: *heterogenous, heterosexual, heterochromia*

hist-, histo-, histio- tissue: *histology, histiocyte*

homeo-, homo- unchanging, the same: *hemeostasis, homosexual*

hydr-, hydro- water: *hydrolysis, hydrocephalus*

hyper- above, over, excessive: *hyperesthesia, hyperglycemia, hypertrophy*

hypo- deficient, below, beneath: *hypochondrium, hypodermic, hypogastrium*

hyster-, hystero- uterus: *hysterectomy*

-ia state of: *myopia, hypochondria, ischemia*

-iatrics, -trics medical specialty: *pediatrics, obstetrics*

idio- self, one's own, separate, distinct: *idiopathic, idiosyncrasy*

im-, in- in, into, lacking: *implantation, inanimate, infiltration*

infra- below: *infraspinous, infracortical*

inter- between: *intercostal, interstitial*

intra- within a part or structure: *intracranial, intracellular, intraocular*

-ism state of: *alcoholism, hyperthyroidism*

iso- equal: *isotonic, isometric*

-itis inflammation: *dermatitis, keratitis, neuritis*

juxta- next to: *juxtaglomerular*

karyo- nucleus: *karyotype, karyoplasm*

kerat-, kerato- cornea of the eye, certain horny tissues: *keratin, keratitis, keratoplasty*

lacri- tear: *lacrimal*

lact-, lacto- milk: *lactation, lactogenic*

later- side: *lateral*

leuk-, leuko- (also written as *leuc-, leuco-*) white: *leukocyte, leukoplakia*

lig- bind: *ligament, ligature*

lith-, litho- stones (calculi): *lithiasis, lithotripsy*

-logy, -ology study of: *physiology, gynecology*

lyso-, -lysis flowing, loosening, dissolution (dissolving of): *hemolysis, paralysis, lysosome*

macro- large, abnormal length: *macrophage, macroblast.* See also **-mega, megalo-**

mal- disordered, abnormal: *malnutrition, malocclusion, malunion*

malac-, malaco-, -malacia softening: *malacoma, osteomalacia*

mast-, masto- breast: *mastectomy, mastitis*

meg-, mega-, megal-, megalo- unusually or excessively large: *megacolon, megaloblast, megakaryocyte*

men-, meno- physiologic uterine bleeding: *menses, menorrhagia, menopause*

mening-, meningo- membranes covering the brain and spinal cord: *meningitis, meningocele*

mes-, mesa-, meso- middle, midline: *mesencephalon, mesoderm*

meta- change, beyond, after, over, near: *metabolism, metacarpal, metaplasia*

-meter measure: *hemocytometer, sphygmomanometer, spirometer*

metr-, metro-   uterus: *endometrium, metroptosis, metrorrhagia*

micro-   very small: *microscope, microbiology, microsurgery, micrometer*

mono-   single: *monocyte, mononucleosis*

my-, myo-   muscle: *myenteron, myocardium, myometrium*

myc-, mycet-, myco-   fungi: *mycid, mycete, mycology, mycosis, mycelium*

myel-, myelo-   marrow (often used in reference to the spinal cord): *myeloid, myeloblast, osteomyelitis, poliomyelitis*

necr-, necro-   death, corpse: *necrosis*

neo-   new: *neoplasm, neonatal*

neph-, nephro-   kidney: *nephrectomy, nephron*

neur-, neuro-   nerve: *neuron, neuralgia, neuroma*

noct-, nocti-   night: *noctambulation, nocturia, noctiphobia*

nos-, noso-   disease: *nosocomial, nosophobia*

ocul-, oculo-   eye: *oculist, oculomotor, oculomycosis*

odont-, odonto-   tooth, teeth: *odontalgia, orthodontics*

-oid   likeness, resemblance: *lymphoid, myeloid*

olig-, oligo-   few, a deficiency: *oligospermia, oliguria*

-oma   tumor, swelling: *hematoma, sarcoma*

onych-, onycho-   nails: *paronychia, onychoma*

oo-, ovi, ovo-   ovum, egg: *oocyte, oviduct, ovoplasm* (do not confuse with **oophor-**)

oophor-, oophoro-   ovary: *oophorectomy, oophoritis, oophorocystectomy.* See also **ovar-**

ophthalm-, ophthalmo-   eye: *ophthalmia, ophthalmologist, ophthalmoscope*

orth-, ortho-   straight, normal: *orthopedics, orthopnea, orthosis*

oscillo-   to swing to and fro: *oscilloscope*

oss-, osseo-, ossi-, oste-, osteo-   bone, bone tissue: *osseous, ossicle, osteocyte, osteomyelitis*

-ostomy   creation of a mouth or opening by surgery: *colostomy, tracheostomy*

ot-, oto-   ear: *otalgia, otitis, otomycosis*

-otomy   cutting into: *phlebotomy, tracheotomy*

ovar-, ovario-   ovary: *ovariectomy.* See also **oophor-**

ox-, -oxia   pertaining to oxygen: *hypoxemia, hypoxia, anoxia*

para-   near, beyond, apart from, beside: *paramedical, parametrium, parathyroid, parasagittal*

path-, patho-, -pathy   disease, abnormal condition: *pathogen, pathognomonic, pathology, neuropathy*

ped-, pedia-   child, foot: *pedialgia, pedophobia, pediatrician*

-penia   lack of: *leukopenia, thrombocytopenia*

per-   through, excessively: *percutaneous, perfusion*

peri-   around: *pericardium, perichondrium*

-pexy   fixation: *nephropexy, proctopexy*

phag-, phago-   to eat, to ingest: *phage, phagocyte*

-phagia, phagy   eating, swallowing: *aphagia, dysphagia*

-phasia   speech, ability to talk: *phasia, dysphasia*

-phil, -philic   to be fond of, to like (have an affinity for): *eosinophilia, hemophilia, hydrophilic*

phleb-, phlebo-   vein: *phlebitis, phlebotomy*

phob-, -phobia   *fear, dread, abnormal aversion:* phobic, acrophibia, hydrophobia

phot-, photo-   light: *photoreceptor, photophobia*

pile-, pili-, pilo-   hair, resembling hair: *pileous, piliation, pilonidal*

-plasty   molding, surgical formation: *cystoplasty, gastroplasty, kineplasty*

pleur-, pleuro-   side, rib, serous membrane covering the lung and lining the chest cavity: *pleurisy, pleurotomy*

-pnea   air, breathing: *dyspnea, eupnea*

pneum-, pneuma-, pneumo-, pneumon-, pneumato-   lung, air: *pneumectomy, pneumograph, pneumonia*

pod-, podo-   foot: *podiatry, pododynia*

-poiesis   making, forming: *erythropoiesis, hematopoiesis*

polio-   gray: *polioencephalitis, poliomyelitis*

poly-   many: *polyarthritis, polycystic, polycythemia*

post-   behind, after, following: *postnatal, postocular, postpartum*

pre-   before, ahead of: *precancerous, preclinical, prenatal*

presby-   old age: *presbycusis, presbyopia*

pro-   in front of, before: *prodromal, prosencephalon, prolapse, prothrombin*

proct-, procto-   rectum: *proctitis, proctocele, proctologist*

pseud-, pseudo-   false: *pseudoarthrosis, pseudostratified, pseudopod*

psych-, psycho-   mind: *psychosomatic, psychotherapy*

-ptosis   downward displacement, falling, prolapse: *blepharoptosis, enteroptosis, nephroptosis*

pulmo-, pulmono-   lung: *pulmonic, pulmonology*

py-, pyo-   pus: *pyuria, pyogenic, pyorrhea*

pyel-, pyelo-   kidney pelvis: *pyelitis, pyelogram, pyelonephrosis*

rachi-, rachio-   spine: *rachicentesis, rachischis*

radio- emission of rays or radiation: *radioactive, radiography, radiology*

re- again, back: *reabsorption, reaction, regenerate*

ren- kidney: *renal, renopathy*

retro- backward, located behind: *retrocecal, retroperitoneal*

rhin-, rhino- nose: *rhinitis, rhinoplasty*

-rhage, -rhagia* excessive flow: *hemorrhage, menorrhagia*

-rhaphy* suturing of or sewing up of a gap or defect in a part: *herniorrhaphy, gastrorrhaphy, cystorrhaphy*

-rhea* flow, discharge: *diarrhea, gonorrhea, seborrhea*

salping-, salpingo- tube: *salpingitis, salpingoscopy*

scler-, sclero- hardness; *scleroderma, sclerosis*

scolio- twisted, crooked: *scoliosis, scoliosometer*

-scope instrument used to look into or examine a part: *bronchoscope, endoscope, arthroscope*

semi- mild, partial, half: *semipermeable, semicoma*

sep-, septic- poison, rot, decay: *sepsis, septicemia*

-sis condition or process, usually abnormal: *dermatosis, osteoporosis*

somat-, somato- body: *somatic, somatotype*

sono- sound: *sonogram, sonography*

splanchn-, splanchno- internal organs: *splanchnic, splanchnoptosis*

sta-, stat- stop, stand still, remain at rest: *stasis, static, homeostasis*

sten-, steno- contracted, narrowed: *stenosis*

sthen-, stheno-, -sthenia, -sthenic strength: *asthenic, calisthenics, neurasthenia*

stomato- mouth: *stomatitis*

-stomy surgical creation of an opening into a hollow organ or an opening between two organs: *colostomy, tracheostomy, gastroenterostomy*

sub- under, below, near, almost: *subclavian, subcutaneous, subluxation*

super- over, above, excessive: *superego, supernatant, superficial*

supra- location above or over: *supranasal, suprarenal*

sym-, syn- with, together: *symphysis, synapse*

syring-, syringo- fistula, tube, cavity: *syringectomy, syringomyelia*

tacho-, tachy- rapid, fast, swift: *tachycardia, tachypnea*

tars-, tarso- eyelid, foot: *tarsitis, tarsoplasty, tarsoptosis*

-taxia, -taxis order, arrangement: *ataxia, chemotaxis, thermotaxis*

tens- stretch, pull: *extension, tensor*

therm-, thermo-, -thermy heat: *thermalgesia, thermocautery, diathermy, thermometer*

-tomy incision of, cutting: *anatomy, phlebotomy, laparotomy*

tox-, toxic-, toxico- poison: *toxemia, toxicology, toxicosis*

trache-, tracheo- trachea, windpipe: *tracheal, tracheitis, tracheotomy*

trans- across, through, beyond: *transorbital, transpiration, transplant, transport*

tri- three: *triad, triceps*

trich-, tricho- hair: *trichiasis, trichosis, trichology*

-trophic, -trophy nutrition (nurture): *atrophic, hypertrophy*

-tropic turning around, influencing, changing: *corticotropic, gonadotropic, thyrotropic*

ultra- beyond or excessive: *ultrasound, ultraviolent, ultrastructure*

uni- one: *unilateral, uniovular, unicellular*

-uria urine: *glycosuria, hematuria, pyuria*

vas-, vaso- vessel, duct: *vascular, vasectomy, vasodilation*

viscer-, viscero- internal organs, viscera: *visceral, visceroptosis*

xero- dryness: *xeroderma, xerophthalmia, xerosis*

---

*When a suffix beginning with *rh* is added to a word root, the *r* is doubled.

Appendices

Appendix 1. Metric Measurements

UNIT	ABBREVIATION	METRIC EQUIVALENT	U.S. EQUIVALENT
Units of length			
Kilometer	km	1000 meters	0.62 miles; 1.6 km/mile
Meter*	m	100 cm; 1000 mm	39.4 inches, 1.1 yards
Centimeter	cm	$\frac{1}{100}$ m; 0.01 m	0.39 inches; 2.5 cm/inch
Millimeter	mm	$\frac{1}{1000}$ m; 0.001 m	0.039 inches; 25 mm/inch
Micrometer	μm	$\frac{1}{1000}$ mm; 0.001 mm	
Units of weight			
Kilogram	kg	1000 g	2.2 lb
Gram*	g	1000 mg	0.035 oz.; 28.5 g/oz
Milligram	mg	$\frac{1}{1000}$ g; 0.001 g	
Microgram	μg	$\frac{1}{1000}$ mg; 0.001 mg	
Units of volume			
Liter*	L	1000 mL	1.06 qt
Deciliter	dL	$\frac{1}{10}$ L; 0.1 L	
Milliliter	mL	$\frac{1}{1000}$ L; 0.001 L	0.034 oz., 29.4 mL/oz
Microliter	μL	$\frac{1}{1000}$ mL; 0.001 mL	

*Basic unit.

Appendix 2. Celsius–Fahrenheit Temperature Conversion Scale

CELSIUS TO FAHRENHEIT

Use the following formula to convert Celsius readings to Fahrenheit readings:

°F = 9/5°C + 32

For example, if the Celsius reading is 37°

°F = (9/5 × 37) + 32
= 66.6 + 32
= 98.6°F (normal body temperature)

FAHRENHEIT TO CELSIUS

Use the following formula to convert Fahrenheit readings to Celsius readings:

°C = 5/9 (°F − 32)

For example, if the Fahrenheit reading is 68°:

°C = 5/9 (68 − 32)
= 5/9 × 36
= 20°C (a nice spring day)

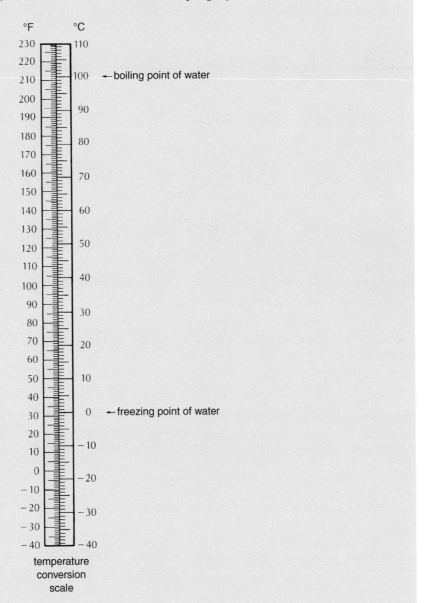

temperature
conversion
scale

Appendix 3. Laboratory Tests

Table 1   Routine Urinalysis

TEST	NORMAL VALUE	CLINICAL SIGNIFICANCE
General characteristics and measurements		
Color	Pale yellow to amber	Color change can be due to concentration or dilution, drugs, metabolic or inflammatory disorders
Odor	Slightly aromatic	Foul odor typical of urinary tract infection, fruity odor in uncontrolled diabetes mellitus
Appearance (clarity)	Clear to slightly hazy	Cloudy urine occurs with infection or after refrigeration; may indicate presence of bacteria, cells, mucus, or crystals
Specific gravity	1.003–1.030 (first morning catch; routine is random)	Decreased in diabetes insipidus, acute renal failure, water intoxication; increased in liver disorders, heart failure, dehydration
pH	4.5–8.0	Acid urine accompanies acidosis, fever, high protein diet; alkaline urine in urinary tract infection, metabolic alkalosis, vegetarian diet
Chemical determinations		
Glucose	Negative	Glucose present in uncontrolled diabetes mellitus, steroid excess
Ketones	Negative	Present in diabetes mellitus and in starvation
Protein	Negative	Present in kidney disorders, such as glomerulonephritis, acute kidney failure
Bilirubin	Negative	Breakdown product of hemoglobin; present in liver disease or in bile blockage
Urobilinogen	0.2–1.0 Ehrlich units /dL	Breakdown product of bilirubin; increased in hemolytic anemias and in liver disease; remains negative in bile obstruction
Blood (occult)	Negative	Detects small amounts of blood cells, hemoglobin, or myoglobin; present in severe trauma, metabolic disorders, bladder infections
Nitrite	Negative	Product of bacterial breakdown of urine; positive result suggests urinary tract infection and needs to be followed up with a culture of the urine
Microscopic		
Red blood cells	0–3 per high-power field	Increased because of bleeding within the urinary tract from trauma, tumors, inflammation, or damage within the kidney
White blood cells	0–4 per high-power field	Increased in infection of the kidney or bladder
Renal epithelial cells	Occasional	Increased number indicates damage to kidney tubules
Casts	None	Hyaline casts normal; large number of abnormal casts indicates inflammation or a systemic disorder
Crystals	Present	Most are normal; may be acid or alkaline
Bacteria	Few	Increased in infection of urinary tract or contamination from infected genitalia
Others		Any yeasts, parasites, mucus, spermatozoa, or other microscopic findings would be reported here

Table 2 Complete Blood Count (CBC)

TEST	NORMAL VALUE*	CLINICAL SIGNIFICANCE
Red blood cell (RBC) count	Men: 4.2–5.4 million/μL Women: 3.6–5.0 million/μL	Decreased in anemia; increased in dehydration, polycythemia
Hemoglobin (Hb)	Men: 13.5–17.5 g/dL Women: 12–16 g/dL	Decreased in anemia, hemorrhage, and hemolytic reactions; increased in dehydration, heart and lung disease
Hematocrit (Hct) or packed cell volume (PCV)	Men: 40%–50% Women: 37%–47%	Decreased in anemia; increased in polycythemia, dehydration
Red blood cell (RBC) indices (examples)		These values, calculated from the RBC count, HGB, and HCT, give information valuable in the diagnosis and classification of anemia
Mean corpuscular volume (MCV)	87–103 μL/red cell	Measures the average size or volume of each RBC: small size (microcytic) in iron-deficiency anemia; large size (macrocytic) typical of pernicious anemia
Mean corpuscular hemoglobin (MCH)	26–34 pg/red cell	Measures the weight of hemoglobin per RBC; useful in differentiating types of anemia in a severely anemic patient
Mean corpuscular hemoglobin concentration (MCHC)	31–37 g/dL	Defines the volume of hemoglobin per RBC; used to determine the color or concentration of hemoglobin per RBC
White blood cell (WBC) count	5,000–10,000/μL	Increased in leukemia and in response to infection, inflammation, and dehydration; decreased in bone marrow suppression
Platelets	150,000–350,000/μL	Increased in many malignant disorders; decreased in disseminated intravascular coagulation (DIC) or toxic drug effects; spontaneous bleeding may occur at platelet counts below 20,000 μL
Differential (Peripheral blood smear)		A stained slide of the blood is needed to perform the differential. The percentages of the different WBCs are estimated, and the slide is microscopically checked for abnormal characteristics in WBCs, RBCs, and platelets.
WBCs		
Segmented neutrophils (SEGs, POLYs)	40%–74%	Increased in bacterial infections; low numbers leave person very susceptible to infection
Immature neutrophils (BANDs)	0%–3%	Increased when neutrophil count increases
Lymphocytes (LYMPHs)	20%–40%	Increased in viral infections; low numbers leave person dangerously susceptible to infection
Monocytes (MONOs)	2%–6%	Increased in specific infections
Eosinophils (EOs)	1%–4%	Increased in allergic disorders
Basophils (BASOs)	0.5%–1%	Increased in allergic disorders

*Values vary depending on instrumentation and type of test.

Table 3 Blood Chemistry Tests

TEST	NORMAL VALUE	CLINICAL SIGNIFICANCE
Basic panel: An overview of electrolytes, waste product management, and metabolism		
Blood urea nitrogen (BUN)	7–18 mg/dL	Increased in renal disease and dehydration; decreased in liver damage and malnutrition
Carbon dioxide (CO_2) (includes bicarbonate)	23–30 mmol/L	Useful to evaluate acid–base balance by measuring total carbon dioxide in the blood: Elevated in vomiting and pulmonary disease; decreased in diabetic acidosis, acute renal failure, and hyperventilation
Chloride (Cl)	98–106 mEq/L	Increased in dehydration, hyperventilation, and congestive heart failure; decreased in vomiting, diarrhea, and fever
Creatinine	0.6–1.2 mg/dL	Produced at a constant rate and excreted by the kidney; increased in kidney disease
Glucose	Fasting: 70–110 mg/dL Random: 85–125 mg/dL	Increased in diabetes and severe illness; decreased in insulin overdose or hypoglycemia
Potassium (K)	3.5–5 mEq/L	Increased in renal failure, extensive cell damage, and acidosis; decreased in vomiting, diarrhea, and excess administration of diuretics or IV fluids
Sodium (Na)	101–111 mEq/L or 135–148 mEq/L (depending on test)	Increased in dehydration and diabetes insipidus; decreased in overload of IV fluids, burns, diarrhea, or vomiting
Additional blood chemistry tests		
Alanine aminotransferase (ALT)	10–40 U/L	Used to diagnose and monitor treatment of liver disease and to monitor the effects of drugs on the liver; increased in myocardia infarction
Albumin	3.8–5.0 g/dL	Albumin holds water in blood; decreased in liver disease and kidney disease
Albumin–globulin ratio (A/G ratio)	Greater than 1	Low A/G ratio signifies a tendency for edema because globulin is less effective than albumin at holding water in the blood
Alkaline phosphatase (ALP)	20–70 U/L (varies by method)	Enzyme of bone metabolism; increased in liver disease and metastatic bone disease
Amylase	21–160 U/L	Used to diagnose and monitor treatment of acute pancreatitis and to detect inflammation of the salivary glands
Aspartate aminotransferase (AST)	0–41 U/L (varies)	Enzyme present in tissues with high metabolic activity; increased in myocardial infarction and liver disease
Bilirubin, total	0.2–1.0 mg/dL	Breakdown product of hemoglobin from red blood cells; increased when excessive red blood cells are being destroyed or in liver disease
Calcium (Ca)	8.8–10.0 mg/dL	Increased in excess parathyroid hormone production and in cancer; decreased in alkalosis, elevated phosphate in renal failure, and excess IV fluids
Cholesterol	120–220 mg/dL desirable range	Screening test used to evaluate risk of heart disease; levels of 200 mg/dL or above indicate increased risk of heart disease and warrant further investigation
Creatine phosphokinase (CPK or CK)	Men: 38–174 U/L Women: 96–140 U/L	Elevated enzyme level indicates myocardial infarction or damage to skeletal muscle. When elevated, specific fractions (isoenzymes) are tested for
Gamma-glutamyl transferase (GGT)	Men: 6–26 U/L Women: 4–18 U/L	Used to diagnose liver disease and to test for chronic alcoholism
Globulins	2.3–3.5 g/dL	Proteins active in immunity; help albumin keep water in blood
Iron, serum (Fe)	Men: 75–175 µg/dL Women: 65–165 µg/dL	Decreased in iron deficiency and anemia; increased in hemolytic conditions
High-density lipoproteins (HDLs)	Men: 30–70 mg/dL Women: 30–85 mg/dL	Used to evaluate the risk of heart disease
Lactic dehydrogenase (LDH or LD)	95–200 U/L (Normal ranges vary greatly)	Enzyme released in many kinds of tissue damage, including myocardial infarction, pulmonary infarction, and liver disease
Lipase	4–24 U/L (varies with test)	Enzyme used to diagnose pancreatitis
Low-density lipoproteins (LDLs)	80–140 mg/dL	Used to evaluate the risk of heart disease

(continued)

Table 3 (continued)		
TEST	NORMAL VALUE	CLINICAL SIGNIFICANCE
Magnesium (Mg)	1.3–2.1 mEq/L	Vital in neuromuscular function; decreased levels may occur in malnutrition, alcoholism, pancreatitis, diarrhea
Phosphorus (P) (inorganic)	2.7–4.5 mg/dL	Evaluated in response to calcium; main store is in bone: elevated in kidney disease; decreased in excess parathyroid hormone
Protein, total	6–8 g/dL	Increased in dehydration, multiple myeloma; decreased in kidney disease, liver disease, poor nutrition, severe burns, excessive bleeding
Serum glutamic oxalacetic transaminase (SGOT)		See Aspartate aminotransferase (AST)
Serum glutamic pyruvic transaminase (SGPT)		See Alanine aminotransferase (ALT)
Thyroxin (T_4)	5–12.5 μg/dL (varies)	Screening test of thyroid function; increased in hyperthyroidism; decreased in myxedema and hypothyroidism
Thyroid-stimulating hormone (TSH)	0.5–6 mIU/L	Produced by pituitary to cause thyroid gland to function; elevated when thyroid gland is not functioning
Triiodothyronine (T_3)	120–195 mg/dL	Elevated in specific types of hyperthyroidism
Triglycerides	Men: 40–160 mg/dL Women: 35–135 mg/dL	An indication of ability to metabolize fats; increased triglycerides and cholesterol indicate high risk of atherosclerosis
Uric acid	Men: 3.5–7.2 mg/dL Women: 2.6–6.0 mg/dL	Produced by breakdown of ingested purines in food and nucleic acids; elevated in kidney disease, gout, and leukemia

Appendix 4. Typical Disease Conditions and Causative Organisms

Table 1 Bacterial Diseases

ORGANISM	DISEASE AND DESCRIPTION
Cocci	
Neisseria gonorrhoeae (gonococcus)	Gonorrhea. Acute inflammation of mucous membranes of the reproductive and urinary tracts (with possible spread to the peritoneum in the female). Systemic infection may cause gonococcal arthritis and endocarditis. Organism also causes ophthalmia neonatorum, an eye inflammation of the newborn.
Neisseria meningitidis (meningococcus)	Epidemic meningitis. Inflammation of the membranes covering brain and spinal cord. A vaccine is available for use in high-risk populations.
Staphylococcus aureus and other staphylococci	Boils, carbuncles, impetigo, osteomyelitis, staphylococcal pneumonia, cystitis, pyelonephritis, empyema, septicemia, toxic shock, and food poisoning. Strains resistant to antibiotics are a cause of infections originating in the hospital, such as wound infections.
Streptococcus pneumoniae (*Diplococcus pneumoniae*)	Pneumonia; inflammation of the alveoli, bronchioles, and bronchi; middle ear infections; meningitis. May be prevented by use of polyvalent pneumococcal vaccine.
Streptococcus pyogenes, Streptococcus hemolyticus, and other streptococci	Septicemia, septic sore throat, scarlet fever, puerperal sepsis, erysipelas, streptococcal pneumonia, rheumatic fever, subacute bacterial endocarditis, acute glomerulonephritis
Bacilli	
Bordetella pertussis	Persussis (whooping cough). Severe infection of the trachea and bronchi. The "whoop" is caused by the effort to recover breath after coughing. All children should be immunized against pertussis.
Brucella abortus (and others)	Brucellosis, or undulant fever. Disease of animals such as cattle and goats transmitted to humans through unpasteurized dairy products or undercooked meat. Acute phase of fever and weight loss; chronic disease with abscess formation and depression
Clostridium botulinum	Botulism. Very severe poisoning caused by eating food in which the organism has been allowed to grow and excrete its toxin. Causes muscle paralysis and may result in death from asphyxiation. Infant botulism results from ingestion of spores. It causes respiratory problems and flaccid paralysis, which usually respond to treatment.
Clostridium perfringens	Gas gangrene. Acute wound infection. Organisms cause death of tissues accompanied by the generation of gas within them.
Clostridium tetani	Tetanus. Acute, often fatal poisoning caused by introduction of the organism into deep wounds. Characterized by severe muscular spasms. Also called *lockjaw*.
Corynebacterium diphtheriae	Diphtheria. Acute inflammation of the throat with the formation of a leathery membranelike growth (pseudomembrane) that can obstruct air passages and cause death by asphyxiation. Toxin produced by this organism can damage heart, nerves, kidneys, and other organs. Disease preventable by appropriate vaccination.
Escherichia coli, Proteus *spp.,* and other colon bacilli	Normal inhabitants of the colon, and usually harmless there. Cause of local and systemic infections, food poisoning, diarrhea (especially in children), septicemia, and septic shock. *E. coli* is a common hospital-acquired infection.
Francisella tularensis	Tularemia, or deer fly fever. Transmitted by contact with an infected animal or bite of a tick or fly. Symptoms are fever, ulceration of the skin, and enlarged lymph nodes.
Haemophilus influenzae type b (Hib)	Severe infections in children under 3 years of age. Causes meningitis, also epiglottitis, septicemia, pneumonia, pericarditis, and septic arthritis. Preschool vaccinations are routine.
Helicobacter pylori	Acute inflammation of the stomach (gastritis), ulcers of the pyloric area of the stomach and of the duodenum.
Legionella pneumophila	Legionnaires' disease (pneumonia). Seen in localized epidemics, may be transmitted by air conditioning towers and by contaminated soil at excavation sites. Not spread person to person. Characterized by high fever, vomiting, diarrhea, cough, and bradycardia. Mild form of the disease called *Pontiac fever*.
Mycobacterium leprae (Hansen's bacillus)	Leprosy. Chronic illness in which hard swellings occur under the skin, particularly of the face, causing a grotesque appearance. In one form of leprosy, the nerves are affected, resulting in loss of sensation in the extremities.

(continued)

Table 1   (continued)

ORGANISM	DISEASE AND DESCRIPTION
Mycobacterium tuberculosis (tubercle bacillus)	Tuberculosis. Infectious disease in which the organism causes primary lesions called *tubercles*. These break down into cheeselike masses of tissue, a process known as *caseation*. Any body organ can be infected, but in adults, the usual site is the lungs. Still one of the most widespread diseases in the world, tuberculosis is treated with chemotherapy; resistant strains of the bacillus have developed.
Pseudomonas aeruginosa	Ubiquitous organism is a frequent cause of wound and urinary infections in debilitated hospitalized patients. Often found in solutions that have been standing for long periods.
Salmonella typhi (and others)	Salmonellosis occurs as enterocolitis, bacteremia, localized infection, or typhoid. Depending on type, presenting symptoms may be fever, diarrhea, or abscesses; complications include intestinal perforation and endocarditis. Carried in water, milk, meat, and other food.
Shigella dysenteriae (and others)	A serious bacillary dysentery. Acute intestinal infection with diarrhea (sometimes bloody); may cause dehydration with electrolyte imbalance or septicemia. Transmitted through fecal–oral route or other poor sanitation.
Yersinia pestis (formerly called *Pasteurella pestis*)	Plague, the "black death" of the Middle Ages. Transmitted by fleas from infected rodents to humans. Symptoms of the most common form are swollen, infected lymph nodes, or *buboes*. Another form may cause pneumonia. All forms may lead to a rapidly fatal septicemia.

Note: the following organisms are smaller than other bacteria and vary in shape. Like viruses, they grow within cells, but they differ from viruses in that they are affected by antibiotics.

Chlamydia oculogenitalis	Inclusion conjunctivitis, acute eye infection. Carried in genital organs, transmitted during birth or through water in inadequately chlorinated swimming pools.
Chlamydia psittaci	Psittacosis, also called *ornithosis*. Disease transmitted by various birds, including parrots, ducks, geese, and turkeys. Primary symptoms are chills, headache, and fever, more severe in older people. The duration may be from 2 to 3 weeks, often with a long convalescence. Antibiotic drugs are effective remedies.
Chlamydia trachomatis	A sexually transmitted disease causing pelvic inflammatory disease and other infections of the reproductive tract. Also causes inclusion conjunctivitis, an acute eye infection, and trachoma, a chronic infection that is a common cause of blindness in underdeveloped areas of the world. Infection of the conjunctiva and cornea characterized by redness, pain, and lacrimation. Antibiotic therapy is effective if begun before there is scarring. The same organism causes lymphogranuloma venereum (LGV), a sexually transmitted disease characterized by swelling of inguinal lymph nodes and accompanied by signs of general infection.
Coxiella burnetti	Q fever. Infection transmitted from cattle, sheep, and goats to humans by contaminated dust and also carried by arthropods. Symptoms are fever, headache, chills, and pneumonitis. This disorder is almost never fatal.
Rickettsia prowazekii	Epidemic typhus. Transmitted to humans by lice; associated with poor hygiene and war. Main symptoms are headache, hypotension, delirium, and a red rash. Frequently fatal in older people.
Rickettsia rickettsii	Rocky Mountain spotted fever. Tick-borne disease occurring throughout the United States. Symptoms are fever, muscle aches, and a rash that may progress to gangrene over bony prominences. The disease is rarely fatal.
Rickettsia typhi	Endemic or murine typhus. A milder disease transmitted to humans from rats by fleas. Symptoms are fever, rash, headache, and cough. The disease is rarely fatal.
Curved rods Vibrio *Vibrio cholerae (Vibrio comma)*	Cholera. Acute infection of the intestine characterized by prolonged vomiting and diarrhea, leading to severe dehydration, electrolyte imbalance, and in some cases, death.
Spirochetes *Borrelia burgdorferi*	Lyme disease, transmitted by the extremely small deer tick. Usually starts with a bulls-eye rash followed by flulike symptoms, at which time antibiotics are effective. May progress to neurologic problems and joint inflammation. A vaccine to prevent Lyme disease has been developed.
Borrelia recurrentis (and others)	Relapsing fever. Generalized infection in which attacks of fever alternate with periods of apparent recovery. Organisms spread by lice, ticks, and other insects.

(continued)

Table 1 (continued)

ORGANISM	DISEASE AND DESCRIPTION
Treponema pallidum	Syphillis. Infectious disease transmitted mainly by sexual intercourse. Untreated syphilis is seen in the following three stages: primary—formation of primary lesion (chancre); secondary—skin eruptions and infectious patches on mucous membranes; tertiary—development of generalized lesions (gummas) and destruction of tissues resulting in aneurysm, heart disease, and degenerative changes in brain, spinal cord, ganglia, and meninges. Also a cause of intrauterine fetal death or stillbirth.
Treponema vincentii (formerly called *Borrelia vincentii*)	Vincent's disease (trench mouth). Infection of the mouth and throat accompanied by formation of a pseudomembrane, with ulceration.

Table 2   Fungal Diseases

DISEASE/ORGANISM	DESCRIPTION
Actinomycosis	"Lumpy jaw," which occurs in cattle and humans. The organisms cause the formation of large masses of tissue, which are often accompanied by abscesses. The lungs and liver may be involved.
Blastomycosis (*Blastomyces dermatitidis*)	A general term for any infection caused by a yeastlike organism. There may be skin tumors and lesions in the lungs, bones, liver, spleen, and kidneys.
Candidiasis (*Candida albicans*)	An infection that can involve the skin and mucous membranes. May cause diaper rash, infection of the nail beds, and infection of the mucous membranes of the mouth (thrush), throat, and vagina.
Coccidioidomycosis (*Coccidioides immitis*)	Also called *San Joaquin Valley fever,* it is another systemic fungal disease. Because it often attacks the lungs, it may be mistaken for tuberculosis.
Histoplasmosis (*Histoplasma capsulatum*)	This fungus may cause a variety of disorders, ranging from mild respiratory symptoms or enlargement of liver, spleen, and lymph nodes to cavities in the lungs with symptoms similar to those of tuberculosis.
Pneumocystis carinii	Pneumonia (PCP). Opportunistic infection in people with a depressed immune system. Invades lungs and causes a foamy exudate to collect in alveoli.

Ringworm
  Tinea capitis
  Tinea corporis
  Tinea pedis
	Common fungal infections of the skin, many of which cause blisters and scaling with discoloration of the affected areas. All are caused by similar organisms from a group of fungi called *dermatophytes.* They are easily transmitted by person to person contact or by contaminated articles.

Table 3 Viral Diseases

ORGANISM	DISEASE AND DESCRIPTION
Cytomegalovirus (CMV)	Common mild infection of the salivary glands. In an immunosuppressed person may cause infection of the retina, lung, and liver, ulceration of GI tract, and inflammation of the brain. Causes severe fetal or neonatal damage.
Hantavirus	Causes pulmonary syndrome with high mortality rate. Spread by inhalation of rodent droppings.
Hepatitis viruses	Cause liver inflammation. Varieties A through G are recognized.
Hepatitis A virus (HAV)	Transmitted by fecal contamination. Does not become chronic or produce carrier state. Infection provides lifelong immunity. Vaccine is available.
Hepatitis B virus (HAB)	Transmitted by direct exchange of blood and body fluids. Can cause rapidly fatal disease or develop into chronic disease and carrier state. Risk of progress to liver cancer. Vaccine is available.
Hepatitis C virus (HCV)	Spread through blood exchange (usually transfusions before 1992 when screening began) or shared needles. May become chronic and lead to cirrhosis, liver failure, cancer. Antiviral drugs may limit infection.
Hepatitis D virus (HDV)	Spread by blood exchange and occurs as coinfection with hepatitis B. Responsible for half of rapidly fatal liver failure cases and also a high rate of chronic disease that progresses to death.
Hepatitis E virus (HEV)	Transmitted by fecal contamination and occurs in epidemics in Middle East and Asia. Resembles hepatitis A. Can be fatal in pregnant women.
Hepatitis F virus (HFV)	Rare type; transmitted from primates to humans
Hepatitis G virus (HGV)	Very mild disease that usually becomes chronic, commonly transmitted by blood and body fluids among IV drug users, often along with hepatitis B or C. Blood test is available.
Herpes simplex virus type 1	Cold sores or fever blisters that appear around the mouth and nose of people with colds or other illnesses accompanied by fever
Herpes simplex virus type 2	Genital herpes. Acute inflammatory disease of the genitalia, often recurring. A very common sexually transmitted disease
Human immunodeficiency virus (HIV)	Acquired immunodeficiency syndrome (AIDS). Fatal disease that infects T lymphocytes of the immune system. Diagnosed by antibody tests, decline in specific (CD4) cells, and presenting disease, including *Candida albicans* infection, *Pneumocystis carinii* pneumonia, Kaposi's sarcoma, persistent swelling of lymph nodes (lymphadenopathy), chronic diarrhea, and wasting. Spread by contact with contaminated body fluids and by transplacental route
Human papillomavirus (HPV)	Genital warts (condylomata acuminata). Sexually transmitted warts of the genital and perianal area in men and women. Associated with cervical dysplasia and cancer
Influenza virus	An epidemic viral infection, marked by chills, fever, muscular pains, and prostration. The most serious complication is bronchopneumonia caused by *Haemophilus influenzae* (a bacillus) or streptococci
Mumps virus	Epidemic parotitis. Acute inflammation with swelling of the parotid salivary glands. Mumps can have many complications, such as orchitis (inflammation of the testes) in young men and meningitis in young children.

(continued)

Table 3 (continued)	
ORGANISM	DISEASE AND DESCRIPTION
Poliovirus	Poliomyelitis. Acute viral infection that may attack the anterior horns of the spinal cord, resulting in paralysis of certain voluntary muscles. North and South America have been declared free of polio as a result of vaccination programs.
Rhabdovirus	Rabies. An acute, fatal disease transmitted to humans through the saliva of an infected animal. Rabies is characterized by violent muscular spasms induced by the slightest sensations. Because the swallowing of water causes spasms of the throat, the disease is also call *hydrophobia* ("fear of water"). The final stage of paralysis ends in death.
Rotavirus	Attacks lining of small intestine causing severe diarrhea in children. A vaccine is available to be administered at 2, 4, and 6 months of age.
Rubella virus	German measles. A less severe form of measles, but especially dangerous during the first 3 months of pregnancy because the disease organism can cause heart defects, deafness, mental deficiency, and other permanent damage in the fetus.
Rubeola virus	Measles. An acute respiratory inflammation followed by fever and a generalized skin rash. Patients are prone to the development of dangerous complications, such as bronchopneumonia and other secondary infections caused by staphylococci and streptococci.
Varicella zoster herpesvirus	Chickenpox (varicella). A usually mild infection, almost completely confined to children, characterized by blisterlike skin eruptions. Vaccine now available.
	Shingles (herpes zoster). A very painful eruption of blisters of the skin that follows the course of certain peripheral nerves. These blisters eventually dry up and form scabs that resemble shingles.
Other viral diseases	
Common cold (coryza)	A viral infection of the upper respiratory tract caused by a wide variety of organisms. May lead to complications, such as pneumonia and influenza.
Viral encephalitis	*Encephalitis* usually is understood to be any brain inflammation accompanied by degenerative tissue changes, and it can have many causes besides viruses. There are several forms of viral encephalitis (Western and Eastern epidemic, equine, St. Louis, Japanese B, etc.), some of which are known to be transmitted from birds and other animals to humans by insects, principally mosquitoes.
Viral pneumonia	Caused by a number of different viruses, such as the influenza and parainfluenza viruses, adenoviruses, and varicella viruses

Table 4 Protozoan Diseases

ORGANISM	DISEASE AND DESCRIPTION
Amebae *Entamoeba histolytica*	Amebic dysentery. Severe ulceration of the wall of the large intestine caused by amebae. Acute diarrhea may be an important symptom. This organism also may cause liver abscesses.
Ciliates *Balantidium coli*	Gastrointestinal disturbances and ulcers of the colon.
Flagellates *Giardia lamblia* *Leishmania donovani* (and others) *Trichomonas vaginalis* *Trypanosoma*	Gastrointestinal disturbances. Kala-azar. In this disease, there is enlargement of the liver and spleen as well as skin lesions. Inflammation and discharge from the vagina of the female. In the male, it involves the urethra and causes painful urination. African sleeping sickness. Disease begins with a high fever, followed by invasion of the brain and spinal cord by the organisms. Usually, the disease ends with continued drowsiness, coma, and death.
Sporozoa *Cryptosporidium* *Plasmodium;* varieties include *vivax, falciparum, malariae* *Toxoplasma gondii*	Cramps and diarrhea that can be long term and severe in people with a weakened immune system, such as those with AIDS. Spread in water and by personal contact in close quarters. Malaria. Characterized by recurrent attacks of chills followed by high fever. Severe attacks of malaria can be fatal because of kidney failure, cerebral disorders, and other complications. Toxoplasmosis. Common infectious disease transmitted by cats and raw meat. Mild forms cause fever and enlargement of lymph nodes. May cause fatal encephalitis in immunosuppressed patients. Infection of a pregnant woman is a cause of fetal stillbirth or congenital damage.

Index

Note: Page numbers followed by *f* indicate figures; those followed by *t* indicate tables.

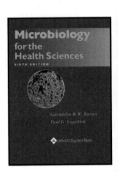
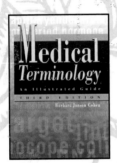
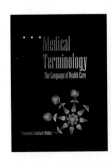